Malignant Effusions:
A Multimodal Approach to Cytologic Diagnosis

Malignant Effusions:
A Multimodal Approach to Cytologic Diagnosis

Carlos W.M. Bedrossian, M.D., FIAC

Professor of Pathology
Wayne State University School of Medicine
Chief of Cytopathology
Detroit Medical Center
Detroit, Michigan

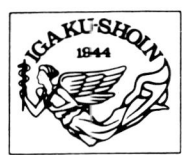

Igaku-Shoin   New York · Tokyo

Published and distributed by

IGAKU-SHOIN Medical Publishers, Inc.
One Madison Avenue, New York, N.Y. 10010

IGAKU-SHOIN Ltd.,
5-24-3 Hongo, Bunkyo-ku, Tokyo 113-91

Library of Congress Cataloging-in-Publication Data

Bedrossian, Carlos W. M.
    Malignant effusions : a multimodal approach to cytologic diagnosis / Carlos W. M. Bedrossian.
        p.   cm.
    Includes bibliographical references and index.
    1. Cancer—Cytodiagnosis.   2. Exudates and transudates.
  3. Cytodiagnosis.   I. Title.
        [DNLM: 1. Cytodiagnosis.   2. Exudates and Transudates.
  3. Neoplasms—diagnosis.   QZ 241 B413m]
        RC270.3.C97B44   1991
        616.99'407582—dc20
        DNLM/DLC
        for Library of Congress   91-7105
                                                                              CIP

ISBN: 0-89640-196-0 (New York)
ISBN: 4-260-14196-1 (Tokyo)

Printed and bound in Hong Kong.

10 9 8 7 6 5 4 3 2 1

To my parents:

HOVANES & APARECIDA

who taught me the love of knowledge
and the value of hard work.

Preface

This is a book about cells, those elusive small structures that hold the secrets of disease. Their occurrence in effusions is not fortuitous, since virtually every major organ is directly or indirectly in contact with a serosal cavity. The rich microvasculature underlying the mesothelium ensures that cells extravasate in just about any pathologic process: inflammation, infection, neoplasia. Effusions also reflect the protean manifestations of systemic diseases and therefore serve as a mirror of the general health.

The entire spectrum of cellular pathology is seen in effusions. However, in this book we will focus on malignant effusions and their mimics. Cytologic diagnosis based upon dichromatic stains is an art requiring daily practice, years of experience and the support of a competent staff. Special stains, the old and the new, add novel dimensions to cytologic interpretation which thus is maximized by a multimodal approach. However, even more sophisticated techniques have not done away with all diagnostic dilemmas in clinical practice. In fact, the explosion of high technology forces one to be judicious and cost effective in the use of these new modalities. This is the balance we have always strived to reach and propose to reflect in this book.

Our purpose is not to promote the use of these various modalities in every case, but rather to stress their feasibility, should the need and opportunity to gain from it arise. Rather than to practice strict cytomorphology by light microscopy and dichromatic stains in a cocoon, we believe in expanding the repertoire of cytology and correlating it with other techniques applied to the diagnosis of disease. However, it is important to integrate the results of these various methods in an eclectic fashion, for maximum gain in understanding and diagnosing disease conditions. This approach is not without its precursors.

Eileen King measured specific gravity and other parameters in effusions as early as the early 1960s. The late Jack Frost was an avid proponent of utilizing special stains in body fluids. Bernard Naylor has combined the use of Papanicolaou's stain in fixed smears and toluidine blue, in wet films for many years. Leopold Koss has stressed the use of electron microscopy, particularly the SEM mode, rather enthusiastically and now propounds image analysis as a wave of the future. Perhaps our choice of this comprehensive approach reflects our formative years in which we studied under Lucien Lison, a Belgian considered the father of histochemistry, who stressed the correlation between cell biology and clinical cytology in his department.

Our interest in effusions dates from the first cytology workshop we ever took, which happened to be on body fluids, conducted by Jack Frost. With him we learned the value of a systematic evaluation of each component of the cell, looking for structural alterations and keeping in mind its functional significance. At the University of Texas in Houston, we started our examination of effusions and other cytologic specimens by EM. Later at Vanderbilt we were impressed by Robert V. Collins multiparameter study of lymphomas and began in earnest to expand our technical repertoire to solid tumors. Most of our immunocytochemical and ultrastructural studies, however, were performed at Saint Louis University, thanks to the generosity of David Lagunoff. You will see this multimodal approach throughout the entire book.

The material to illustrate this text-atlas was collected over twenty years, with the help of innumerable technologists and especially a number of our trainees. It would be impossible to acknowledge each one individually, but Doctors Susan Rollins, Rosa Davila, Felix Martinez, and Sandy Gibson deserve special mention for their significant contributions. Drs. Clyniece Breland and Marianne Prey in St. Louis and Ross Lavoie and Jenise Gyurnek in Detroit assisted in the preparation of workshop packets from which classical examples and rare entities were easily culled. All immunostains were performed by Ursula Bedrossian and Colleen Fahey, who also kept records and slides easily retrievable and always rallied to meet deadlines, often playing the role of typists, and graphic artists. They were also my voice of reason when my enthusiasm led me to unrealistic expectations and goals.

A number of colleagues throughout the world enriched the pages of this text-atlas. I am grateful to Doctor M. Gonzalez-Devesa, from the University of Valencia, Spain for the scanning electron micrographs in chapter 14. At the University of Iowa, Sue Zaleski opened her teaching files to my perusal and located that one more example of a diagnostic oddity, when needed; while Dr. Steve Bonsib made it possible for us to illustrate the ultrastructural features of various neoplasms. Dr. Tony Leong kindly read and commented on the chapter on lymphomas and leukemias. Many colleagues contributed rare cases throughout various chapters. Drs. Ruth Katz and Nour Sneige, from our alma mater, the M.D. Anderson Hospital and Cancer Institute, contributed illustrations of rare infections and other unusual conditions. This was also true of Dr. Prabodh Gupta of the University of Pennsylvania, Dr. De-nise Hidvegi of Northwestern University in Chicago and Kim Geisinger of Wake Forest University in Winston-Salem.

Despite the vicissitudes of the Gulf War, my military tour of duty at the AFIP allowed me the opportunity to study cases of rare infections to which Dr. Larry Ash, from the University of California in Los Angeles, also contributed interesting cases. Special thanks are also due to Diane Solomon, who made my stay in Washington, D.C. lighter by opening the doors of the National Cancer Institute to me and making available some of their interesting cases. Last, but not least, many thanks to Angel Blankenship for typing and retyping the manuscript and Terri Steinke for formatting and laser printing the final product and to Lila Maron and George Schall of Igaku-Shoin for their patience and helpful assistance. My greatest gratitude, however, goes to my wife, who tolerated my late hours and was always there to pitch in whenever and wherever I needed help the most and who always provided loving emotional support. I hope the labor of so many will bear fruit and this volume will assist you in your daily practice of cytopathology.

Carlos W.M. Bedrossian, M.D., FIAC

Foreword

By the first decade of the twentieth century, published accounts already existed on the finding of cancer cells in various fluids of the human body, including those from the serous cavities. Subsequently, however, clinicians seemed to have placed little reliance on cytologic examination of pleural, peritoneal and pericardial fluids in the management of their patients despite that the finding of cancer cells in these fluids has always carried the gravest prognostic significance. It was not until the late 1940s, following the publications of Papanicolaou and Traut on the cytologic diagnosis of uterine cancer, that the wide applicability of cytology to the diagnosis of cancer was finally recognized, culminating in the latter day surge of interest in fine needle apiration cytology as well as the application of a variety of ancillary techniques to cytologic specimens. As a result, there can be few clinicians or pathologists who remain unaware of or indifferent to the potential and practicality of diagnosing neoplastic and non-neoplastic diseases by cytologic examination of serous fluids.

Although the literature on the cytologic examination of serous fluids now spans almost 150 years, very few books have been devoted solely to the subject, especially books that adopt an up-to-date multimodal approach. Not only is there a place for a comprehensive account of the cytopathology of serous fluids based on the tried and tested conventional techniques, but there is also a need for an account that includes modern diagnostic techniques that have proven their worth in other aspects of anatomic pathology. This book fills the need.

Dr. Bedrossian is a seasoned cytopathologist whose broad background in general pathology has served him well in dealing with the demands and difficulties of cytopathology. Not only is he a capable diagnostician, he is also an experienced teacher and author who has shared his knowledge and expertise with numerous students in the United States and abroad. His expansive interests in the cytopathology of serous fluids is reflected in the scope of this monograph, which includes discussion of a wide range of conditions, both neoplastic and non-neoplastic, studied by a multimodal approach.

For those who are about to embark on the cytopathology of pleural, peritoneal and pericardial fluids as well as those who already have experience in the field, this book will serve as an invaluable guide and reference.

Bernard Naylor
Professor of Pathology
The University of Michigan
Ann Arbor, Michigan

Contents

1 Introduction *1*

2 Clinicopathologic Correlations *9*

3 Multimodal Approach *18*

4 Serosal Reaction to Injury *26*

5 Inflammatory Processes *52*

6 Infectious Diseases *73*

7 Iatrogenic, Organ-related, and Systemic Processes *85*

8 Mesothelioma *101*

9 Epithelial Malignancies *120*

10 Nonepithelial Neoplasms *148*

11 Leukemia and Lymphoma *160*

12 Small Blue Round Cell Tumors *177*

13 In Search of the Primary Site *190*

14 Electron Microscopy *211*

15 Immunocytochemistry *244*

16 Ancillary Techniques *260*

Index *269*

CHAPTER ONE

Introduction

THE BODY CAVITIES

Body cavities first appear as spaces within the lateral and cardiogenic mesoderms of the developing embryo. Soon thereafter their lining by a serous membrane can be appreciated. All serous membranes consist of a single row of flat mesothelial cells on the surface and a submesothelial layer of connective tissue underneath. A plexus of blood vessels and lymphatic channels is present in the submesothelial layer surrounded, above and below, by a thin elastic band. The space between the parietal and visceral serosae measures 5 to 10 μm wide under physiologic circumstances and as such it contains only a minimal amount of fluid. The lymphatic lacunae open onto the mesothelial surface via narrow gaps or stoma so that the body cavities are, in effect, an extension of the lymphatic system. They act, therefore, as a reservoir for fluid extravasation whenever the absorptive capacity of the lymphatics has been exceeded. The resulting phenomenon, known as effusion, leads to an abnormal accumulation of fluid in the body cavities. Under normal circumstances each pleural cavity can hold 1.5 liters of fluid, and the peritoneal cavity up to 2.0 liters. The pericardial sac, however, cannot hold more than 600 mL of fluid without the danger of cardiac tamponade.

NORMAL ANATOMY AND HISTOLOGY

The pleural membranes surround both lungs and also cover the inner surfaces of the thoracic cavity. The pleura reflects itself over pulmonary fissures and the bronchovascular sheath of the hilum. The fusion of the pleura and the pericardium delimits the lateral boundaries of the mediastinum. The pericardium surrounding the heart, known as epicardium, is lined by unusually flat mesothelial cells. Interiorly, the parietal layer of the pericardium and the pleura line the dome of the diaphragm. The concave surface of the diaphragm is lined by the parietal peritoneum, which also covers all other internal surfaces of the abdominal cavity. Here too, the peritoneal membrane reflects over the abdominal organs in the form of the visceral peritoneum of the liver, spleen, and intestines. Because important disease processes may affect the retroperitoneum, it should also be remembered that only a very thin layer of parietal peritoneum separates this space from the abdominal cavity.

The parietal peritoneum blends imperceptibly with the pelvic peritoneum only to reflect over the fallopian tubes and the ovaries. The cul-de-sacs represented by the dependent portions of the pelvic space are important sources of cytologic specimens. During exploratory surgery, not only the cul-de-sacs but the mesenteric recesses and the lateral gutters may be washed, brushed, or otherwise sampled for cytologic examination (Fig. 1.1). The most frequent mode of samplings, however, is represented by therapeutic taps to alleviate symptoms related to fluid accumulation. The peritoneal space may hold up to 15 to 20 L of fluid, while each pleural cavity may accumulate 3 L. As already stated, the pericardial sac cannot hold more than 600 mL without the danger of cardiac tamponade.

PATHOPHYSIOLOGY

To best interpret the abnormalities detected in an effusion, one should be familiar with the physiologic events that lead to its accumulation. Starling's principle applies to the formation of edema within the interstitial space of the serous membranes (Fig. 1.2). So long as hydrostatic and colloid osmotic pressures of the blood are in equilibrium, fluid remains in the intraluminal compartment of the microvasculature. Any break in this delicate

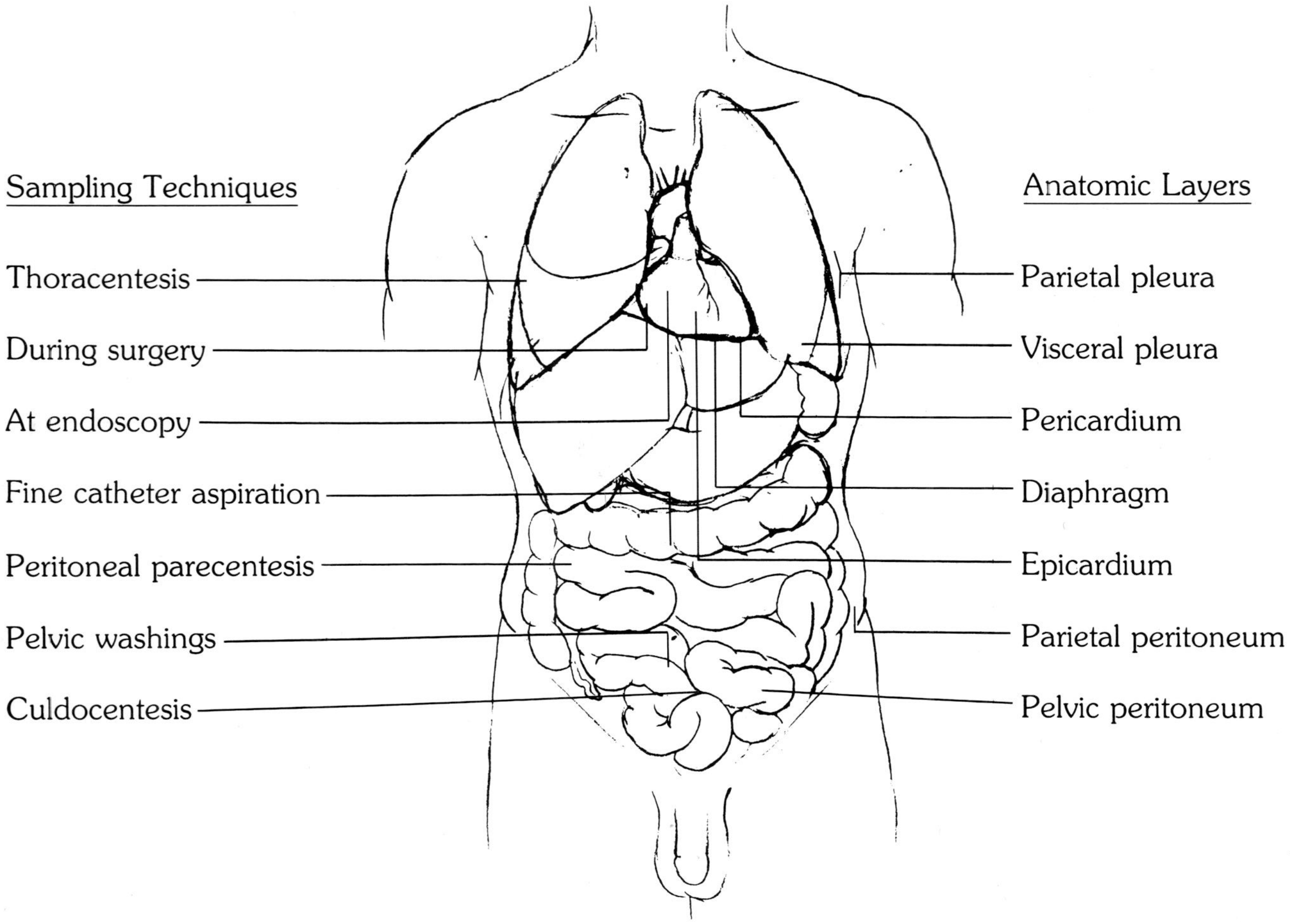

Sampling Techniques

Thoracentesis

During surgery

At endoscopy

Fine catheter aspiration

Peritoneal parecentesis

Pelvic washings

Culdocentesis

Anatomic Layers

Parietal pleura

Visceral pleura

Pericardium

Diaphragm

Epicardium

Parietal peritoneum

Pelvic peritoneum

FIGURE 1.1 Anatomy of the body cavities.

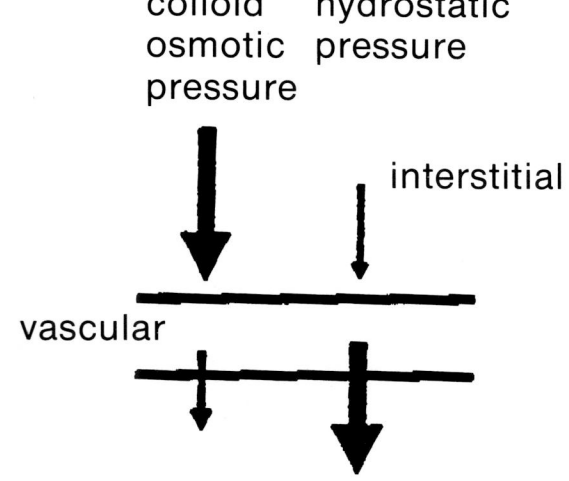

colloid   hydrostatic
osmotic   pressure
pressure

interstitial

vascular

FIGURE 1.2 Starling's Law of fluid extravasation.

balance leads to interstitial edema followed by effusion. The fluid is usually formed by the parietal layer and reabsorbed by the visceral layer of the serous membrane. Important causes of increased hydrostatic pressure include heart failure and localized forms of vascular obstruction. A decrease in colloid osmotic pressure may be caused by hypoalbuminemia secondary to starvation, renal disease, or cirrhosis.

Effusions may form because of regional (organ-related) abnormalities in response to a more generalized (systemic) process. Sometimes the effusion is caused by a direct interaction between the diseased organ and the overlying serosal membrane. At other times the systemic effect follows well understood pathophysiologic mechanisms as, for example, in cardiac failure leading to edema of many organs. In other organ-related effusions the organ linked to the manifestation is identified but little is known about the mechanism involved. Pancreatic ascites, the pleural effusion that occurs in cases of cirrhosis is one such condition. Nephrogenic effusion may be explained by hypoproteinemia, the same mechanism responsible for the anasarca that accompanies malnutrition. However, very little is known to explain Meig's syndrome.

In the collagen diseases a generalized inflammatory process affects the microvasculature of many organ systems. Although each condition has preferential sites of involvement, all have at least some effect on the serosal membranes. Rheumatoid arthritis is the one collagen disease most frequently accompanied by pleural effusion, which appears to be mediated by an increased capillary permeability. Another form of generalized but transient inflammatory response is drug hypersensitivity, which may also cause exudative effusions. In some generalized inflammatory conditions the response is mainly vascular with passage of leukocytes into the serous effusion. In others, particularly in processes of long duration, there is an associated reactive proliferation of the mesothelial cells. Extravasation of fluid may also be caused by localized inflammatory response to the serosal membrane secondary to infection or other pathologic processes affecting an underlying organ. In such cases vasodilation and hyperpermeability of the microvasculature allow the extravasation primarily of plasma and a few circulating white blood cells. Neoplasms may obstruct the lymphatic blood vessels of the serosal surfaces or break the integrity of their walls. In such destructive processes, red blood cells and other cellular blood elements extravasate with the plasma. Neoplastic and reactive mesothelial cells are also swept into the effusion, leading to a mixed population of cells that require sorting out by the cytopathologist for correct diagnosis.

In sarcoidosis the multiplicity of granulomata in the lymph nodes interferes with lymphatic flow. If the interference with lymphatic flow is severe, lymph fails to enter the systemic circulation and accumulates in the pleural space resulting in chylothorax, also common consequence of lymphangioleiomyomatosis, a rare pulmonary disease of obscure etiology. Other conditions associated with effusion due to decreased lymphatic flow include Milroy's (Meig's) disease and the yellow nail syndrome.

TRANSUDATES AND EXUDATES

An effusion is classically divided into exudate and transudate on the basis of its specific gravity, protein content, and other biochemical parameters (Table 1.1). Transudates represent filtrates of blood across a physiologically intact vasculature. Exudates on the other hand are associated with damage to the vascular wall. Because of the wider gaps present in an injured vessel a larger number of cells is present in exudates than in transudates. As these cells degenerate or die, the specific gravity of the exudate increases and greater amounts of protein and enzymes, among which is lactate dehydrogenase (LDH), are released from dead cells. Of all biochemical parameters, the LDH ratio between the serosal fluid and the plasma is the most reliable criterion to distinguish between exudate and transudate. Light determined that in exudates the pleural fluid : plasma LDH ratio is greater than 0.6 and the same ratio for total protein is greater than 0.5. It is possible to perform certain simple biochemical tests in the cytology laboratory. These include pH, total protein (Rivalta's test), specific gravity, and a few others. It is more feasible, however, to obtain the results from more sophisticated analyses performed in the biochemistry laboratory and to correlate them with the cytologic examination. Correlation between the cytologic and hematologic examination of the same specimen is also fruitful. Supravital staining is useful in determining the viability of tumor cells, particularly if the effusion is

TABLE 1.1 Differences Between Transudate and Exudate

Characteristics	Transudate	Exudate
Appearance	Clear	Cloudy
Specific gravity	<1.015	>1.015
Total protein	<3.0	>3.0
Pleural fluid : plasma LDH	<0.6	>0.6
Coagulation	Does not coagulate	Coagulates on standing
Bacteriology	Usually sterile	May yield bacterial growth
Cellularity	Sparse, predominantly mesothelial	Highly cellular, predominantly inflammatory

tapped to monitor the effect of chemotherapy. The practice of using the unused portion of specimens intended for microbiologic examination for cytologic evaluation is counterproductive and should be discouraged.

PATHOLOGIC CLASSIFICATION

Effusions may also be classified according to their predominant pathogenetic mechanism (Table 1.2). This may be useful in discerning the cause of the effusion by clinical means. In practice, however, a combination of mechanisms usually contributes to the extravasation of fluid and cells that ultimately constitute the effusion. Consequently, no fast rules can be applied to every individual case, and careful clinicopathologic correlation is ultimately needed to arrive at a correct diagnosis. For example, not every malignancy is accompanied by an exudative effusion, a more common result of inflammatory processes. However, certain malignant processes may contain such a high number of neoplastic cells as to render the exudative effusion opalescent and even allow visualization of clumps of tumor cells with the naked eye. A transudate will form in a cancerous patient if hypoalbuminemia results from cachexia or

---

TABLE 1.2 Pathogenetic Mechanisms of Effusion

TRANSUDATES
Increased hydrostatic pressure
   Congestive heart failure
   Venous thrombosis
   Pulmonary embolism and infarct
   Postpartum pleural effusion
Decreased oncotic pressure
   Hypoalbuminemia
   Liver cirrhosis
   Advanced renal disease
EXUDATES
Increased capillary permeability
   Pneumonia
   Pancreatitis
   Retroperitoneal abscess
   Radiation therapy
Decreased lymphatic drainage
   Chylothorax
   Sarcoidosis
Increased capillary permeability with decreased lymphatic
   drainage
   Tuberculosis
   Malignancy

---

from widespread metastasis to the liver. Conversely, if congestive heart failure leads to pneumonia, the resulting pleural effusion is exudative rather than a transudate. The most common mechanism of effusion in malignancy is obstruction of the lymphatic drainage by metastatic seeding of neoplastic cells along the rich vascular plexuses of the serosal membranes.

Depending on the nature of its cellular elements and its gross appearance, an effusion may be classified into different diagnostic categories (Table 1.3). This classification is extremely arbitrary, however, and serves only to narrow the range of differential diagnoses during initial evaluation. Certain types of effusion can be easily identified by noncytologic means; for example, infectious effusions may be grossly purulent and foul smelling. Cultures or microbiologic stains may be required to identify the etiologic agent. The fat droplets in a chylous effusion may require biochemical means for their recognition.

It is obvious that the mesothelial membranes cover a vast surface area and come into close contact with every major organ throughout the three main cavities of the body. Because of their continuity with the lymphatic system, these cavities are commonly the seat of metastasis from tumors located at distant sites. The extensive surface area renders these serosal membranes susceptible to primary neoplasms and other proliferative lesions affecting the mesothelium. Consequently every effort should be made to extract the highest diagnostic yield from a number of laboratory methods applicable to the study of effusions.

Even though some gross appearances are highly characteristic of certain disease conditions, most diagnoses have to be confirmed by more precise laboratory methods, including microscopy (Table 1.4). A combination of methods is usually needed to narrow down the differential diagnosis, and by employing them in a logical sequence a cost-effective strategy can be followed. Over the years clinicians have formed rather entrenched opinions about the usefulness of the different methods, and it is gratifying to realize that cytology ranks among the most useful, rendering helpful information in the majority of cases.

The departure point in the evaluation of effusions is the distinction between exudate and transudate. Transudates are seldom if ever submitted for microscopic examination. Exudates, chylous effusions, and hemorrhagic effusions on the other hand are often submitted for cytologic and biochemical analysis. It is up to the clinician to consider each clinical scenario situating cytology in relation to other diagnostic methods applicable to the examination of effusions.

TABLE 1.3 Pathologic Types of Effusions

Type	Gross appearance	Microscopic appearance	Significance
Serous	watery, clear	hypocellular	transudate
Chylous	milky, white	fat-filled cells	lymph retention
Pseudochylous	milky, green	foamy cells	cholesterol crystals
Cirrhotic	watery, brown	atypical cells	transudate, bilirubin
Eosinophilic	watery, silky	eosinophils	allergic process
Inflammatory	yellowish, white	neutrophils, lymphocytes	collagen disease
Infectious	greenish, smelly	lymphocytes	tuberculosis
Hemorrhagic	brownish, silky	malignant cells	carcinoma
Hemorrhagic	brownish, viscid	malignant cells	mesothelioma
Pigmented	chocolate, brown	malignant cells	melanoma

TABLE 1.4 Laboratory Evaluation of Body Fluids

BIOCHEMICAL
Total protein
pH
Glucose
Amylase
LDH (pleural fluid:plasma)
Total lipid
Cholesterol
Ammonia
Hyaluronic acid
Special (CEA, ACE, C3–C4, etc)
MORPHOLOGIC
Cytologic examination (Papanicolaou, Diff-Quik)
Cell counts and differential (Wright–Giemsa)
Supravital stains (Sudan black; TPT)
LDH isoenzyme stain
Histochemistry ("special" stains)
Immunocytochemistry (monoclonal antibodies)
Electron microscopy (transmission/scanning)
QUANTITATIVE
Flow cytometry (surface markers, DNA ploidy studies)
Morphometry
Image analysis
AgNOr Counts
MICROBIOLOGIC
Cultures
Gram's stain
IMMUNOLOGIC
Rheumatoid factor
Complement
Anti-nuclear antibody (A.N.A.)
OTHER
Cytogenetics
"Living cytology" (tissue culture)
Pleural brushing
Peritoneal washes (2nd-look operation)

MICROSCOPIC EXAMINATION

A quick microscopic examination of the effusion with Diff-Quik or any of the Romanowsky-type stains can render very useful information and is often performed on a stat basis. Diff-Quik and a rapid Papanicolaou stain can be used in the cytology laboratory to triage the effusion for further handling, particularly the need for flow cytometry and marker studies in lymphoma is suspected. Naylor uses a wet film stained by toluidine blue for the same purpose. The viability of tumor cells can be ascertained by supravital stains such as Sudan black, methylene blue, or the TPT stain. The Wright–Giemsa stain is the preferred method for the performance of absolute and differential cell counts in the United States, whereas the May–Grünwald–Giemsa (MGG) method is favored in Europe. Overtly purulent fluids can be examined by the Gram stain, PAS, and silver stain for microorganisms. In every case with lymphocytosis the diagnosis of tuberculosis should be considered and the fluid examined by an AFB stain such as Ziehl–Nielsen or the auramine–rhodamine method, as well as being submitted for appropriate cultures.

In general, transudates have a total leukocyte count of 1000 cells/mL or less whereas exudates have more than 1000 cells/mL. An RBC count greater than 12,000 cells/mL is indicative of either malignancy or pulmonary infarction, although a traumatic tap may also lead to a hemorrhagic effusion. However, Naylor has seen a serosanguinous effusion in only half of his cases of malignancy. A finding of hemosiderin-laden macrophages under microscopic examination reinforces the suspicion that a significant pathologic condition explains the RBC extravasation. The LDH isozyme stain can be applied to the microscopic examination of effusions. According to Takahashi, the H subunit predominates in mesothelial cells and macrophages, and the M subunit predominates in malignant (adenocarcinomatous) cells. The so-called AgNOR stain has been used to impregnate the nucleolar organizer region with silver and is reportedly helpful in distinguishing mesothelioma from mesothelial hyperplasia.

BIOCHEMICAL ANALYSIS

Total protein measurements are helpful in distinguishing between transudate and exudate but aid little in the detection of malignancy. In infections the protein level is elevated to greater than 3 g/dL except in infected ascites. Because of the large volume attained by ascites, the available protein is not sufficient to raise the protein level to that of exudates. Electrophoresis is able to identify specific immunoglobulins in the fluid, but it correlates poorly with the cell types and the underlying disease processes responsible for the effusion. Lipoproteins and lipids are elevated in chylous effusions. Orosomucoid, an alpha$_1$ acid glycoprotein of molecular weight 45 kd, is helpful in identifying nonmalignant effusions. Elevated levels of fibrinogen degradation products are noted in malignant effusion, but the usefulness of this finding is limited by the elevated levels found in pulmonary infarction and infections.

A decreased level of glucose in the exudate is noted in malignant effusion but its diagnostic usefulness is limited because such a decrease is also found in bacterial infections, tuberculosis, and rheumatoid arthritis. A decrease of the pH in pleural fluid is associated with malignancy but also accompanies empyema, collagen diseases, esophageal rupture, and tuberculous pleuritis. Certain enzymes have attained modest specificity in the diagnosis of benign and malignant disorders. Amylase is elevated in pancreatic disorders and esophageal rupture and only rarely in lung carcinoma. High levels of LDH characterize exudates, a large proportion of which are due to malignant disorders. In benign exudates the proportion of LDH isoenzymes is the same as that in the serum. A large proportion of malignant effusions show a predominance of the LD5 fraction, the isoenzyme that corresponds to the M subunit demonstrable by histochemical stains. An elevation of alkaline phosphatase is noted in association with pulmonary infarction. An elevation of the BB isoenzyme of creatine kinase (CK-BB) has been associated with malignant effusion, especially metastatic prostatic carcinoma. Lysozyme activity

is greater in the effusions of patients with tuberculosis than in carcinoma and the connective tissue diseases. Angiotensin-converting enzyme can be measured in pleural effusions, but its level correlates poorly with the serum level of patients with sarcoidosis and other pulmonary disorders.

TUMOR MARKERS

Distinction should be made between substances detected immunocytochemically in cells and those measured biochemically in the effusion. Substances known as tumor markers are biochemical indicators of malignant transformation, either by their sudden appearance as an abnormal product not commonly found or as an increased concentration in the body fluid. The ideal tumor marker would be

1. Released only by transformed tumor cells, or by the host, in response to neoplastic state
2. Produced at levels proportional to the state of differentiation of the tumor cells, or detectable even in small amounts so that early neoplastic residual primaries and small recurrences could be easily detected
3. Related to certain cell types and thus useful in tumor classification
4. Susceptible to the effects of therapy so that an increase or decrease could be useful in the monitoring of treatment
5. Easily reproducible or measurable in specimens obtained in a noninvasive fashion in such substances as body fluids, serum, or effusions.

Many tumor markers are in existence (Table 1.5), but none fulfill the criteria of the ideal tumor marker. Some of these markers are gaining popularity for clinical use with different degrees of success and semispecificity, and they are gradually finding their way into the pathologist's armamentarium. We and others have searched for them regularly by immunocytochemistry in cytologic specimens, particularly fine-needle aspirations and effusions as discussed in chapter 15. Other authors have investigated the value of measuring their level in the fluids accumulated in serous cavities.

Carcinoembryonic antigen (CEA) is one of the earliest markers described in association with malignancy. This glycoprotein component of the glycocalyx of epithelial cells is expressed by a very large number of carcinomas. The marker has been found elevated in the

TABLE 1.5	Categories of Tumor Markers

HORMONES
Human chorionic gonadotropin
Antidiuretic hormone
Parathyroid hormone
Calcitonin
Insulin-like growth factors
Catecholamines and metabolites
ONCOFETAL ANTIGENS
Alpha-fetoprotein
Carcinoembryonic antigen
ISOENZYMES
Prostatic acid phosphatase
Neuron-specific enolase
Regan ALP isoenzyme
LDH-1
SPECIFIC PROTEINS
Immunoglobulins
Prostate-specific antigen
Alpha-lactalbumin
Beta$_2$-microglobulin
MUCINS AND OTHER GLYCOPROTEINS
CA-125
CA-19-9
CA-15-3
ONCOGENES AND THEIR PRODUCTS
src
N-myc
H-ras
OTHERS
Polyamines
Sialic acid
Glycolipids

Modified from: Virji MA, Mercer DW, Herberman RB. Tumor markers in cancer diagnosis and prognosis. *CA.* 32:107; 1988. With permission.

serum of patients with carcinoma arising in a variety of primary sites and has also been measured in pleural fluid. Approximately 50 to 60% of malignant effusions are associated with an elevation of CEA. Elevation is noted only exceptionally in empyema and tuberculosis, and consistently low levels are found in mesothelioma.

Elevated levels of hyaluronic acid have been encountered in pleural fluid and ascites of patients with mesothelioma. Electrophoretic analysis of mesotheliomatous tissue also reveals elevated levels of glycosaminoglycans, most often hyaluronic acid. Some adenocarcinomas, however, can show elevated levels of hyaluronic acid, and hyaluronic acid is not elevated in all cases of mesothelioma.

BIBLIOGRAPHY

The Body Cavities: Anatomy, Histology and Pathophysiology

Black LF. The pleural space and pleural fluid. *Mayo Clin Proc.* 1972;47:493–506.

Sahebjami H, Loudon RG. Pleural effusion: Pathophysiology and clinical features. *Semin Roentgenol.* 1977;12:269–275.

Transudates and Exudates

Light RW, MacGregor MI, Luchsinger PC, et al. Pleural effusions: The diagnostic separation of transudates and exudates. *Ann Intern Med.* 1972;77:507–513.

Melsom RD. Diagnostic reliability of pleural fluid protein estimation. *J R Soc Med.* 1979;72:823–825.

Pathologic Classification

Bynum LJ, Wilson JE. Characteristics of pleural effusions associated with pulmonary embolism. *Arch Intern Med.* 1976; 136:159–162.

Hughson WG, Friedman PJ, Feigin DS, et al. Postpartum pleural effusion: A common radiologic finding. *Ann Intern Med.* 1982;97:856–858.

Light RW, George RB. Incidence and significance of pleural effusion after abdominal surgery. *Chest.* 1976;65:621–625.

Light RW, Girard WM, Jenkinson SF, et al. Parapneumonic effusions. *Am J Med.* 1980;69:507–512.

Biochemical Analysis

Arai H, Kang KY, Sato H, et al. Significance of the quantification and demonstration of hyaluronic acid in tissue specimens for the diagnosis of a pleural mesothelioma. *Am Rev Respir Dis.* 1979;120:529–532.

Bedrossian CWM, Stein DA, Miller WC, et al. Angiotensin-converting enzyme levels in pleural effusion. *Arch Pathol Lab Med.* 1981;105:345–347.

Boyer RD, Kahn AM, Reynolds TB. Diagnostic value of ascitic fluid lactic dehydrogenase, protein and WBC levels. *Arch Intern Med.* 1978;138:1103–1105.

Ervin PE, Wibell L. The serum levels and urinary excretion of α_2-microglobulin in apparently healthy subjects. *Scan J Clin Lab Invest.* 1972;29:69–74.

Hellstrom PE, Friman C, Teppo L. Malignant mesothelioma of 17 years duration with high pleural fluid concentration of hyaluronate. *Scand J Respir Dis.* 1977;58:97–102.

Kim YD, Weber GF, Tomita JT, et al. Galactosyltransferase variant in pleural effusion. *Clin Chem.* 1982;28:1133–1136.

Lee YN. Alkaline phosphatase in intestinal perforation. *JAMA.* 1969;208:361.

Peterman TA, Speicher CI. Evaluating pleural effusions: A two-stage laboratory approach. *JAMA.* 1984;252:1051–1053.

Riska H, Pettersson T, Froseth B, et al. β₂-Microglobulin in pleural effusions. *Acta Med Scand.* 1982;211:45–50.

Rudman D, Chawla RK, DelRio AE, et al. Orosomucoid content of pleural and peritoneal effusions. *J Clin Invest.* 1974;54:147–155.

Seriff NS, Cohen ML, Samuel P, et al. Chylothorax: Diagnosis by lipoprotein electrophoresis of serum and pleural fluid. *Thorax.* 1977;32:98–100.

Sherr HP, Light RW, Merson MH, et al. Origin of pleural fluid amylase in esophageal rupture. *Ann Intern Med.* 1972;76:985–986.

Sileo AV, Chawla SK, LoPresti PA. Pancreatic ascites: Diagnostic importance of ascitic lipase. *Dig Dis Sci.* 1975;20:1110–1114.

Teloh HA. The clinical pathology of pleural fluids. *Ann Clin Lab Sci.* 1973;3:98–107.

Waxler B, Eisenstein R, Battifora H. Electrophoresis of tissue gylcosaminoglycans as an aid in the diagnosis of mesotheliomas. *Cancer.* 1979;44:221–227.

Westrom L, Skude G, Mardh PA. Amylases of the genital tract. II: Peritoneal fluid isoamylases in acute salpingitis. *Am J Obstet Gynecol.* 1976;126:657–660.

Tumor Markers

Coleman D, Omerod M. Tumor markers in clinical cytology. In: Koss L, Coleman D, eds. *Advances in Clinical Cytology.* New York: Masson Publishers; 1984, pp 33–47.

Lin CW, Inglis NR, Rule AH, et al. Histaminase and other tumor markers in malignant effusion fluids. *Cancer Res.* 1979;39(12):4894–4899.

Yam L, Janckila A. Immunocytodiagnosis of carcinocythemia in disseminated breast cancer. *Acta Cytol.* 1987;31(1):68–72.

CEA in Effusions

Pinto MM, Bernstein LH, Brugan DA, et al. Measurement of CA 125, CEA and α-fetoprotein in ovarian cyst fluid: Diagnostic adjunct to cytology. *Diagn Cytopathol.* 1990;6(3):160–163.

CHAPTER TWO

Clinicopathologic Correlations

HISTORICAL DEVELOPMENT

The first cytologic description of mesothelial cells in effusions is attributed to Reinhardt, who in 1847 commented on the morphologic transformation exhibited by free cells in the exudate. Shortly thereafter, Bennett documented the first example of metastatic malignancy, an ovarian carcinoma that spread to the peritoneal fluid and was diagnosed by paracentesis. Later in the nineteenth century both Reincke and Beneke reported on gynecologic malignancies diagnosed by cytologic examination of the ascitic fluid. The early reports on pleural effusion described the cytologic features of pleurisy, empyema, and pulmonary infarction. Paul Ehrlich, of later fame in the field of chemistry, wrote a paper in 1880 entitled "Contribution to the Etiology and Histology of Pleural Effusions." He is believed to have described the first malignant cases noted in effusions examined by the cytologic technique of staining air-dried smears. At the turn of the century, attention focused on the significance of mitotic figures in effusions, which became the subject of hot debate among investigators. Likewise, controversy engulfed the meaning of lymphocytosis in tuberculous pleural effusions. For a long time effusions were divided into three major categories: (1) "Idiopathic," which in fact included tuberculosis, characterized by lymphocytosis and an absence of mesothelial cells; (2) "mechanical," as found in cardiac failure, renal disease, and malignancy; and (3) "infective," including the purulent exudates and eosinophilic pleural effusions. The difficulty in distinguishing malignant cells from mesothelial cells was fully appreciated, and the large sheets of cells were called "placards endotheliaux."

In the early 1930s, supravital methods of stain were very popular for verifying the viability of cells suspended in the effusion. Quensel was the major proponent of the method, which later became supplanted by phase contrast microscopy. The cell block technique was first attempted in 1896 and by the 1920s was firmly entrenched in the armamentarium of the cytopathologist. Some of the early trials at quantitation were performed in effusions in an attempt to distinguish mesothelial and tumor cells. These efforts persist to the present.

CLINICAL APPLICATIONS

Clinicopathologic correlations remain the backbone of successful cytologic evaluation of effusions. A good clinical history is crucial because malignancy constitutes the etiology of the effusion in less than 50% of the cases. Approximately 46% of patients with malignant effusions have no previously known primary site of the neoplasm. This makes the examination of an effusion not only a challenge to the diagnostic acumen of cytopathologists but an anxiously regarded piece of information as well. The number of specimens submitted to the cytopathology laboratory as well as their proportion varies from institution to institution. Over a 10-year period at St. Louis University, 2470 samples of serous fluids were submitted for examination, including pelvic washes. Of these, 619 were malignant for an overall rate of positivity of about 25%. This number is low in relation to other institutions where a greater number of cancer patients are regularly seen (Table 2.1).

In general, effusions fall into four major diagnostic groups: patients with previously diagnosed malignancy, patients with a newly developed effusion in whom malignancy is a diagnostic possibility, pleural or peritoneal effusion in patients with a history of asbestos exposure and suspicion of mesothelioma, and patients in whom routine methods fail to establish a diagnosis.

In patients with known malignancy, the objective is

TABLE 2.1 Malignant Effusions and Pelvic Washes Diagnosed at St. Louis University over a 10-Year Period (1980–1989)

Type of specimen	1980	1981	1982	1983	1984	1985	1986	1987	1988	1989	Total
Pleural effusion	21/122 17%	57/144 40%	21/85 25%	29/131 22%	17/113 15%	32/208 15%	26/157 16%	17/139 12%	23/146 12%	19/121 16%	262/1253 21%
Ascites	15/37 40%	33/61 33%	15/42 15%	20/38 52%	13/57 23%	16/58 27.5%	13/47 27%	10/44 23%	12/50 24%	14/48 29%	161/482 31.5%
Pelvic washes	7/22 32%	15/26 57%	22/57 38.5%	30/91 33%	15/97 15%	19/91 21%	17/88 19%	20/73 27%	14/68 20.5%	12/59 20%	171/678 25%
Pericardial effusion	1/2 50%	2/8 25%	2/8 25%	2/3 66%	0/4 0%	2/7 28.5%	3/7 43%	6/10 60%	4/8 50%	3/7 43%	25/57 44%
Total	44/183	107/39	60/192	81/263	45/271	69/370	59/299	53/266	53/272	48/235	519/2470 25%

to establish whether the effusion is due to a spread of neoplasia to the serous space. Malignant cells in the effusion can be identified with those in the primary site simply by comparing the cytologic preparations with the pathologic material previously derived from the original neoplasm. If the morphology shows variation, another primary site should be clinically investigated. In these cases a wide variety of special stains and immunologic markers can be applied to both sites. Even if individual members of the immunocytochemical panel are nonspecific, an exact match of positivity in the two sites is strong evidence of metastasis from that primary site.

In newly developed effusions the first task at hand is to establish whether a malignancy is present. The clinical picture invariably offers some clues about the origin of the malignant cells, but accurate information is not always available to the cytopathologist. These data must be obtained through a process greatly facilitated by open communication with the clinical colleague. A complete clinical history including a thorough review of systems and a radiologic profile including the results of the CT scans are crucial in this regard. Sometimes the clinical data are noncontributory. However, the cytopathologist can considerably narrow the differential diagnosis by an intelligent combination of cytomorphologic criteria and an assortment of special studies.

These studies are a must if the suspicion is mesothelioma. The same is true of effusions that resist repeated attempts at diagnosis by the conventional techniques. Consequently, every precaution should be taken to handle the specimen properly so that the required tests can be applied.

DIAGNOSTIC YIELD

Koss suggests extreme caution in rendering a diagnosis of malignancy in the absence of solid clinical grounds. His guidelines to avoid pitfalls and the overdiagnosis of malignancy are as follows:

- An accurate clinical history must point in the direction of cancer.
- If the protein level is less than 3g% the diagnosis of cancer is less likely.
- A diagnosis of cancer should be avoided if the morphology of the cells is not optimal.
- A diagnosis of cancer should be avoided if the cellular and nuclear sizes are monotonous.
- Cancer is very unlikely if nuclear size is below the upper unit of normal (25 μm in diameter) and the nucleus does not appear enlarged for the size of the cell.
- A diagnosis of cancer should not be rendered if there are no structural nuclear abnormalities affecting either the nuclear envelope, the chromatinic content, or the nucleoli.
- Cancer is unlikely if there is evidence of inflammatory processes with numerous polys and macrophages noted against a necrotic background resulting from cell death.

Lymphomas are unique in that the monotony of the cell population in effusions is often the first clue to the diagnosis. We have seen examples of carcinomas in which the neoplastic cells had to be diligently sought amidst a very heavy inflammatory exudate. In our ex-

TABLE 2.2 Analysis of 6001 Specimens of Pleural and Peritoneal Fluids

Total cases	6001
Total with malignant disease	(2558)
Cytology positive	1489
Cytology negative	860
Total without malignant disease	(3443)
Cytology positive	10
Cytology negative	3340
Sensitivity	0.58
Specificity	0.97
Predicted positive value	0.99
Predicted negative value	0.80

Modified from: Naylor B. Pleural, peritoneal and pericardial fluids. In: Bibbo M, ed. *Comprehensive Cytopathology.* Philadelphia: WB Saunders; 1990: chap 22, 541–614. (Based on the work by Spriggs and Boddington.) With permission.

TABLE 2.3 Etiology of Pleural Effusions

	Percent
Malignancy	45
Congestive heart failure	12
Infectious	22
Tuberculosis	(10)
Bacterial	(9)
Viral	(1)
Fungal	(<1)
Empyema	(1)
Parasitic	(<1)
Indeterminant	10
Pulmonary embolus or infarct	3
Cirrhosis	2
Collagen disease	1
Other	5

From: Hausheer F, Yarbro J. Diagnosis and treatment of malignant pleural effusions. *Semin Oncol.* 1985;12(1):54–75. With permission.

perience a reliable deterrent to a malignant diagnosis is the absence of a distinct two-cell population in the effusion. Only when the malignant cells clearly stand out from their mesothelial neighbors are we willing to render a diagnosis of metastatic malignancy.

The largest series of effusions analyzed for diagnostic accuracy is that of Spriggs and Boddington, who culled the statistical results of six large published series. Their analysis showed a sensitivity of 58% and a specificity of 97% in a total of 6001 effusions, mainly from pleural and peritoneal specimens (Table 2.2).

PLEURAL EFFUSION

Pleural fluid is the most common of the three serous effusions routinely submitted to the cytology laboratory. A review of recent large series showed that about half of these were suspicious for malignancy which was confirmed in about 45% of the cases as summarized by Hausheer and depicted in Table 2.3. At our institution, ovarian carcinoma in the female and gastrointestinal carcinoma in the male were the most frequent sources of malignancy found in the ascitic fluid.

The pleural space is the best studied because of the high frequency with which effusion occurs in this location. Consequently, a considerable amount of information is available regarding the frequency of malignancy and the primary origin of neoplasms in such specimens (Table 2.4). It would serve the cytopatholo-

gist well to become acquainted with the prevalence of various diagnoses in his or her own body of work. Familiarity with the disease conditions one is searching for facilitates the discovery of an answer in difficult cases.

In our own material, breast cancer in the female and lung cancer in the male ranked first in pleural effusions, but pulmonary carcinoma is rapidly overtaking breast cancer in the female as well. Lung tumors lead the list in most series. The cause of pleural effusions in lung carcinoma varies from patient to patient but usually includes one or more of the following: hilar lymph node involvement, neoplastic seeding of the parietal or visceral pleura, and liver metastasis. Tuberculosis leads the list of infections causing pleural effusion and should be suspected in an elderly patient with lymphocytosis of the pleural fluid. In children a pleural effusion with a high lymphocyte count is suggestive of viral infection. With the higher prevalence of immunosuppression among hospitalized patients, rarer opportunistic pathogens such as viruses, protozoa, fungi and helminths are to be expected in pleural effusions. Indeed, parasites such as echinococcus, strongyloides and filaria have been infrequently observed in pleural and peritoneal effusions. An amebic abscess of the liver or the lung may break into the pleural spaces and give rise to a hemorrhagic pleural effusion. Other rare infectious agents include Pneumocystis, Leishmania and Giardia, which have been detected in body fluids and will be discussed in chapter 6.

TABLE 2.4   Malignancy in Pleural Effusions

Site of Origin	Percentage in Various Series			
	Johnston	Monte	Sears	Hsu
MALE				
Lung	49.1	51.4	25.4	61.7
Lymphoma/leukemia	21.1	11.4	22.4	10.2
GI tract	7.0	11.4	5.6	11.8
Mesothelioma	1.0	5.7	6.8	. . .
Miscellaneous	10.5	14.2	24.5	4.2
Unknown	10.9	5.7	15.0	9.5
FEMALE				
Breast	37.4	52.7	38.1	20.7
Female genital tract	20.3	9.8	11.9	13.2
Lung	15.0	20.8	14.7	46.2
Lymphoma/leukemia	8.0	3.2	11.1	4.9
GI tract	4.3	4.3	3.6	6.6
Mesothelioma	. . .	2.1	1.6	. . .
Miscellaneous	5.9	5.4	7.5	0.4
Unknown	9.1	1.0	11.3	7.4

PERICARDIAL FLUID

Pericardial fluid constitutes less than one percent of the serous effusions examined in a cytology laboratory. At St. Louis University 57 cases (2%) of serous effusions were of pericardial origin and 25 of these (44%) were positive for malignancy (see Table 2.1). Most of these effusions are exudates, but transudates may result from congestive heart failure or collagen vascular diseases affecting the pericardium. Other rare nonmalignant disorders resulting in pericardial effusions include sarcoidosis, which often results in a transudate, and lymphangioleiomyomatosis, which may lead to chylopericardium. More common causes of chylopericardium include trauma, thrombosis of vessels in the chest, tuberculosis, cystic hygroma, and lymphangiectasis. A lymphocytic predominance (T cells) in the pericardial effusion most frequently represents a viral or a tuberculous process, but less frequently is a sign of lymphoma. The most common type of pericardial effusion, however, is an exudate, and most exudates reflect a metastatic neoplasm. Only one large series reported by Zipf and Johnston tabulated the most common sources of metastatic malignancies detected in pericardial effusions for males and females (Table 2.5). Rare cases of mesothelial papilloma and primary mesotheliomas have also been described in the pericardium. In our own experience, carcinomas of breast and lung and lymphomas are the most commonly encountered malignancies in the pericardial fluid.

ASCITIC FLUID

Ascites is a common complication of neoplastic and nonneoplastic diseases, but ascitic fluid is not examined cytologically as frequently as pleural effusions. This is because cirrhosis of the liver and congestive heart failure are the most common causes of ascites and do not

TABLE 2.5   Sources of Malignancy in Pericardial Fluid

Diagnostic Features	Percentage
Positive cytology	27.6
Site of origin:	
Breast	33.3
Colon	20.0
Lung	20.0
Lymphoma/leukemia	6.6
Miscellaneous	6.6
Unknown	13.3

Modified from: Zipf RE, Johnston WW. The role of cytology in the evaluation of pericardial effusions. *Chest.* 1972;62:593–596. With permission.

TABLE 2.6 Sources of Malignancy in Ascitic Fluid

Site of Origin	Percentage in Two Series	
	Monte	Sears
MALE		
Lung	4.7	9.5
GI tract	42.8	23.8
Miscellaneous	38.0	46.4
Unknown	14.2	16.6
FEMALE		
Female genital tract	61.0	50.6
Breast	10.3	17.6
GI tract	9.0	9.7
Lung	0.0	1.7
Miscellaneous	15.5	13.2
Unknown	3.8	8.3

necessitate cytologic evaluation for a clinical diagnosis. Malignancy, the third most common cause of ascites, can be easily diagnosed by cytologic examination of peritoneal fluid. The most commonly encountered neoplasms are depicted on Table 2.6. A number of techniques for peritoneal sampling during surgery or at laparoscopy have expanded the usefulness of cytology in the study of peritoneal fluid. In particular, so-called second-look operations for tumors of the ovary are popular sources of peritoneal fluid for cytologic examination. The method lends itself well to the monitoring of therapeutic outcome in ovarian cancer.

CULDOCENTESIS AND PERITONEAL WASHINGS

Culdocentesis had a brief popularity as a screening method for uterine adenocarcinoma. However, the method has been a major failure in the detection of early ovarian carcinoma. These tumors remain a diagnostic challenge because of the inaccessibility of the ovary to physical examination, the difficulties in radiologic visualization, and the late development of signs and symptoms. Not infrequently, the first sign of ovarian carcinoma is pelvic discomfort and accumulation of a small amount of fluid in the cul de sac. In these cases, culdocentesis is indicated, leading to the identification of a mixture of mesothelial and nonmesothelial cells. Schwinn recommends the plan outlined in Figure 2.1

for the follow-up of patients with abnormal cells in culdocentesis fluid.

If peritoneal washings are to be effective in symptomatic women, close cooperation must exist between the gynecologist and the cytology laboratory. Peritoneal washings during surgery for the removal of ovarian carcinoma have shown some promise as a diagnostic tool, however, the accuracy of the method has not been clearly established. The method is less reliable for the detection of implants during second-look operations, but so is its alternative, random biopsies of peritoneal surfaces. A problem in culdocentesis and peritoneal washings is the reactivity of mesothelial cells and the difficulty in distinguishing them from malignant cells. This phenomenon is particularly acute in peritoneal washings that yield sheets of mesothelial cells affected by instrumentation. Samples from the pelvic cavity, the lateral gutters and the diaphragmatic surface are obtained. Of these, the ones deriving from the most dependent portions cause the greatest difficulties because of cellular degeneration.

REPORTING OF RESULTS

Cytopathology has gained respectability as a reliable diagnostic method, and interpretation of cytologic samples should be handled in the same fashion as any consultative report rendered by the pathologist. Consequently, equivocal wording or imprecise terminology has no place in the repertoire of the cytopathologist. The report should be based on concise clinical data including laboratory and radiologic findings. The gross description is crucial in effusions and can be a clue to the underlying disease process. The descriptive terms used in the microscopic portion of the report should be both cytologically accurate and compatible with the histopathologic terminology used for resected surgical specimens. Whenever applicable, comment and recommendation may be used to clarify the diagnostic interpretation. The examples depicted in Table 2.7 show the terminology used most often in our practice.

FOLLOW-UP

Because of the seriousness implied by a diagnosis of malignant effusion, every such event should be followed up by clinical inquiry of cytologic–histologic correlation. This is also crucial in cases reported as suspi-

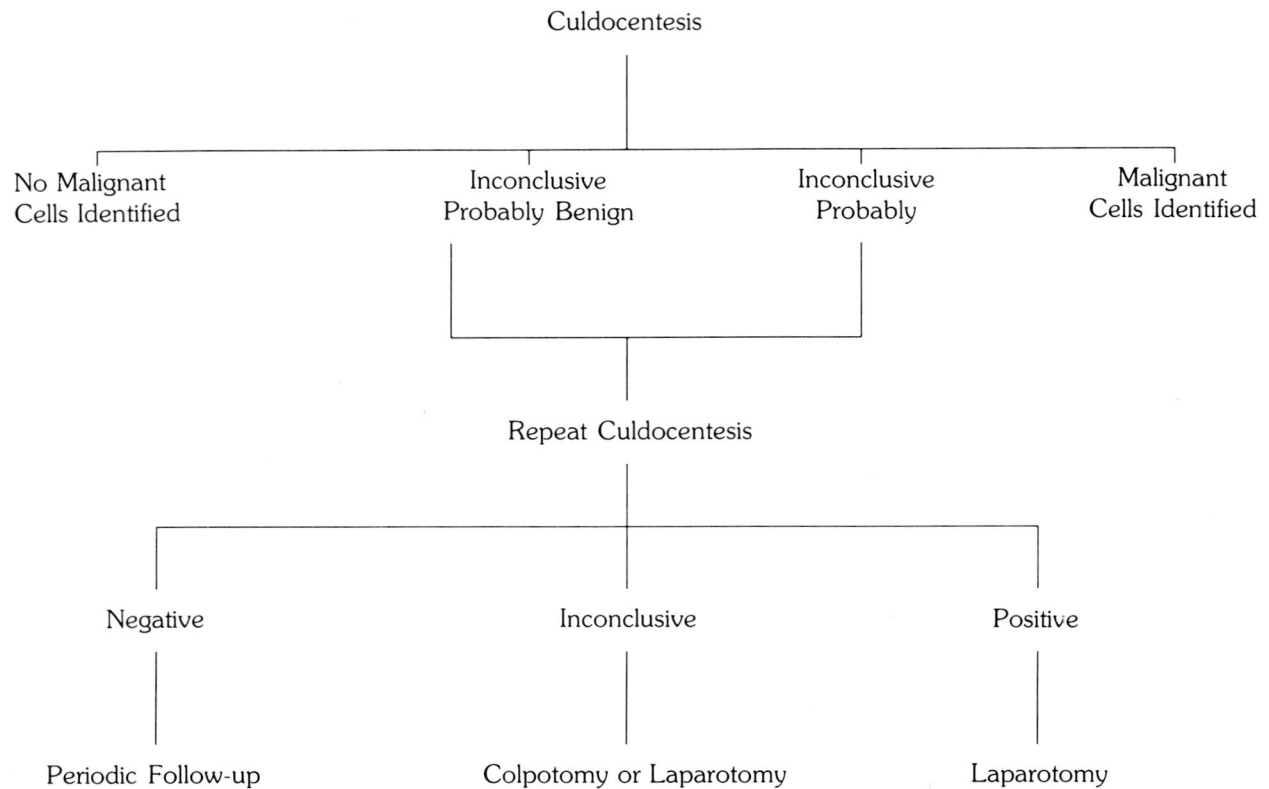

Culdocentesis

No Malignant Cells Identified | Inconclusive Probably Benign | Inconclusive Probably | Malignant Cells Identified

Repeat Culdocentesis

Negative | Inconclusive | Positive

Periodic Follow-up | Colpotomy or Laparotomy | Laparotomy

FIGURE 2.1   Schema for the follow-up of culdocentesis results. Close communication between clinician and pathologist are crucial to maximize results. (From Schwinn CP, Bernstein C, Samona W, Culdocentesis. In Wied G, et al (eds), Compendium on Diagnostic Cytology: Tutorials of Cytology. Chicago, IL, 1988:216–227. With permission.)

cious for malignancy. A letter to the clinician may suffice if the surgical procedure is not performed at the same institution. A comparison between the histologic and cytologic preparations permits the correlation of morphologic findings and clarifies any diagnostic discrepancy. It is very useful to examine new cytologic material along with the existing histologic sections of the primary tumor when these are available in advance.

QUALITY ASSURANCE

The measures outlined above go a long way to improve diagnostic accuracy in the interpretation of cytologic specimens of effusions. However, other measures such as rescreening of positive cases, intradepartmental consultations among not only cytotechnologists but also attending cytopathologists, and the use of referral centers for difficult cases can also be of help in assuring good

results. Discussion of difficult cases and illustration of confirmatory special studies increase the level of confidence of the staff. In practice, the most common sources of error are poorly preserved or poorly processed specimens, which lead to degeneration or overstaining of cytologic preparations. Providing heparinized containers avoids the clotting of specimens and the collection of specimens in the wrong containers. These errors can be prevented by monitoring the collection and preparation of cytologic specimens, in particular the technical quality of filters, cell blocks, and staining methods. Dryness of filters and poor cellularity of cell blocks are problems that require constant monitoring and prompt correction. Preventive maintenance of centrifuges, cytospins, and filtering apparatuses protects against overblown and fragmented cells. A microscope with impeccable optics and a clean lens system is indispensable for the subtle appreciation of the cytologic morphology. The reliability of screeners in identifying significant changes can be monitored by the so-called

TABLE 2.7 Examples of Cytopathologic Interpretation of Various Effusions

Specimen	Diagnosis	Comment	Recommendation
Pleural fluid	Negative for tumor cells	Marked inflammation Compatible with empyema	Suggests bacteriologic culture
Pericardial fluid	Negative for tumor cells	Acute inflammation Microorganisms with characteristics of cocci	Suggests bacteriologic culture
Peritoneal fluid	Negative for tumor cells	Numerous cholesterol crystals, compatible with pseudochylous ascites	. . .
Pleural fluid	Negative for tumor cells	Mesothelial hyperplasia Compatible with history of recent pulmonary emboli	. . .
Pleural fluid	Suspicious for tumor cells	Rather atypical but degenerated cells noted	Suggest repeat cytology if effusion reaccumulates
Ascites	Positive for tumor cells	Monotonous population of atypical lymphocytes, compatible with lymphoma Marker studies to follow	Suggest submit specimen for flow cytometry
Ascites	Positive for tumor cells	Adenocarcinoma present Cells positive for CEA Unable to identify source	Specimen submitted for further markers to identify primary site
Ascites	Positive for tumor cells	Adenocarcinoma present Cells positive for PSA	Suggest biopsy of prostate

buddy system between two cytotechnologists or a pyramidal hierarchy among the screening staff. Continuing education sessions to familiarize the screeners with the lesions more likely to occur in the serosal cavities also constitute a very effective quality assurance measure. Of particular merit is the use of test samples with an unknown diagnosis provided by several professional organizations.

BIBLIOGRAPHY

Historic Development

Bahremberg LPH. On the diagnostic results of microscopical examination of the ascitic fluid in two cases of carcinoma involving the peritoneum. *Cleve Med Gazette.* 1896;11:274–278.

Beneke R. Uber freies wachsthun metastatischer geschwulstelemente in serosen hohlen. *Dtsch Arch Klin Med* 1899;64:237–241.

Bennett JH. *On Cancerous and Cancroid Growths.* Edinburgh: Sutherland and Know; 1849.

Ellis EB. Cancer cells in pleural fluid. *Bull Int Assoc Med Museums.* 1922;8:126.

Erlich P. Beitrage zur atiologie and histologie pleuritischer exsudate. *Charite-Annalen.* 1882;7:199–203.

Light RW. Pleural effusions: Symposium on pulmonary disease. *Med Clin North Am.* 1977;61:1339–1352.

Lucke A, Klebs E. Beitrag zur ovariotomie and zur Kenntni's der abdominalgeschwulste. *Virchows Arch [A].* 1867;41:1–6.

Mandlebaum FS. The diagnosis of malignant tumors by paraffin sections of centrifuged exudates. *J Lab Clin Med* 1917;2:580.

Quensel U. Für Frage der Zytodiagnostik der Ergüsse seroser höhlen: Methodologische and pathologisch-anatomische Bemerkungen. *Acta Med Scand.* 1928;68:427–457.

Reincke J. Zowei falle von Krebsimpfung in punctionskanalen bei carcinomatoser peritonitis. *Virchows Arch [A].* 1870;51:391.

Reinhardt B. Uber die sogenannte spalbarkeit der Zellenkerne. *Virchows Arch [A].* 1847;1:528.

Saphir O. Cytologic diagnosis of cancer from pleural and peritoneal fluids. *Am J Clin Pathol.* 1949;19:309–314.

Warren LF. The diagnostic value of mitotic figures in the cells of serous exudates. *Arch Intern Med.* 1911;8:648–653.

Clinical Applications

Byrd RB. Current concepts in diagnosing the cause of pleural effusion. *Geriatrics.* 1977;10:44–48.

Hausheer F, Yarbro J. Diagnosis and treatment of malignant pleural effusions. *Semin Oncol.* 1985;12:54–75.

Johnson W. The cytologic diagnosis of cancer in serous effusions. *Acta Cytol.* 1966;10(3):161–172.

Monte SA, Hormoz E, Lang WR. Positive effusion cytology as the initial presentation of malignancy. *Acta Cytol.* 1987;31:448–452.

Sahn SA. The differential diagnosis of pleural effusions. *West J Med.* 1982;137:99–108.

Soplo JA. Pleural effusions: Guide to diagnosis. *Hosp Med.* 1986;86–92.

Irani DR, Underwood RD, Johnson EH, Greenberg SD. Malignant pleural effusions: A clinical cytopathologic study. *Arch Int Med* 1987;147:1133–1136.

Van de Molengraft FJJM, Vooijs GP. The interval between the diagnosis of malignancy and the development of effusions with reference to the role of cytologic diagnosis. *Acta Cytol.* 1988;32:183–187.

Diagnostic Yield

Berge T, Hellstein S. Cytological diagnosis of cancer cells in pleural and ascitic fluid. *Acta Cytol.* 1966;10(2):138–140.

Cardozo PL. Critical evaluation of 3,000 cytologic analyses of pleural fluid, ascitic fluid and pericardial fluid. *Acta Cytol.* 1966;10:455–460.

Hsu C, Path MRC. Cytologic detection of malignancy in pleural effusion: A review of 5,255 samples from 3,811 patients. *Diagn Cytopathol.* 1987;3:8–12.

Jarvi O, Kunnas R, Tyrkko J. The accuracy and significance of cytologic cancer diagnosis of pleural effusions. *Acta Cytol.* 1972;16:152–157.

Johnston W. The malignant pleural effusion: A review of cytopathologic diagnoses of 584 specimens from 472 consecutive patients. *Cancer.* 1985;56:905–909.

King DT, Neiberg RK. The use of cytology in the evaluation of pleural effusions. *Am Clin Lab Sci.* 1973;9:18–23.

Prakash UBS, Reiman HM. Comparison of needle biopsy with cytologic analysis for the evaluation of pleural effusion: Analysis of 414 cases. *Mayo Clin Proc.* 1985;60(3):158–164.

Sears D, Hajdu SI. The cytologic diagnosis of malignant neoplasms in pleural and peritoneal effusions. *Acta Cytol.* 1987; 31:85–97.

Bottles K, Reznicek MJ, Holly EA, et al. Cytologic criteria used to diagnose adenocarcinoma in pleural effusions mod. *Pathol* 1991;4:677–681.

Pleural Effusion

Dines DE, Elvebach LR, McCall JT. Zinc, copper and iron content of pleural fluid in benign and neoplastic disease. *Thorax.* 1972;27:368–370.

Doust JY, Kohout E. Alkaline phosphatase in pleural effusions. *Isr J Med Sci.* 1973;9:1588–1590.

Freidman MA, Slater E. Malignant pleural effusions. *Cancer Treat Rev.* 1978;5:49–66.

Good JT, Taryle DA, Maulitz RM, et al. The diagnostic value of pleural fluid pH. *Chest* 1980;78:55–59.

Houston MC. Pleural effusion: Diagnostic value of measurements of PO_2, PCO_2, and pH. *South Med J.* 1981;74:585–589.

Klockars M. Pleural fluid lysozyme in human disease. *Arch Intern Med.* 1979;139:73–77.

Light R, Ball WC Jr. Lactate dehydrogenase isoenzymes in pleural effusions. *Am Rev Respir Dis.* 1973;108:660–664.

Light RW, Ball WC Jr. Glucose and amylase in pleural effusions. *JAMA.* 1973;225:257–260.

Pettersson T, Weber TH, Ojala K. Creatine kinase isoenzyme BB as a tumor marker in pleural effusions. *Clin Chem.* 1981;27:1147–1148.

Potts DE, Levin DC, Sahn SA. Pleural fluid pH in parapneumonic effusions. *Chest.* 1976;70:328–331.

Prakash UBS. Malignant pleural effusions. *Postgrad Med.* 1986;80(5):201–207.

Prakash UBS, Dines DE. Thoracentesis, pleural biopsy, and pleuroscopy. *Semin Respir Med.* 1981;3(1):42–53.

Sahn SA. Malignant pleural effusions. *Clin Chest Med.* 1985;6(1):113–125.

Vladutin AO, Adler RH, Brason FW. Diagnostic value of biochemical analysis of pleural effusions. *Am J Clin Pathol.* 1979;71:210–214.

Winkelman M, Pfitzer. Blind pleural biopsy in combination with cytology of pleural effusions. *Acta Cytol.* 1981;254(4):373–376.

Pericardial Fluid

Chai BL, da Costa JL, Ransome GA. Cardiac tamponade due to pericardial effusion. *Thorax.* 1973;28:657–659.

Krikorian JG, Hancock EW. Pericardiocentesis. *Am J Med.* 1978;65:808–814.

Paradis IL, Caldwell EJ. Diagnostic approach to pleural effusion. *J Maine Med Assoc.* 1977;10:378–382.

Pinto M. Malignant pericardial effusion and cardiac tamponade. *Acta Cytol.* 1986;30:657–661.

Ramsey SL, Tweendale DN, Bryant LR, et al. Cytologic features of pericardial mesothelium. *Acta Cytol.* 1970;14:283–290.

Reyes CV, Strinden C, Banerji M. The role of cytology in neoplastic cardiac tamponade. *Acta Cytol.* 1982;26:299–302.

Zipf RE, Johnston WW. The role of cytology in the evaluation of pericardial effusions. *Chest.* 1972;62:593–596.

Peritoneal Fluid

Bercovici B, Gallely R. The cytology of the human peritoneal fluid. *Acta Cytol.* 1978;22(3):124–127.

Brook I, Altman RS, Lachman WW, et al. Measurement of lactate in ascitic fluid: An aid in the diagnosis of peritonitis with particular relevance to spontaneous bacterial peritonitis of the cirrhotic. *Dig Dis Sci.* 1981;26:1089–1094.

Bruno B, Gallily R. The cytology of the human peritoneal fluid. *Acta Cytol.* 1978;22:124–127.

Coupland G. Pancreatic ascites in childhood. *J Pediatr Surg.* 1970;5:570.

Craig R, Sparberg M, Ivanovich P, Rice L. Nephrogenic ascites. *Arch Intern Med.* 1974;134:276–279.

Delaney HM, Moss CM, Carnevale N. The use of enzyme analysis of pertoneal blood in the clinical assessment of abdominal organ injury. *Surg Gynecol Obstet.* 1976;142:161–167.

Donowitz M, Kerstein MD, Spiro HM. Pancreatic ascites. *Medicine.* 1974;53:183–195.

Franco AE, Levine HD, Hall AP. Rheumatoid pericarditis. Report of 17 cases diagnosed clinically. *Ann Intern Med.* 1972;77:837–844.

Gitlin N, Stauffer JL, Silvestri RC. The pH of ascitic fluid in the diagnosis of spontaneous bacterial peritonitis in alcoholic cirrhosis. *Hepatology.* 1982;2:408–411.

Greene LS, Levine R, Gross MJ, et al. Distinguishing between malignant and cirrhotic ascites by computerized step-wise discrimination functional analysis of its biochemistry. *Am J Gastroenterol.* 1978;70:448–454.

Keettel WC, Pixley EE, Buchshaum AJ. Experience with peritoneal cytology in the management of gynecologic malignancies. *Am J Obstet Gynecol.* 1974;120:174–182.

Mansberger AR Jr. The value of peritoneal fluid ammonia levels in the differential diagnosis of the acute abdomen. *Ann Surg.* 1962;155:998–1010.

Marsan C. A propos du cyto-diagnostic des ascites. *Gastroenterol Clin Biol.* 1980;4:636–639.

Rush BF Jr, Host WR, Fewel J, et al. Intestinal ischemia and some organic substances in serum and abdominal fluid. *Arch Surg.* 1972;105:151–157.

Sawer BA, Jamieson WG, Durand D. The significance of elevated peritoneal fluid phosphate level in intestinal infarction. *Surg Gynecol Obstet.* 1978;146:43–45.

CHAPTER THREE

Multimodal Approach

Clinicians map out their own diagnostic strategies by choosing to send specimens to different kinds of laboratories: cytology, chemistry, microbiology, hematology. Pathologists on the other hand must choose the method they apply to the specimens they receive. The use of special techniques considerably expands the usefulness of cytopathology in arriving at correct diagnoses. Very often this expanded methodology enables the observation of features that further classify the disease process or may even influence treatment. For this reason we subscribe to a multimodal approach that maximizes the effectiveness of our study of specimens sent for cytologic examination. Not every case gets examined by all modalities depicted in the diagram. The challenge is to use the ancillary techniques in a cost-effective and target-appropriate manner. As we will see in this chapter, the success of this approach relies on a commitment to technical excellence from collection of the specimen to reporting of the results.

COLLECTION PROCEDURES

Effusions may be tapped for therapeutic or diagnostic purposes. It is also possible to sample the mesothelium by fine catheter aspiration of the peritoneal cavity in the absence of effusion. During surgery it is possible to obtain fluid from the serous cavities by aspiration, brushings, and localized washings of suspicious areas, if the amount of effusion fluid is small. Extensive sampling of subdiaphragmatic mesothelium and the lateral gutters of the abdominal cavity usually accompanies pelvic washings during so-called second-look operations (Table 3.1).

Large pleural and pericardial effusions are most frequently tapped because of symptoms such as shortness of breath or impending tamponade. Smaller effusions are detected on physical examination and tapped exclu-

sively for diagnostic purposes. The effusion should be tapped in its most dependent portion with an 18-gauge needle and withdrawn into an ACD-treated vacuum tube or a heparinized container. Up to 1000 mL of fluid are transferred promptly to the laboratory where the condition of the specimen is described and multiple aliquots may be processed separately according to the diagram shown in Figure 3.1. A 5.0 mL aliquot is stained immediately with Tolnidine blue for triage purposes, as popularized by Naylor. Depending on the findings in this initial evaluation, aliquots may also be submitted to the microbiology, immunopathology, cell biology, or cytogenetics laboratory.

In our practice we have developed experience with morphometry, special stains, immunocytochemistry, electron microscopy, and flow cytometry. However, as it will be stressed in Chapter 16, effusions lend themselves well to the application of a number of other ancillary procedures such as cell image analysis, tissue culture, gene rearrangement studies, in situ hybridization, and the polymerase chain reaction among many.

If the effusion cannot be sent immediately for examination it can be refrigerated at 4°C but not frozen. Once in the laboratory, effusions may be kept refrigerated for days without loss of cellular detail in subsequent examinations. Unless the effusion is rather hypocellular, direct cytocentrifugation yields thick smears, too crowded for adequate examination. For this reason we prefer smears obtained by centrifuging 5.0-mL aliquots of the effusion at 2500 rpm for 30 minutes followed by resuspension. The cell pellet is sampled with a cotton swab. A minimum of four smears are postfixed in 95% alcohol and are stained by Papanicolaou's method. At least two air-dried smears are prepared from the centrifugate and stained by the MGG method. These preparations are particularly useful in the classification of lymphomas and leukemias because they are easily comparable to preexisting hematologic material. They also allow for identification of nonhematologic

18

TABLE 3.1 Collection of Specimens from the Serous Cavities

Tapping of effusion:
  Thoracentesis
  Peritoneal paracentesis
  Pericardial centesis
During surgery:
  Direct brushings
  Localized washings
  Pelvic washings
At endoscopy:
  Laparoscopy
  Thoracoscopy
  Pericardioscopy
Other:
  Fine catheter aspiration
  Drainage of dialysate
  Peritoneal catheter
  Drainage of chest tube

malignancies, and it is not uncommon for the cytologist to be called upon to interpret studies initially ordered for cell counts by the hematology laboratory.

CYTOPREPARATORY METHODS

Several methods are available to concentrate the cells from effusions. These include centrifugation followed by smear preparation from the sediment, sedimentation by a gradient method, cytocentrifugation, and membrane filtration (Table 3.2).

All effusions submitted to our laboratory for cytologic evaluation are examined by a membrane filtration technique. We used Gelman filters exclusively for the past 3 years but recently reverted to millipore because Gelman filters became scarce. Regardless of the filter used, care should be exercised not to exceed the optimal vacuum in order not to burst the cells under study. There are three commercial sources of filters suitable for the processing of effusions: Millipore (Millipore Filter Corporation, Bedford, MA 01730), Nucleopore (Wallabs, P.O. Box 455, Fairfax, CA 94565), and Gelman (Scientific Products, McGraw Park, IL 60085). Our filters are cut in half and stained by Papanicolaou's method (occasionally by Diff-Quik). When only a rare group of significant cells are present, filters may be destained and utilized for immunocytochemistry. Only when the effusion is a very clear transudate do we use

the cytocentrifugation method. This method yields small cell spreads, approximately 6 mm in diameter, which facilitates screening. However, it is very difficult to judge the cellularity of specimens because the thick preparations resulting from cytocentrifugation are difficult to interpret because of cellular overlap.

CELL BLOCK TECHNIQUES

For cell block preparation, one of the cell pellets obtained by centrifugation is mixed with a drop of plasma and 0.2 mL of thrombin. The resulting clot is postfixed overnight in a mixture of B-5 and formalin, embedded in paraffin, and sectioned as a cell block. These blocks may also be obtained by collecting the specimen in colloidin-coated tubes and creating a "colloidin bag" to concentrate the cells.

We routinely use H&E on cell block preparations together with PAS-D and mucicarmine in all malignant cases. Other special stains such as Fontana–Masson or Grimelius may be added to the selection if needed. For immunocytochemistry, unstained sections from the cell blocks are first deparaffinized. They are incubated with the appropriate antibody and the reaction developed by DAB according to the peroxidase–antiperoxidase method. The most useful panel for solid tumors includes CEA, EMA, cytokeratin, vimentin, and Leu M1. For lymphomas or leukemias, LN1, LN2, LN3, and UCHL-1 work well in B-5 fixed paraffin-embedded cell blocks. The distinction between mesothelioma and carcinoma and the elucidation of the primary site and the phenotyping of lymphomas are all possible in cell blocks and will be discussed in detail in subsequent chapters.

ROUTINE STAINS

In cases where leukemia or lymphoma is suspected, air-dried smears and freshly collected unfixed cells are submitted for histochemical analysis and cell surface marker studies. For the latter, cells are resuspended in balance salt solution and cytocentrifuged. The slides thus prepared are air dried, placed in acetone for 10 seconds, air dried again and then frozen. In this manner T- and B-cell subsets can be stained and even quantitated. Cytocentrifuged smears are also stained by MGG for morphologic assurance that the sample is representative of the lesion under scrutiny (Table 3.3).

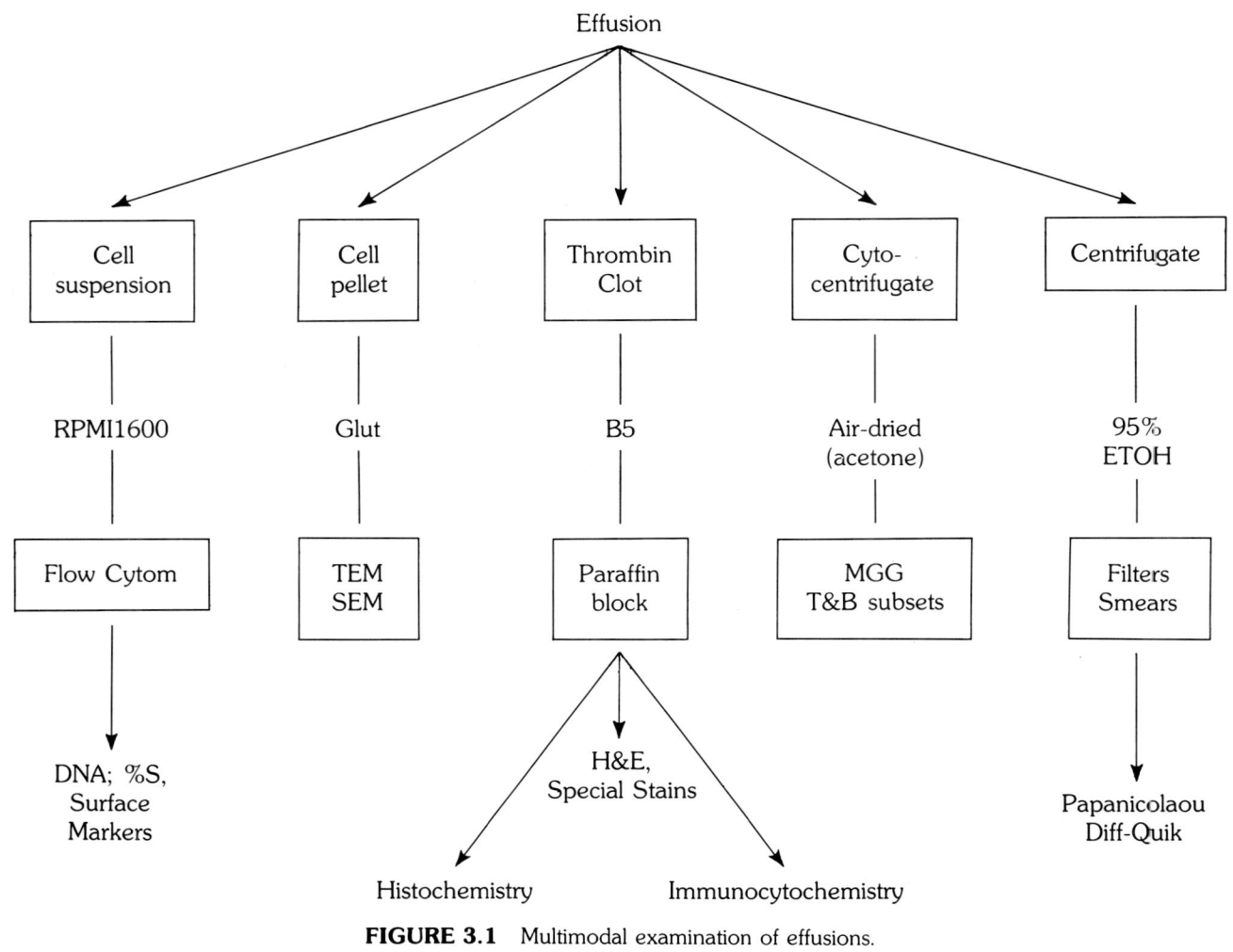

FIGURE 3.1 Multimodal examination of effusions.

TABLE 3.2 Cytopreparatory Techniques in the Study of Effusion

Concentration of cells:
 Sedimentation
 Centrifugation
 Cytocentrifugation
 Membrane filtration
Preparation of slides:
 Smears
 Stripes
 Cytospins
 Filters
Cell block preparation:
 Inclusion in agar
 Plasma–thrombin
 Colloidin bag

SPECIAL STAINS

Several studies have demonstrated the utility of special stains in the study of effusions. These span the demonstration of microorganisms in infected exudates, the elucidation of hematopoietic lineage in lymphoma and leukemia, and the demonstration of secretory products in solid tumors. The Brown and Brenn stain is a modified Gram stain that works well in tissue sections and in cell blocks. The Ziehl–Nielsen stain demonstrates acid fast bacilli, but its low yield makes culture a necessity to confirm the diagnosis of tuberculosis. Fungal microorganisms can be demonstrated by silver impregnation methods such as the GMG and Grocott's stain. The PAS stain is positive in budding yeasts and the thick capsule of cryptococcus can be stained by alcian blue and mucicarmine stains. In effusions due to *Legionella*

TABLE 3.3 Comparison between Two Major Categories of Stains Used Routinely in Cytology

	Papanicolaou's Method[a]	Romanowsky's Stains[b]
Nuclear features	Size and shape of cells: closer to tissue specimens	Size and shape of cells: enlarged and defined owing to air drying
	Excellent demonstration of nuclear detail	Poor demonstration of nuclear detail
	Nucleoli: crisp and well visualized	Nucleoli: pale, difficult to discern
Cytoplasmic contents	Cytoplasm: occasionally visible, often nonspecific	Texture of cytoplasm well visualized
	Cell grouping: well defined (eg, tridimensionality)	Cell grouping: poorly visualized, often overstained
Extracellular material	*Extremely poor demonstration*	*Frequently visible; specific identification often possible*

[a]Only one variation (Schorr's) enjoys some popularity.
[b]Several variations exist: MGG, Wright, Giemsa, Diff-Quik.

the Dieterle stain can be used to demonstrate the microorganisms.

A useful application of special stains is the distinction between mesothelial cells, macrophages, and epithelial cells. The positivity for PAS in mesothelial cells is along the cell periphery. Macrophages usually give a negative PAS reaction, but when present the positivity is in granules of various sizes distributed unevenly throughout the cytoplasm. The PAS positivity of macrophages is not abolished by diastase digestion, indicating its lysosomal nature. In mesothelial cells the PAS-positive material proves to be glycogen, which is removable by digestion with diastase. The positivity in epithelial cells is punctate, ranging from small droplets to large vacuoles that push the nuclei aside, and since it corresponds to mucin it is not removable by diastase digestion. Renal cell carcinoma and other glycogen-rich tumors show punctate PAS positivity removable by diastase digestion.

A vast number of special stains are available, based on chemical, physical, and immunologic principles that are useful in cytology (Table 3.4). In practice, however, only a few of them are used in effusion cytology, particularly the ones that identify secretory products and others that define the antigenic make-up of the cells. One should not overlook histochemistry-based special stains and assume that only immunocytochemistry or other sophisticated methods are capable of solving difficult diagnostic dilemmas (Table 3.5).

TABLE 3.4 Principles Responsible for the Selective Affinity of Various Stains for Different Cellular Products

Electrostatic attraction
Covalent binding
Colloid precipitation
Dye solubility
Vital staining
Metachromasia
Antigen–antibody reaction
Chemical affinity
DNA/RNA hybridization
Matrix impregnation
Resistance to chemical digestion
Light polarization

TABLE 3.5 Special Stains Applicable to the Study of Cell Blocks or Smears from the Sediment of Effusions

Stain	Substance Demonstrated	Applications
PAS	Glycogen particles	Mesothelioma vs adenocarcinoma
PAS-D	Mucosubstances	Identification of adenocarcinoma
Alcian blue	Acid mucosubstances	Mesothelioma vs adenocarcinoma
Alcian blue–H	Hyaluronic acid	Identification of mesothelioma
Mucicarmine	Neutral mucosubstances	Identification of adenocarcinoma
Grocott's	Capsule of various fungi	South American & North American blastomycosis
GMS	Wall of certain fungi	*Pneumocystis carinii*
Churukian's	Neuroendocrine granules	Identification of neuroendocrine differentiation

PAS-D: PAS with diastase digestion.
Alcian blue–H: Alcian blue with hyaluronidase digestion.

Mucin-producing neoplasms are positive for muci-carmine and alcian blue as cytoplasmic vacuoles of varying sizes and shapes. Colloidal iron, on the other hand, is positive in an apical distribution typical of adenocarcinoma. Digestion of alcian blue positivity by hyaluronidase indicates hyaluronic acid production, typical of mesothelioma. The stain works better in histologic sections than in cytologic preparations, but even in the tissues the method is sensitive to the duration of fixation. Long fixation leads to elution of hyaluronic acid into effusions where it can be measured or characterized by electrophoresis.

Neuroendocrine tumors can demonstrate argentaffin or argyrophil activity, but they are difficult to interpret in small cellular samples. The granules in Grimelius stain are rather small and only demonstrable in highly granulated tumors such as carcinoids and endocrine neoplasms. The Seveier–Munger and Churukian methods are more sensitive for the demonstration of granules in tumors with only a fraction of neuroendocrine activity.

It is possible to combine special stains with immunocytochemical methods to better define the localization of antigenic sites. An example of this is the combination of alcian blue with CEA, which is very useful in revealing the immunoarchitecture of cell groupings. In well differentiated adenocarcinomas, the CEA positivity is diffuse throughout the cytoplasm while alcian blue positivity is strongest within the vacuoles. In poorly differentiated carcinomas the alcian blue positivity is distributed as a crown around the glycoceal apex of the cell. CEA positivity may actually be stronger in these tumors than in well differentiated adenocarcinomas. Another useful combination is that of chromogranin and mucicarmine, which can demonstrate adenocarcinoids.

IMMUNOCYTOCHEMISTRY

All specimens suspicious for mesothelioma are examined by the cell block technique and submitted for immunocytochemistry. A carefully selected immunocytochemical panel may also be applied to cytologic specimens in an attempt to discern the primary origin of the malignant effusion. Cell blocks are ideally suited for using immunocytochemistry in effusions. Among the advantages:

- Architectural relationships among cells are preserved, thus allowing the recognition of positivity in diagnostically important structures such as acini, papillae, and gland formations.

- Serial sections are obtainable and results of different markers in the same or closely related groups of cells provide useful information.
- Cells of interest are concentrated in a small area, permitting economical use of antibodies.
- Histotechnologists accustomed to performing immunocytochemistry of tissue sections consider immunostaining easier to perform in cell blocks than in smears.
- Results are easily compared to those obtained in histologic sections of the same neoplasm.
- There is less danger of loss of cells if care is taken to use an adhesive solution to glue the paraffin section of the cell block onto the slide.

Even though edge effect may be a problem in cell clusters in the cell blocks, this is also noted in smears of cytologic material. It is important to keep in mind that there are no magical markers and that only a few antibodies are highly specific. The best approach therefore is to use panels derived from a menu of antibodies of high and low specificity (Table 3.6). Immunocytochemistry has its greatest applications in the following circumstances:

- Differential diagnosis between carcinoma and mesothelioma
- Elucidation of the primary site of metastatic tumors
- Defining the phenotype of lymphomas and leukemia
- Characterization of sarcomas and other non-epithelial neoplasms and
- Classification of small, blue, round cell tumors.

The method is of no help in distinguishing a benign from a malignant effusion, a task best accomplished by expert cytologic examination.

ELECTRON MICROSCOPY

An additional cellular sample is centrifuged at a slower speed (1500 rpm) with the pellet being fixed in glutaraldehyde for electron microscopy (Table 3.7). Ultrastructural evaluation yields excellent information in these cases and appears to be the most reliable technique for confirming the diagnosis of mesothelioma. Mesothelial cells have slender, bushy microvilli when compared with the short and stubby epithelial cells. There are several techniques to concentrate cells for electron microscopy. We prefer simple centrifugation yielding a pellet that can easily be incorporated into the routine work schedule of the electron microscopy laboratory.

TABLE 3.6 Clinically Helpful Tumor Markers Detectable in Cells or Measurable in the Plasma and in Body Fluids

Marker	Associated Neoplasms	Specificity
Thyro-globulin	Thyroid	High
PSA, PSAP	Prostate	High
GFAP	Astrocytoma	High
Calcitonin	Medullary carcinoma of thyroid	High
BhCG	Trophoblastic neoplasm	High
Immuno-globulins	Multiple myeloma	High
Surfactant apoprotein	Bronchioloalveolar carcinoma	High
HMB-45	Melanoma	High
ER/PR	Breast, prostate	Moderate
Du-Pan 2	Pancreas, other carcinomas	Moderate
CA-125	Ovary, other carcinomas	Moderate
α_1AT/α_1ACT	Histiocytic tumors, liver neoplasms	Moderate
Ber Ep 4	Carcinoma, various sites	Moderate
CEA	Colon, lung, breast, other carcinomas	Low
EMA	Carcinoma, mesothelioma	Low
B 72.3	Breast, other carcinomas	Low
Vimentin	Sarcoma, carcinomas	Low
NSE	Neuroendocrine tumors, other neoplasms	Low
S100 Protein	Neurogenic tumors, melanoma	Low

It's not easy to convert all the cytologic features observed from light microscopy to electron microscopy. Cytology in effect looks at intact cells squashed between the glass slide and the coverslip. Transmission electron microscopy looks at very thin sections through the entire cell and scanning electron microscopy looks only at the cell surface coated with heavy metals. By simultaneous scanning and Back-scatter electron imaging (BEI) visualization of cells, however, a close approximation between light microscopy and electron microscopy is possible. The value of electron microscopy in the study of effusions is discussed and illustrated in chapter 14.

FLOW CYTOMETRY

For flow cytometry 15 mL of the fluid are centrifuged at 1500 rpm, resuspended in RPMI-1600, and stained with a mixture of propidium iodine and ethydium bromide. Up to 1000 cells per second are then read in an

TABLE 3.7 Cytopreparatory Technique for the Study of Effusions by Transmission Electron Microscopy

1. Centrifuge 20–50 mL of fluid for 10 min at 1000 rpm.
2. Remove supernatant; resuspend cells in 10 volumes distilled water for no more than 60 s.
3. Promptly restore isotonicity with cacodylate buffer, adjusting the pH to 7.4.
4. Centrifuge for 10 min at 1000 rpm to form cell-rich suspension.
5. Remove supernatant and add 1 mL of 2% glutaraldehyde; allow fixation for 1 hour.
6. Centrifuge for 10 min at 2100 rpm to form pellet; wash in buffer overnight.
7. Process routinely as a small sample of solid tissue.
8. Select thick sections stained with toluidine blue; view and photograph under electron microscope.

ICP-22-Ortho Fluorograph for cell cycle analysis. The DNA content is expressed as an index (DI) to the DNA readout of chicken embryo cells or human leukocytes. The number of cells in the proliferative phase of the cell cycle (S phase) is expressed as a percentage. It is possible to perform analysis by flow cytometry for T-cell and B-cell surface markers. This technique is extremely useful in the classification of lymphomas as well as for CEA, alpha fetoprotein, and other antigens of assistance in the classification of nonhematopoietic solid neoplasms.

BIBLIOGRAPHY

Collection Procedures

Barrett D, King E, Hasson PL. Collection and cytopreparatory techniques for serous effusions and cerebrospinal fluids: part 1. *Lab Med.* 1978;9:9–22.

Bejui-Thivolet F, Guerin JC, Salk M, et al. Apport du brossage par thoracoscopie au diagnostic des affections pleurales. *Ann Pathol.* 1984;4:195–201.

Clare N, Rone R. Detection of malignancy in body fluids. *Lab Med.* 1986;17(3):147–150.

Li CY, Lazcano-Villareal O, Pierre RV, et al. Immunocytochemical identification of cells in serous effusions: Technical considerations. *Am J Clin Pathol.* 1987;88(6):696–706.

Nathan N, Van Deth A. Comparative evaluation of diagnostic cytological features of malignancy in GMA sections, paraffin sections and smears. *Pathology.* 1985;17:467–473.

Spriggs AI. A simple density gradient method for removing red cells from hemorrhagic serous fluids. *Acta Cytol.* 1975; 5:470–472.

Stewart RJ, Gupta RK. Fine-catheter aspiration cytology of peritoneal cavity: A new system with potential for oncologic diagnosis. *Diagn Cytopathol.* 1987;3:339–341.

Van Driel-Kulker A, et al. A preparation technique for exfoliated and aspirated cells allowing different staining procedures. *Anal Quant Cytol.* 1980;2:243–246.

Wentland S. An expanded Saccomano cytopreparatory technique for processing a medical cytology specimen. 23rd Annual Scientific Meeting of the American Society of Cytology; November 1975.

Cytopreparation

Burrows S, Carpenter E, Warren LS. Centrifuges cover glass method for cytologic study of body fluids. *Acta Cytol.* 1968; 12:404–405.

Dekker A, Bupp PA. Cytology of serous effusions: A comparative study of this slightly different preparative method. *Acta Cytol.* 1976;20:394–399.

Niwayama G, Walker B, Neal C. Modified filter preparation for effusion cytology. *Cytotechnol Bull.* 1978;22:225–226.

Plowden K, Gill G. Pitfalls in cytopreparation with membrane filters. *Cytotechnol Bull.* 1975;12:6–7.

Stark E, Wurster U. Preparation procedure for cerebrospinal fluid that yields cytologic samples suitable for all types of staining, including immunologic and enzymatic methods. *Acta Cytol.* 1987;31(3):374–376.

Cell Block Techniques

Bedrossian UK, Fahey CA. The colloidin-bag technique for the preparation of cell blocks. *Lab Med.* 1993;24(2):94–96.

De Girolami E. Applications of plasma-thrombin cell block in diagnostic cytology. *Pathol Annu.* 1977;12:91–100.

Dekker A, Bupp PA. Cytology of serous effusions. An investigation into the usefulness of cell blocks versus smears. *Am J Clin Pathol.* 1978;70(6):855–860.

Di Sant'Angnese P, De Mesy Jensen K, Bonfiglio T, et al. Plastic embedded semi-thin sections of fine needle aspiration biopsies with dibasic staining. *Acta Cytol.* 1985;29(3):477–483.

Krogerus LA, Anderson LC. A simple method for the preparation of paraffin-embedded cell blocks from fine needle aspirates, effusions and brushings. *Acta Cytol.* 1988;32(4):585–587.

Yam LT, Janckilla AJ. A simple method for preparing smears from bloody effusions for cytodiagnosis. *Acta Cytol.* 1983; 27:114–118.

Routine Stains

Wittekind D, Hilgarth M, Kretschmen V, et al. The new and reproducible Papanicolaou stain. *Anal Quant Cytol.* 1982; 4(4):286–294.

Special Stains

Apibal S, Sestapruks P, Bunyaratvy A. Use of tartaric acid resistance of B. Glucoronidase for the characterization action of cancer cells in pleural effusions. *Acta Cytol.* 1987;31 (15):611–614.

Ayres JG, Crocker JG, Skilbeck NQ: Differentiation of malignant from normal and reactive mesothelial cells by argyrophil technique for nucleolar organizer region associated proteins. *Thorax.* 1988;43:366–370.

Boon M, Veldhuizen R, Ruinaard C, et al. Qualitative distinctive differences between the vacuoles of mesothelioma cells and of cells from metastatic carcinoma exfoliate in pleural fluid. *Acta Cytol.* 1984;28(4):443–449.

Cibas E, Corson J, Pinkus G. The distinction of adenocarcinoma from malignant mesothelioma in cell blocks of effusions. *Hum Pathol.* 1987;18:67–74.

Das D, Gupta S, Ayyagara S, et al. Pleural effusions in non-Hodgkin's lymphoma. *Acta Cytol.* 1987;31(2):119–124.

Glick A, Paniker K, Flerner J, et al. Acute leukemia of adults. *Am J Clin Pathol.* 1980;73(4):459–470.

O'Hara M, Cousar J, Glick A, et al. Multiparanete approach to the diagnosis of hematopoietic lymphoid neoplasms in body fluids. *Diagn Cytopathol.* 1985;1(1):33–38.

Sachdeva R, Kline T. Aspiration biopsy cytology and special stains. *Acta Cytol.* 1981;25(6):678–683.

Immunocytochemistry

Banner BF, Warren WH, Gould VE. Cytomorphology and marker expression of malignant neuroendocrine cells in pleural effusions. *Acta Cytol.* 1986;30:99.

Bedrossian CWM. Immunocytochemistry. In Astarita RC, ed. *Practical Cytopathology.* New York, Churchill Livingstone; 1990:403–457.

Duggan MA, Masters CB, Alexander F. Immunohistochemical differentiation of malignant mesothelioma, mesothelial hyperplasia and metastatic adenocarcinoma in serous effusions, utilizing staining of carcinoembryonic antigen, keratin and vimentin. *Acta Cytol.* 1987;31:807.

Ghosh AK, Butler EB. Immunological staining reactions of anti-carcinoembryonic antigen, CA and anti–human milk fat globule monoclonal antibodies on benign and malignant exfoliated mesothelial cells. *J Clin Pathol.* 1987;40:1424.

Ghosh A, Spriggs A, Taylor-Papadimitriou J, et al. Immunocytochemical staining of cells in pleural and peritoneal effusions with a panel of monoclonal antibodies. *J Clin Pathol.* 1983; 36:1154–1164.

Nadji M. The potential value of immunoperoxidase techniques in diagnostic cytology. *Acta Cytol.* 1980;24:442–447.

To A, Dearnaley D, Ormerod M, et al. Indirect immunoalkaline phosphatase staining of cytologic smears of serous effusions for tumor marker studies. *Acta Cytol.* 1983;27(2):109–113.

E. M. Technique

Lorenzetti E, Albedi F, Nardi F. Use of the cytocentrifuge for electron microscopy investigations. *Acta Cytol.* 1986; 30(1):70–74.

Odselius R, Falt K, Sandell L. A simple method for processing cytologic samples obtained from body cavity fluids and by fine needle aspiration biopsy for ultrastructural studies. *Acta Cytol.* 1987;31(2):194–198.

Yamamoto Y, Yasumura K, Murakoshi M, et al. Application of immuno-electron microscopy to the cytologic study of benign and malignant mammary lesions. *Acta Cytol.* 1985; 29(3):257–261.

Bedrossian CWM. Electron microscopy: the neglected tool of cytopathology. *Diagn Cytopathol.* 1992;8:IV–VII.

Scanning Electron Microscopy

Bahr G, Bibbo M, Mikel U, et al. Correlation of light and scanning electron microscopy. A new method for exfoliative cytology. *Acta Cytol.* 1976;20(3):239–242.

Berliner JA, Janssen M, McLatchie C. The use of scanning electron microscopy in the diagnosis of malignancy in human serous effusions. *Scanning Electron Microsc.* 1978; 2: 797–802.

Domagala W, Woyke S. Transmission and scanning electron microscopic studies of cells in effusions. *Acta Cytol.* 1975; 19:214–224.

Kaneshima S, Kiyasu Y, Kudo H, et al. An application of scanning electron microscopy to cytodiagnosis of pleural and peritoneal fluids. *Acta Cytol.* 1978;22(6):490–499.

Beals TF. Scanning electron microscopy of body fluids. *Diagn Cytopathol* 1992;8:266–271.

Transmission Electron Microscopy

Gondos B, McIntosh K, Renston RH, et al. Application of electron microscopy in the definitive diagnosis of effusions. *Acta Cytol.* 1978; 22:297–304.

Hultgren S, Hidvegi D. Improved transmission electron microscopy technique for the study of cytologic material. *Acta Cytol.* 1985;29(2):179–183.

Kaps M, Burkhardt E. An improved method for electron microscopic observation of cerebrospinal fluid cells. *Acta Cytol.* 1985;29(3):484–486.

Wuerker RB, Guglietti LC, Nations ED. Comparison on light and transmission electron microscopy in the definitive diagnosis of effusions. *Acta Cytol.* 1983;22:297–304.

Flow Cytometry and Image Analysis

Bedrossian CWM, Masood S. Immunocytochemistry applied to cytologic specimens in Leong AS-Y, ed. Applied Immunohistochemistry for the Surgical Pathologist. London, Edward Arnold, 1994, pp 341–376.

Goerttler K, Stohr M. Automated cytology. *Arch Pathol Lab Med.* 1982;106:657–661.

Hedley DW, Philips J, Rugg CA, et al. Measurement of cellular DNA content as an adjunct to diagnostic cytology in malignant effusions. *Eur J Cancer Clin Oncol.* 1984;20(6):749–752.

Ryan DH, Fallon MA, Horan PK. Flow cytometry in the clinical laboratory. *Clin Chim Acta.* 1988;171:125–174.

Stonesifer KJ, Xiang J, Wilkinson EJ, et al. Flow cytometric analysis and cytopathology of body cavity fluids. *Acta Cytol.* 1987;31(2):125–130.

Unger KM, Raber M, Bedrossian CWM, et al. Analysis of pleural effusions using automated flow cytometry. *Cancer.* 1983;52:873–877.

CHAPTER FOUR

Serosal Reaction to Injury

The major cause of false-positive and false-negative cytologic results in effusions is poor technique. Specimens that are only perfunctorily examined yield a minimal number of cells and malignancy is missed. As tedious as it may be, a large amount of fluid must be aliquoted out and centrifuged, and the sediment of many small aliquots must be represented in the slides ultimately examined under the microscope. For excellence in cytologic detail, processing must be prompt or the fluid must be refrigerated immediately upon collection. The longer the interval between collection and processing, the greater the degeneration affecting the cells and the greater the difficulty in appreciating fine cytologic detail.

NORMAL CELL POPULATIONS

An effusion does not occur in the absence of disease. Consequently, as previously stated, the so-called body cavities are in reality virtual spaces practically devoid of fluid. In the early stages of fluid accumulation the effusion contains only a small number of cells. The vast majority of these cells are mesothelial in origin, but a few resident peritoneal macrophages are also represented along with a few lymphocytes. At this point, the mesothelial cells in the fluid are extremely bland. They are found mostly singly with occasional clumping or rouleau formation. The cell size varies slightly (15–20 microns) and the shape is mainly cuboidal while in place and oval when exfoliated. The cells show centrally placed nuclei and a relatively small amount of cytoplasm, the peripheral band of which is paler staining than the immediate perinuclear area. In pristine condition, bushy microvilli in the form of a brush border are noted along the entire perimeter of the cell's free surface. In long-standing effusions the microvilli are frequently lost. In persistent exudates the mesothelial cells are more reactive, having the appearance of cell groups containing as many as 20 to 40 individual cells in pseudoacinar, rosettelike or cell ball–like arrangement. In smaller groups the articulation between two neighboring cells can be best appreciated and shows a cleft or "window" created by the pinchlike positioning of a cell in relation to another. Although the quiescent mesothelial cells of persistent exudates may be quite large (40–50 microns), their nuclei lack an irregular distribution of the chromatin granules and the nucleoli are rather inconspicuous. The dominant picture is one of monotony due to the regular size and shape of the mesothelial cells.

RESIDENT MACROPHAGES

Macrophages are ubiquitous in the serous cavities, particularly the peritoneum where, after deriving from bone marrow monocytes, they may take up residence for up to several days. However, macrophages are wandering cells, and they may leave a serosal cavity via the lymphatic vessels. The morphologic distinction between mesothelial cells and macrophages can be quite difficult. This is due to the propensity of mesothelial cells to undergo foamy vacuolization (Fig. 4.1). Biologically, transition forms between histiocytes and mesothelial cells have been observed. Phagocytosis is not a good criterion to distinguish these two types of cells, because recently arrived macrophages may not exhibit any engulfed material. Indeed, when compared to alveolar macrophages, pleural and pericardial macrophages are more quiescent and lack phagocytic debris. In addition, mesothelial cells are quite capable of phagocytosis and may indeed take up carbon, gobble up dead cells, and ingest degenerating debris. Under phase contrast microscopy, mesothelial cells are not so actively phagocytic as macrophages. Foamy cells and cells containing hemosiderin, bile, or bacteria are usually considered

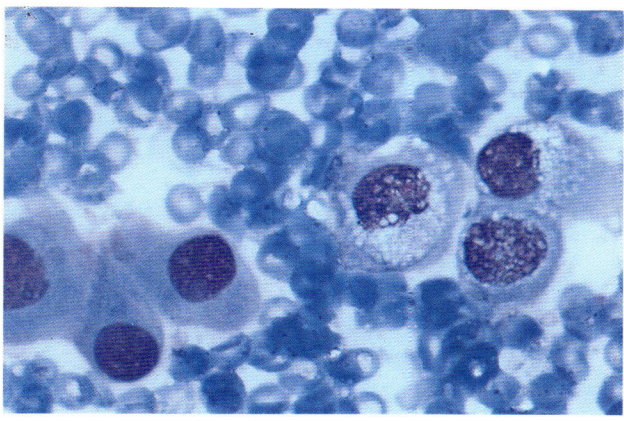

FIGURE 4.1 Contrast between mesothelial cells in peritoneal fluid. Intact mesothelial cells (*left*) snow bluish, homogeneous cytoplasm, while their neighbors (*right*) display vacuoles. (MGG × 180)

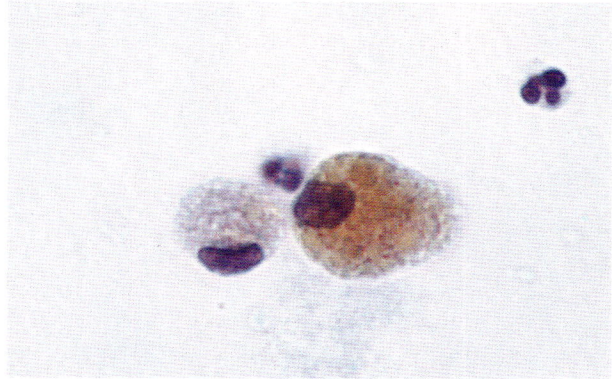

FIGURE 4.3 Peritoneal macrophages. Note the position of the nuclei and the vacuolization and pigmentation of the cytoplasm. (Pap × 180)

macrophages (Fig. 4.2). The MGG stain is helpful in the distinction of the two cell types because the difference between blue cells (mesothelial cells) and paler cells (macrophages) is more noticeable than the difference of color and texture of the two cell types when stained by Papanicolaou's method (Fig. 4.3).

When compared to quiescent mesothelial cells, recently arrived macrophages are slightly larger, ranging in diameter from 20 to 25 microns. However, just like mesothelial cells, macrophages are rather reactive and soon increase their size in response to various stimuli.

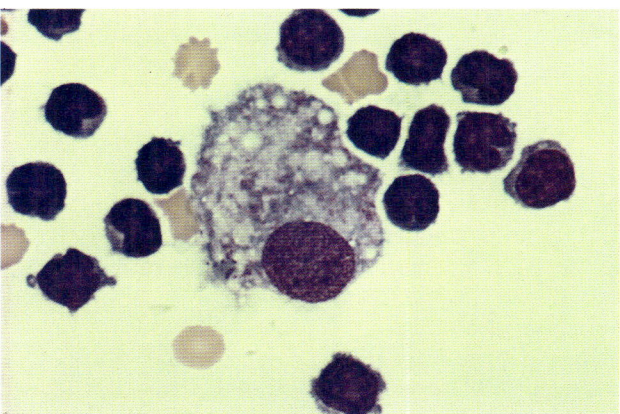

FIGURE 4.2 Typical macrophages with a mixture of granules and vacuoles. While occurring in all serosal spaces, they are more common in the peritoneal cavity. (MGG × 180)

Macrophages may balloon up to very large, signet ring–like degenerated forms measuring as much as 50 to 80 microns. The nuclei of macrophages are often kidney-shaped and eccentric, or they may appear perfectly round or oval near the center of the cell. Occasionally the nuclei attain an irregular shape and aggregate the chromatin beneath their nuclear membrane (Fig. 4.4). Nucleoli are single and small. These cells tend to proliferate rapidly in the peritoneal fluid so that up to 90% of the mitosis in such fluid is accounted for by macrophages. Not infrequently, these cells are multinucleated (Fig. 4.5). Of all cytologic features, the absence of a clear ecto–endoplasmic demarcation most typically characterizes macrophages. The cytoplasm is usually lacy and cyanophilic and, not uncommonly, vacuolated. Upon adjusting the focus of the microscope, birefringent particles are noted in the cytoplasm, which may also contain lipofuscin. In hemorrhagic effusions macrophages engulf hemosiderin; but they may also engulf anthracotic pigment (Fig. 4.6). When macrophages degenerate, their rich lysosomal content may lead to the formation of bright eosinophilic inclusions. Other material sometimes noted in the cytoplasm of macrophages includes intact RBCs, fragments of macrophages and other inflammatory cells, and bile pigment, particularly in patients who have had repeated peritoneal taps or recent abdominal surgery.

Both macrophages and mesothelial cells may become very large, but macrophages may reach true giant cell proportions (Langhans cells) rarely attained by mesothelial cells (Fig. 4.7). Macrophages are positive for A1AT and lysozyme, whereas mesothelial cells are invariably negative. Ultrastructural examination reveals a large number of lysosomes in macrophages but only

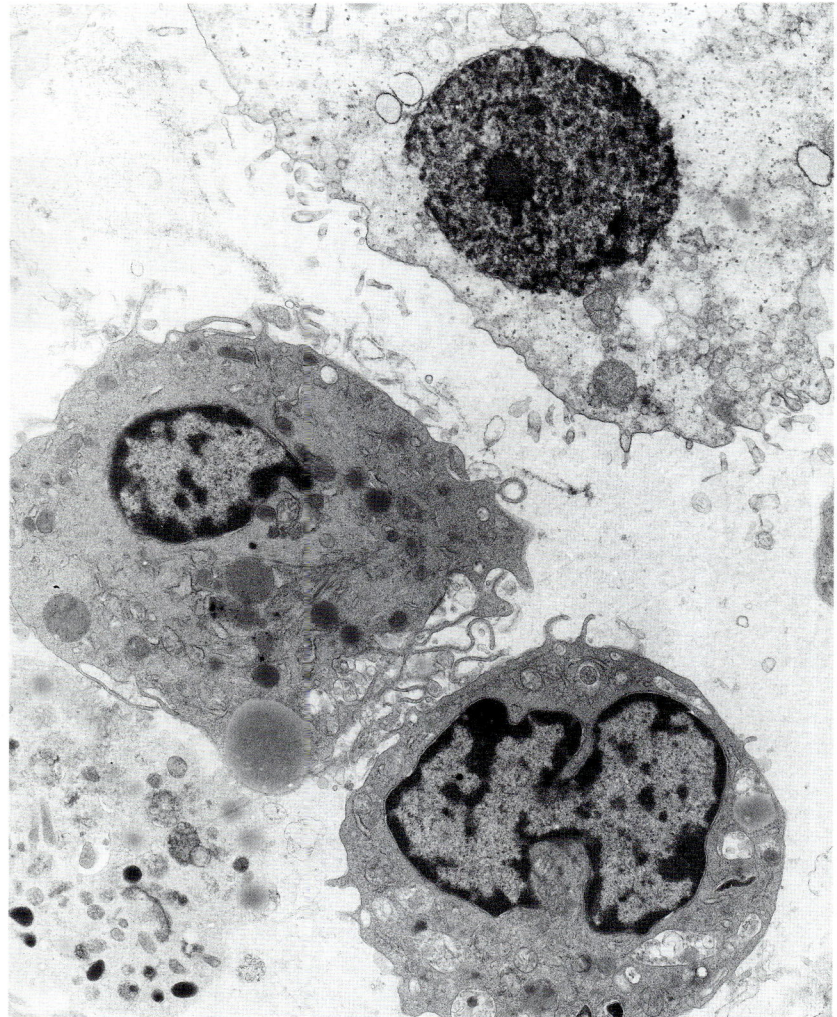

FIGURE 4.4   Macrophages in peritoneal fluid. Notice the lipid droplets in the cytoplasm and the ruffle-like pseudopodia on the cell surface. (EM × 9,750.)

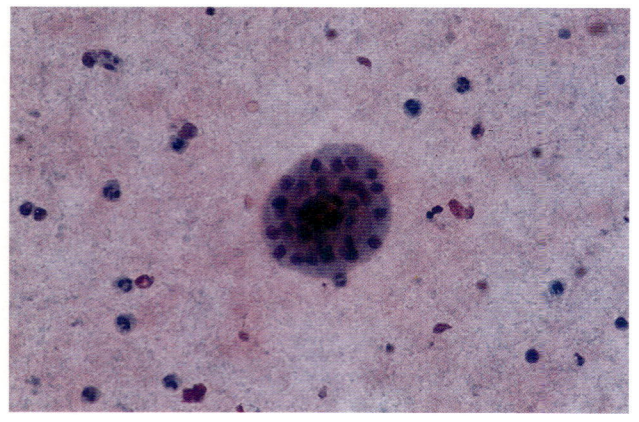

a few in mesothelial cells. The cell surface of macrophages exhibits cytoplasmic processes of varied length and thickness known as pseudopods, in sharp contrast to the slender uniform-caliber microvilli of mesothelial cells (Fig. 4.8). Macrophages also display a large Golgi apparatus, lysosomes, multivesicular bodies, vacuoles, and lipid inclusions in the cytoplasm (Fig. 4.9). The distinctive differences between these surface charac-

FIGURE 4.5   Multinucleated histiocyte in a peritoneal wash. Phagocytized debris is barely discerned in the center of the cell. (Pap × 60)

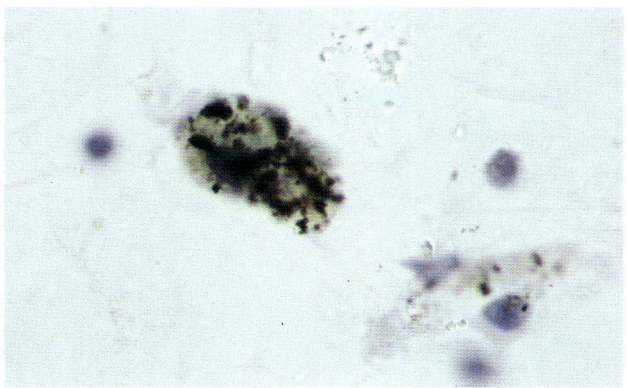

FIGURE 4.6   Anthracotic, pigmented cell in the pleural fluid of a patient with black lung disease. Note nonpigmented mesothelial cells in the backgound. (Pap × 90)

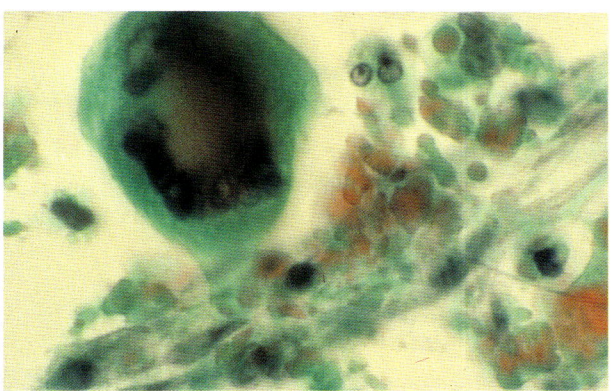

FIGURE 4.7   Multinucleated histiocyte in pleural fluid. Contrast the size of the giant cell with that of mesothelial cells in the background. (Pap × 400) (Courtesy D. Hidvegi, M.D.)

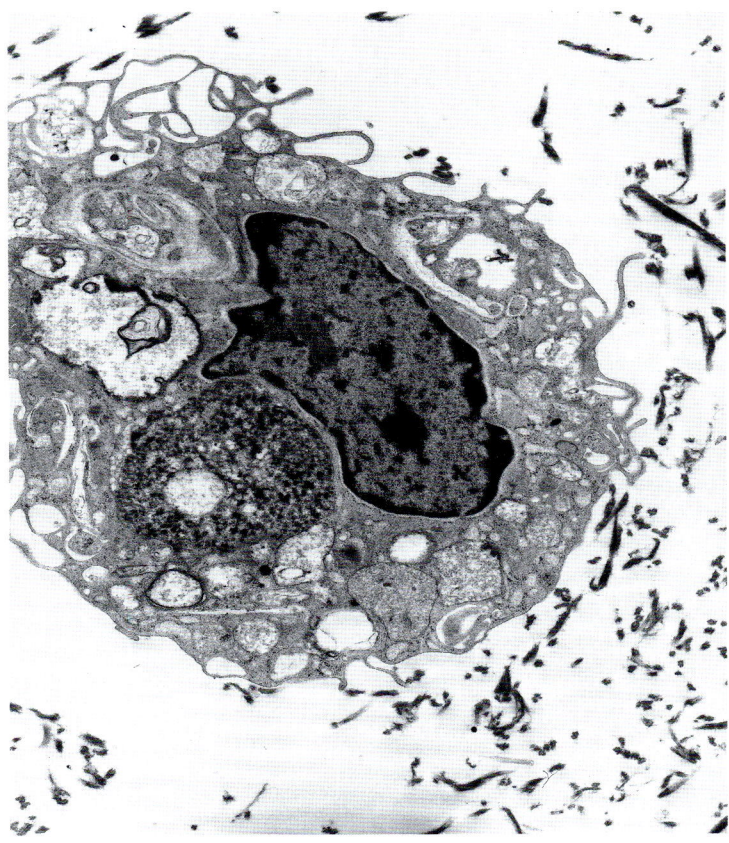

FIGURE 4.8   Macrophage with numerous phagolysosomes in cytoplasm. Notice also pseudopod-like projections on the surface of the cell. (EM × 13,000)

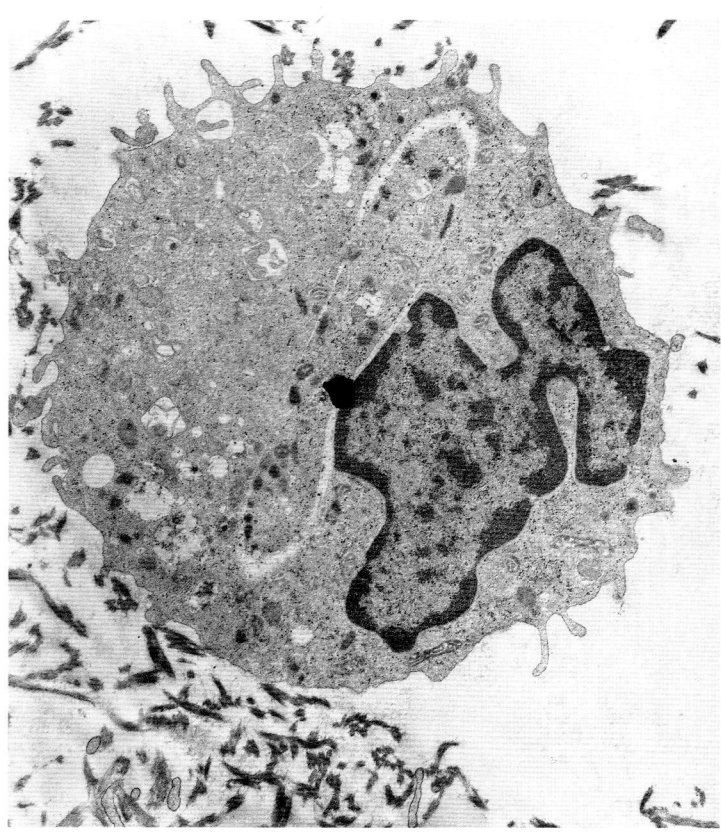

FIGURE 4.9   Elongated, partially digested structure in the paranuclear area of a macrophage. Notice irregular shape and coarseness of the nuclear envelope. Pseudopods are much shorter and thicker than those depicted in Figure 4.8. (EM × 16,500)

teristics can be elegantly demonstrated by scanning electron microscopy. Table 4.1 summarizes additional features that are helpful in the distinction between mesothelial cells, and macrophages. It is very seldom that one needs to resort to either immunocytochemistry or electron microscopy in routine diagnostic work to recognize macrophages. However, a basic knowledge of their function and ultrastructure assists in their recognition when unusual morphology is encountered in cytologic samples.

The number of macrophages in an effusion is extremely variable and appears to increase in both non-malignant and malignant conditions. The macrophages interact closely with other cells, including neoplastic cells, to which they intimately attach by means of pseudopods. An in vivo LE-cell phenomenon has also been documented in effusions. Macrophages are increased in histiocytosis, in metabolic abnormalities such as storage diseases, and as a result of chronic inflammation or in-

fection. They may also increase in number resulting in hemorrhage or infarction as a response to foreign substances that gain access to the serous cavity. Following their accumulation, macrophages gradually decrease in number. Individual cells ingest debris, reducing it to phagolysosomes and undigestible lipid droplets responsible for the granularity of these cells under light microscopy.

MESOTHELIAL CELLS

In their native state mesothelial cells are low cuboidal, arranged in pavement-like rows, lining the serosal membranes. If one touches a mesothelial surface with a glass slide or scrapes it with a spatula, mesothelial cells appear in sheets, closely apposed to one another (Fig. 4.10). Such an unencumbered situation is seldom

TABLE 4.1 Comparison of Single Cells in Effusions

	Mesothelial Cells	Macrophages
Shape of cells	Round to oval	Irregular
Size of cells	15–20 μ (qui-escent)	20–25 μ (young)
	40–50 μ (re-active)	60–80 μ (re-active)
NUCLEUS		
Shape	Round to oval	Kidney-shaped
Location of nuclei	Central	Peripheral
Chromatin pattern	Variable	Finely granular
Nucleoli	Distinct	Indistinct
Nuclear membrane	Regular	Regular
CYTOPLASM		
Pap stain	Basophilic or acidophilic; ecto–endo-plasmic demarcation	Cyanophilic, lacy; phagocy-tosed debris
PAS stain	Peripheral posi-tivity (glycogen)	Punctate posi-tivity, (lysosomes)
Mucicarmine stain	Negative	Negative
Immunoperoxidase	Keratin +	Keratin −
	CEA −	CEA −
	α1 AT −	α1 AT +
	Lysozyme −	Lysozyme +
Oil red stain	Few scattered granules	Rosettelike for-mation

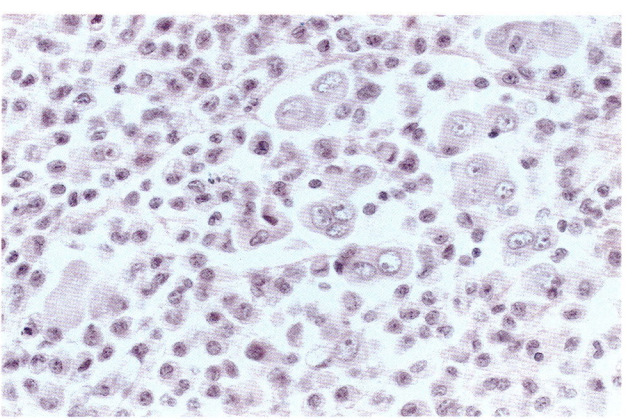

FIGURE 4.11 Clinical specimen from same case as Figure 4.10. The cell block shows a variegated population of reactive mesothelial cells against a background of inflammatory cells. (H&E × 90)

found in clinical specimens containing mesothelial cells. The majority of these are mononuclear but a few multinucleated cells are also noted (Fig. 4.11). The nuclei of normal mesothelial cells are regular in shape and relatively uniform in size, although they may show grooves or be slightly hyperchromatic. Only one sex chromatin body is seen in female patients, and the chromatin granules are small as well as evenly distributed. The nucleoli are small and rounded but may be multiple (Fig. 4.12). Mitotic figures are extremely rare because exfoliated

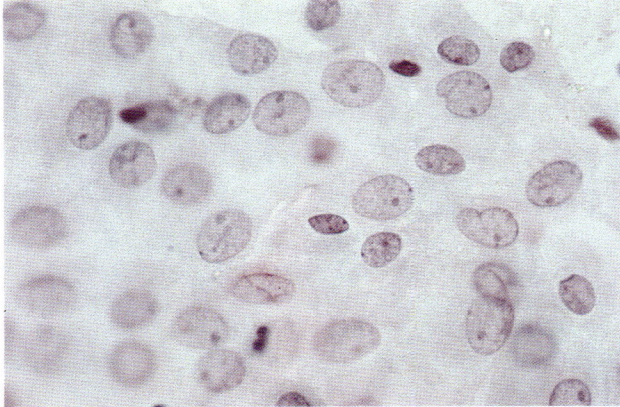

FIGURE 4.10 Sheet of normal mesothelial cells obtained by the imprint method. Nuclei of regular size and shape display small nucleoli and are surrounded by pale, lacy cytoplasm. Oval-shaped bare nuclei may derive from submesothelial cells (Pap × 180)

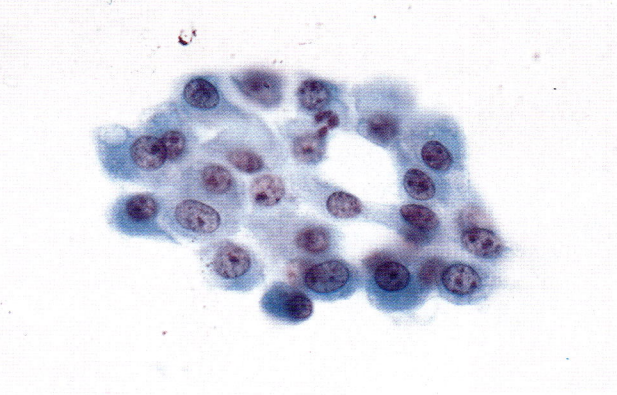

FIGURE 4.12 Normal sheet of mesothelial cells about to break off. Most cells show small nucleoli. Note the peripheral vacuolization and stretching of the cytoplasm, leaving gaps between the cells. (Pap × 120)

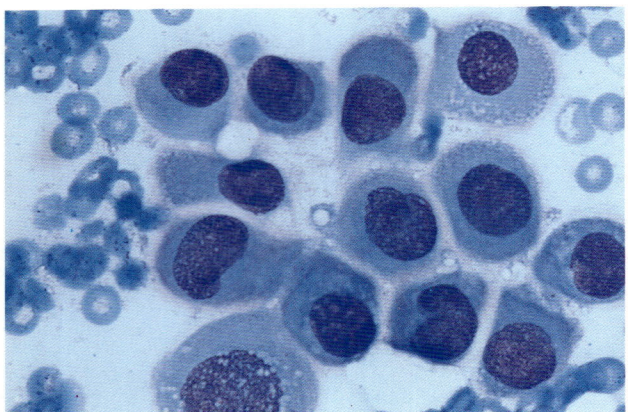

FIGURE 4.13 Greater separation between mesothelial cells with a barely apparent mosaic pattern. Note the ruffles on the face of the cells and occasional peripheral vacuole. (MGG× 180)

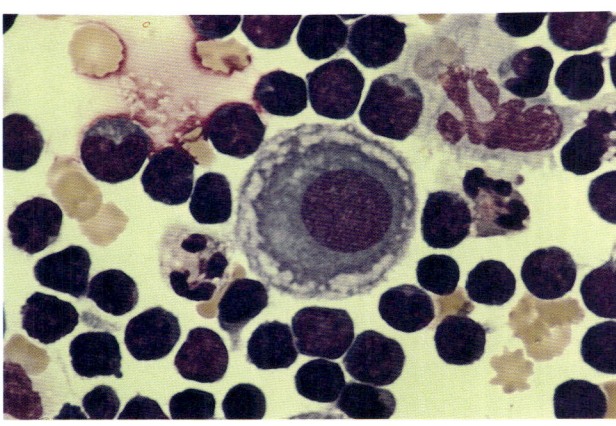

FIGURE 4.15 Peripheral vacuolization of MGG-stained mesothelial cells, a pattern not displayed by vacuolated epithelial cells. (MGG × 180)

cells tend to complete already initiated cell divisions. The number of mitotic figures is of no consequence for the diagnosis of malignancy unless they are grossly abnormal.

Mesothelial cells may have a fuzzy border or show ruffles on their free surfaces, reflecting their richness in microvilli (Fig. 4.13). However, in most clinical specimens these microvilli are markedly attenuated or impossible to appreciate. Mesothelial cells stain very intensively with the Diff-Quik stain, which helps distinguish them from macrophages. The ecto—endoplasmic demarcation is also appreciable with this stain. Mesothe-

lial cells give a positive reaction with PAS stain but not with mucin stains (Fig. 4.14). The PAS-positive material corresponds to discrete vacuoles containing glycogen. The vacuoles may be coalesced but more typically they appear as a string of beads located just beneath the cell membrane (Fig. 4.15). Mesothelial cells may occasionally reveal a granular appearance to the cytoplasm. These are not readily appreciable with Papanicolaou's stain but are easily noted with the Diff-Quik stain. With the Diff-Quik stain mesothelial cells may display a perinuclear halo, caused by shrinkage and condensation of their cytoplasm (Fig. 4.16).

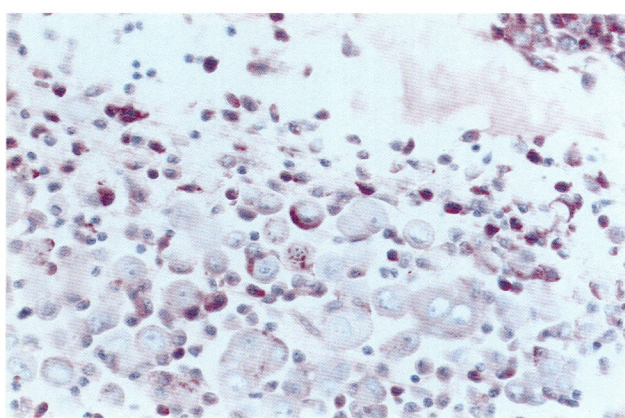

FIGURE 4.14 Peripheral vacuolization of mesothelial cells accentuated by the PAS stain. Coalesced peripheral vacuoles containing glycogen are pathognomonic for mesothelial cells. (PAS × 90)

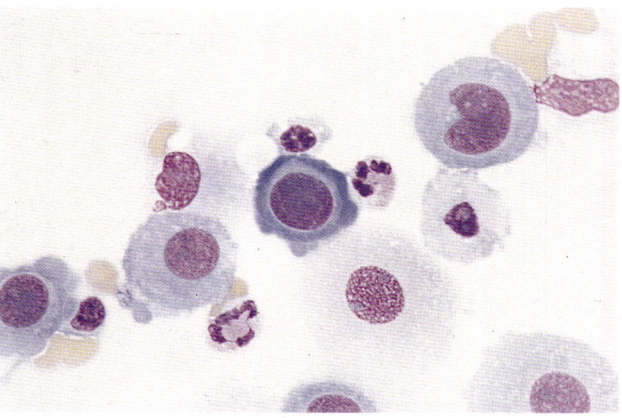

FIGURE 4.16 Variability in the appearance of mesothelial cells. The cell at the center shows a perinuclear halo and is surrounded by pale and bluish mesothelial cells. (MGG × 90)

Mesothelial cells tend to degenerate rapidly and attain a hypervacuolated configuration. In these situations it is not uncommon for mesothelial cells to acquire a signet-ring–like appearance, difficult to distinguish from degenerated macrophages. They are easily distinguished from neoplastic signet-ring cells by their non-malignant-appearing nuclei. Malignant signet-ring cells vary in size and shape, may form cell clusters, and are positive for mucin secretion. The nuclei of malignant signet-ring cells often show macronucleoli, a feature not observed in degenerating signet-ring–like mesothelial cells. Because their malignant nuclei are actually enlarged, they may attain a crescent shape due to the pushing of the large vacuole but they never flatten to the extent noted in signet ring–like degenerated cells. By electron miscroscopy it is possible to demonstrate that the signet-ring shape of degenerating mesothelial cells or macrophages may be due to deformity rather than to vacuolization of the cytoplasm. In these cases the cytoplasm is deeply indented and when the excavation is seen en face it gives the illusion of a large vacuole. Electron microscopy is also useful in demonstrating the surface characteristics and the relationship between mesothelial cells that allow their distinction from other cell types (Fig. 4.17).

MESOTHELIAL INJURY AND REPAIR

The sequence of events leading to effusion in mesothelial injury has been studied experimentally. By looking at surgical specimens in the absence of effusion, it is possible to observe quiescent mesothelium. Excoriation of a mesothelial surface is followed immediately by the vascular events typical of inflammation, and shortly thereafter, by the exfoliation of mesothelial cells. Within a few hours of fluid accumulation, the surface of the denuded area is covered by a deposit of fibrin, polymorphonuclear leukocytes, and mononuclear cells. If the extravasated effusion is tapped at this point it will reflect a variegated cell population composed of mesothelial cells, macrophages and lymphocytes. Mesothelial cells often appear as immature doublets and do not reveal a florid endowment of microvilli (Fig. 4.18). The number of macrophages increases after 1 day and fibroblasts appear in 2 to 3 days. Within 5 to 8 days normal-appearing mesothelial cells are again in place and the integrity of the serosal membrane is restored. These recently regenerated cells appear as orderly rows of cuboidal cells with a fuzzy apex, typical of their mesothelial origin.

If the injury persists the mesothelium exhibits a chronic response that remains a challenge to the diagnostic ability of the pathologist because the cells will be enlarged and look like their surface microvilli. In this regard the mesothelium should be considered as a biphasic histologic unit in its propensity to chronic response to injury. As such, the spindle-shaped cells of the submesothelial layer undergo hyperplasia. Not uncommonly, the submesothelial layer shows increased vascularity in response to injury; rarely, spindle-shaped mesothelial cells appear in the effusion. As previously noted, mesothelial cells tend to exfoliate but they are also capable of an active regenerative response. These cells may undergo degeneration and metaplasia, but it is hyperplasia that causes most diagnostic difficulties. Scraping during surgical manipulation, the effect of an underlying disease process, even poorly understood stimuli such as distant foci of inflammation and cirrhosis of the liver, all lead to a common pathway culminating in mesothelial hyperplasia. These mechanisms are summarized in Table 4.2 and discussed in more detail in Chapter 7.

Once free floating in an effusion, viable mesothelial cells receive oxygen, nutrients, and protection from degeneration for up to several days. For this reason one not uncommonly encounters proliferating groups, binucleate cells and occasional mitosis, often in metaphase. Even in specimens refrigerated before being sent to the laboratory the cells may appear very crisp and show clasplike articulations and intercellular clefts or windows between two cells; these findings should not be confused with signs of degeneration (Fig. 4.19). Individual reactive mesothelial cells may show protrusion of the cytoplasmic contents as if they were about to initiate an ameboid movement (Fig. 4.20). Occasionally, mesothelial cells may elongate, leaving trails of cytoplasm behind, again suggesting that they are attempting to spread, as they do in culture flasks.

The borders of mesothelial cells are fuzzy because of the microvilli, which may occupy the entire circumference of the cell or project only focally as a tuft of hair. The microvilli are extremely fragile and may not be easily recognized in effusion. It is possible also that they disappear as a result of deformity events due to functional changes of the cells. In cases accompanied by tissue destruction, as in infarction, radiation, necrotizing infection, and traumatic irritation, a few spindle-shaped elements may be found in the effusion. They represent either fibroblasts or spindle-shaped mesothelial cells from the submesothelial layer. It is important to recognize them as such so as not to confuse them with neoplastic cells. Fibroblastlike cells from the submesothelial layer play an integral part in the serosal response to injury by way of proliferation and laying down of colla-

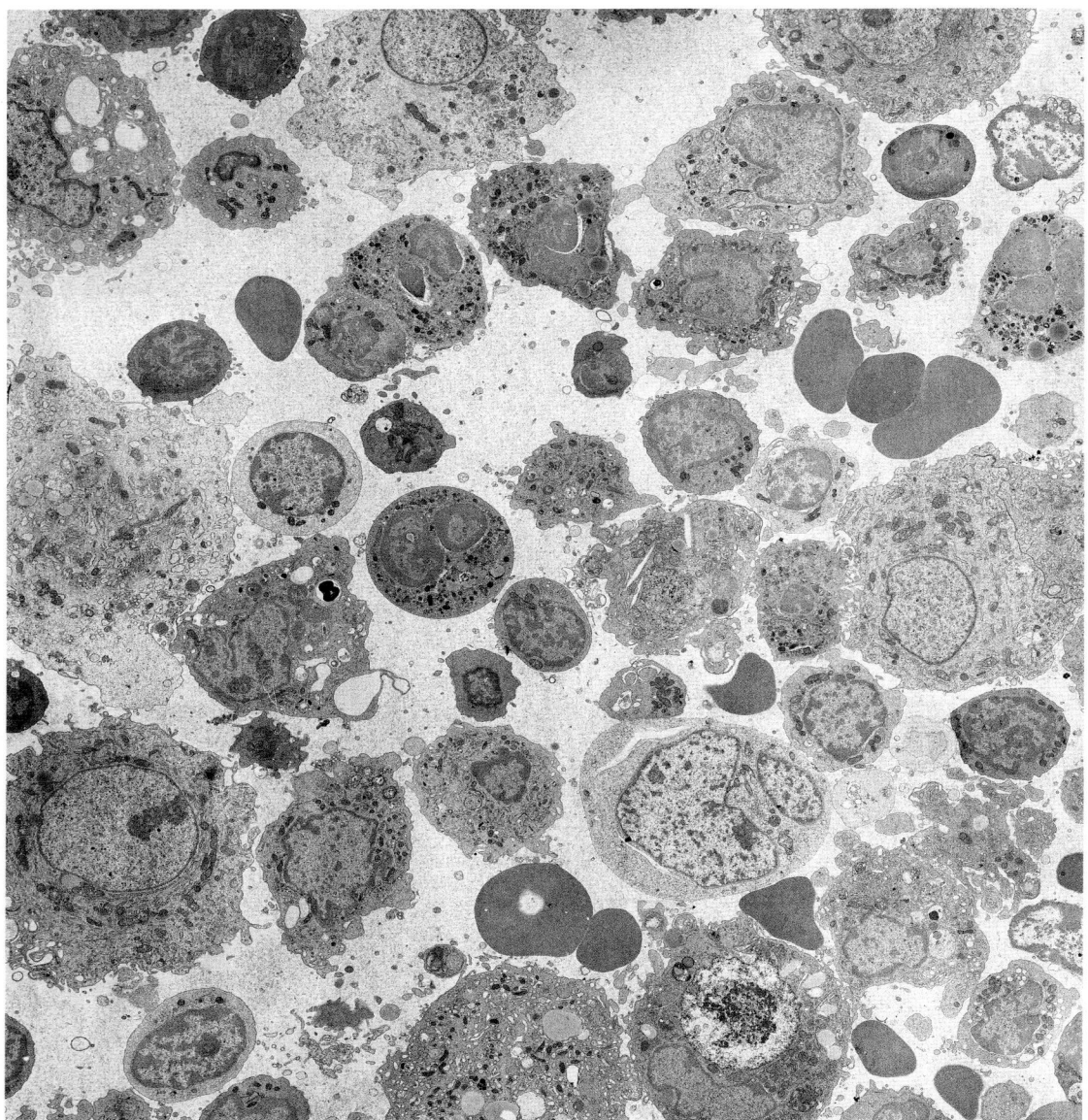

FIGURE 4.17   Mesothelial cells collected at start of second look operation. Despite slight trauma, notice admixture of mesothelial cells, macrophages and lymphocytes. (EM × 7,375)

gen. Even in effusions with bizarre cells of possible submesothelial cells it is always possible to recognize mesothelial cells with their typical, clasplike articulations with one another (Fig. 4.21). The surface mesothelial cells themselves may transform into fibroblasts, a phenomenon that can be observed in tissue culture and has been explored for diagnostic purposes.

Mechanical trauma in the form of sustained rubbing or pressure applied to a mesothelium-covered surface may lead to a localized area of fibrosis, particularly in the pleura. If the underlying lung shows interstitial fibrosis and the pleura contains areas of inflammation, a localized mesothelioma is ruled out even though the underlying pulmonary lesion can be ascribed to asbes-

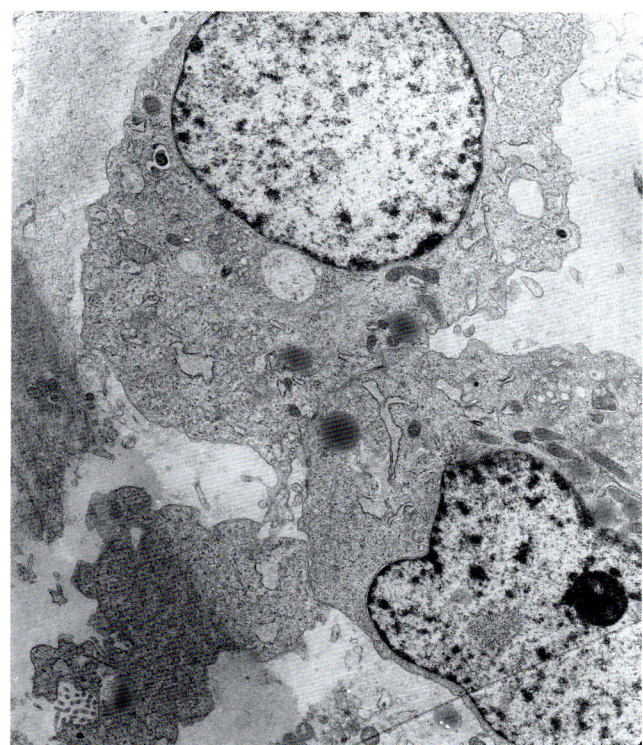

FIGURE 4.18 Doublet of nonreactive mesothelial cells. Notice absence of window and sparsity of microvilli (EM × 12,000)

TABLE 4.2 Common Causes of Mesothelial Hyperplasia

Heart disease (cardiac failure)
Infection (pneumonia, lung abscess)
Infarction (pulmonary embolism, thrombosis)
Liver disease (hepatitis, cirrhosis)
Collagen disease (rheumatic fever, lupus erythematosus)
Renal disease (uremia)
Pancreatic disease (pancreatic ascites)
Radiation (split field, tandem ovoids)
Chemotherapy (bleomycin, cytoxan)
Traumatic irritation (hemodialysis, surgery)
Chronic inflammation (PID, pleuritis)
Underlying neoplasms (fibroids, hamartoma)
Foreign substance (talc, asbestos)

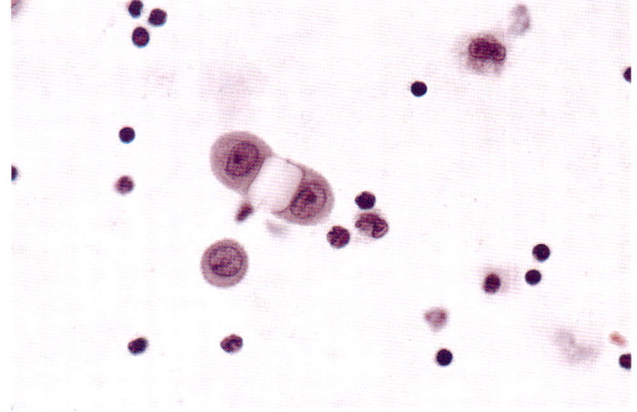

FIGURE 4.19 Window between two mesothelial cells occupied by microvilli. The microvilli prevent these cells from clasping one another. (Pap × 60)

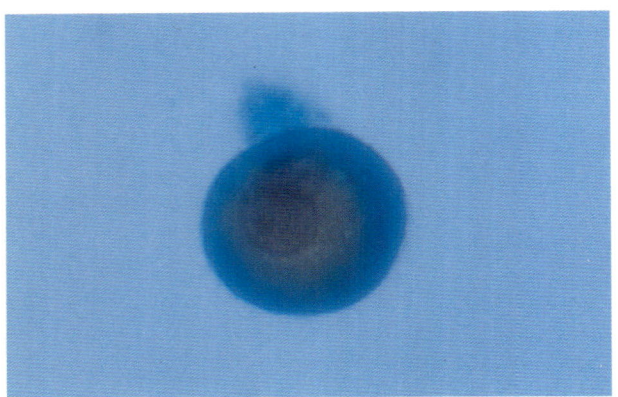

FIGURE 4.20 Cytoplasmic protrusion from single mesothelial cells. The cytoplasm is rather dense and partially orangeophilic. Only tufts of microvilli project from the cell. (Pap × 90)

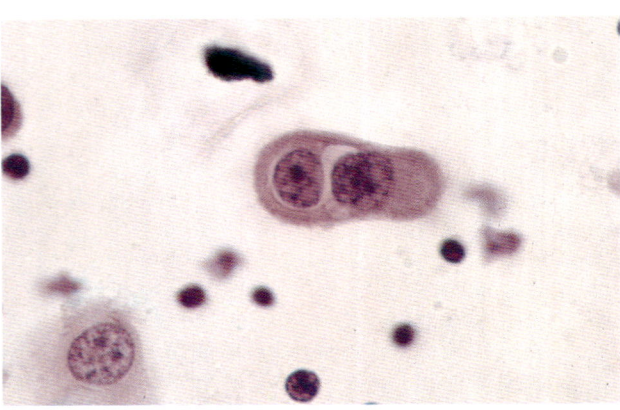

FIGURE 4.22 One mesothelial cell clasping another. In contrast to Figure 4.21, the pinched portion of cytoplasm is pushed away from the clasping cell. (Pap × 60)

tosis. In localized fibrous mesothelioma the underlying lung may be completely uninvolved, and there is no inflammatory response of the pleura. Inflammatory cells are seldom seen in pleural plaques, a unique form of fibrosis ascribable to asbestos exposure. Localized proliferation of mesothelial cells in the form of benign papillary excrescences is extremely rare. It is still controversial whether these lesions should be considered a mesothelioma. In biopsies from inflamed tissue, infoldings of the proliferating mesothelial cells may mimic adenocarcinoma. This same resemblance is reflected in cytologic specimens, but long-standing localized areas

of fibrosis and pleural plaques shed relatively few mesothelial cells. The fibrous component of the lesion is seldom represented in the effusion. The resulting effusion is minimal in volume, and the only cells present are reactive mesothelial cells in rather small numbers. A tell-tale piece of evidence of the origin from the surface mesothelium is the presence of a mesothelial cell clasping another showing a bulbous pinched out portion of cytoplasm (Fig. 4.22). Other features commonly seen in mesothelial cells are depicted in Table 4.3. One must search for these clues when trying to identify the cells as mesothelial in origin because they are not present in every mesothelial cell doublet.

MESOTHELIAL HYPERPLASIA

Much larger effusions are formed in response to pneumonia, pulmonary infarction, malignant disease, chronic inflammation, and systemic processes such as the collagen–vascular diseases. In these long-standing processes a greatly increased number of mesothelial cells appear hyperplastic and are accompanied by a large number of macrophages and a variable number of lymphocytes. Hyperplastic mesothelial cells differ little from their quiescent counterparts except for their larger size and more prominent nucleoli (Fig. 4.23). Occasional quiescent sheets of mesothelial cells are noted in long-standing effusions, but reactive and hyperplastic mesothelial cells make up the majority of rather cellular specimens. Hyperplastic mesothelial cells attain a re-

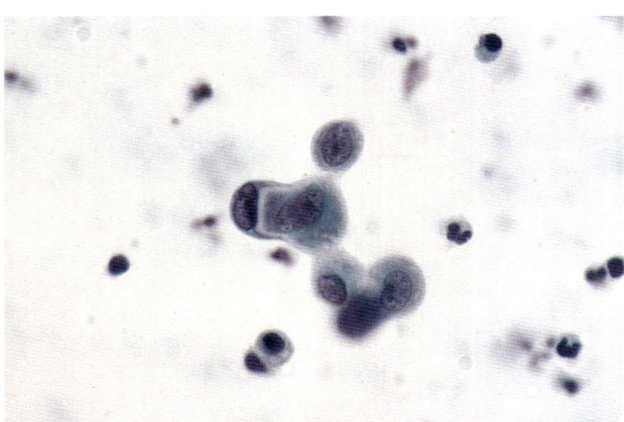

FIGURE 4.21 Typical of clasplike articulation between two mesothelial cells. The clasping cell, seen sideways, surrounds a reactive cell, which appears en face. (Pap × 60)

TABLE 4.3 Distinctive Cytologic Characteristics of Mesothelial Cells

"QUIESCENT" MESOTHELIAL CELLS
 Occur in sheets, closely apposed to one another
 Tendency to break off in small groups
 Fuzzy border due to microvilli
 Mononuclear or binucleated elements
 Occasional mitosis, often in metaphase
 Monotonous, oval to round nuclei
 Inconspicuous nucleoli
 Evenly distributed chromatin
 Moderate amount of translucent cytoplasm
 Peripheral vacuoles containing glycogen
"REACTIVE" MESOTHELIAL CELLS
 Doublets or triplets with windows between the cells
 Occasional papillary groups
 Multinucleation, anisonucleosis
 Abundant cytoplasm with ecto–endoplasmic demarcation
 Connections by clasplike "articulation"
 Cytoplasmic protrusions distal to cellular connection
 Engulfment of neutrophils or other mesothelial cells
 Signet-ring–like ballooning of cytoplasm
 Discrete inclusions of proteineous material

TABLE 4.4 Contrasting Appearance of Reactive and Hyperplastic Mesothelial Cells

Reactive	Hyperplastic
May form cell balls in occasional papillary groups	Frequently exfoliate in papillary groups of proliferating cells
Tendency to break up in doublets and triplets	Groups may contain larger numbers of cells
Mononuclear or binuclear cells predominate	May contain multinucleated cells showing anisonucleosis
Only a thin rim of cytoplasm surrounds bland nuclei	Cytoplasm is enlarged, leading to a very low nuclear:-cytoplasmic ratio
Monotonous, round to oval nuclei display inconspicuous nucleoli	Nuclei with prominent nucleoli, and mitosis often in metaphase
Individual cells with little variation of size and shape	Marked variation of size, shape, texture, and tinctorial properties of the cytoplasm

markable morphologic diversity, which allow for their distinction from reactive mesothelial cells (Table 4.4). In long standing effusions the microvilli may be inconspicuous or totally absent, and the cells must be differentiated from malignant cells of metastatic origin (Fig. 4.24). Even at the ultrastructural level the cells show only sparse microvilli (Fig. 4.25). However, close scrutiny discloses the clasplike arrangement typical of mesothelial cells (Fig. 4.26).

Mesothelial cells in long-standing effusions display characteristics that identify these as mesothelial in origin, but also show evidence of a chronic reactive process. Thus, they may show increased cytoplasmic staining around the nucleus. This accentuation of the usual

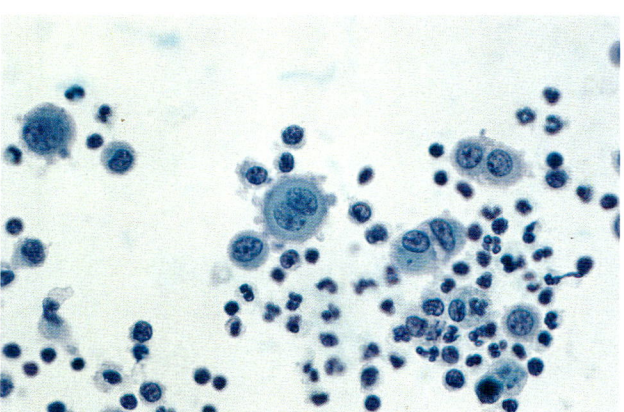

FIGURE 4.23 Reactive mesothelial cells surrounded by inflammatory cells. Notice bleb formation and coalescence of microvilli affecting hyperplastic cells. (Pap × 60)

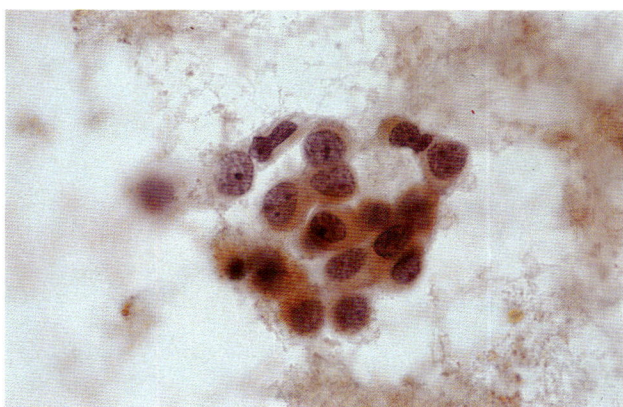

FIGURE 4.24 Newly regenerated mesothelial cells. Persistent injury leads to immature-appearing mesothelial cells with hyperchromatic nuclei and prominent nucleoli. (Pap × 90)

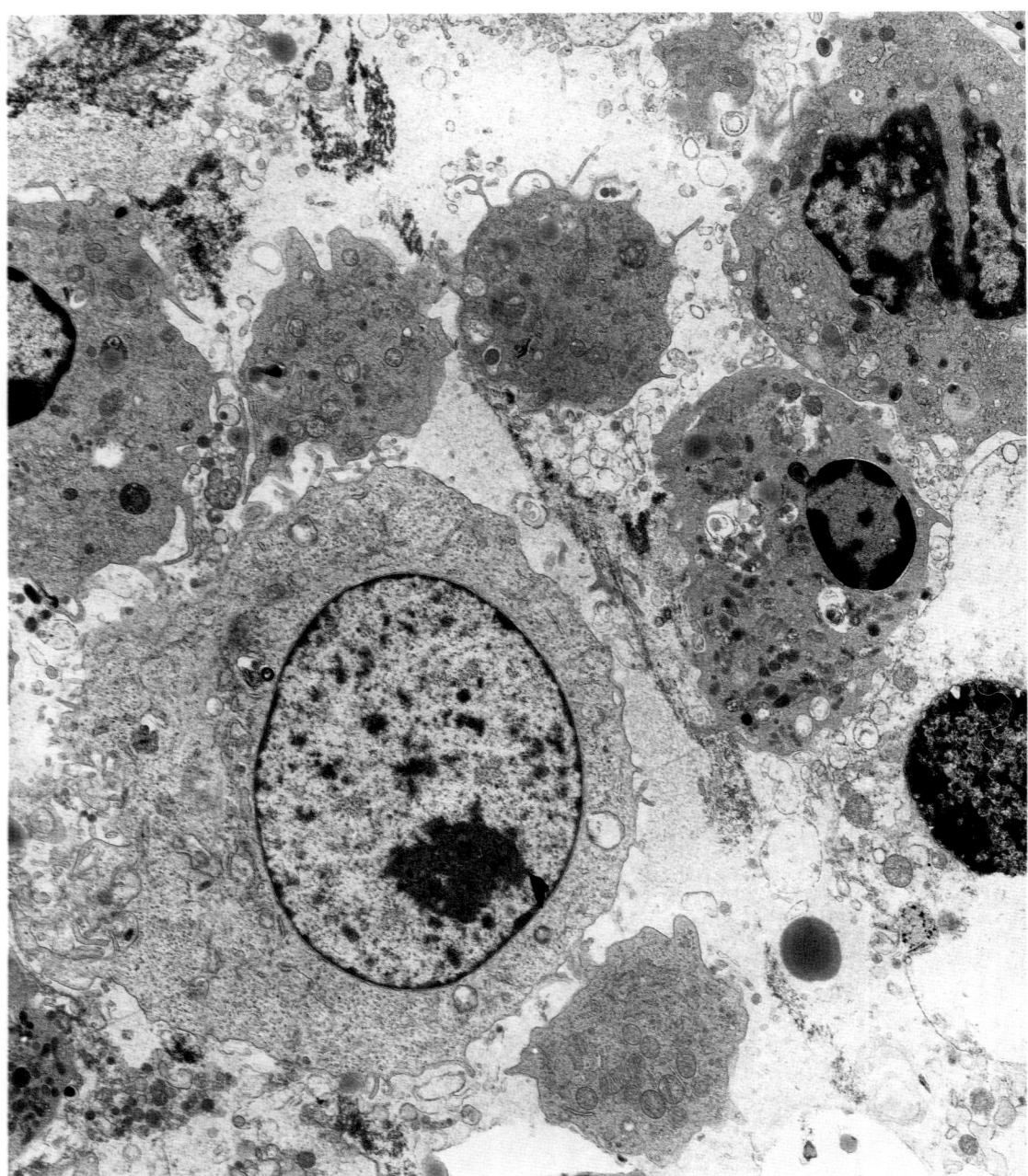

FIGURE 4.25   Reactive mesothelial cell from pleural effusion. The cell is much larger than neighboring histiocytes. Notice delicate nuclear envelope and large nucleolus. (EM × 9,500)

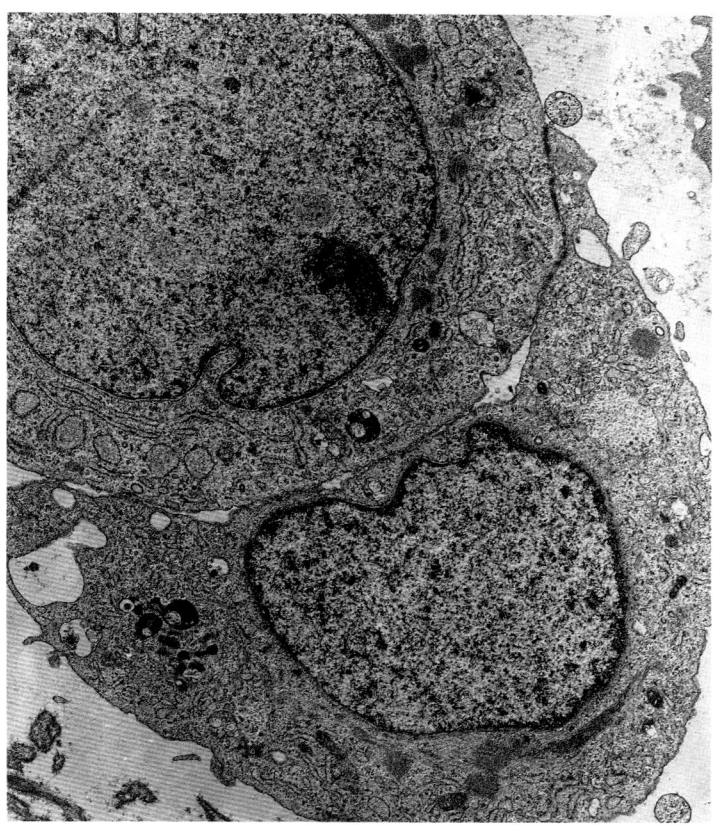

FIGURE 4.26 Mesothelial cell clasping another. Dark bundles of intermediate filaments surround bland-appearing nuclei. (EM × 16,500)

endoplasmic–ectoplasmic demarcation may occur either by a greater density of intermediate filaments around the nucleus or the appearance of a collar of vacuolelike spaces along the periphery of the cell. By electron microscopy the clear peripheral area corresponds to true glycogen-containing vacuoles (Fig. 4.27). However, clear spaces may also be formed by adherence of the slender microvilli leading to bleb-like structures at the periphery of the cell (Fig. 4.28). True vacuoles may coalesce and render the cytoplasm extremely clear and result in a signet ring–like appearance. When the vacuolization is restricted to the cytoplasm, the process is most likely part of the spectrum represented by reactive mesothelial hyperplasia. In the absence of degeneration, more extensive vacuolization that extends also to the nuclei warrants a search for the cause of the abnormality. In such cases, a history of radiation and chemotherapy should be ruled out. Another cause for extensive vacuolization is amiodarone

therapy, which may induce cytoplasmic foaminess or single large inclusions that are shown by electron microscopy to represent conglomerates of phospholipid (Fig. 4.29). These are strongly PAS-positive but should not be confused with mucin, which occurs only in adenocarcinomatous cells.

A strongly characteristic feature of hyperplastic mesothelial cells, which enables their easy distinction from macrophages and epithelial cells, is their frequent occurrence in doublets, triplets, or short rows of cells articulated to one another in a distinctive fashion (Fig. 4.30). One member of the doublet acquires a clasplike appearance while the other cell may have another neatly tucked in its concavity or may even attempt to engulf companion cells (Fig. 4.31). Very often this partially surrounded member of the doublet exhibits a protrusion of the cytoplasm opposite to the edge nearest to the embracing cell. By electron microscopy, truly engulfed cells exhibit markedly electron-dense cytoplasm

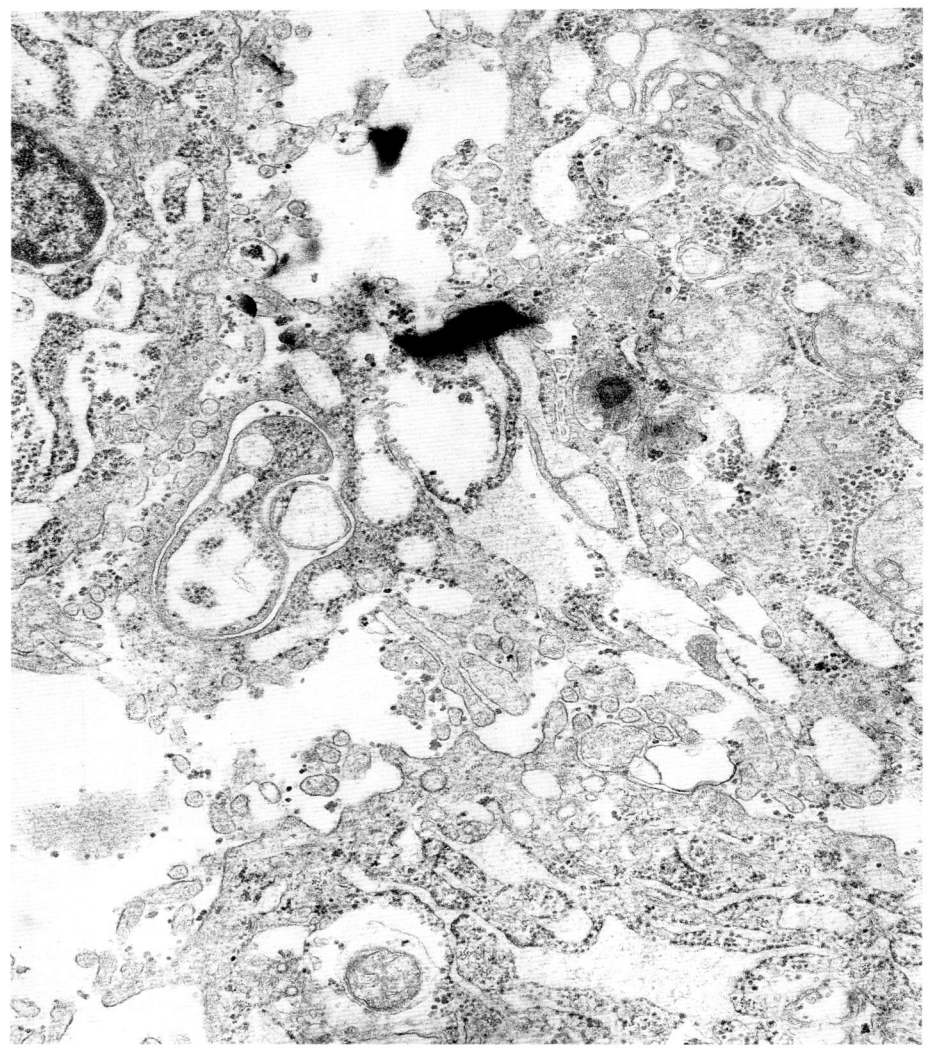

FIGURE 4.27 Boundary between neighboring mesothelial cells. Notice glycogen in granular form and clear spaces deriving from glycogen removal during fixation. (EM × 38,750)

or overt signs of degeneration; in contrast, cells that simply lie in the cytoplasmic excavation of another have intact organelles typical of viable cells. (Fig. 4.32). Mesothelial cells may also appear as tandem-like rows. By electron microscopy, mesothelial cells in the row may be still displaying their typical articulations among the members of the train (Fig. 4.33) associated with macrophages and lymphocytes touching one another by their respective cytoplasmic projections (Fig. 4.34). No exact significance has been ascertained for this phenomenon, even though an increased number of gap junctions have been found in between mesothelial cells.

The tendency of mesothelial cells to hold together in effusions is responsible for the appearance of triplets, and other multiple arrangements, not indicative of malignancy (Fig. 4.35).

Mesothelilal cells often appear paired with one member of the doublet demonstrating a cytoplasmic protrusion or a tuft of microvilli projecting from the cell surface. The clefts between mesothelial cells that appear as windows in cytologic preparations are not empty at the ultrastructural level. By electron microscopy they are shown to contain tightly intertwined, long, slender microvilli, below the resolution power of light mi-

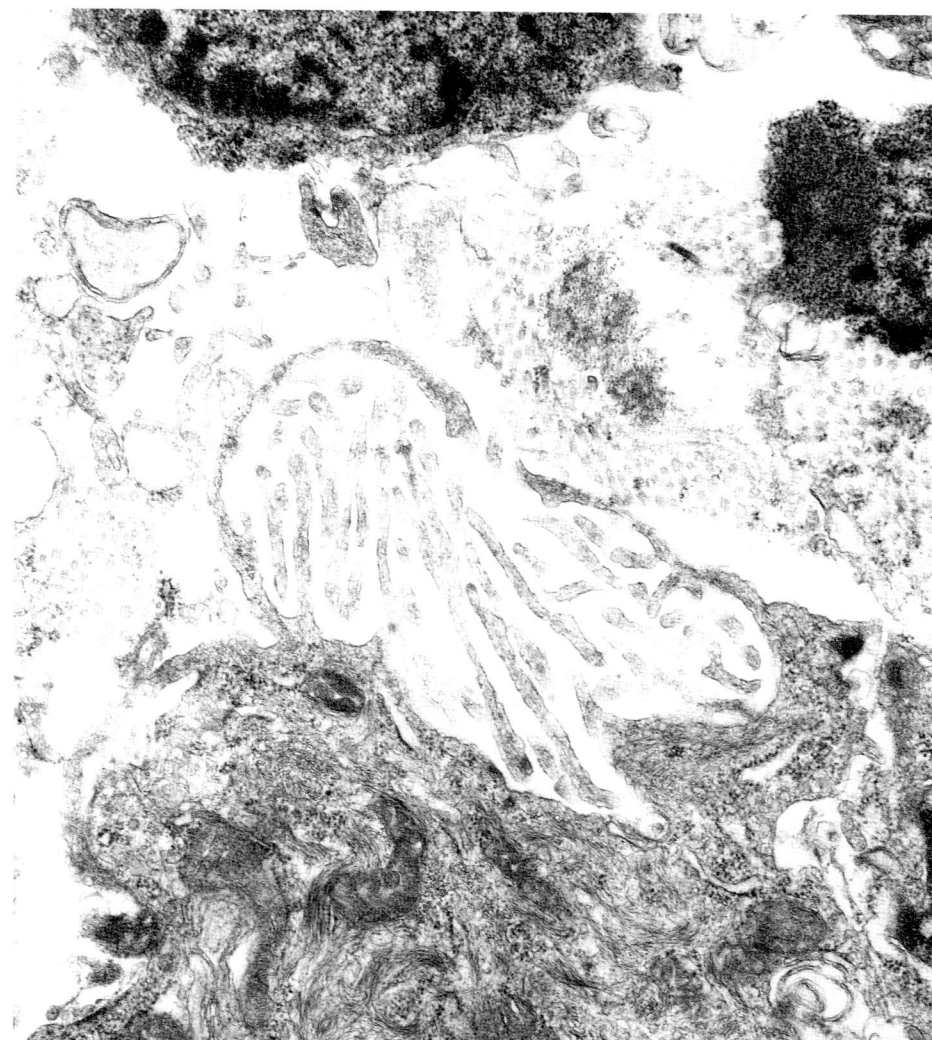

FIGURE 4.28 Artificial space surrounding microvilli on surface of mesothelial cell. Together with clear spaces shown in Figure 4.27 structures such as this contribute to the peripheral "vacuolization" of mesothelial cells. (EM× 36,000)

croscopy (Fig. 4.36). Nuclear hyperchromasia, a high nuclear:chromatin ratio, binucleation, and prominent nucleolization are features of hyperplastic mesothelial cells that need careful scrutiny to avoid a false-positive interpretation. Another possible pitfall is the presence of mitosis, a normal feature of reactive mesothelial cells that should not be mistaken for malignancy (Fig. 4.37).

Mesothelial cells may engulf other cells as well as particulate matter such as talc or starch; they may also be penetrated by neutrophils, particularly in long-standing effusions. From the conceptual point of view,

the term "reactive" may be objectionable if abused to mean any abnormal mesothelial cells. Likewise, the recognition of "hyperplastic" mesothelial cells is a rather subjective endeavor. In practice, the cells that appear in effusion—a physiological abnormality of the serosal cavities—display a spectrum of appearances different from those seen in their quiescent state of lining the serosal surfaces. Just as a normal lymph node is a reactive one, "normal" mesothelial cells—ie, cells found in nonmalignant effusions—are reactive to the cause of the effusion. Reactive mesothelial cells acquire a num-

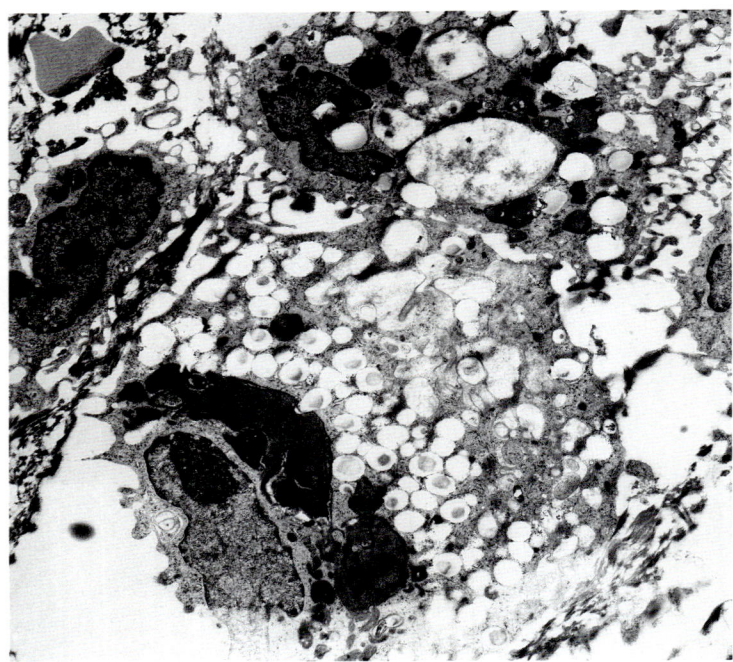

FIGURE 4.29 Mesothelial cell engorged with phospholipid in Amiodarone toxicity. Notice also large lipid inclusion in golgi portion of the cytoplasm. (EM× 28,000)

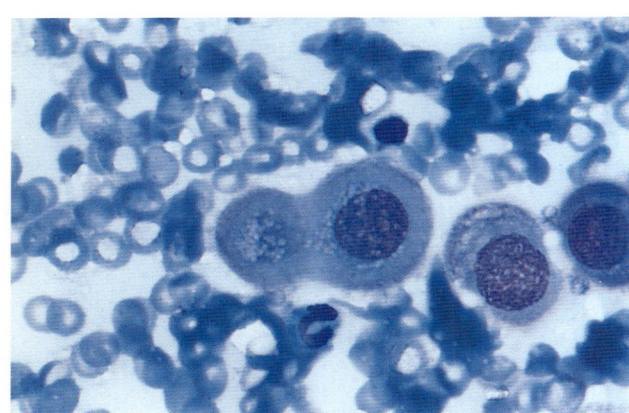

FIGURE 4.30 Doublet of mesothelial cells, a common occurrence in long-standing effusions. The cells show fine vacuolization of the cytoplasm, an indication of their normal glycogen content. (MGG× 180)

ber of characteristics that should not be misinterpreted to represent preneoplastic or neoplastic transformation. Even though these characteristics may be ascribable to hyperplasia, they may be rather florid and worrisome in mesothelial cells. The spectrum of these changes is responsible for the expression "the many faces of mesothelial hyperplasia" used in describing the morphologic diversity of mesothelial cells.

Short of a biopsy, it is not possible to ascertain the exact origin of mesothelial hyperplasia, but it may be safely assumed that a vast majority derive from nonneoplastic conditions leading to mesothelial cell hyperplasias and hypertrophies. Unlike hyperplasias affecting other sites such as the female genital tract and the lung, the progression of these hyperplasias into neoplastic processes has not been well documented in either clinical material or experimental models. From the morphologic point of view, however, there comes a point where the cytologic abnormalities of mesothelial cells assume such magnitude that one wonders about the possibility of malignancy. We reserve the term "atypical" mesothelial cells to distinguish these from their hyperplastic counterparts, recognizing that this is a rather subjective exercise.

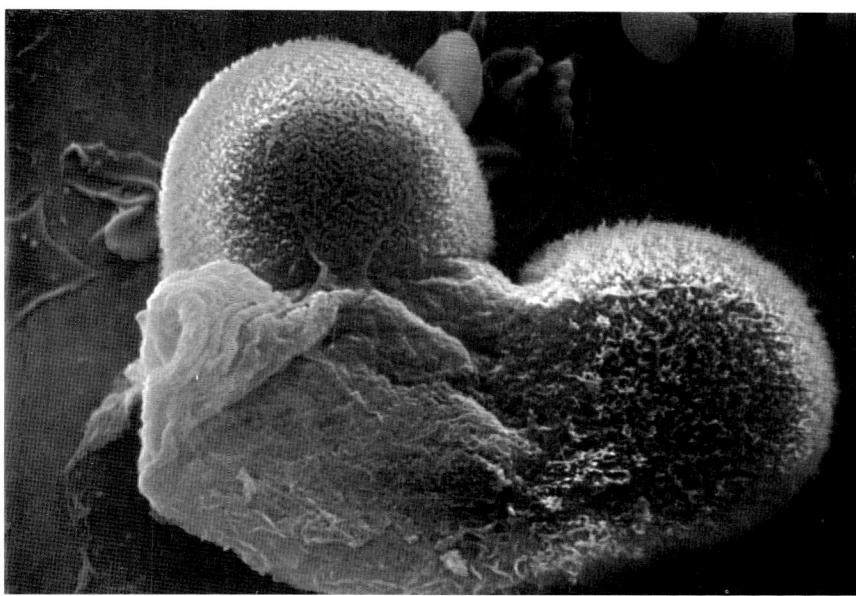

FIGURE 4.31 Scanning electron microscopy of mesothelial cell doublet. Intertwined microvilli create a bulging space between the two cells. (EM × 6,000)

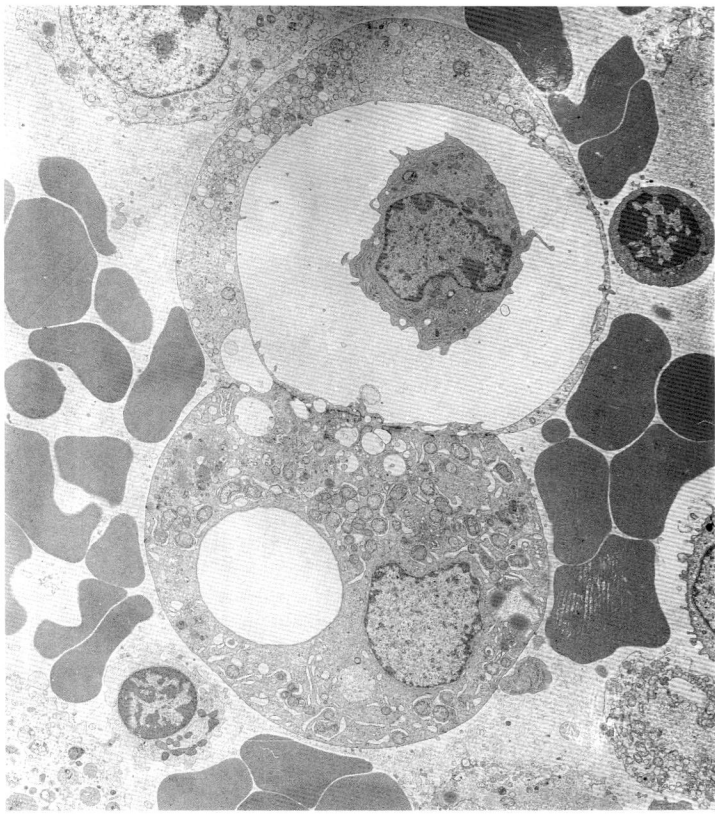

FIGURE 4.32 Mesothelial cell doublet with a rather concave member of the pair. The plane of section is such that a plasma cell appears to be inside of the concave cell. (EM × 5,500)

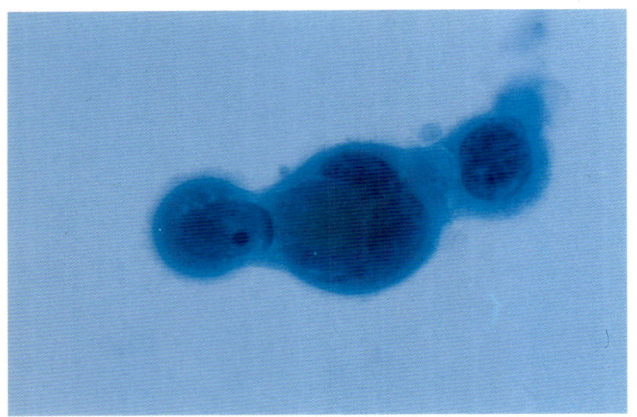

FIGURE 4.33 Tandem arrangement of several mesothelial cells. Notice the pinching articulation (*center*) and the windows filled by microvilli (*right of center*). The fuzzy border corresponds to the florid microvilli of mesothelial cells. (Pap × 90)

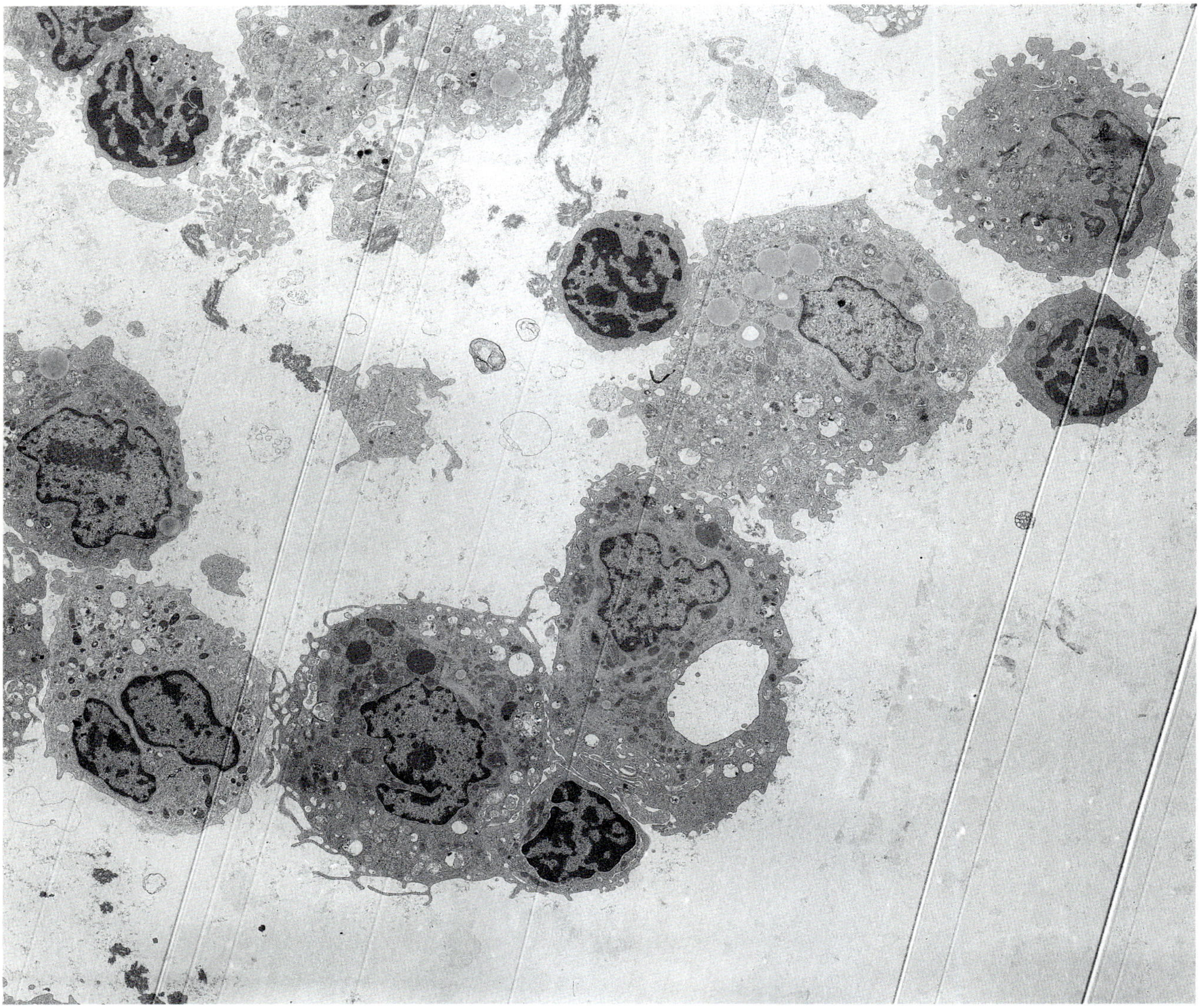

FIGURE 4.34 Tandem arrangement of mesothelial cells. Notice also accompanying lymphocytes and macrophages, with surface projections entangled with those of mesothelial cells. (EM × 4,125)

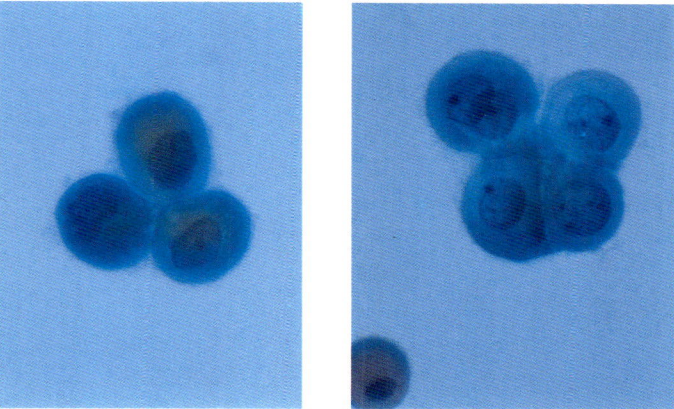

FIGURE 4.35 Multiple grouping of mesothelial cells. (*left*) Triplet of cells with ecto–endoplasmic variation of cytoplasmic density. (Pap × 90) (*right*) Quartet of mesothelial cells, one of which is binucleated. (Pap × 60)

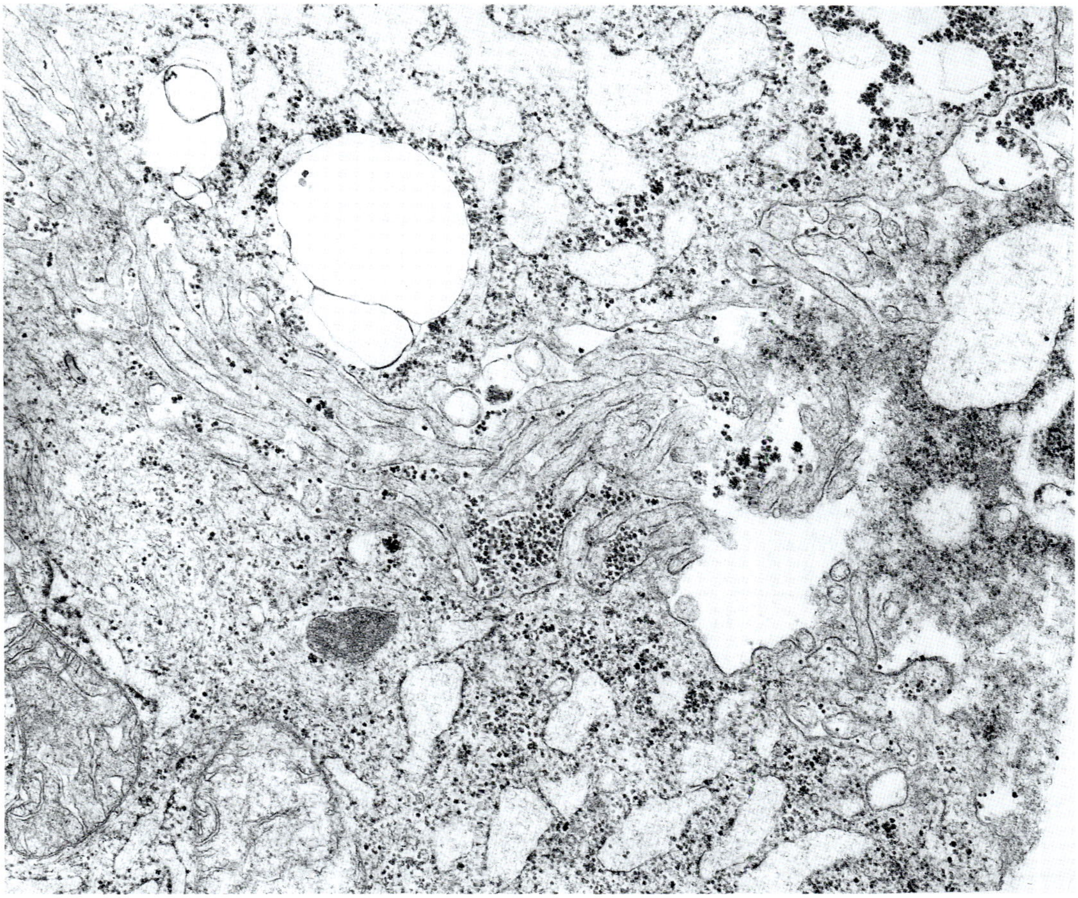

FIGURE 4.36 Compacted microvilli between adjacent mesothelial cells. By light microscopy this would appear as a clear window. Notice dilated endoplasmic reticulum as well as glycogen vacuoles and particles in the cytoplasm of the cells. (EM × 6,000)

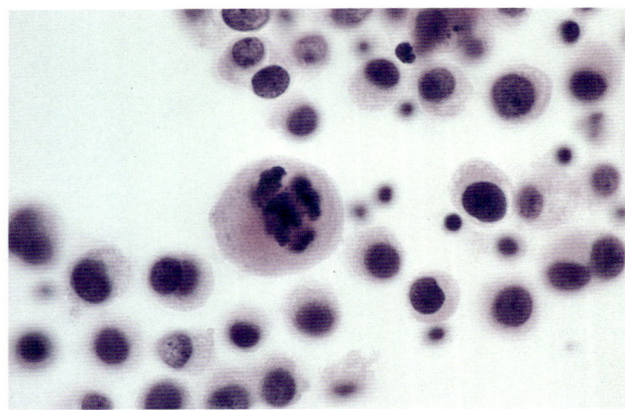

FIGURE 4.37 Mitosis of mesothelial cells. This normal feature of these active proliferating cells should not be taken as evidence of malignancy. (Pap × 120)

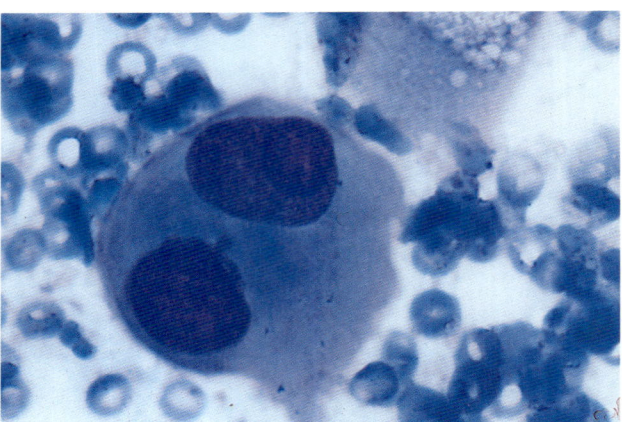

FIGURE 4.38 Binucleate mesothelial cell. The two nuclei lack definition of their chromatinic material. (MGG × 180)

DIFFICULTIES IN INTERPRETATION

As it has been stressed, mesothelial cells tend to proliferate and often occur in multiples with identifiably separate nuclei and cytoplasm. However, the nuclei have a limited range of response and should not be directly responsible for the rendering of an atypical or suspicious diagnosis. Because the repertoire of nuclear responses is limited, hyperplastic mesothelial cells may show hyperchromasia, chromatin clumping and prominent nucleoli. Not infrequently mesothelial cells are binucleated, with bland-appearing chromatin and totally inconspicuous nucleoli (Fig. 4.38). The nuclear features are better demonstrated in Pap-stained preparations, particularly where there is good cell preservation (Fig. 4.39) Multinucleation should not be considered a sign of atypia even though the pattern of multinucleation may be unusual, such as represented by all nuclei lined along the cell periphery (Fig. 4.40). The presence of nuclei in a horseshoe-like distribution should not lead to the misinterpretation of mesothelial cells as multinucleated histiocytes (Fig. 4.41).

The boundary between merely hyperplastic and "atypical" mesothelial cells is imprecise. Cytologic abnormalities suspicious for malignancy are characterized by very large groups of cells. These groups exhibit scalloped borders, attempted molding between cells, and marked hyperchromasia of nuclei. The nuclear: cytoplasmic ratio is high, the chromatin clumps are coarse, and nucleoli may be very prominent. However,

TABLE 4.5 Alien Cells and Extraneous Material Sometimes Found in Effusions

Liver cells or fragments
Fragments of lung parenchyma
Skin tags
Vegetable matter
Starch granules
Skeletal muscle fibers
Esophageal mucosa
Cholesterol crystals
Detached ciliary tufts
Colonic mucosa
Fragments of cartilage
Feces droplets
Endometrial cells from reflux or endometriosis
Fallopian tubal epithelium
Cells from ovarian cysts

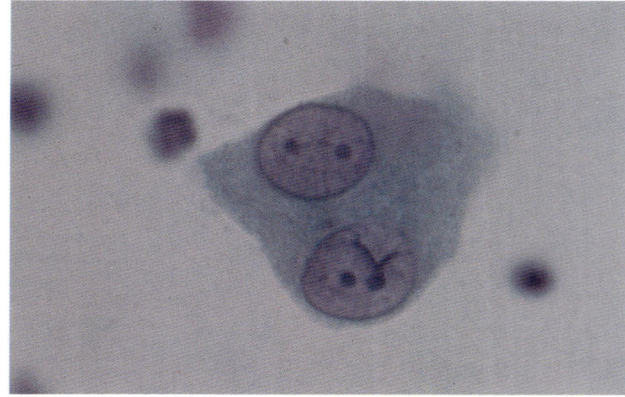

FIGURE 4.39 Pap-stained binucleate cell. The Papanicolaou stain delineates well the delicate nuclear membrane and the inconspicuous nucleoli. (Pap × 90)

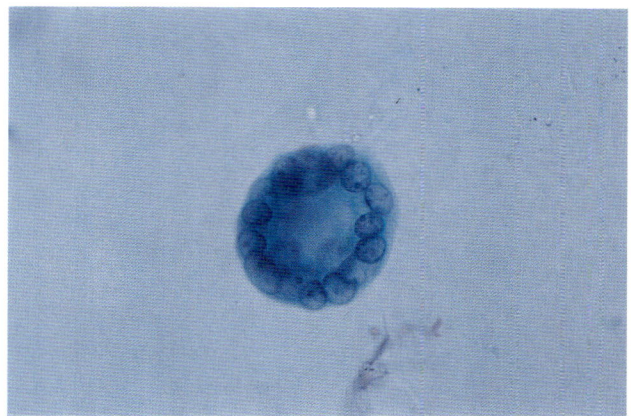

FIGURE 4.40   Multinucleated mesothelial cell. In this example, all nuclei are lined up at the periphery of the cytoplasm. Note absence of secretory or engulfed material in the center of the cell. (Pap × 180)

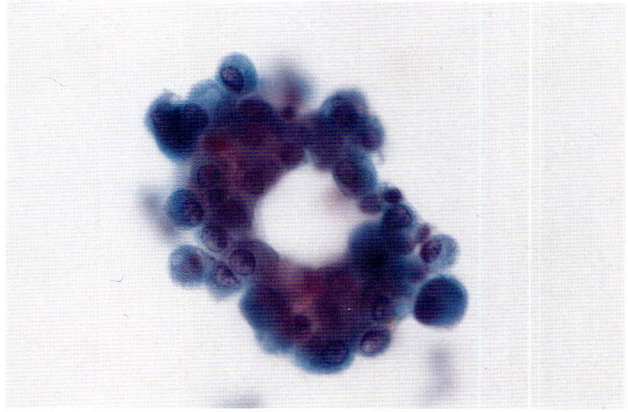

FIGURE 4.42   Pseudoacinar arrangement of reactive mesothelial cells. The group simulates a lumen, but the cells lack the polarity seen in adenocarcinoma. (Pap × 200)

these cells still bear some resemblance to their slightly less abnormal neighbors and, in fact, the entire spectrum from perfectly normal mesothelial cells to very atypical elements can be found in the same smear. Only when there is the distinct impression that the abnormal cells constitute an alien cell population should one more seriously suspect a metastatic malignancy. Such distinction can be accentuated by special stains and immunocytochemistry or by growing the cells in tissue culture. The distinction between mesothelial hyperplasia and mesothelioma is more problematic because one cannot count on the recognition of a two-cell population for its appreciation.

Distinguishing mesothelial hyperplasia from carcinoma may be very difficult even in a biopsy specimen. Not only do the cells from the surface proliferate upward but they appear also to dip into the submesothelial layer. Fibroblastlike cells of the submesothelial layer also react to the injury and may acquire an epitheloid appearance. In cytologic specimens, mesothelial cells may acquire a pseudoacinar configuration (Fig. 4.42). However, the absence of true molding among the cells should be sufficient to rule out malignancy. Additionally the nuclear characteristics of mesothelial cells simulating a lumen appear strictly benign (Fig. 4.43). In the presence of only a few cells suspicious for malignancy, greater attention should be paid to the overwhelming number of accompanying benign-appearing cells. If they show the cytologic features of mesothelial cells, the process is benign. Florid microvilli are good evidence of mesothelial origin, but absence of a fuzzy border is not sufficient to negate the mesothelial identity of a cell (Fig. 4.44). The character of the atypical mesothelial hyperplasia is not sufficiently specific to allow a diagnosis of the underlying etiology. Particularly difficult to analyze is the atypical hyperplasia that occurs in association with cirrhosis or following a pulmonary infarct. In both of these processes the shape of the mesothelial cells is considerably altered so that elongated, squared-off, and rather bizarre forms can be found in the effusion. Extensive bleb formation may occur in cirrhosis, but is not specific for this condition (Fig. 4.45). The cytologic atypia is not restricted to the contiguous body

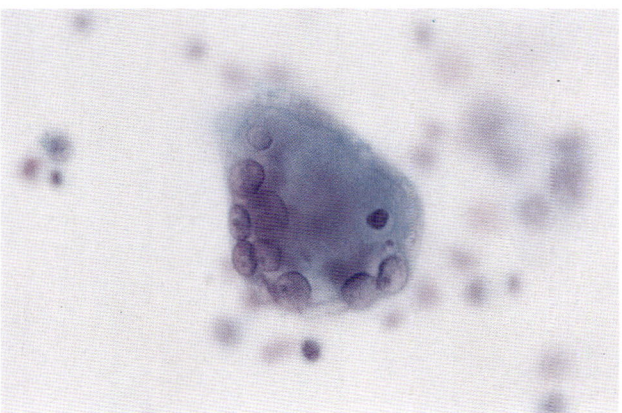

FIGURE 4.41   Multinucleated mesothelial cell. Several nuclei of similar size and shape share a large expanse of cytoplasm. No phagocytized debris is noted in the cytoplasm, except for the remnant of degenerating lymphocyte. (Pap × 200)

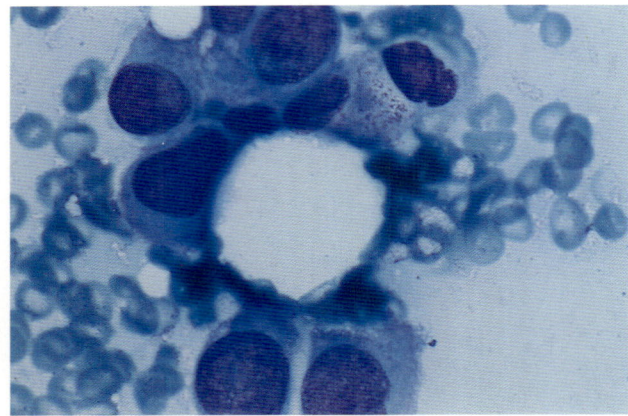

FIGURE 4.43   Diff-Quik stain of the fluid showning a pseudoacinus. The artifactually produced lumen lacks any secretion and the mesothelial cells are obviously benign. (MGG 180)

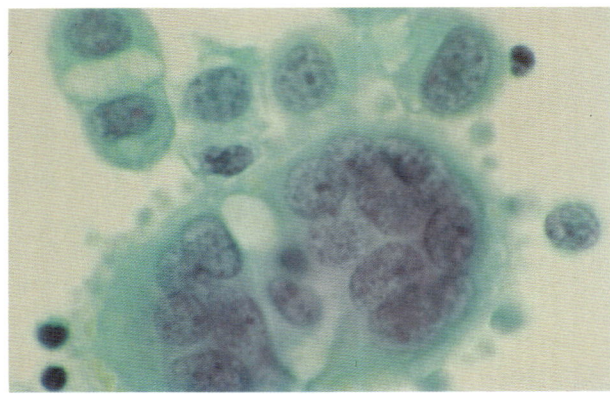

FIGURE 4.44   Bizarre, multinucleated mesothelial cells with microvilli appearing as blebs. Notice typical articulations and windows among neighboring mesothelial cells. (Pap × 240)

cavity, so that cirrhosis is accompanied by atypical cells in the pleural cavity and pulmonary infarct may lead to atypical cells in the ascitic fluid. In Meig's syndrome, by mechanism unknown, primary ovarian neoplasms are accompanied by pleural effusion containing reactive mesothelial cells. These and other nonneoplastic conditions are further discussed in Chapter 7.

ALIEN CELLS

A number of foreign materials may appear in effusion specimens as a result of the trajectory of the needle traversing neighboring structures of the spontaneous appearance of cells resulting from a variety of physiologic mechanisms. As depicted in Table 4.5, alien cells may provene from various origins. Solid organs like the liver and hollow viscera such as the esophagus and the intestines may be pierced, yielding portions of parenchyma or mucosa that may be troublesome to the inexperienced examiner. Vegetable matter derived from foodstuff or feces may be noted in ascites or cul-de-sac aspirates (Fig. 4.46). Sheets of liver cells have been confused with mesothelial cells and even carcinoma. Individual hepatocytes may resemble macrophages, particularly if they contain lipofuscin (confusable with hemosiderin) or fat (confusable with phagocytic vacuoles). Long standing effusions may demonstrate cells from the female genital tract that accumulate in the cul-de-sac and undergo degeneration. Detached ciliary tufts (DCTs), probably derived from the fallopian tube, are

an odd curiosity since they are motile by phase contrast microscopy and in wet films stained by toluidine blue (Fig. 4.47). Serosanguinous effusions accumulate hemosiderin-laden macrophages and crystals of hematoidin. Any long-standing effusion may lead to cholesterol crystals, responsible for the golden brown shimmer characteristic of pseudochylous effusions. Other crystals and substances appear as a result of toxic, iatrogenic, and systemic processes and are discussed separately in Chapter 7. Many of these structures are easily identified and cause little difficulty in interpretation, but some,

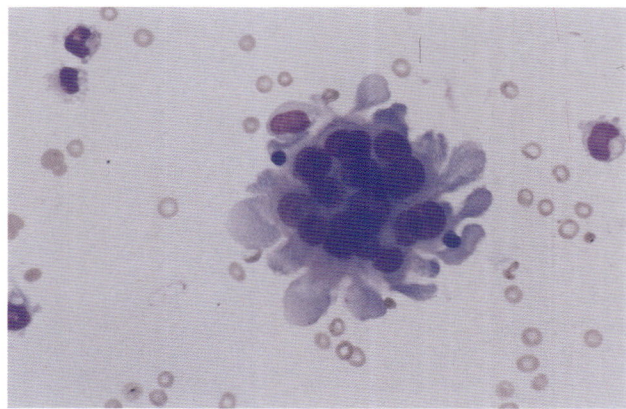

FIGURE 4.45   Bleb formation on the surface of giant mesothelial cells. This phenomenon occurs in both benign and malignant cells, but its exact mechanism and significance are unknown. (MGG × 180) (Courtesy Dr. A.Y. Leong)

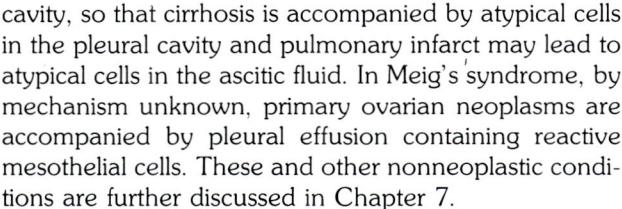

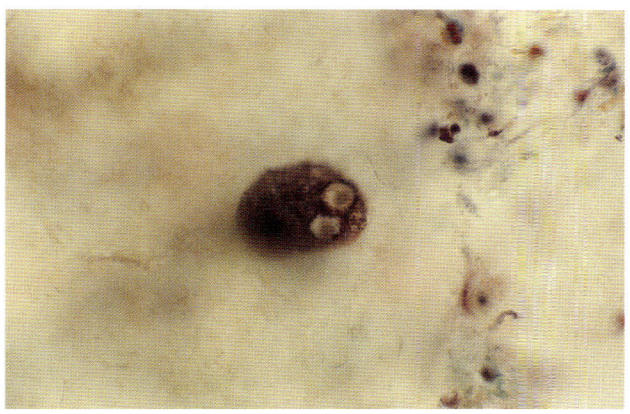

FIGURE 4.46 Vegetable matter in cul-de-sac aspirate submitted for suspicion of bowel perforation. (Pap × 100)

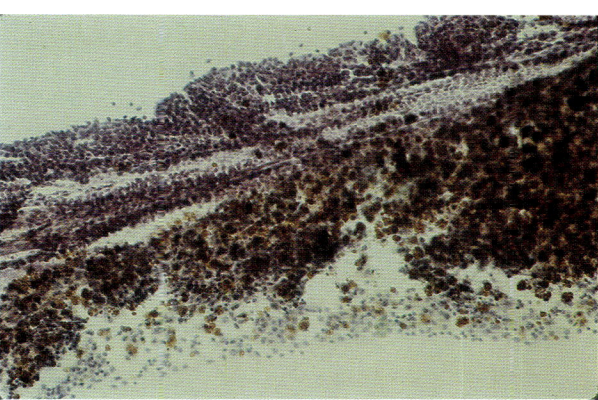

FIGURE 4.48 Pelvic washings in woman with pain during menstrual cycle. Note sheets of cells against a bloody background. (Pap × 40) (Courtesy Dr. D. Hidvegi)

such as the cells derived from the female genital tract, may be confused with malignancy (Table 4.5).

UTERINE CELLS

A certain level of reflux occurs during menstruation, particularly in IUD wearers, whereby cells of intrauterine origin gain access to the cul-de-sac by way of the fallopian tube. The occurrence of reflux is substantiated by histologic section of perisalpyngeal tissues that show

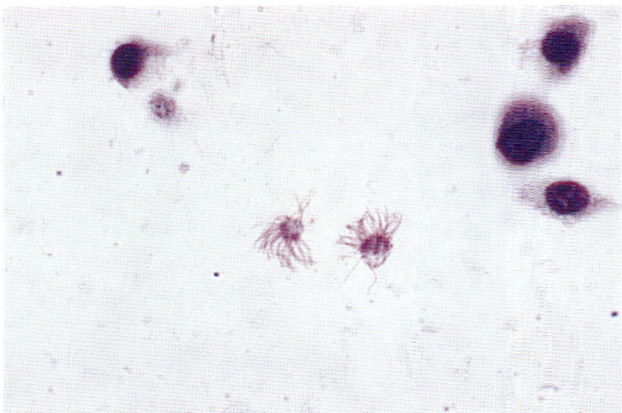

FIGURE 4.47 Detached ciliary tufts (DCTs) in a peritoneal washing. These structures are believed to represent the effect of mechanical abrasion. (MGG × 120) (Courtesy Dr. P. Gupta)

implants of endocervical or endometrial cells, or both, and may indeed be the basis of endometriosis. Sheets of dark blue cells in peritoneal fluid should not be confused with the presence of malignancy. In full-blown endometriosis these cells are extremely numerous, forming large sheets and papillary groups of cells that may overwhelm the background mesothelial cells (Fig. 4.48). In peritoneal washes obtained during second-look operations, the findings of large numbers of small, dark blue cells may be a source of diagnostic difficulties. Unless a history of endometriosis is available, these cells are easily confused with lymphocytes. A helpful clue to endometriosis is the presence of blood and hemosiderin laden macrophages associated with endometrial cells. In endometriosis the cells may be considerably small and compact, forming morulalike groups of extremely dark cells. Occasionally it is possible even to distinguish between stromal and epithelial endometrial cells if the architecture of the endometrial tuft is well preserved or if histiocytes are identified amid the endometrial cells. The use of cell blocks facilitate the diagnosis of endometriosis by demonstrating the relationship between epithelial lining cells and stromal cells. Cells of endosalpingiosis have also been encountered in ascitic fluid and are more frequently noted in cul-de-sac aspirates.

OTHER CONTAMINANTS

Aspiration of fluid from the dependent portion of the cul-de-sac is not without mishaps. An improperly placed needle may aspirate fecal contents from the intestine,

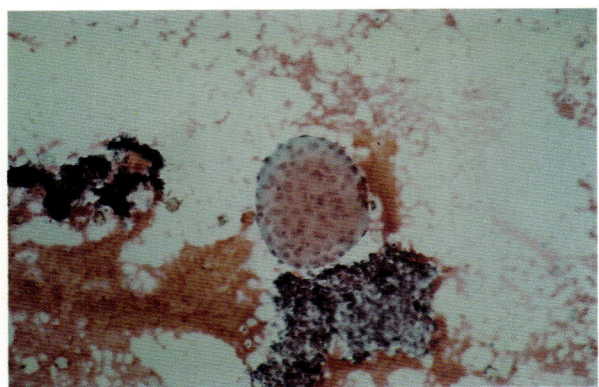

FIGURE 4.49 Peritoneal washing. Note rounded fragment of ovarian stroma. Also present is a sheet of dark-staining, surface epithelial cells against a bloody background. (Pap × 90) (Courtesy Dr. D. Hidvegi)

fluid and cells from an ovarian cyst that may have been mistaken for ascites, or cells from the occluded end of the fallopian tube. These situations are not necessarily known at the time ascitic fluid or cul-de-sac aspirates are submitted for cytologic evaluation, and the cells identified may be mistaken for malignancy. Cells from the ovarian stroma and cells from the surface and granulosa layers have both been observed in ascitic fluid (Fig. 4.49). The greatest difficulty arises when repeated surgery has caused brittle fibrotic knots along the omentum and the surfaces of pelvic organs. In these cases, papillary fragments with a fibrous core, psammoma bodies, and omental fat may be aspirated during cul-de-sac aspiration or peritoneal washings. Spriggs and Boddington have documented rare examples of stomach contents, squamous cells of esophageal origin, and cells arising in teratoma of the ovary contaminating pleural and peritoneal effusions. Naylor has seen vegetable fibers, lung parenchyma, epidermis, skin appendages, and portions of cartilage which he attributes to a misdirected needle during aspiration of fluid from the serosal cavities.

BIBLIOGRAPHY

Normal Cell Populations

Blaustein A. Peritoneal mesothelium and ovarian surface cells—shared characteristics. Int J Gynecol Pathol. 1984; 3(4):361–375.

Koss L. *Effusions in the Absence of Cancer: Diagnosis Cytology and its Histopathologic Bases,* 4th Ed. Philadelphia, J.B. Lippincott; 1992:1082–1115.

Luse J, Regan J. A histo-cytological study of effusions, I: Effusions not associated with malignant tumors. *Cancer* 1954; 7:1155–1166.

McGowan L. Morphology of mesothelial cells in peritoneal fluid from normal women. *Acta Cytol.* 1974;18:205–209.

Resident Macrophages

Beelen RH, Fluitsma DM. What is the relevance of exudate-resident macrophages? *Immunobiology.* 1982;161(3–4): 266–273.

Gaulier A, Jouret-Mourin A, Marsan C. Peritoneal endometriosis. Report of a case with cytologic, cytochemical and histopathologic study. *Acta Cytol.* 1983;27(4):446–449.

Katz DR. Macrophages from malignant effusions. J Pathol. 1981;134(4):279–290.

Lubinski J. Distribution pattern of concanavalin A on carcinoma cells, histiocyte and mesothelial cells from effusions. *Acta Cytol.* 1987;31(2):99–103.

Radzum H, Bommes M, Henselmans M, et al. Resident human peritoneal macrophages: A monocytic cell line. *Acta Cytol.* 1982;26(3):363–366.

Mesothelial Cells

Domagala W, Koss LG. Surface configuration of mesothelial cells in effusions. A comparative light microscopic and scanning electron microscopic study. *Virchows Arch [B].* 1979; 30:321.

Takahashi M. *Effusions in Body Cavities in Takahasi—an Atlas of Cancer Cytology.* New York: Igaku-Shoin; 1979: 409–458.

*Mesothelial Injury and Repair
Reactive Mesothelial Cells*

Ryan G, Groberty J, Majno G. Mesothelial injury and recovery. Am J Pathol. 1973;71:93–112.

Whitaker D, Papadimitriou J. Mesothelial healing morphological and kinetic investigations. *J Pathol.* 1985;145:159–175.

Agostoni A, Marasini B. Orosomucoid contents of pleural and peritoneal effusions of various etiologies. *Am J Clin Pathol.* 1977;67:146–148.

Marshall RJ, Herbert A, Brayer SG, et al. Use of antibodies to carcinoembryonic antigen and human milk fat globule to distinguish carcinoma, mesothelioma, and reactive mesothelium. *J Clin Pathol.* 1984;37:1215–1221.

Stoebner P, Miech G, Sengel A, et al. Notions d'ultrastructure pleurale, I: L'hyperphasie mesotheliale. *Presse Med.* 1970;78:1179–1183.

Vladutiu A, Brason FW, Adler RH. Differential diagnosis of pleural effusions. *Chest.* 1981;79(3):297–301.

Hyperplastic Mesothelial Cells
Atypical Mesothelial Hyperplasia

Becker S, Pepin D, Rosenthal D. Mesothelial papilloma. A case of mistaken identity in a pericardial effusion. *Acta Cytol.* 1976;20:266–268.

Duggan M, Masters C, Alexander F. Immunohistochemical differentiation of malignant mesothelioma, mesothelial hyperplasia and metastatic adenocarcinoma in serous effusions, utilizing staining for carcinoembryonic antigen, keratin and vimentin. *Acta Cytol* 1987;31:814–817.

Gondos B, Lai C, King E. Distinction between atypical mesothelial cells and malignant cells by scanning electron microscopy. *Acta Cytol.* 1979;23(4):321–326.

Jouret-Mourin A, Gaulie A, et al. Diagnostic cytologique et anatomo-pathologique de l'endometriose peritoneale. *Gynecologie.* 1981;32:459–464.

Kutty CPK, Remeniuk E, Varkey B. Malignant-appearing cells in pleural effusion due to pancreatitis: Case report and literature review. *Acta Cytol.* 1981;25:412–416.

Alien Cells, Uterine Cells, and other Contaminants

Carlson GJ, Samuelson JJ, Dehner LP. Cytologic diagnosis of florid peritoneal endosalpingosis. *Acta Cytol.* 1986;30:494.

Hibbard LT, Schumann WR, Goldstein GF. Thoracic endometriosis: A review and report of two cases. *Am J Obstet Gynecol.* 1981;140:227–232.

Naylor B: Pleural, peritoneal and pericardial fluids. In Bibbo M, ed. Comprehensive cytopathology. WB Saunders; Philadelphia: 1991, 541–614.

Spriggs AL, Boddington MM: Atlas of serous fluid cytopathology, London: Kluwer Academic Publishers; 1989, 120–122.

Zaatari G, Gupta P, Bhagavan B. Cytopathology of pleural endometriosis. *Acta Cytol.* 1982;26(2):227–232.

CHAPTER FIVE

Inflammatory Processes

As noted in the preceding chapter, mesothelial cells are extremely sensitive to any pathologic process affecting the serosal membrane. The resulting mesothelial hyperplasia represents a nonspecific reaction to injury and offers little insight about the underlying cause of the process. This cause is varied, encompassing mechanical, neoplastic and inflammatory etiology. The etiology of the inflammatory effusion usually requires a careful history as well as specialized studies to be elucidated. However, observation of the number and types of the inflammatory cells may offer some clues about the causative agent of the process. It is therefore important to recognize the several kinds of inflammatory cells in an effusion and not to confuse them with mesothelial or malignant cells.

Inflammatory processes account for almost half of all clinically significant effusions. The vast majority of transudates are caused by circulatory abnormalities, either of a generalized (cardiogenic) nature or secondary to localized (inflammatory) disturbances of the microvasculature. Even though most exudates derive from malignant processes they are commonly accompanied by an inflammatory response. In fact, many cases lack malignant cells but are accompanied by the vascular events of inflammation, of which an effusion is the most dramatic. The inflammatory response has been classically divided into acute and chronic on the basis of time and the cells involved in the process. This division is arbitrary, and the cellular composition of the inflammatory response can be altered by the immunologic status of the patient and the effect of the treatment. In exudates, resident macrophages and lymphocytes commonly increase in number, regardless of the cause of the effusion. Other cell types, such as neutrophils, plasma cells, eosinophils, and multinucleated giant cells, are linked to slightly more specific processes.

PURULENT EXUDATES

The presence of polymononuclear leukocytes in an effusion indicates an acute inflammatory response. Usually neutrophils are the predominant cell of the exudate. A small number of basophils may also accompany an effusion of long duration, whereas the presence of eosinophils denotes a special form of inflammatory response that will be discussed separately. Both eosinophils and basophils are difficult to recognize by Papanicolaou's stain but are easily demonstrated by Romanowsky's stains such as MGG or Diff Quik. Acute inflammatory exudates result from a number of causes including perforation of a viscus; transcoelomic spread of infection; pelvic inflammatory disease; pneumonia; lung abscess; and rheumatic carditis. Occasionally they are the result of direct bacterial seeding such as in tuberculous pleuritis and bacterial pericarditis. Surgical intervention may also be accompanied by an acute inflammatory exudate in any of the three body cavities. Coronary artery bypass, in particular, is accompanied by such effusion, which is described in greater detail under iatrogenic effusions in chapter 7. It is important not to overlook a malignant process in effusions containing mainly neutrophils. Very commonly, the necrotizing nature of the tumor leads to the appearance of many neutrophils or eosinophils in the effusion.

Neutrophils in post-pneumonic effusions combine their typical multilobed nuclei with an unusual abundance of granulations in the cytoplasm (Fig. 5.1). Only exceptionally one encounters infective agents phagocytized by neutrophils. However, the finding of engulfed cellular debris and granular material is a rather common occurrence (Fig. 5.2). Frankly purulent exudates are characterized by a large number of neutrophils and a highly necrotic background indicative of a more destructive form of acute inflammation (Fig. 5.3). They

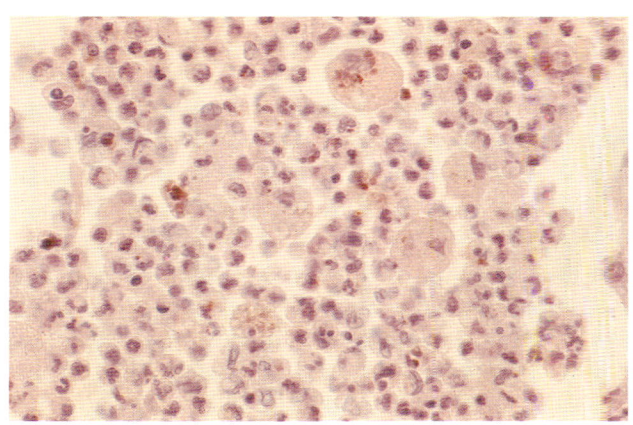

FIGURE 5.1 Purulent exudate from a case of empyema. Along with a few hemosiderin-laden macrophages and degenerating mesothelial cells, note the many polymorphonuclear leukocytes (PMNs). (H&E × 40)

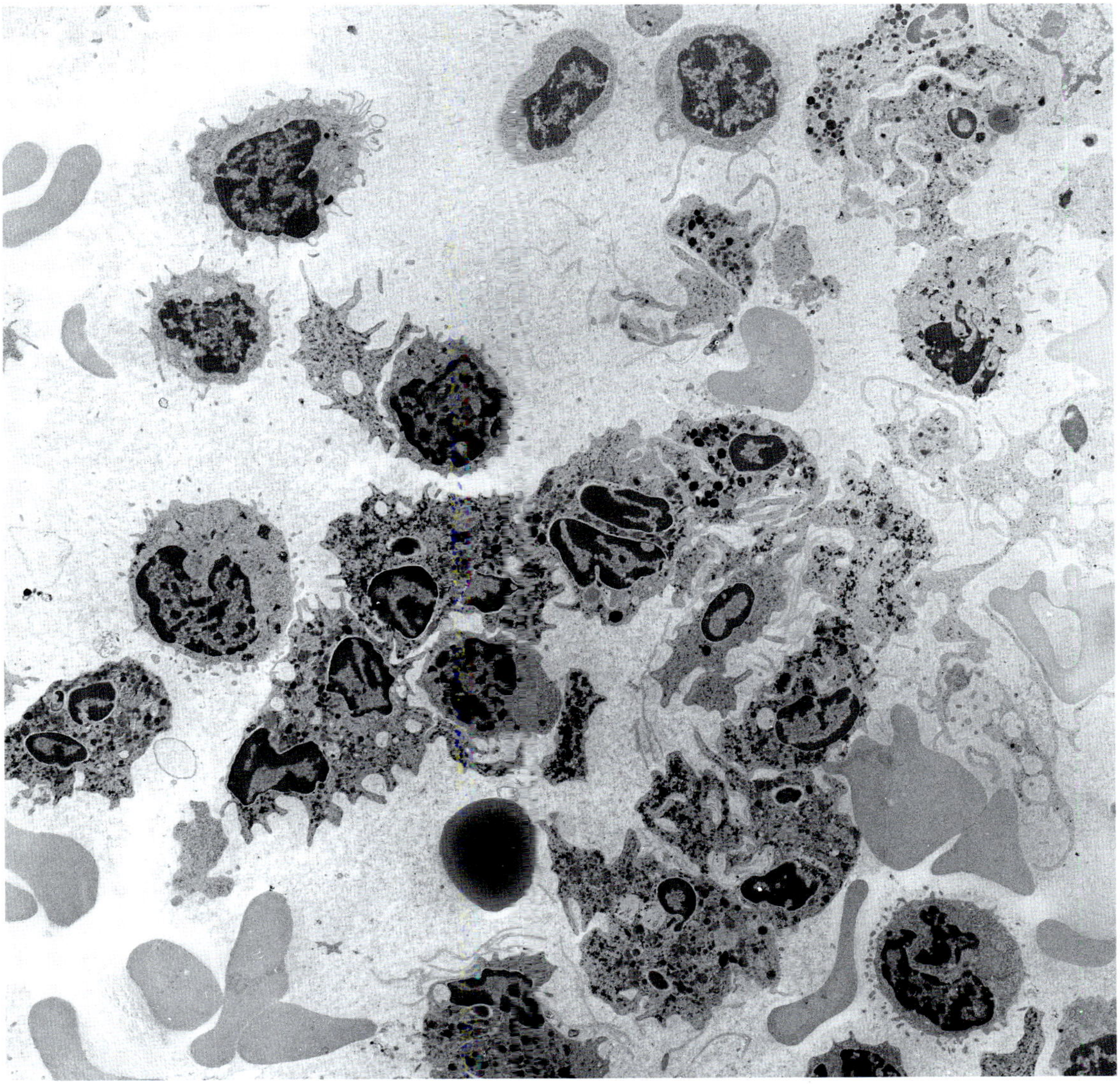

FIGURE 5.2 Purulent pleural effusion secondary to pneumonia. Notice large number of leukocytes with irregular nuclei and rather granular cytoplasm. (EM × 7,125).

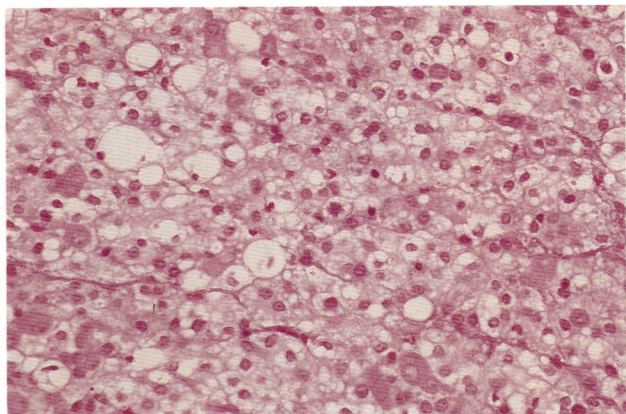

FIGURE 5.3 Resolving empyema. Only a few viable cells remain, trapped in a fibrinous meshwork. Large clear spaces are artifactual, resulting from ambient air entering the cell block during processing. (H&E × 40).

are usually the result of ruptured abscesses that cause empyema and parapneumonic loculation of the pleural space. A moderate number of neutrophils accompany fibrinopurulent effusions such as those secondary to pneumonia. As the process progresses, intact cells are cleared by enzymatic digestion. With resolution of the process, a more fibrinous exudate is all that remains, even though the effusion may persist for some time (Fig. 5.3). Subphrenic and hepatic abscesses may also lead to purulent peritonitis, but the pericardial sac is only rarely affected by a purulent tamponade. This site, however, is commonly involved in viral pericarditis, and the pericardium may become secondarily infected by bacteria, with the appearance of neutrophils in association of a lymphocytic response (Fig. 5.4). In malignant processes accompanied by tissue destruction, variable numbers of neutrophils may appear in the effusion (Fig. 5.5).

LYMPHOCYTIC PREDOMINANCE

An effusion with a predominance of lymphocytes should raise the suspicion of pulmonary tuberculosis without pleural involvement. However, the list of causes of lymphocyte-rich effusions is quite extensive (Table 5.1). Of these, collagen diseases are commonly associated with lymphocytes in the pleural fluid ranging from a few in number to marked lymphocytosis. (Fig. 5.6). When the pleura is affected by granulomas, giant cells are associated with macrophages and neutrophils. In children, viruses account for the majority of pleural effu-

sions with a predominance of lymphocytes. Sometimes the lymphocytes occur in such large numbers that the possibility of lymphoma is entertained in the differential diagnosis (Fig. 5.7). However, caution in rendering a diagnosis of lymphoma should be exercised when

- There is a mixture of lymphocytes showing various degrees of maturation.
- There is evidence of inflammation including a fibrinous background and occasional neutrophils, eosinophils, and plasma cells.
- One finds tingible body macrophages admixed with the lymphocytes
- The nuclei of the lymphocytes are not atypical.
- There is no evidence of generalized lymphadenopathy.
- The lymphocytes give evidence of polyconality.

A monotony of lymphocytes without cytologic atypia may cause more diagnostic difficulties than atypical lymphocytes with great morphologic diversity (Fig. 5.8). A monotonous population suggests clonality and is more consistent with lymphoma.

The polymorphous cell population of reactive processes often contain atypical lymphocytes (Fig. 5.9). Clonality can easily be established by immunostaining for **kappa** and **lambda** in cell blocks. Positivity for both heavy chains excludes the diagnosis of lymphoma (Fig. 5.10). Immunocytochemistry is also helpful in identifying B and T lymphocytes and distinguishing lymphocytes from malignant, blue round cells of non-lymphoid origin (Figs. 5.11 and 5.12).

It is imprudent at best to make the diagnosis of lymphoma on the basis of cytologic atypia alone, particularly in institutions where flow cytometry and immunophenotyping are available. A good rule of thumb is to back off from the diagnosis when lymphoma is contemplated for the first time and to order flow cytometry and marker studies when in doubt. If a good cell block is available, immunostaining for kappa and lambda chains may quickly establish the clonality of the process. Table 5.1 lists common causes of lymphocytic predominance. Other markers may establish T-cell or B-cell origin of the process.

PLASMA CELLS

One should be cautious not to assume the presence of plasma cells as evidence of benignness in a lymphocyte-rich effusion, since occasionally plasmacytomas may involve a serosal space (Fig. 5.13). Neoplastic

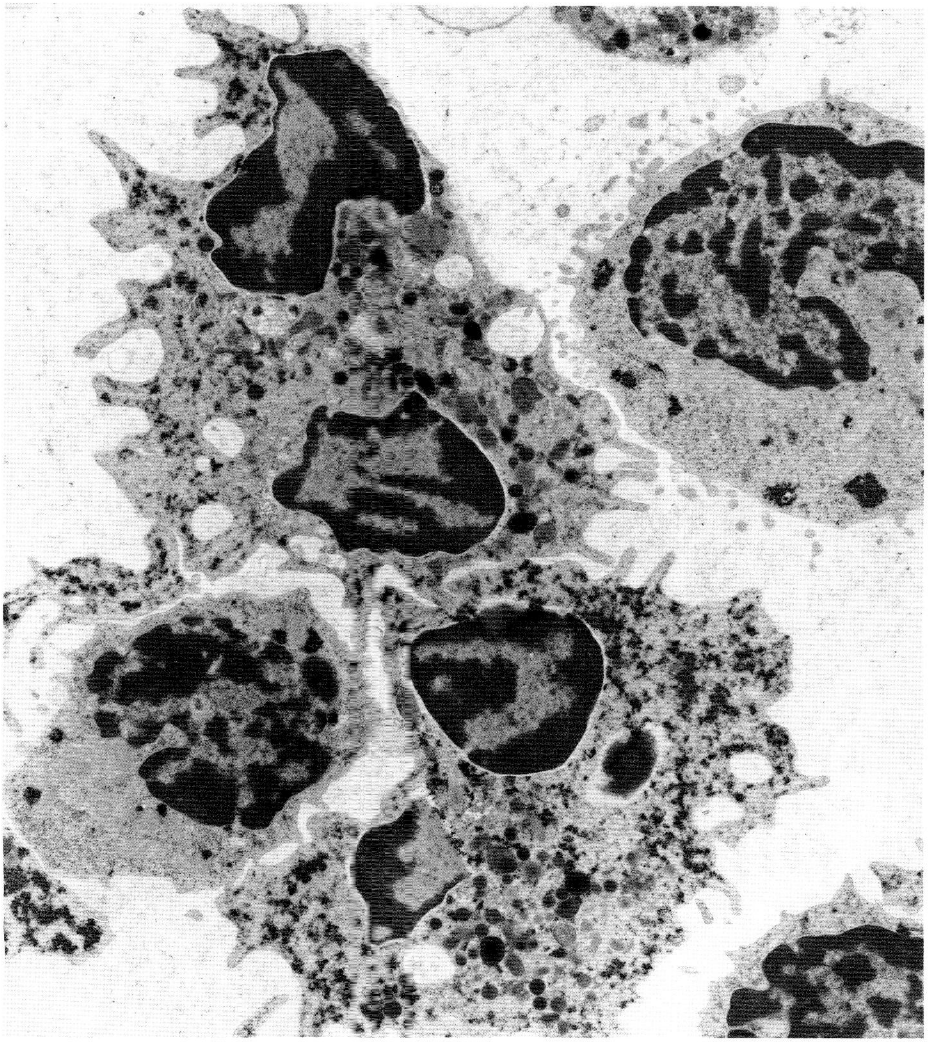

FIGURE 5.4   Viral pericarditis with lymphocytes and neutrophils showing engulfed cellular debris. Broad cytoplasmic pseudopods contrast with ruffles from neighboring lymphocytes. (EM × 13,000).

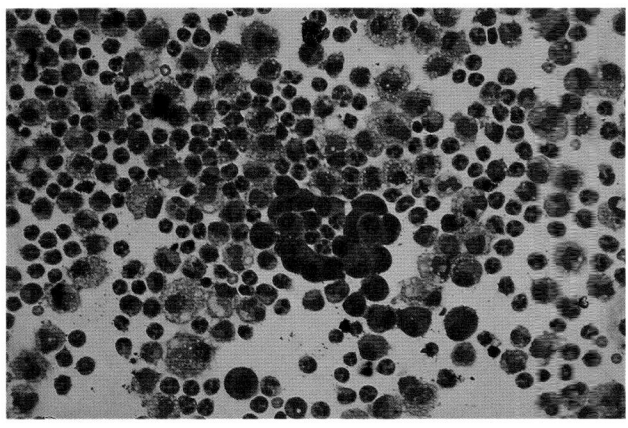

FIGURE 5.5   Neutrophils in a malignant effusion. Dark malignant cells are surrounded by degenerating, vacuolated mesothelial cells, macrophages and a large number of PMNS. (MGG × 40).

TABLE 5.1   Common Causes of Lymphocytic
Predominance in Effusions

Tuberculosis
Viral infections
Bronchogenic carcinoma
Collagen vascular disease
Sarcoidosis
Cardiac surgery
Chylous effusion
Infectious mononucleosis
Yellow-nail syndrome

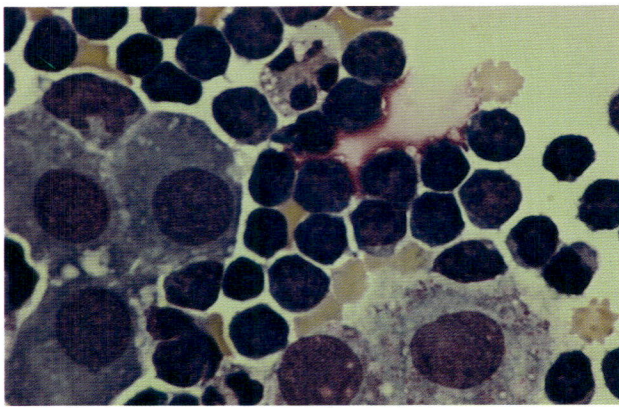

FIGURE 5.7   Effusion showing lymphocytosis. Note the dark, block-like chromatin of mature lymphocytes, in sharp contrast to reactive mesothelial cells. (MGG × 120).

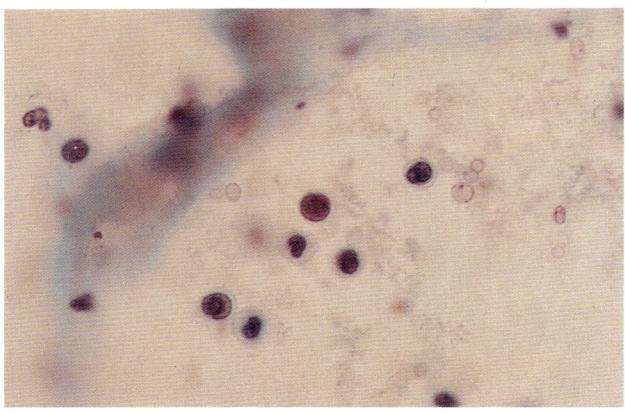

FIGURE 5.6   Reactive lymphocytes in an effusion from a patient with rheumatoid arthritis. A few immature forms of lymphocytes are noted, along with amorphous debris and ghosts of RBCs. (Pap × 60).

plasma cells lose their classical morphology and may necessitate ancillary studies to elucidate their true nature. Methyl green pyronin is a useful stain to identify plasma cells that are rich in kappa and lambda light chains by immunocytochemistry. Ultrastructurally, plasma cells are easily recognized by their parallel stacks of rough endoplasmic reticulum in the cytoplasm (Fig. 5.14). Any time there is a predominance of plasma cells in an effusion, amyloidosis should be suspected. Occasionally, proteinaceous material with amyloid-like properties may be demonstrated in the cytologic specimen (Fig. 5.15). The exact source of the amyloid in the effusion cannot be always detected and its identification may require polarization microscopy (Fig. 5.16). In our only example of this condition, a massive amyloid tumor of the lung had broken into the pleural space near the apex (Fig. 5.17).

EOSINOPHILIC EFFUSIONS

Accumulation of eosinophils in an effusion should bring about clinical suspicion of an allergic disease or hypersensitivity to drugs. In tropical countries, the possibility of parasitic infestation should be ruled out. However, in over half of the cases no cause can be elicited for the effusion, which may also result from overlooked trauma to the chest. Other common causes of eosinophilic pleural effusion include collagen diseases (21% of the cases), tuberculosis (19%), and cancer (9%). Of the malignancies, Hodgkin's disease is most commonly accompanied by an eosinophilic pleural effusion. Table 5.2 lists common causes of eosinophilic effusions.

The finding of pleural effusion does not necessarily imply a peripheral blood eosinophilia. The latter is more commonly formed in association with eosinophilic effusion due to allergy and hypersensitivity as well as helminthiasis. The degree of eosinophilia in the effusion can be extremely high, up to 42% of the cell count. In reactive eosinophilic pleuritis there is no peripheral eosinophilia. Eosinophils are easily recognized in cell blocks, but are not easily identified in Papanicolaou-stained preparations where they can be recognized by their bilobed nuclei (Figs. 5.18 and 5.19). Ultrastructurally, equatorial bands across the granules pathognomonic for polymorphonuclear eosinophils (Fig. 5.20). In general, there is an associated lymphocytosis reinforcing a possible immunologic basis for the eosinophilic effusion. Mast cells are sometimes associated with eosinophilic pleural effusion, but their role is not clear.

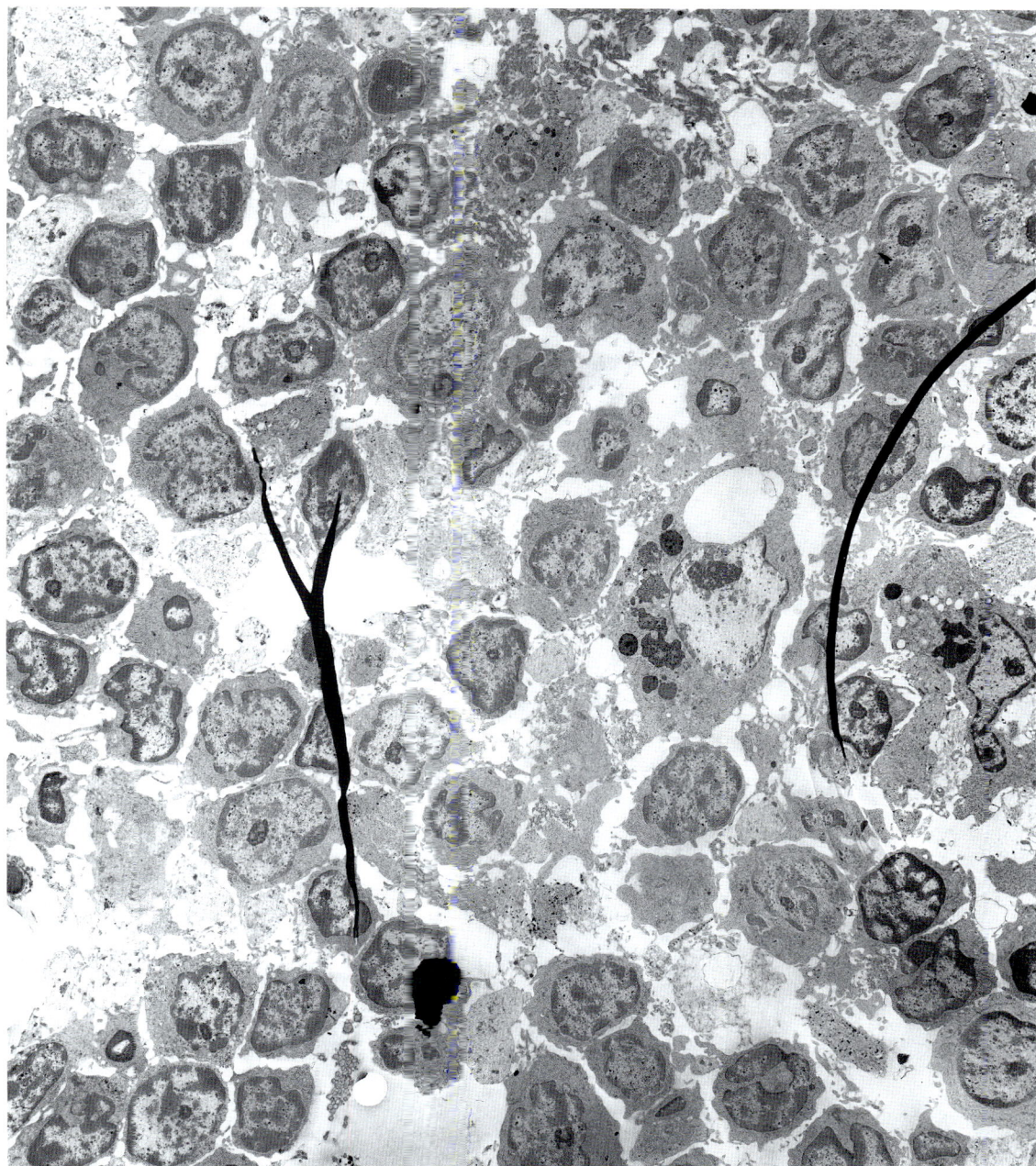

FIGURE 5.8 Large number of lymphocytes with wide range of nuclear size and shape in effusion secondary to tuberculosis. Activated lymphocytes and macrophages attest to the mixed cell population indicative of a benign process. (EM × 5,000).

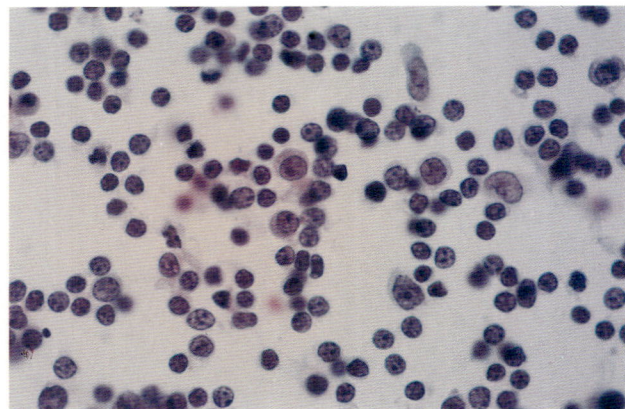

FIGURE 5.9   Florid lymphocytic effusion. The mixture of cell types and the different stages of lymphocyte maturation attest to the polyclonality of the effusion. Tuberculosis was suspected but not proved in this case (Pap × 40).

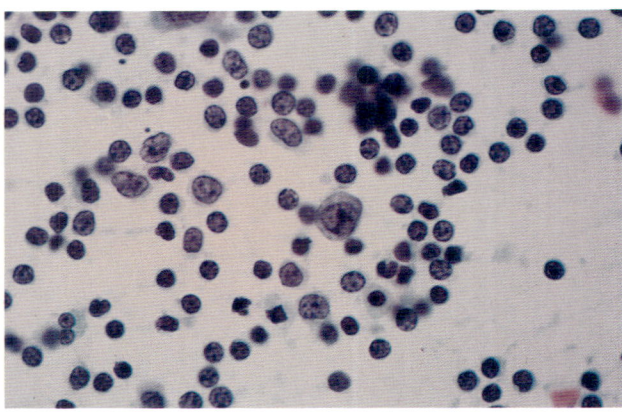

FIGURE 5.11   Persistent lymphocytic effusion. Numerous lymphocytes and rare, intermixed partially clumped dark cells of questionable origin. Since the patient was known to suffer from oat cell carcinoma, marker studies were ordered. (Pap × 90)

Depending on the longevity of the effusion and the cytopreparatory technique used, Charcot–Leyden crystals can be identified in eosinophilic effusion (Fig. 5.21). The eosinophilic granules are better demonstrated with the MGG stain than with Papanicolaou's stain. With MGG, eosinophils stain bluish gray and display bilobed nuclei, while the granules acquire a bright red eosinophilia (Fig. 5.22).

COLLAGEN VASCULAR DISEASES

A number of conditions affect multisystem organs, causing an inflammatory response of their microvasculature and their accompanying connective tissue stroma. These conditions have been loosely grouped under the all-inclusive terms connective tissue disorders or collagen vascular diseases. By far the most common form

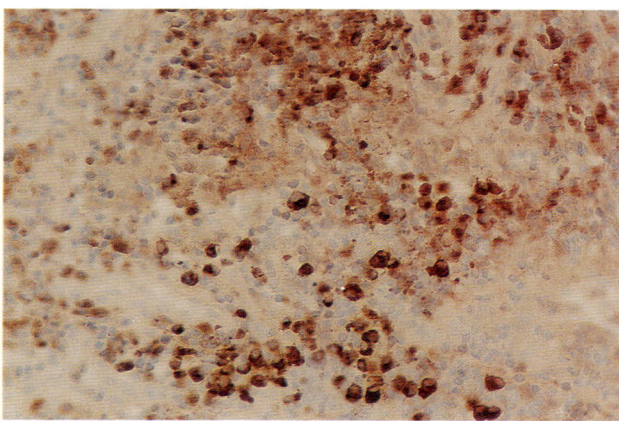

FIGURE 5.10   Same fluid as Fig 5.9. Many lymphocytes marked with antibody against kappa chains. The same was true of lambda chains, an indication of the polyclonality of the process. [Peroxidose anti-peroxidose (P.A.P.) × 40].

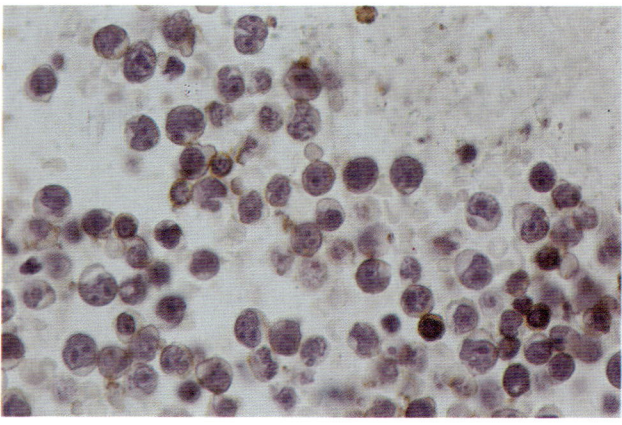

FIGURE 5.12   Lymphocytes are weakly positive with leukocyte common antigen; this excludes an epithelial origin for the cells. (P.A.P. × 75).

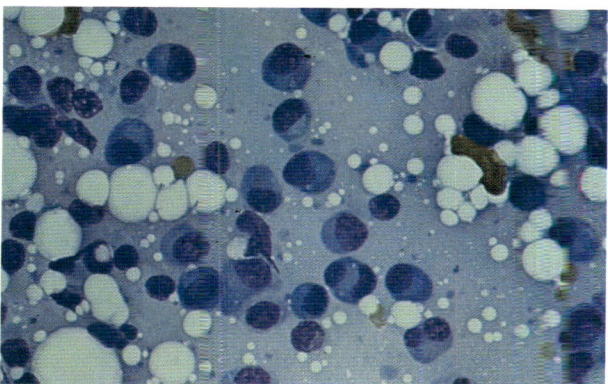

FIGURE 5.13   Plasmacytic process in a pleural effusion suspected of being reactive. The marker studies showed positivity only for kappa chains, thus establishing the diagnosis of plasmacytoma. (MGG × 90).

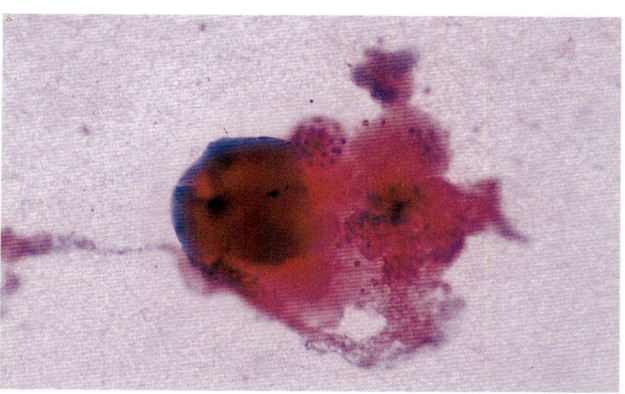

FIGURE 5.15   Amyloid-like substance from a pleural effusion in patient with amyloidosis. Without immunocytochemistry and/or electron microscopy, it is not possible to identify amyloid. (Pap × 40).

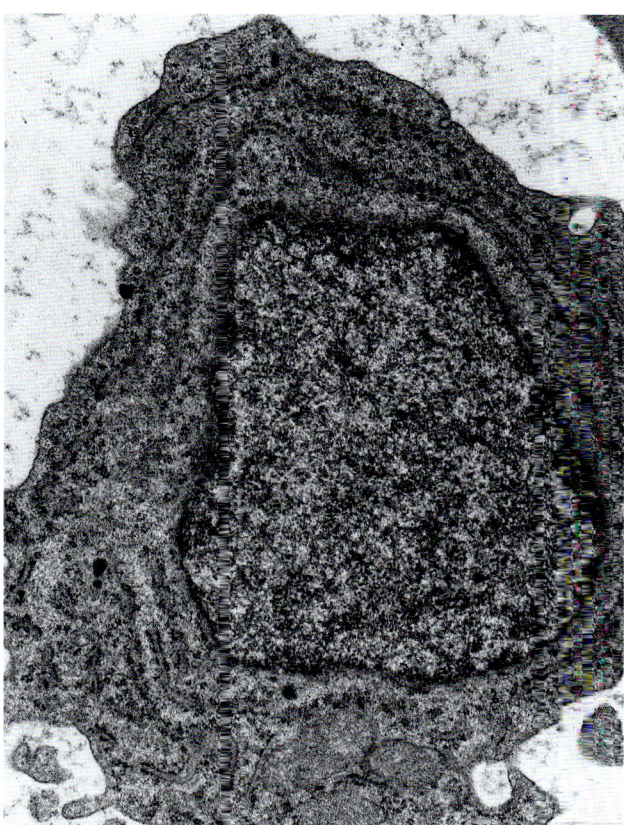

FIGURE 5.14   Plasma cell with parallel stacks of rough endoplasmic reticulum. Notice bland distribution of chromatin and squared-off shape of the cell (EM × 6,000).

of presentation is pleural effusion in patients with rheumatoid arthritis (RA), which has a characteristic cytologic appearance. The effusion is long standing and contains a large amount of proteinaceous debris which tends to dull the serous membrane (Fig. 5.23). The proteinaceous material forms granular aggregates detectable under low magnification by their eosinophilic coloration (Fig. 5.24). The combination of unusually elongated cells, multinucleated giant cells, and an eosinophilic amorphous background is pathognomonic for rheumatoid arthritis (Fig. 5.25). As with other effusions of long duration there is also an elevated number of inflammatory cells, including neutrophilis, lymphocytes and foamy histiocytes (Fig. 5.26). The nuclei of the giant cells are not grouped preferentially but show a wavy contour and prominent nucleoli (Fig 5.27). Occasionally the pleural fluid demonstrates granulocytes containing cytoplasmic inclusions (so-called RA cells), but only when they are shown to liberate rheumatoid factor should they be considered diagnostic of rheumatoid arthritis. Both glucose and the pH are decreased, which may account for the raw, inflamed appearance of the serous surfaces where the eosinophilic necrotic debris and elongated mesothelial cells can be identified.

Rheumatoid nodules have been found in the pleural biopsy specimens of patients with rheumatoid effusion so that the eosinophilic granular material may actually derive from the necrobiotic center of the nodules. It is not clear whether some of the elongated giant cells noted in effusions correspond to the palisading histiocytes of the nodules, but ultrastructurally, they are obvi-

TABLE 5.2   Common Causes of Eosinophilic Effusions

Pleural Effusions	Pericardial Effusions	Peritoneal Effusions
Pneumothorax	Pulmonary eosinophilia	Allergic reaction
Thoracic trauma	Hypersensitivity reaction	Parasitic infestation
Löffler's pneumonia	Hodgkin's disease	Eosinophilic gastroenteritis
Autoimmune disease	Non-Hodgkin's lymphoma	Peritoneal dialysis
Viral pneumonia		
Bacterial pneumonia		
Tuberculosis		
Fungal infection		
Pneumonic state		
Pulmonary infarct		
Hemothorax		
Hodgkin's disease		
Metastatic disease		
Lung carcinoma		
Allergic reaction		
Strongyloides stercoralis		
Hydatid disease		

ously of histiocytic origin (Fig. 5.28). Because these cells are degenerated, their pyknotic nuclei may be a cause of alarm and should not be misinterpreted as malignant. The large multinucleated giant cells also have been clearly identified as histiocytic in origin by immunocytochemistry and electron microscopy (Fig. 5.29). The rheumatoid factor is commonly positive in pleural effusions from patients with rheumatoid arthritis but appears nonspecific, since it is elevated in other collagen vascular diseases as well as other inflammatory conditions. It is not clear whether this factor corresponds to the amorphous granular debris typical of rheumatoid effusions (Fig. 5.30). Cholesterol crystals can be visualized under polarized light in cases of long-standing effusions secondary to rheumatoid arthritis. Less commonly, rheumatoid arthritis of long duration leads to pseudochylous effusions rich in cholesterol, which creates characteristic clefts in cell blocks.

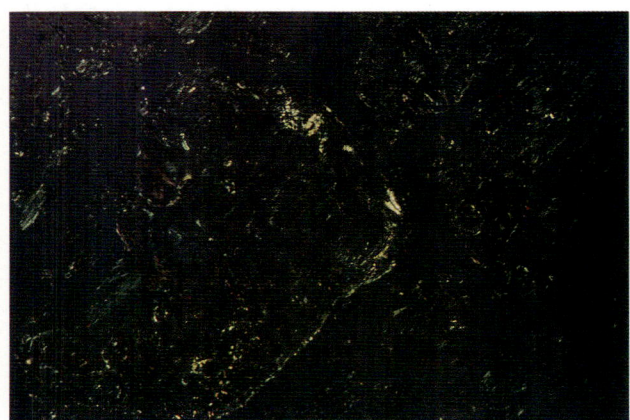

FIGURE 5.16   Amyloid stained with Congo-red and examined under polarized light. The typical birefringence of amyloid is readily appreciated. (Congo Red × 60)

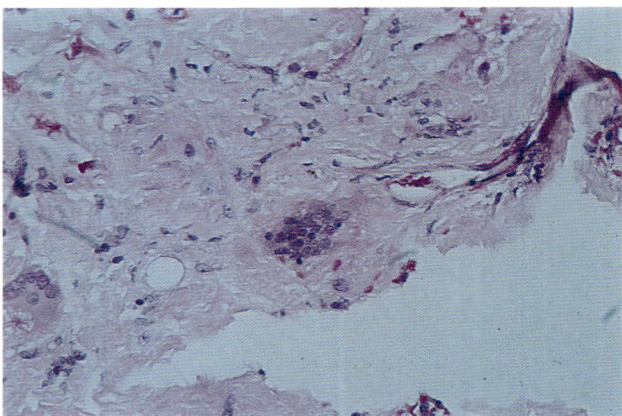

FIGURE 5.17   Biopsy of the lung from patient with amyloidosis. Note the break in the integrity of the visceral pleura, and direct contact with the pleural cavity. (H&E × 40)

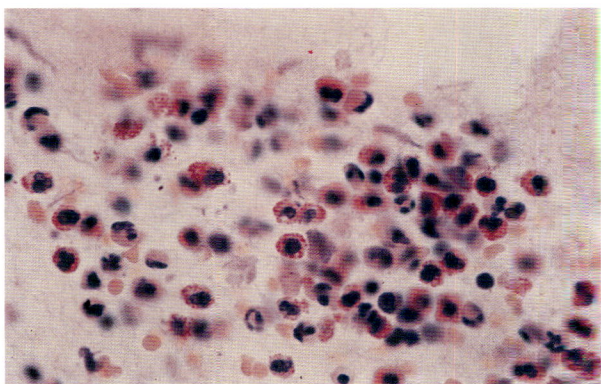

FIGURE 5.18 Cell block from same effusion as Fig 5.19. With the H&E stain the eosinophilia is readily appreciated. (H&E × 90)

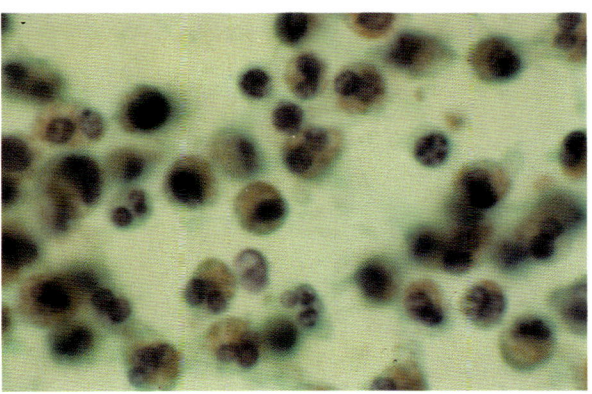

FIGURE 5.19 Eosinophilic pleural effusion. Notice bilobed nuclei and absence of frank eosinophilia with the Pap stain (Pap × 120)

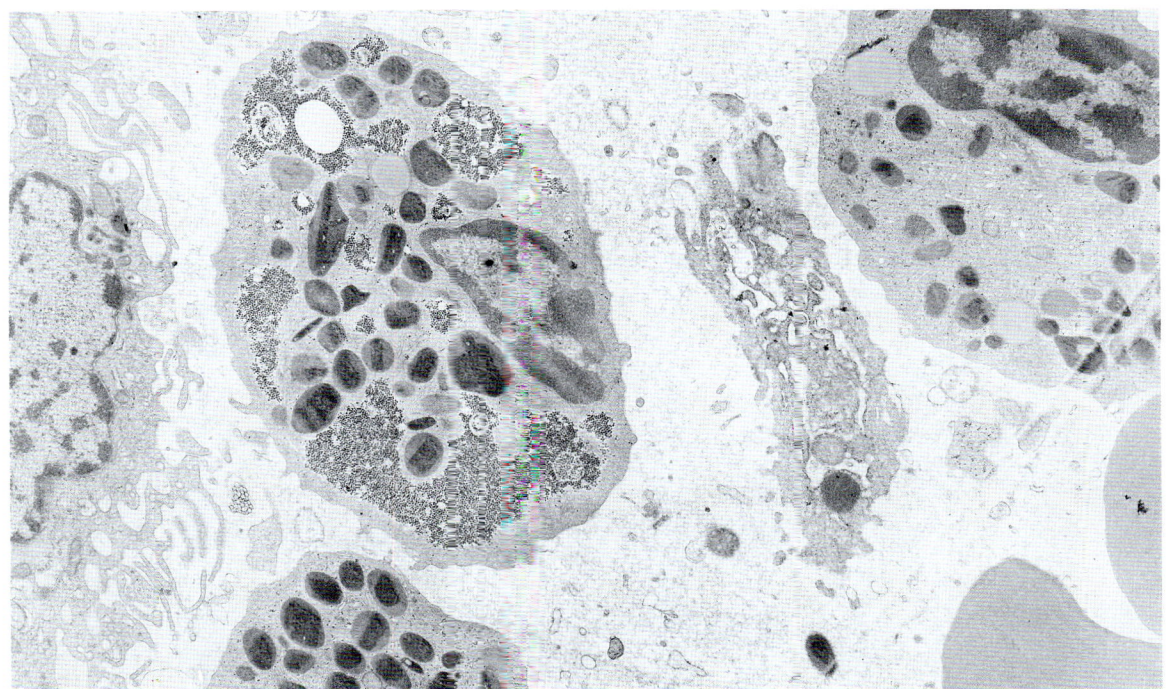

FIGURE 5.20 Eosinophil from pleural effusion resulting from chest trauma. Notice bilobed nucleus and typical banded granules in the cytoplasm. (EM × 6,750)

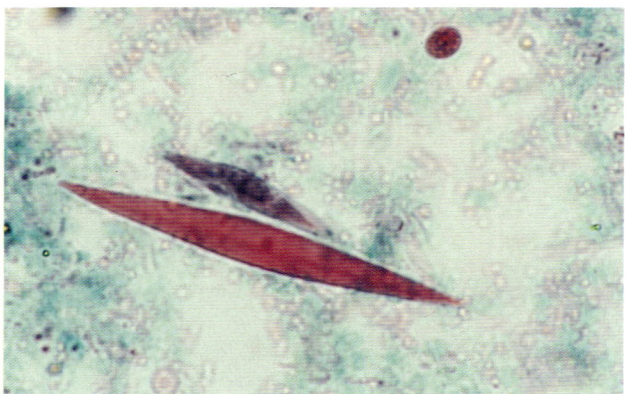

FIGURE 5.21   Charcot-Leyden crystals from a long-standing eosinophilic pleural effusion. These spindle-shaped crystals may only partially stain with Papanicolaou's method and tend to fragment. (Pap× 120)

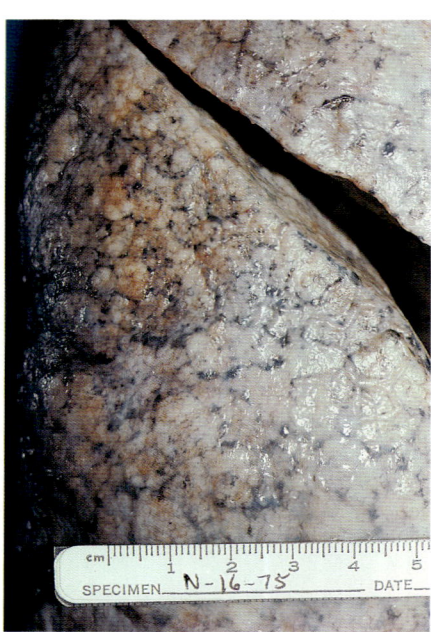

FIGURE 5.23   Surface of the lung in rheumatoid pleuritis. The dull "sugar-coating" of the pleura is characteristic of long-standing rheumatoid pleuritis.

Systemic lupus erythematous (SLE) is another collagen vascular disease that may be specifically diagnosed in cytologic specimens. This is possible when in vivo LE cells are noted in effusions, their characteristic structure being better demonstrated with the MGG stain than with Papanicolaou's stain (Fig. 5.31). LE cells are leukocytes whose cytoplasm contains altered, homogeneously degenerated material that stains purplish-blue by Papanicolaou's method. In contrast, tart cells engulf nuclear material in which the chromatinic structure is not totally disintegrated and there is still some resemblance to nuclei (Fig. 5.32). The finding of both of these structures should trigger antinuclear antibody tests for confirmation of the LE diagnosis. Care should be taken not to confuse true LE cells with nonspecific debris in the cytoplasm of degenerating cells. In general, the mesothelial hyperplasia is less pronounced in LE than in rheumatoid arthritis and the other collagen vascular

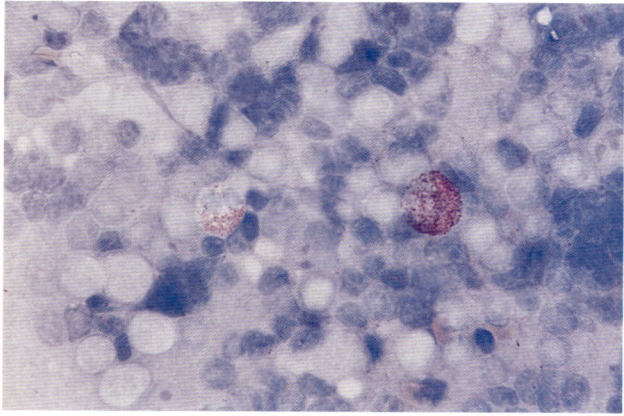

FIGURE 5.22   Eosinophils and a mast cell in a pleural effusion secondary to Hodgkin's diease. The Romanowsky-type stains are superior to the Pap stain for the identification of cells of lymphohistiocytic lineage. (MGG× 90)

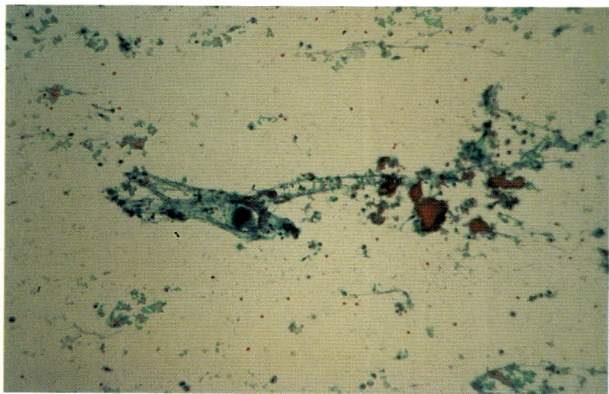

FIGURE 5.24   Pleural effusion in rheumatoid arthritis. Notice inflammatory cells in the vicinity of clumps of granular, eosinophilic debris. (Pap× 40)

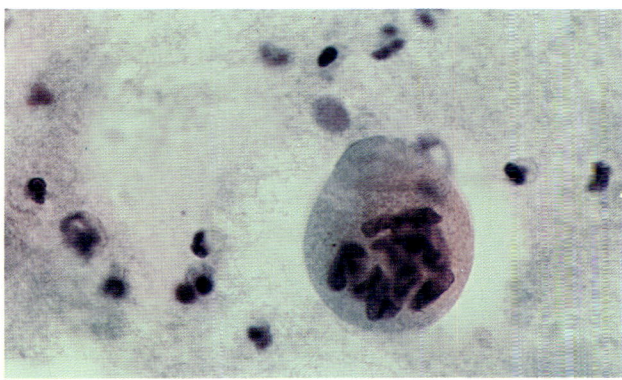

FIGURE 5.25 Pleural effusion from a patient with rheumatoid arthritis. The combination of giant cells and inflammatory cells in a proteinaceous granular milieu is typical of this condition. (Pap × 120) (Figs. 5.25 and 5.26, courtesy of Doug King)

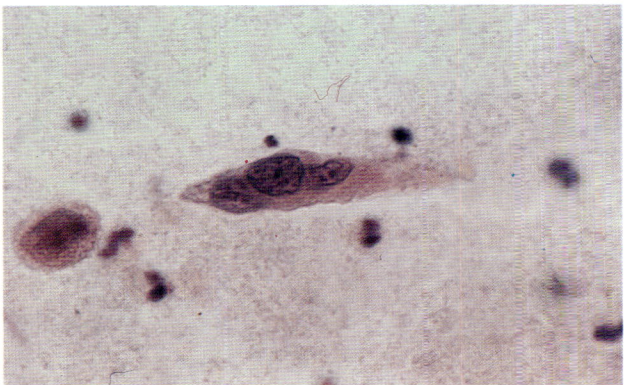

FIGURE 5.26 Rheumatoid pleural effusion. Note the elongated, multinucleated macrophage against a background of amorphous granular material. (Pap × 90)

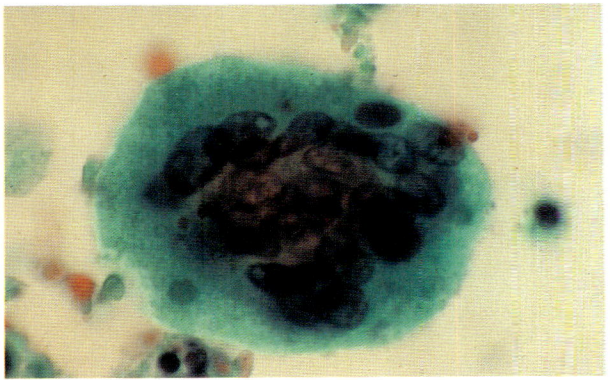

FIGURE 5.27 Giant cell from rheumatoid arthritis. The nuclei are crowded and show a wavey border. (Pap × 600)

diseases. The inflammatory response is similar, with a predominance of lymphocytes, few plasma cells, and only a rare eosinophil. The antinuclear antibody assay and other serologic factors are usually positive in the collagen vascular diseases, but differential diagnosis of the several subtypes often necessitates correlation with clinical and laboratory data.

GRANULOMATOUS INFLAMMATION

Tuberculosis is the prototype of granulomatous disorders, but fungi and other bacteria may also be accompanied by granuloma formation (Fig. 5.33). In these cases occasional giant cells may be found in the effusion, but most often the chronic inflammatory component dominates the cytologic picture and may be indistinguishable from chronic nonspecific serositis (Fig. 5.34). In granulomata many macrophages, plasma cells, and plump cells of difficult interpretation are noted against a backdrop of mesothelial hyperplasia. The plump histiocytes oftentimes hug together in an epithelioid fashion (Fig. 5.35). In the presence of giant cells careful examination of the background is warranted to identify the offending agent. In tuberculous empyema the caseous character of the necrotic material may be still appreciated in a thick fluid milieu (Fig. 5.36).

In sarcoidosis there is no necrotic material in the background but the epithelioid histiocytes are virtually identical to those seen in tuberculosis (Fig. 5.37). Neither giant cells nor the asteroid bodies of sarcoidosis are specific enough to warrant a differential diagnosis without careful clinicopathologic correlation. Elevation of ACE in the pleural fluid would be supportive of the diagnosis of sarcoidosis. Fungal infections may incite granulomatous reactions but their distinction from those caused by tuberculosis requires the identification of hyphae or yeast forms of fungus in the effusions. This is best accomplished by special staining even though the Pap stain may be adequate in many cases as discussed in Chapter 6. The character of the mesothelial hyperplasia is of no help in distinguishing granulomatous from other causes of effusion.

GIANT CELL REACTIONS

Occasionally, giant cells dominate the cytologic picture with inflammatory cells and mesothelial cells playing a minor role. The first difficulty following the finding of

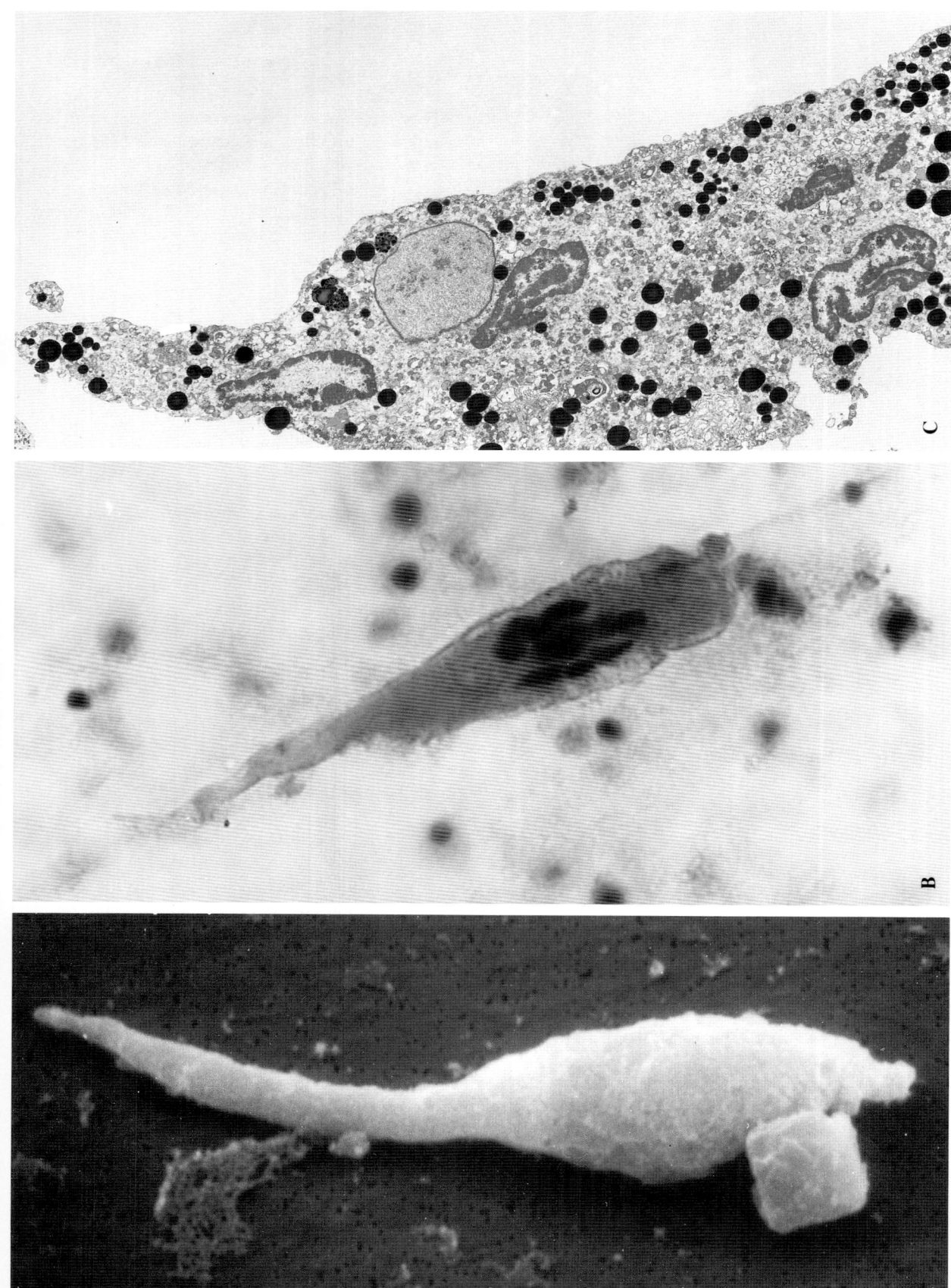

FIGURE 5.28 Elongated giant cells from rheumatoid arthritis shown by SEM (A); light microscopy (B); and TEM (C). Notice similarity of cytoplasmic contents with plump giant cells shown in Figure 5.29. (Figs. 5.28 through 5.30 courtesy Dr. K. Geisinger)

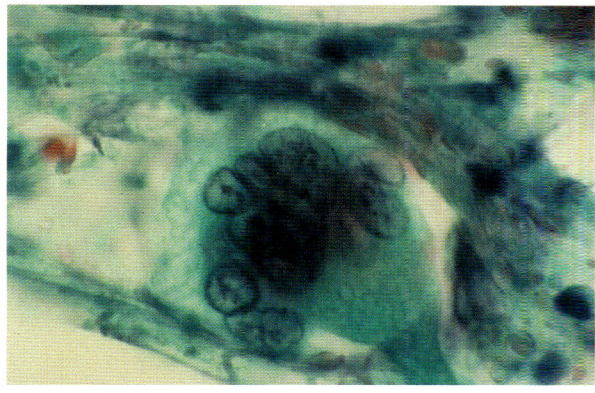

A

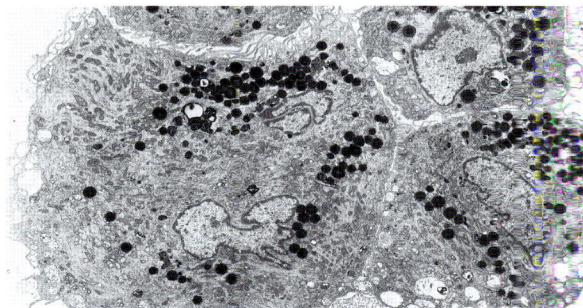

B

FIGURE 5.29 Multinucleated giant cells in reumatoic arthritis. (*A*) The nuclei are grooved and eccentrically located. (Pap × 500) (*B*) By EM notice ruffled surfaces as well as lysozomes and lipid droplets in the cytoplasm. (EM × 9,750).

giant cells in an effusion is to determine their exact nature. Multinucleation may occur in any cellular elements such as mesothelial cells and macrophages, and this phenomenon should be distinguished from giant cells of epithelial and mesenchymal origin. The classical configurations of Langhans', Touton's, and foreign-body giant cells may all be found in an effusion but are of little clinical significance. Langhans' cells are not specific for tuberculosis as they can be found not only in sarcoidosis but also in miscellaneous granulomatous conditions. Special stains are helpful in demonstrating AFB in tuberculosis, but the yield of these and of cultures of serous fluids is lower than in sputum specimens. Foreign bodies affecting the soft tissues surrounding the serous cavities may also be accompanied by giant cells of histiocytic origin. When foreign substances are present in the serous fluid they may be engulfed by both

macrophages and mesothelial cells, which are thus capable of phagocytosis. A simple panel of immunostains resolves most diagnostic dilemmas, α_1AT/α_1ACT are positive in giant cells of histiocytic origin; multinucleated mesothelial cells may lose part of their keratin positivity but they do not acquire α_1AT/α_1ACT or lysozyme positivity. Neoplastic cells of epithelial and mesenchymal origin are positive for CEA and vimentin, respectively, even though they may also express a variety of other markers.

Myelometaplasia is usually accompanied by megakaryocytes scattered along the mesothelial surfaces. These cells are recognizable by their characteristic cytomorphology, but they may be confused with other multinucleated elements, including malignant giant cells, especially when degenerated and pyknotic (Fig. 5.38). Identification of megakaryocytes may be especially difficult in markedly bloody effusions (Fig. 5.39). The use of Factor VIII–related antigen as a marker facilitates the recognition of these cells as megakaryocytes (Fig. 5.40). AIDS has been known to induce effusions with an unusual cytologic picture. Polykaryocytes of putative megakaryocytic origin have been noted in some cases (Fig. 5.41). Other AIDS-related effusions have been accompanied by giant cells of conventional histiocytic origin.

CHYLOUS EFFUSIONS

The diagnosis of chylous effusion is easily established by biochemical examination and can even be accomplished by visual means under gross examination (Fig. 5.42). The characteristic cytologic feature is the presence of foamy macrophages, hypervacuolated and reactive mesothelial cells, and a viscous lipid-rich material in the background. Ultrastructurally, macrophages show lipid in their degenerated cytoplasm (Fig 5.43). If the effusion is of long duration lymphocytes, plasma cells, and atypical mesothelial cells are also noted. In recurrent cases attempts at obliterating the effusion may have been made in the past. In these cases one may find talcum powder with the characteristic maltese cross or another crystalline sclerosing agent recognizable with polarized light. Occasionally, the underlying disease process responsible for the chylous effusion may be apparent as in the case of malignancy-associated chylous ascites, which can be accompanied by tumor cells. True chylous effusions should be differentiated from pseudochylous effusions, as depicted in Table 5.3.

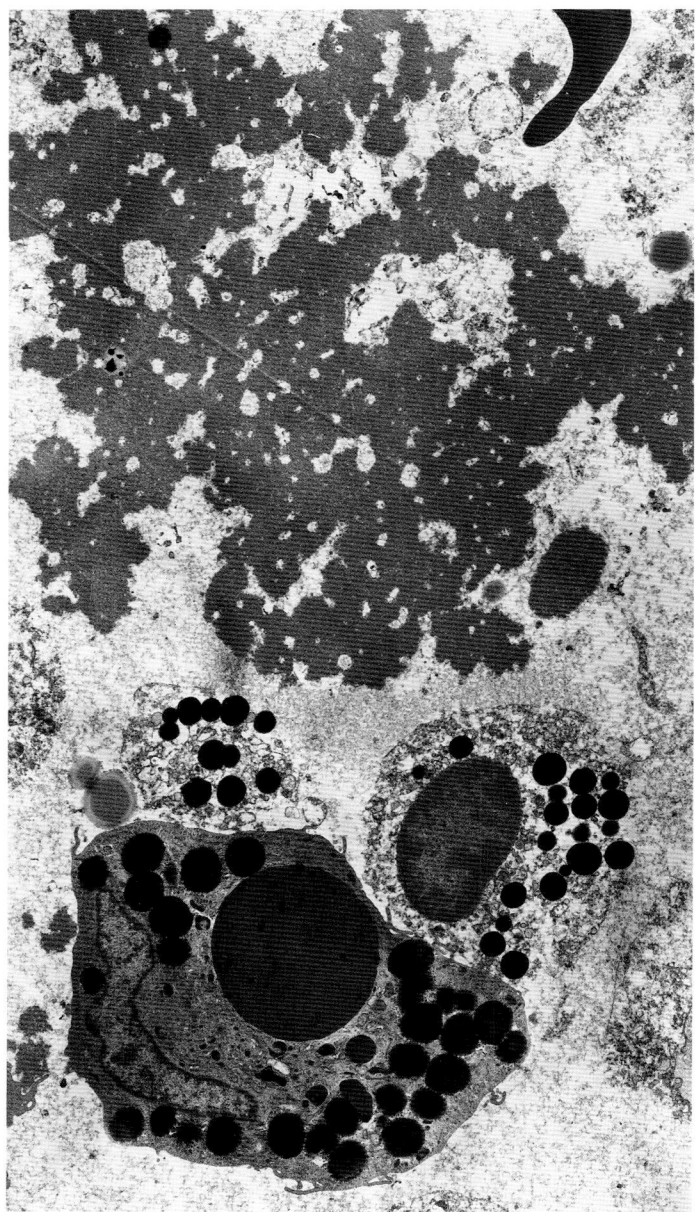

FIGURE 5.30   Granular amorphous material in the vicinity of histiocytes. The large lipid droplets are responsible for the foamy appearance of their cytoplasm. (EM × 6,000).

SEROSANGUINOUS EFFUSION

As little as 2 mL of blood in 500 mL of a pleural effusion is sufficient to turn it rosy pink, and a slightly larger amount may impart a bloody appearance to it. In contrast, a considerable amount of blood may go unde- tected in 10 L of ascitic fluid. Blood from a traumatic tap will clot in a few mintues if left nonheparinized. In truly hemorrhagic effusions due to underlying malig- nancy or another pathologic process, no clot will form. The most common cause of serosanguinous effusion is malignancy, followed by tuberculosis and lymphoma. Of the neoplasms, mesotheliomas usually present as hemorrhagic effusions, but many nonmalignant pro-

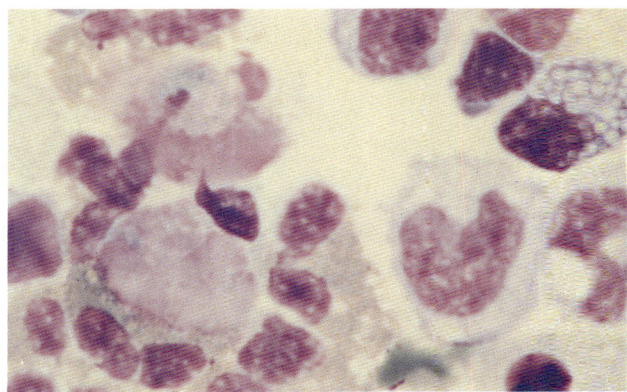

FIGURE 5.31 LE cell in an effusion secondary to systemic lupus erythematosus. The amorphous material stains pale red, rather than dark blue as in Papanicolaou-stained preparation. (MGG × 240)

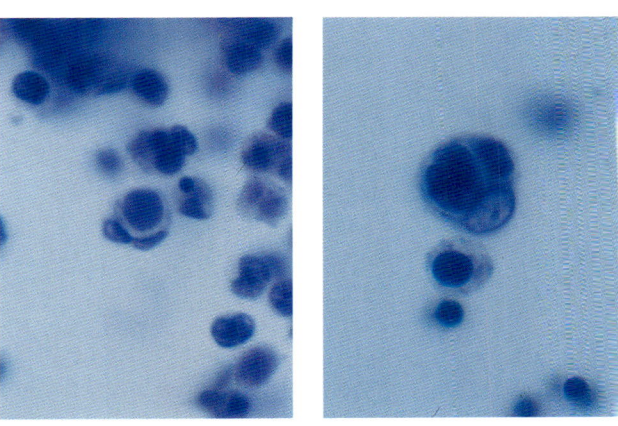

A **B**

FIGURE 5.32 LE-related effusion. (A) The LE cell in the center engulfs a hematoxylin body. (Pap × 120) (B) The tart cell engulfs dark staining chromatinic debris (Pap × 120)

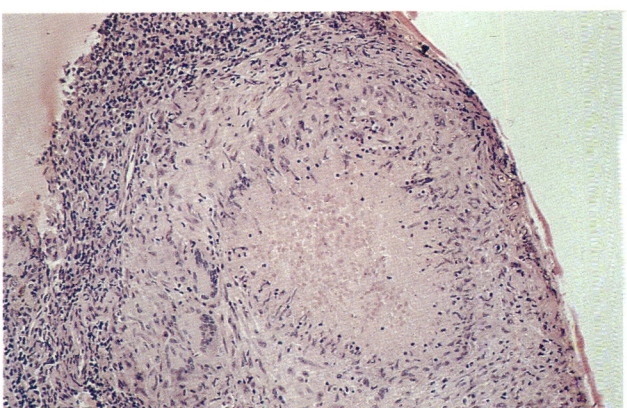

FIGURE 5.33 Typical granuloma in a histologic section. The necrotic center surrounded by inflammatory cells sometimes may appear intact in a cell block preparation. (H&E × 40)

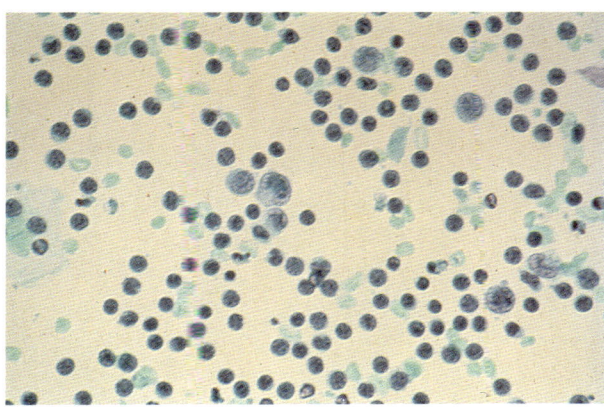

FIGURE 5.34 Granulomatous pleural effusion in tuberculosis. Reactive lymphocytosis and a paucity of mesothelial cells are typical of Tb. (Pap × 90)

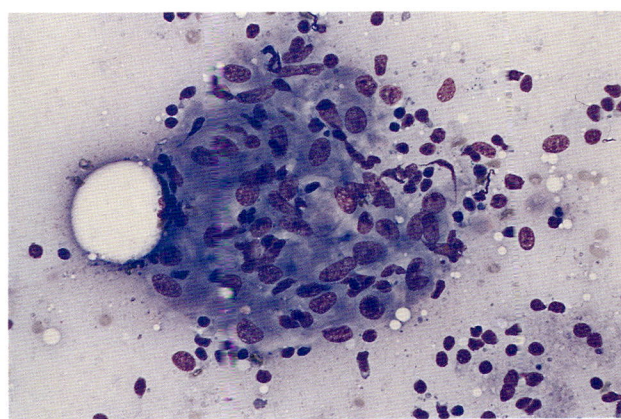

FIGURE 5.35 Plump epithelioid histiocytes in granulomatous tissue fragment. Short of bacteriologic special stains, the etiology of the process cannot be elucidated. (MGG × 60)

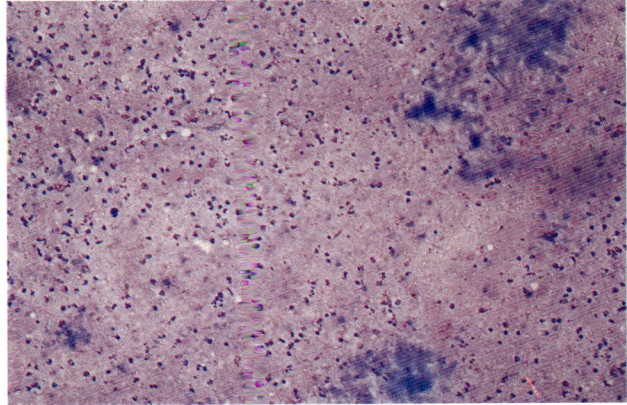

FIGURE 5.36 Granular necrotic material in tuberculous empyema. The predominantly lymphocytic cell population is in keeping with the long-standing nature of the process. (MGG × 40)

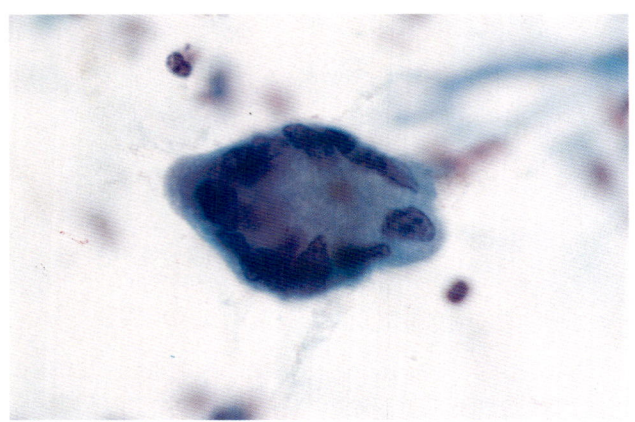

FIGURE 5.37 Giant cell from a case of sarcoidosis. Notice slightly elongated nuclei distributed along the periphery of the cell. (Pap× 120)

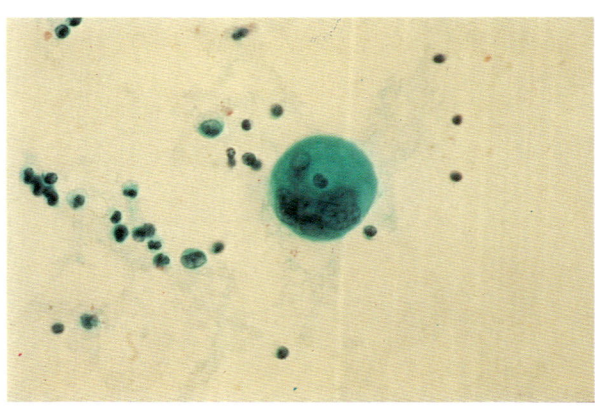

FIGURE 5.38 Megakaryocyte in ascitic fluid. Notice eccentrically located, crowded nuclei (Pap× 90)

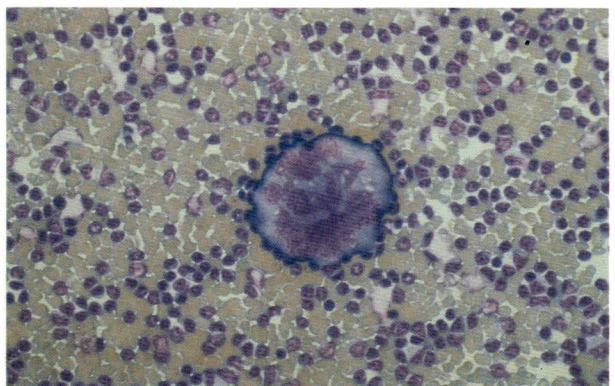

FIGURE 5-39 Megakaryocyte in a smear stained by Diff-Quik. The cell is surrounded by numerous blood cells extravasated during manipulation (MGG× 90)

TABLE 5.3 Comparison between Chylous and Pseudochylous Effusion

Characteristic	Chylous Effusion	Pseudochylous Effusion
Immediate appearance	Color and consistency of milk	Variable, "gold paint" or greenish
Appearance upon standing	Creamy top layer, thick bottom	Crystalline appearance settles to bottom
pH	Alkaline	Variable
Microscopic examination	Predominance of lymphocytes	Variable inflammatory reaction
Cytologic features	Fine lipid droplets in macrophages and mesothelial cells	Cholesterol crystals and fat droplets, mainly in macrophages
Odor	Odorless	May be foul
Microbiologic findings	Sterile	Usually sterile
Etiology	Trauma, neoplasia, tuberculosis	Rheumatoid arthritis, tuberculosis, myxedema
Pathogenesis	Obstruction to thoracic duct	Chronic inflammation
Oral ingestion of lipophilic dye	Dye appears in effusion	No dye appears in effusion

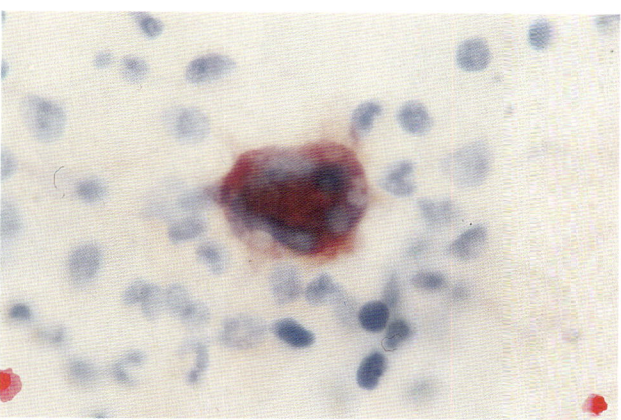

FIGURE 5.40 Factor VIII staining of cells from the fluid shown in Figure 5.39. Positivity for this marker excludes mesothelial, epithelial, and histiocytic origin and confirms the cells' identity as megakaryocytes. (P.A.P. × 90) (Courtesy Dr. R. Katz)

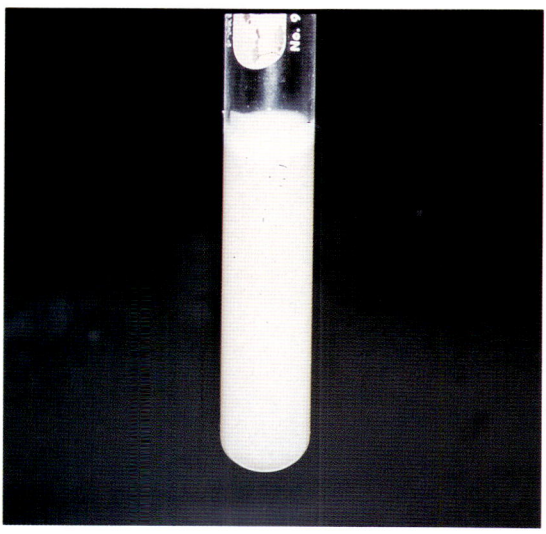

FIGURE 5.42 Milky appearance of chylous effusion. No cytologic evaluation is necessary for the diagnosis of overt cause such as this example.

cesses can also be accompanied by serosanguinous effusion. The RBCs in hemorrhagic effusion following pulmonary infarct tend to clump and appear as biconcave disks under microscopic examination. In wet films, they may produce the rouleaux phenomenon. They degenerate rapidly and swell into pale, spherical structures, or they may partially preserve their discoid shape. After erythrophagocytosis RBCs initially occupy clear vacuoles in the cytoplasm of macrophages. Subsequently, as their breakdown generates hemosiderin, the cytoplasm of macrophages turns dark brown because

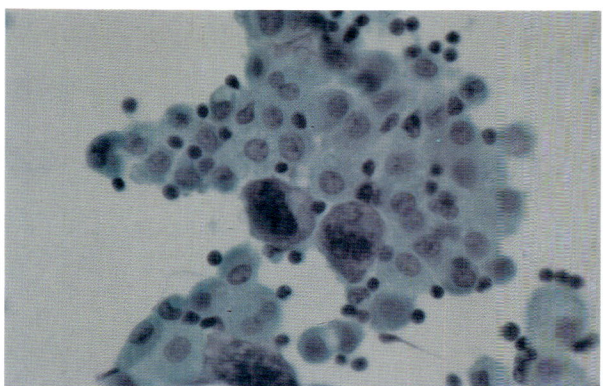

FIGURE 5.41 Polykaryons in an effusion secondary to AIDS. Multinucleated giant cells are noted, along with sheets of mesothelial cells. (Pap × 90) (Courtesy Dr. D. Hidvegi)

of the presence of irregular clumps of pigment. Later still, the yellowish brown color of the accumulated particles indicates the formation of hematoidin pigment. The last residue of RBCs within the cytoplasm of macrophages is iron, not visible by itself but easily demonstrable with the Prussian blue reaction. The most troublesome appearance of the RBC residues is the hemosiderin stage, because of its resemblance to fragmented ferruginous bodies. Only when intact fibrous cores are clearly identifiable as such should these bodies be equated with asbestos. Other products of blood degeneration include Heinz bodies in the cytoplasm of RBCs and free-floating hematoidin crystals, sometimes found in long-standing hemorrhagic effusions.

GRANULATION TISSUE

The granulation response should not be confused with granuloma formation. Granulation tissue is characterized by sprouting capillaries that contain RBCs and may display plump endothelial cells in their walls. Plasma cells, lymphocytes, and macrophages are noted in the background, but again they are not distinctive enough to warrant a specific diagnosis. The only pathognomonic feature is the presence of cellular spherules with a prominent vascular core and mesothelial cells in their

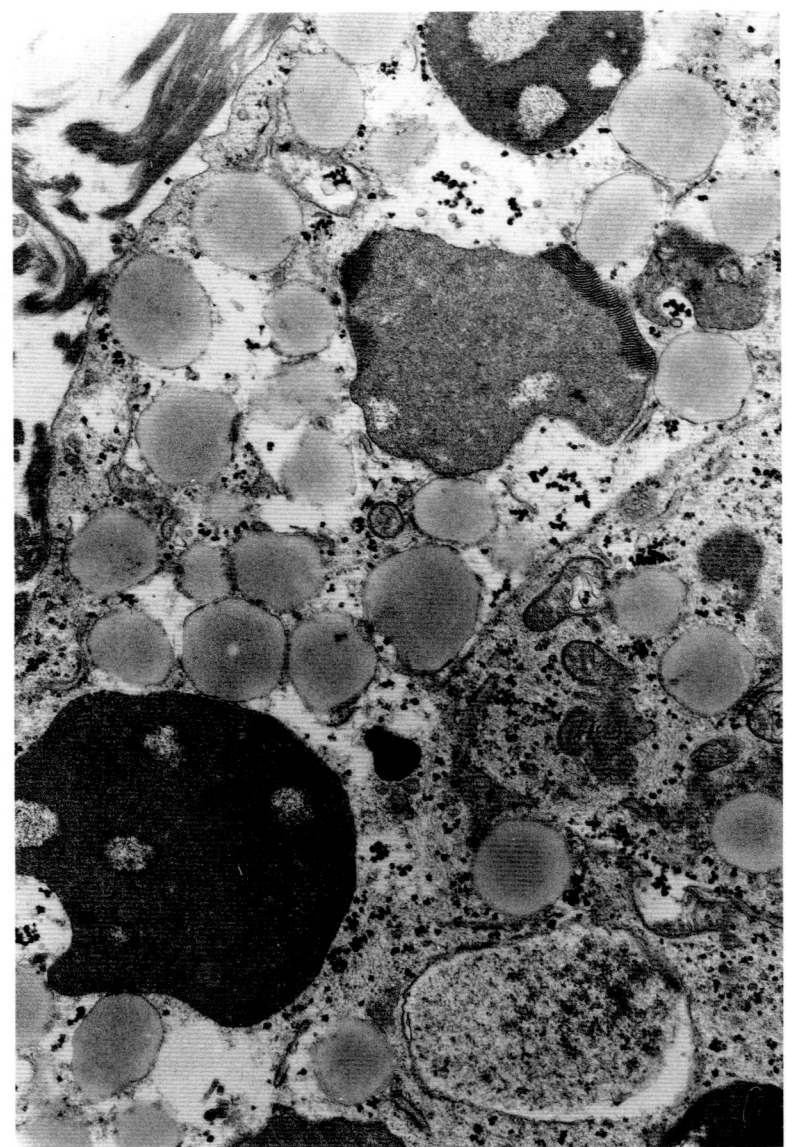

FIGURE 5.43   Histiocyte from chylous effusion. The cytoplasm is replete with lipid and the nuclei are rather pyknotic. (EM× 28,000).

outer layer. Occasionally, the cellular spherules are degenerated and appear composed of dark-staining fibroblasts surrounded by neutrophils. These findings occur following an acute inflammatory process or trauma to the chest resulting in hemothorax. It is best to request repeat cytologic evaluations if effusions such as these reaccumulate, rather than trying to interpret the findings as "atypical" or "suspicious" for malignancy.

BIBLIOGRAPHY

Polymorphonuclear Leukocytes

Perera MR, Kirk A, Noone P. Presentation diagnosis and management of liver abscess. *Lancet.* 1980;3:629–632.

Pettersson T, Riska H. Diagnostic value of total and differential leukocyte counts in pleural effusions. *Acta Med Scand.* 1981;210:129–135.

Wandall JH. Function of polymorphonuclear neutrophilic leukocytes. Comparison of leukocytes from blood and exudate in healthy volunteers. *Acta Pathol Microbiol Immunol Scand.* 1982;90(1):7–13.

Lymphocytes and Plasma Cells

Higby DJ, Ohnuma T. Plasmacytoma cell ascites. *NY State J Med.* 1975;75:1074–1076.

Lopes-Cardozo E, Harting MC. On the function of lymphocytes in malignant effusions. *Acta Cytol.* 1972;16:307–313.

Perou ML, Littman MS. Diagnostic study of serous effusions with emphasis on some unusual findings. *Am J Clin Pathol.* 1955;25:467–479.

Spriggs AI, Boddington MM. Absence of mesothelial cells from tuberculous pleural effusions. *Thorax.* 1960;15:169–171.

Yam LT. Diagnostic significance of lymphocytes in pleural effusions. *Ann Intern Med.* 1967;66:972–982.

Eosinophilic Effusions

Adams HW, Mainz DL. Eosinophilic ascites. *Am J Dig Dis.* 1977;22:40–43.

Adelman M, Albelda SM, Gottlieb J, et al. Diagnostic utility of pleural fluid eosinophilia. *Am J Med.* 1984;77:915–922.

Askin FB, McCann BG, Kuhn C. Reactive eosinophilic pleuritis. *Arch Pathol Lab Med.* 1977;101:187–192.

Bertolig D, Anata C, Agosti E. Mast cells in eosinophilic pleural effusions. *Acta Cytol.* 1981;25(4):431–432.

Bower G. Eosinophilic pleural effusion. A condition with multiple causes. *Am Rev Respir Dis.* 1967;95:746–751.

Contino CA, Vance JW. Eosinophilic pleural effusion. *NY State J Med.* 1966;2044–2048.

Curran WS, Wilson JN, Shoop JD. Eosinophilic pleural effusion bronchiectasis. *Rocky Mountain Med J.* 1968;65:49–53.

Farah MG, Nassar VH, Shahid M. Marked eosinophilia and eosinophilic pleural effusion in Hodgkin's disease. Report of a case with review of literature. *J Med Liban.* 1973;26:513–521.

Hunt CE, Papermaster TC, Nelson EH, et al. Eosinophilic peritonitis. Report of two cases. *Lancet.* 1967;87:473–475.

Krishman S, Statsinger A, Kleinman M, et al. Eosinophilic pleural effusions with Charcot-Leyden crystals. *Acta Cytol.* 1983;27(5):529–532.

Veress J, Koss L, Schrieber K. Eosinophilic pleural effusion with Charcot-Leyden crystals. *Acta Cytol.* 1983;27:529–532.

Rheumatoid Arthritis

Boddington MM, Spriggs AI, Morton JA, et al. Cyto-diagnosis of rheumatoid pleural effusions. *J Clin Pathol.* 1971;24:95–106.

Geisinger K, Vance R, Prater T, et al. Rheumatoid pleural effusion: A transmission and scanning electron microscopic evaluation. *Acta Cytol.* 1985;29:239–247.

Keagle M, Marcks K, Kaiser J. Cytologic manifestations of rheumatoid arthritis in pleural effusion. A case report. *Acta Cytol.* 1981;25(1):33–36.

Levine H, Szanto M, Grieble HC, et al. Rheumatoid factor in nonrheumatoid pleural effusions. *Ann Intern Med.* 1968;69:487–492.

Montes S, Guarda L. Cytology of pleural effusions in rheumatoid arthritis. *Diagn Cytopathol.* 1988;4:71–73.

Nosanchuck JA, Naylor B. A unique cytologic picture in pleural fluid from patients with rheumatoid arthritis. *Amer J Clin Pathol* 1968;50:330–335.

Richards AJ, Koehler BE, Broder I, et al. Rheumatoid pericarditis: Comparison of immunologic characteristics of pericardial fluid, synovial fluid and serum. *J Rheumatol.* 1976;3:275–282.

Systemic Sclerosis and Polyarteritis Nodosa

Kinney E, Wynn J. Hinton DM, et al. Pericardial-fluid complement: Normal values. *Am J Clin Pathol.* 1979;72:972–973.

McWhorter JE, Leroy EC. Pericardial disease in scleroderma (systemic sclerosis. *Am J Med.* 1974;57:566–575.

Siguier F, Godeau P, Herreman G. Les pericardites sclerodermiques (a propos de trois observations). *Bull Soc Med Hop Paris.* 1967;118:1299–1312.

Spieler P, Hell M. Rheumatische Rorperhohlemergüsse im Verlauf von chronischer Polyarteritis. *Schweiz Med Wochenschr.* 1984;114:1110–1117.

Lupus Erythematosus

Carel RS, Shapiro MS, Shoham D, et al. Lupus erythematosus cells in pleural effusion. *Chest.* 1977;72:670–672.

Goldenberg DL, Left G, Grayzel AI. Pericardial tamponade in systemic lupus erythematosus with absent hemolytic complement activity in pericardial fluid. *NY State J Med.* 1975;75:910–912.

Good JT, King TE, Antony BV, et al. Lupus pleuritides: Clinical features and pleural fluid characteristics with special reference to pleural fluid antinuclear antibodies. *Chest.* 1983;84:714–718.

Kelley S, McGarry P, Hutson Y. Atypical cells in pleural fluid characteristic of systemic lupus erythematosus. *Acta Cytol.* 1971;15:357–362

Keshgegian AA. Lupus erythematosus cells in pleural fluid. *Am J Clin Pathol.* 1978;69:570–571.

Mertzger AL, Coyne M, Lee S. In vivo LE cell formation in peritonitis due to SLE. *J Rheumatol.* 1974;1:130.

Osamura RY, Shioya S, Hauda K, et al. Lupus erythematosus cells in pleural fluid: Cytologic diagnosis in two patients. *Acta Cytol.* 1977;21:215–217.

Reda MG, Baigelman W. Pleural effusion in systemic lupus erythematosus. *Acta Ctyol.* 1980;24:555–557.

Small P, Frank H, Kreisman H, et al. An immunological evaluation of pleural effusions in systemic lupus erythematosus. *Ann Allergy.* 1982;49:101–103.

Granulomatous Inflammation

Chusid EL, Vieira LOBD, Siltzbach LE. Sarcoidosis of the pleura. In: Iway K, Hosada Y, eds. *Proceedings of the Sixth International Conference on Sarcoidosis.* Tokyo: University Press; 1972:373–378.

Levine H, Metzger W, Kay L. Diagnosis of tuberculous pleurisy by culture of pleural biopsy specimen. *Arch Intern Med.* 1970;126:269–271.

Kinney E, Murthy R, Ascunce G, et al. Pericardial effusions in sarcoidosis. *Chest.* 1979;76:476–478.

Papowitz AJ, Li JK. Abdominal sarcoidosis with ascites. *Chest.* 1971;59:692–695.

Poppius H, Kokkola K. Diagnosis and differential diagnosis in tuberculous pleurisy. *Scand J Respir Dis.* 1968;63:105–110.

Sharma OP, Gordonson J. Pleural effusion in sarcoidosis: A report of six cases. *Thorax.* 1975;30:95–101.

Shiff AD, Blatt CJ, Colp C. Recurrent pericardial effusion secondary to sarcoidosis of the pericardium. *N Engl J Med.* 1969;281:141–143.

Chylous Effusion

Bruno MS, Ober WB. Recurrent chylous ascites. *NY State J Med.* 1970;70:282–290.

Fawal IA, Kirkland L, Dykes R, et al. Chronic primary chylopericardium. Report of a case and review of the literature. *Circulation.* 1967;25:777–782.

Lesser GT, Bruno MS, Enselberg K. Chylous ascites. *Arch Intern Med.* 1970;125:1073–1077.

Lieberman J, Agliozzo C. Intrapleural nitrogen mustard for treating chylous effusion of pulmonary lymphangioleiomyomatoses. *Cancer.* 1967;33:777–782.

Serosanguinous Effusion

Bartziota E, Naylor B. Megakaryocytes in a hemorrhagic pleural effusion caused by anticoagulant overdose. *Acta Cytol.* 1986;30:163–165.

Broghamer W, Richardson M, Faurest S. Malignancy-associated serosanguinous pleural effusions. *Acta Cytol.* 1984;28(1):46–50.

Buja LM, Friedman CA, Roberts WC. Hemorrhagic pericarditis in uremia. Clinicopathologic studies in six patients. *Arch Pathol.* 90:325–330.

Dekker A, Graham T, Bupp PA. The occurrence of sickle cells in pleural fluid. Report of a patient with sickle cell disease. *Acta Cytol.* 1975;19:251–254.

Miriajanian A, Ambruoso VN, Derby BM, et al. Massive bilateral hemorrhagic pleural effusions in chronic relapsing pancreatitis. *Arch Surg.* 1969;98:62–66.

CHAPTER SIX

Infectious Diseases

Infectious diseases account for less than 50% of the diagnoses in cytologic specimens from the serosal cavities, yet these preparations are always challenging to the cytopathologist. Virtually all infective agents have been demonstrated in effusions by bacteriologic means but relatively few lend themselves to cytologic detection. Viruses cause profound cytomorphologic alterations in mesothelial cells and can be diagnosed cytologically with relative ease, but this not true of bacteria. Fungi and protozoa are of sufficient size and display enough cytologic distinctiveness to warrant identification provided they are present in sufficient numbers. It is worth remembering that fungi are, in essence, living vegetable cells, and protozoa are one-celled organisms and as such are a legitimate object of cytologic examination. For confirmation, however, the cytologic diagnosis should be followed by appropriate bacteriologic techniques such as culture and sensitivity tests. The advantage of the cytologic method is its simplicity and cost-effectiveness and the rapidity with which the diagnosis can be rendered as opposed to the long time it takes to obtain cultures.

Among infections, tuberculosis leads the list and should be suspected if the pleural effusion is from an elderly patient and exhibits lymphocytosis. In children a pleural effusion with a high lymphocyte count is suggestive of virus infection. With the greater prevalence of immunosuppression among hospitalized patients, rarer opportunistic pathogens such as protozoa and helminths are to be expected in pleural effusions. Strongyloides stercoralis has been infrequently observed in peritoneal effusions. An amebic abscess of the liver or the lung may break into the pleural spaces and give rise to a hemorrhagic pleural effusion. Other rare infectious agents include Echinococcus and Giardia, which have been detected in body fluids. Cell blocks are ideally suited for special stains such as PAS, AFB, GMS, and Giemsa in cases of suspected infections. Microbiologic cultures should be obtained in all effusions from patients with infectious diseases. Handling of specimens under a hood and other precautionary measures should be taken to protect cytotechnologists handling infected specimens.

VIRAL INFECTIONS

Viruses only seldom gain access to the serosal cavities and do so only in the immunosuppressed host. Three members of the herpesvirus family have been known to infect the serosal spaces: herpes simplex virus (HSV), cytomegalovirus (CMV) and herpes zoster virus (HZV).

HSV induces multinucleation molding and profound alteration of the chromatin distribution in the nuclei. In one form of infection, the chromatin granules and the viral particles are finely dispersed, leading to the so-called ground glass appearance. In the other, the chromatin granules, together with the viral particles, are tightly clumped in the form of a distinct intranuclear inclusion (Fig. 6.1). Whether the latter represents primary infection as opposed to recurrent infection is still a matter of debate.

CMV causes enlargement of the cell without multinucleation. The viral particles occupy most of the nucleus in the form of a large inclusion, surrounded by a clear halo leading to an "owl's eye" appearance (Fig. 6.2). Smaller inclusions pepper the cytoplasm and stain purplish with Papanicolaou's method. The virus may be positively identified by in situ hybridization using a rather specific probe, but results are dubious with immunocytochemistry. Electron microscopy demonstrates well both the nuclear and the cytoplasmic inclusions, the latter in the form of viral particles arranged in bunches and displaying rather electron dense cores (Fig. 6.3).

HZV belongs to the zoster-vaccinia group and bears a striking morphologic resemblance to HSV (Fig. 6.4). Only one documented case of varicella pleuritys has

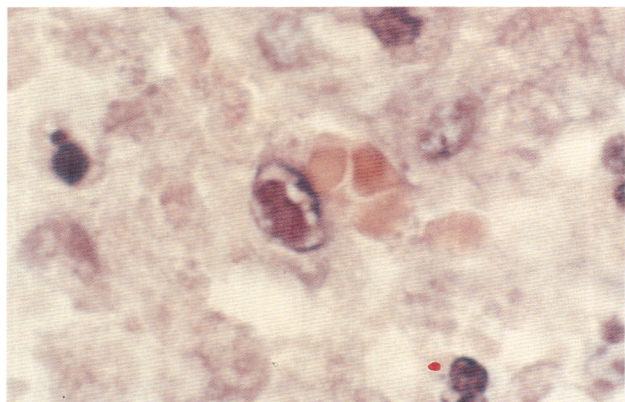

FIGURE 6.1   Cell block showing Herpetic virocyte with a discrete inclusion. The patient was elderly, debilitated patient who also had herpetic tracheobronchitis and stomatitis. (H&E × 90)

been reported in an immunosuppressed cancer patient, confirmed by immunocytochemistry and electron microscopy (Fig. 6.5).

BACTERIAL INFECTIONS

Bacteria are rather small and stain too faintly with Papanicolaou's method for precise identification. However, when first suspected by cytologic examination, the

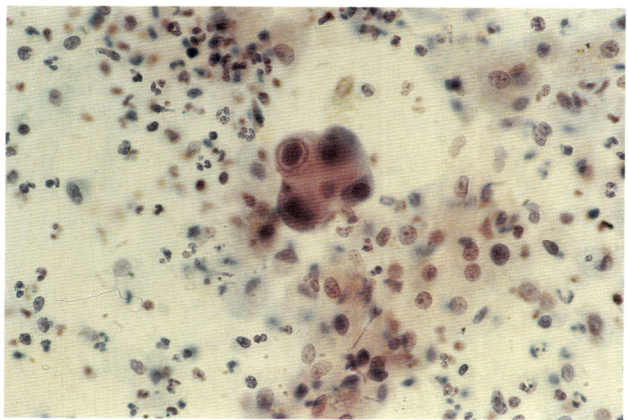

FIGURE 6.2   Pericardial effusion in a renal transplant patient, presumably secondary to uremia. Note the group of reactive mesothelial cells, one of which shows a discrete inclusion surrounded by a halo, typical of cytomegalovirus. (Pap × 60)

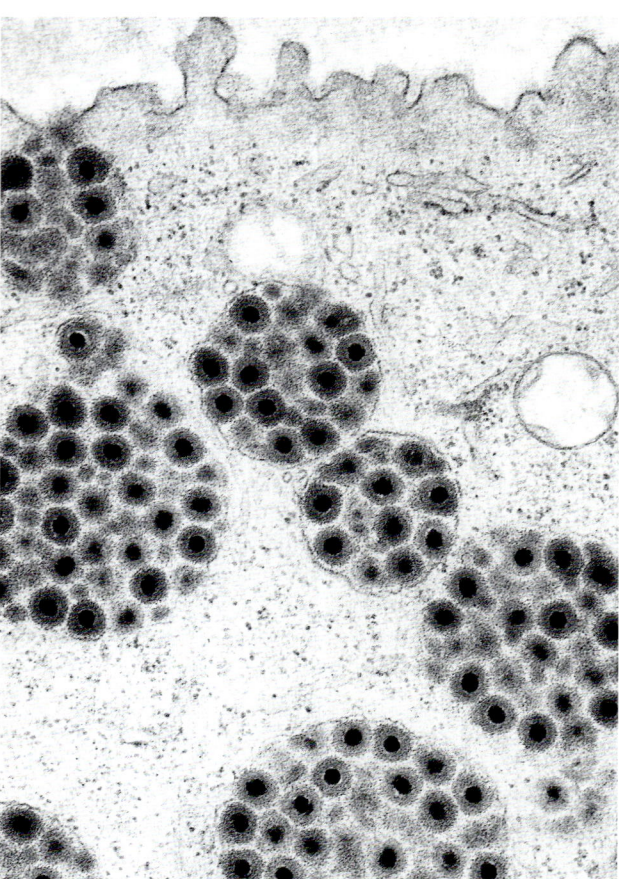

FIGURE 6.3   Electron micrograph of virocyte affected by CMV. Viral inclusions with an electron dense core are typical of the herpesviruses. (EM × 12,000)

cause of the infection may be pursued by bacteriologic stains such as Gram's, AFB, or immunofluorescence. As a terminal event in perforation of the bowel or as a result of bronchopleural fistulae, bacterial infection may be fulminant and as such easily recognized by the overwhelming number of organisms growing in the effusion. Less severe forms of infection require familiarity with the morphologic characteristics of the bacterium.

Pneumococci appear as intracellular diplococci which stain pale gray with the MGG stain. Only rarely have they been documented in pleural effusion. *Neisseria gonorrheae* shares a similar morphology and has been identified in cul-de-sac aspirates in pelvic inflammatory disease (Fig. 6.6). *Hemophilus* organisms are rather small but may be recognized by Papanicolaou's method because of their tendency to cling to the surface of cells. Gram-stain is most commonly utilized in its identification (Fig. 6.7). The AIDS epidemic is responsi-

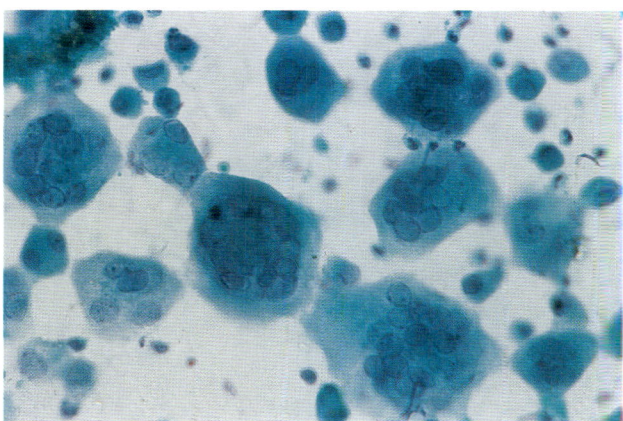

FIGURE 6.4   Pleural effusion from a terminally ill cancer patient. Multinucleated mesothelial cells display the "ground glass"-appearing nuclei typical of herpesvirus infection. (Pap × 240) (Figs. 6.4 and 6.5, courtesy R. Katz, MD)

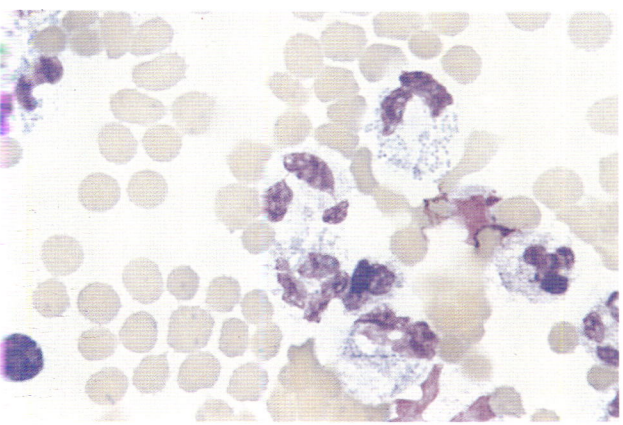

FIGURE 6.6   Culdocentesis in a patient with pelvic inflammatory disease. There were numerous neutrophils with gram-negative diplococci in the cytoplasm. The patient developed peritonitis, and culture revealed *Neisseria gonorrhoeae* as the culprit. (MGG × 60)

ble for a resurgence of tuberculosis and mycobacteria may sometimes be diagnosed in the pleural or pericardial fluid of AIDS victims (Fig. 6.8).

Staphylococci grow easily in the pleural fluid, forming grapelike conglomerates of coccoid bacteria. Anaerobes cannot be distinguished morphologically from other gram-negative rods, and have been documented in pleural effusions obtained at autopsy of patients succumbing from septicemia.

FUNGUSLIKE BACTERIA

Certain bacteria grow very large, and their filamentous nature resembles that of the fungi. *Nocardia* is one of these (Fig. 6.9). It is characterized by AFB-positive threads that are markedly matted and may form the cores of spherules which appear to float freely in the effusion. They may be surrounded by a crown of ne-

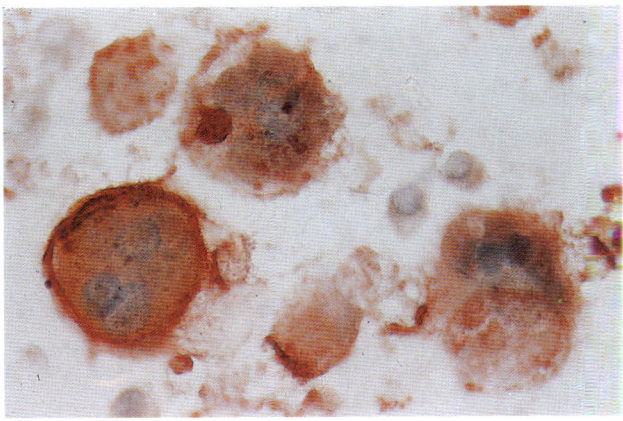

FIGURE 6.5   Same specimen as the one shown in Figure 6.4. Immunostaining against varicella zoster showed positivity for this member of the herpesvirus family, confirmed by electron microscopy. (P.A.P. × 240)

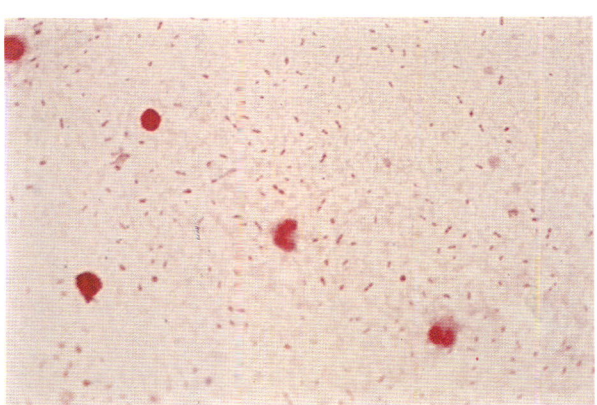

FIGURE 6.7   Culdocentesis in a patient with severe pelvic inflammatory disease. The cul-de-sac contained 50 mL of grossly purulent fluid, and the Gram's stain revealed thread forms of a coccobacillum that upon culture was identified as *Gardnerella vaginalis*. (Gram × 40)

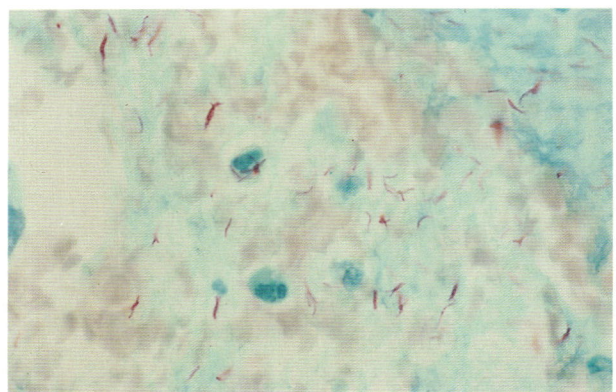

FIGURE 6.8   Peritoneal fluid from a patient with AIDS. Virtually acellular fluid revealed only amorphous debris with the Papanicolaou stain. The Ziehl-Nielsen stain shows *Mycobacterium tuberculosis* bacilli arranged in threads. (Z-N × 60)

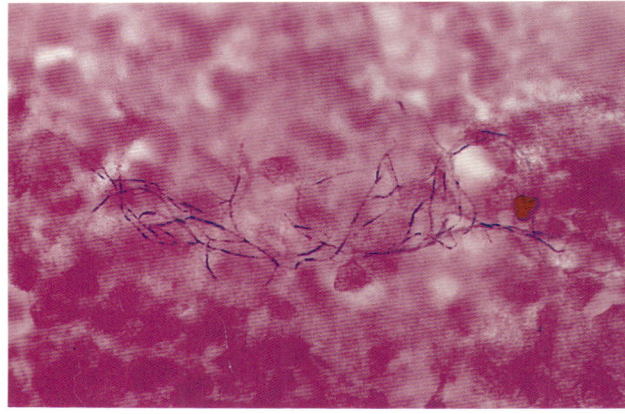

FIGURE 6.10   Same specimen as the one shown in Figure 6.9 stained by Groccott's method. Note the filamentous branching pattern of *Nocardia asteroides*, well demonstrated by silver impregnation. (Grocott's × 40)

crotic tissue but they seldom form sulfur granules, which are characteristic of actinomycosis. These structures can be visualized grossly along the pleural surfaces at autopsy. Sediment from pleural fluid may show colonies of the Nocardia microorganisms that give a positive reaction both to AFB and Groccott's methods (Fig. 6.10). Actinomyces resembles nocardia and may cause microabscesses along the serosal membranes of severely immunosuppressed or malnourished patients (Fig. 6.11).

OPPORTUNISTIC FUNGI

The immunosuppressed host is an easy victim of infections with opportunistic pathogens that cause little harm to the immunocompetent. Among these, the fungi have a tendency toward widespread involvement, including the invasion of serosal cavities. In candidiasis, pseudohyphae can be identified by Papanicolaou's stain but they appear only as an indistinct pale gray. Special

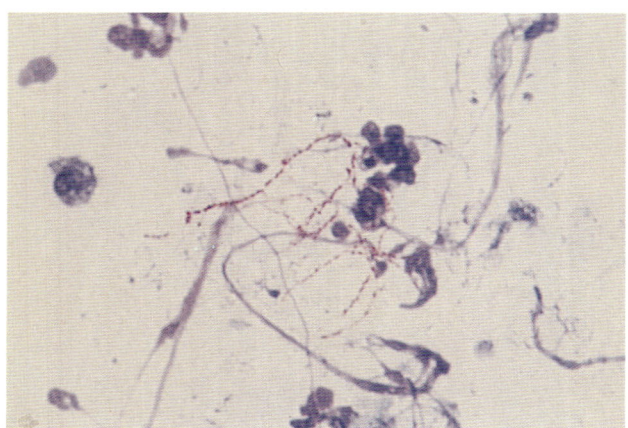

FIGURE 6.9   Filamentous, AFB-positive bacteria in a pleural effusion from a patient with AIDS. Matted organisms in the center elicited a minimum inflammatory response due to immunosuppression. (MGG × 40)

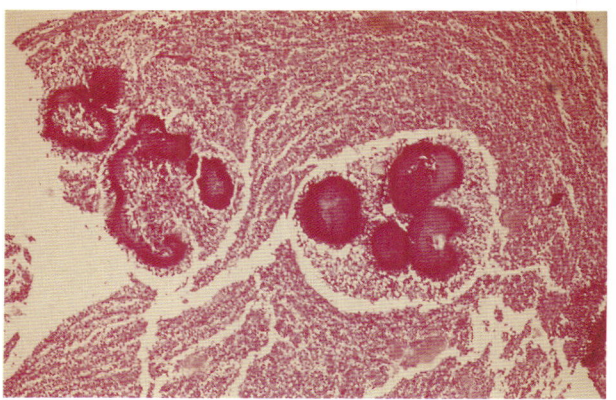

FIGURE 6.11   Cell block peritoneal fluid from an immunosuppressed transplant recipient. Numerous rounded colonies of *Actinomyces israelii* that grossly resemble sulfur granules are noted. (H&E × 40)

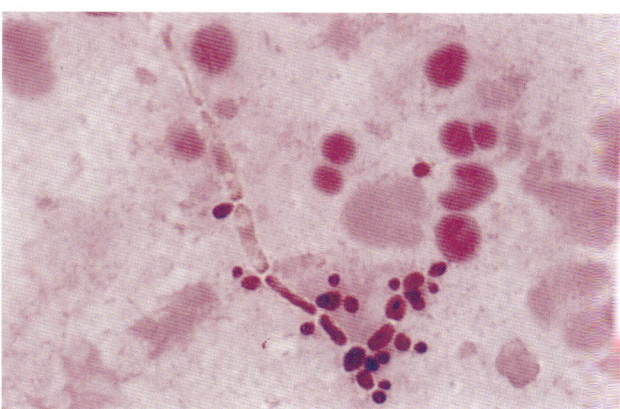

FIGURE 6.12   Ascites from a transplant patient undergoing chronic peritoneal dialysis. Both yeast and pseudohyphae of *Candida* species are noted with Gram's stain. (Gram × 90)

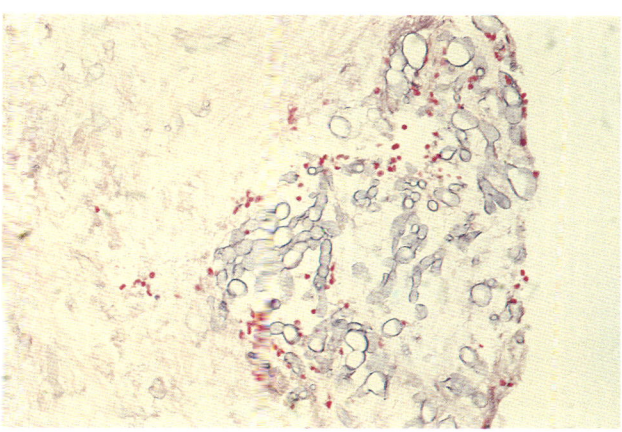

FIGURE 6.14   Pleural surface of the lung covered by an exudate. The GMS stain demonstrates nonseptate hyphae, some sectioned longitudinally and some transversely. The irregularity of the caliber is typical of *Zygomyces*. (GMS × 50)

stains such as Gram's method easily identify the microorganism, including pseudohyphae and yeast elements (Fig. 6.12).

Aspergillus is characterized by true septation, and 45°-angle dichotomous branching, well demonstrated by silver stain. Aspergillus hyphae may be seen in H&E-stained cell blocks (Fig. 6.13). Aspergillus is frequently associated with crystals of calcium oxalate. These are best visualized under polarized light where they appear as strongly birefringent rosettelike and sheaflike structures. Septate mycelia and budding forms of conidiophores may occasionally appear in the effusion, but full-blown fruiting conidiophores are only demonstrated in cultured material. The hyphae of mucormycosis are also septate, but they vary widely in caliber and in length and their branching pattern is haphazard (Fig. 6.14). These organisms have been observed colonizing the mesothelial surfaces at autopsy, a ready target for identifying microorganisms by the use imprint method (Fig. 6.15).

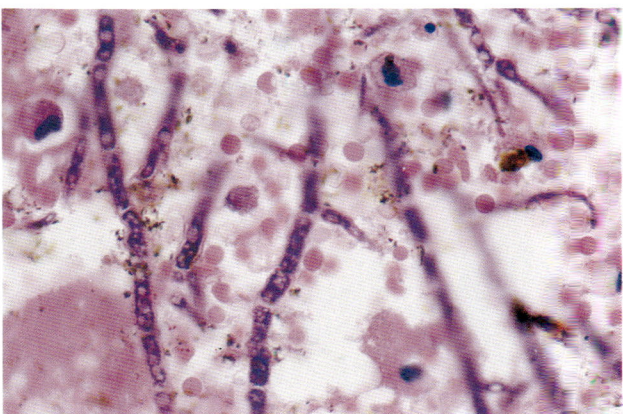

FIGURE 6.13   Cell block of peritoneal fluid from an immunosuppressed host. Amid necrotic debris, the walls of *Aspergillus* hyphae are well delineated, and the fungus demonstrates its typical septation and branching pattern. (H&E × 120)

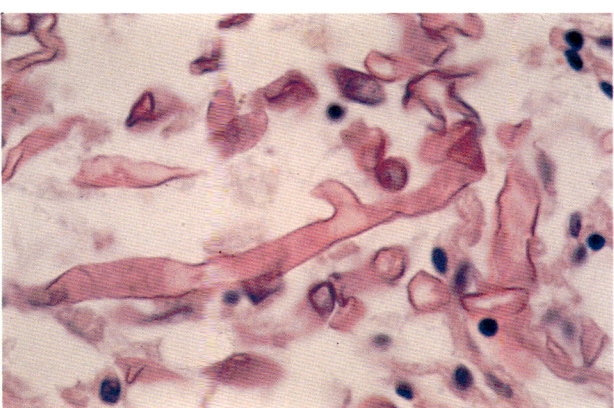

FIGURE 6.15   Direct imprint smear from the lesion shown in Figure 6.14 stained by Papanicolaou's method. Note *Zygomyces*, with an irregular branching pattern, and variable caliber of the hyphae. (Pap × 120)

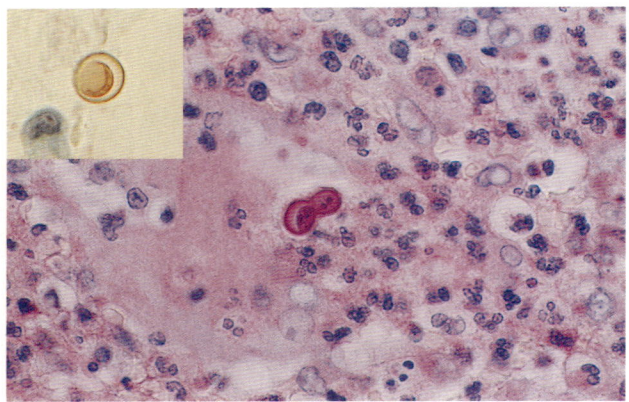

FIGURE 6.16 Cell block of sediment from pericardial fluid. Note the budding *Blastomyces* organism staining positive by PAS. (PAS× 90) *Insert: Pap-stained Blastomyces in the sputum, with the typical internal halo in relation to the wall resulting from shrinkage of the yeast.* (Pap× 90)

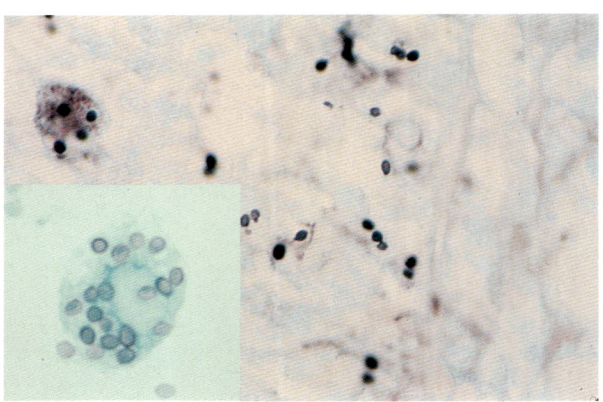

FIGURE 6.17 *Histoplasma capsulatum* in pericardial fluid. The GMS stain demonstrates small, rounded yeast forms. Note the yeast forms within the macrophage. (GMS× 40) Insert: Sputum from the same patient. Note the macrophage, with numerous *H. capsulatum* organisms in the cytoplasm. (MGG× 60)

PATHOGENIC FUNGI

The advent of modern antifungal therapy considerably reduced the prevalence of fungus related effusions, already not so frequent in mycotic infections. However, in endemic areas, pleural and pericardial effusions and, less commonly, the peritoneal fluid, have been known to harbor fungi. Although pleuritic chest pain is prominent in blastomycosis, pleural effusions are rare and when present are small. In advanced untreated blastomycosis, the hilar lymph nodes are affected by cavitary lesions from which Blastomyces may reach the pericardial fluid (Fig. 6.16).

Pleurisy due to *Histoplasma capsulatum* may occur in cavitary histoplasmosis affecting elderly patients with chronic obstructive pulmonary disease. However, the fungus is much more commonly identified in effusions from patients suffering from disseminated histoplasmosis, due to overt or covert immunosuppression. The yeast forms of H. Capsulatum are typically found within microphages in a variety of specimens including sputum, urine and serous effusions (Fig. 6.17).

Cryptococcus neoformans also occurs in disseminated fashion among immunosuppressed hosts and has been identified in pleural effusions. However, unlike histoplasmosis, cryptococcosis yields predominantly extracellular forms. The fungi are surrounded by a thick capsule which fails to take a variety of routine stains. As a result, cryptococcus is easily recognized by its negative image in preparations stained with MGG (Fig. 6.18). Up to 10 percent of patients with acute coccidiomycosis

present with pleural effusions. Repeated examinations of the pleural fluid may be unsuccessful in identifying *coccidioides immitis*. However, in some instances, degenerated spherules containing endospores can be identified and should not be confused with other yeast-forming fungi (Fig. 6.19). South American blastomycosis, a condition caused by *Paracoccidioides braziliensis* is endemic in central Brazil. Not infrequently, malnourished victims of this mycosis, particularly children, are also immunocompromised. The ensuing pleuropulmonary disease can result in pleural effusion where

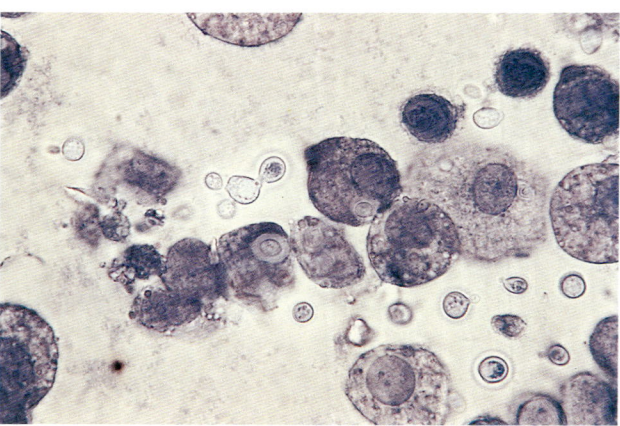

FIGURE 6.18 Pleural fluid stained by MGG. The negative image of the thick capsule, which fails to take Romanowsky-type stains, and the partial staining of the yeast are typical of *Cryptococcus neoformans*. (MGG× 120)

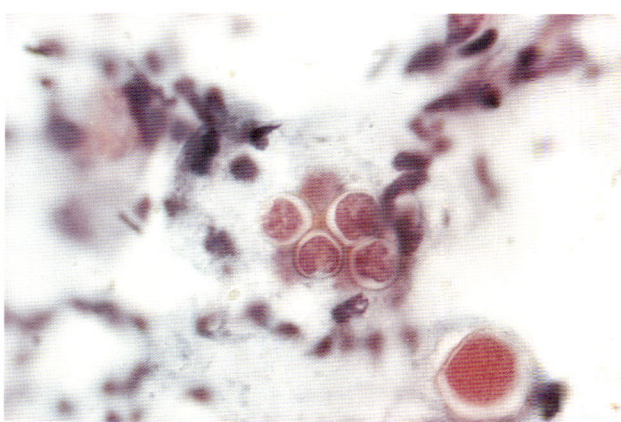

FIGURE 6.19 *Coccidioides immitis* in pleural fluid. Partially degenerated endospores lack a surrounding capsule. In situations like these, individual spores resemble the yeast form of *Blastomyces*. (Pap × 90)

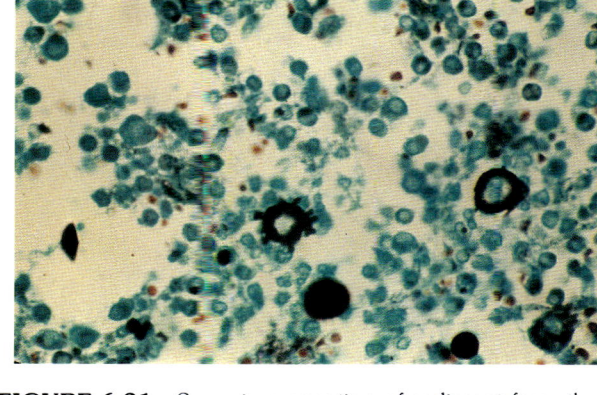

FIGURE 6.21 Silver impregnation of sediment from the same specimen shown in Figure 6.20. Note the variably sized yeast forms with multiple buds along their circumference. (GMS × 120)

the typical microorganism can be identified with the PAS stain (Fig. 6.20). By silver impregnation, the ''Captain's Wheel'' appearance of the yeast form is characteristic (Fig. 6.21).

PROTOZOAL INFECTIONS

Pneumocystis carinii pneumonia is reaching near epidemic proportions among AIDS victims who may har-

bor the organism in histiocytes that make their way into pleural fluid (Fig. 6.22). The infection is changing in character from a frothy pneumonia characterized by the presence of foamy alveolar casts in distal air spaces to destructive forms of pulmonary involvement. Small colonies of *P. carinii* resembling the foamy casts are sometimes noted in pleural effusions (Fig. 6.23). These can be stained by the same stains used in BAL for the demonstration of *P. carinii*; including silver impregnation by Groccott's metheramine (Fig. 6.24). Cavitary, granulomatous, and extrapulmonary involvement are now

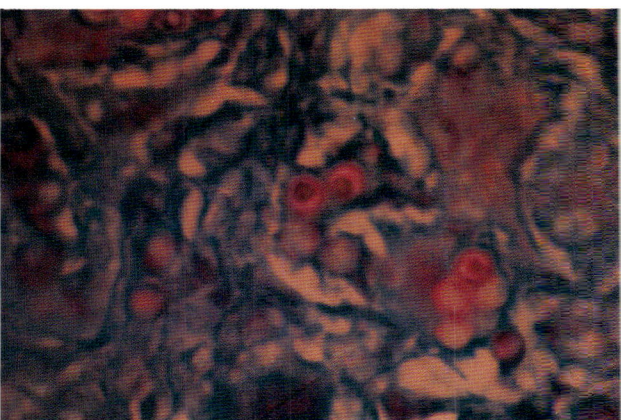

FIGURE 6.20 South American blastomycosis in pleural fluid from a Brazilian national. The lesions are similar to those induced by *Blastomyces dermatitidis*, but *Paracoccidioides brasiliensis* sprouts multiple daughter cells responsible for the spoked wheel budding pattern. (PAS stain, × 400)

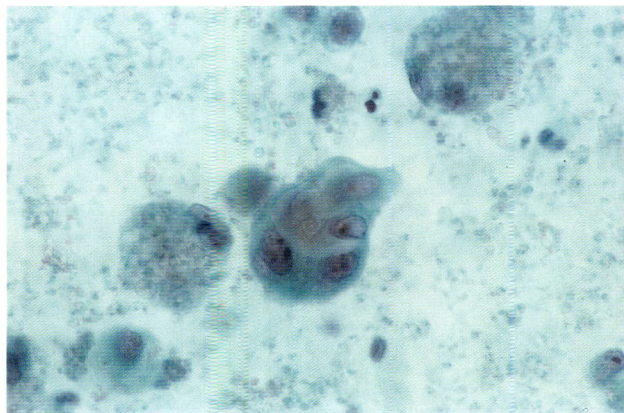

FIGURE 6.22 Pleural effusion from a patient with AIDS treated at NCI. Note the several trophozoitic forms of *Pneumocystis carinii* in the cytoplasm of the macrophages. (Pap × 120) (Courtesy L. Elwood, MD)

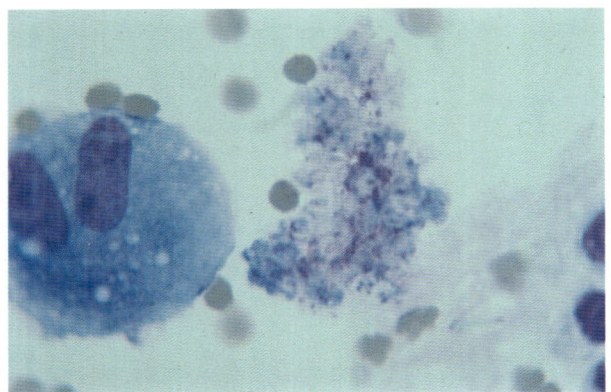

FIGURE 6.23 Pneumocystis in peritoneal fluid. Note that the colony of *Pneumocystis* resembles the foamy alveolar casts seen in bronchoalveolar lavage specimens. (MGG × 120) (Courtesy D. Hidvegi, MD)

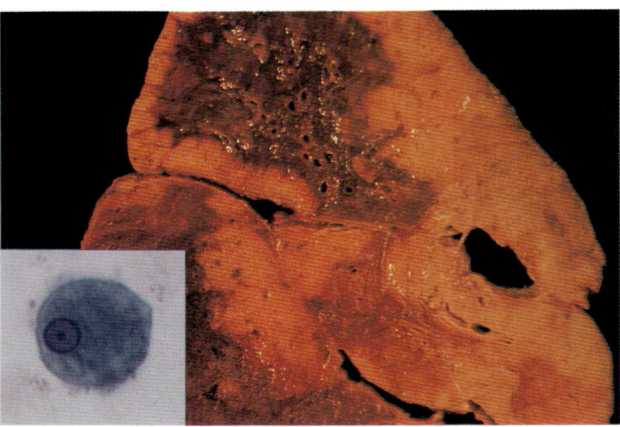

FIGURE 6.25 Amebic abscess in a lung that ruptured and released a thick exudate into both the right pleural and peritoneal spaces. The insert shows a trophozoite of *Entamoeba histolytica*.

commonplace and there have also been more recent cases documented in peritoneal and pericardial effusions.

Amebiasis of the colon and liver may perforate into the peritoneal space. Amebic abscesses of both the liver and the lungs may rupture into the pleural cavities. The resulting exudate is rather thick and purulent, and intact amebas are difficult to identify (Fig. 6.25). Examples of empyema secondary to trichomoniasis have been described in the literature. The organisms are difficult to recognize with Papanicolaou stain but can be demonstrated well with MGG. Giardia lamblia may rarely gain access to the peritoneal space (Fig. 6.26). Leishmaniasis occurs in pleural effusion (Fig. 6.27). Toxo-

plasmosis in the AIDS victim may cause infections in unusual locations such as the lung and the liver. Further dissemination of the infection rarely results in occurrence of the protozoa in effusions (Fig. 6.28).

HELMINTHIC INFECTIONS

Verminosis is the most common of infectious diseases in third world countries. However, with people's migra-

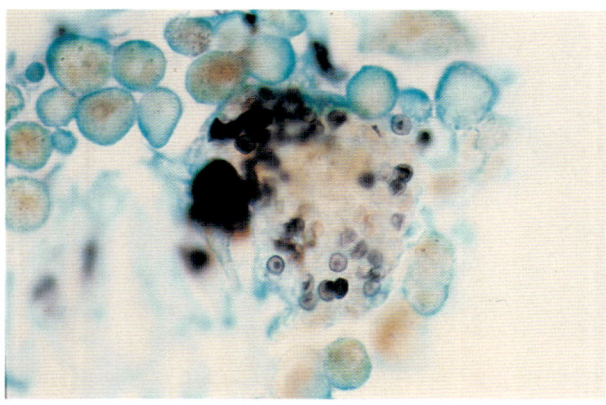

FIGURE 6.24 GMS stain of the fluid showning Pneumocystis. Numerous cyst forms with various shapes and curved walls are noted. (GMS × 80)

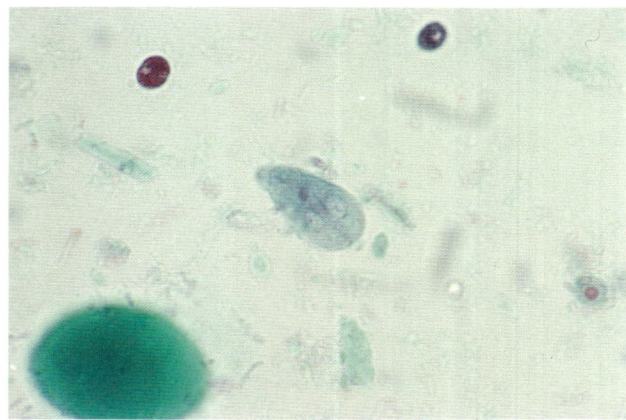

FIGURE 6.26 Trophozoite of *Giardia lamblia*. Note the "owl's eye" and the poorly preserved tail. The organism presumably gained access to the peritoneal fluid through a perforation of the bowel wall. (Trichrome × 60) (Courtesy Dr. L. Ash)

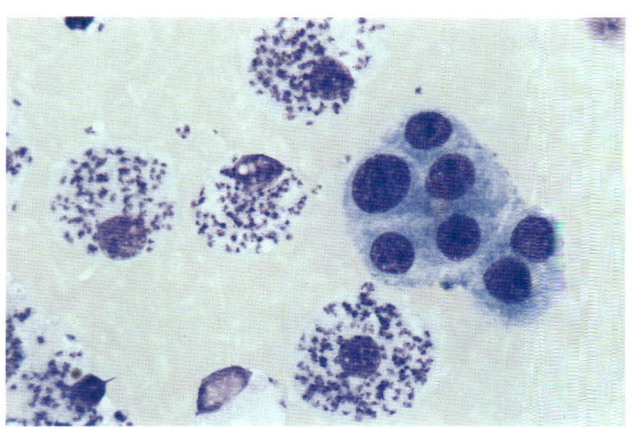

FIGURE 6.27 Leishmaniasis in a pleural effusion. Numerous microorganisms are seen in the cytoplasm of a macrophage. Note also the group of reactive mesothelial cell (MGG × 120) (Courtesy D. King, CT)

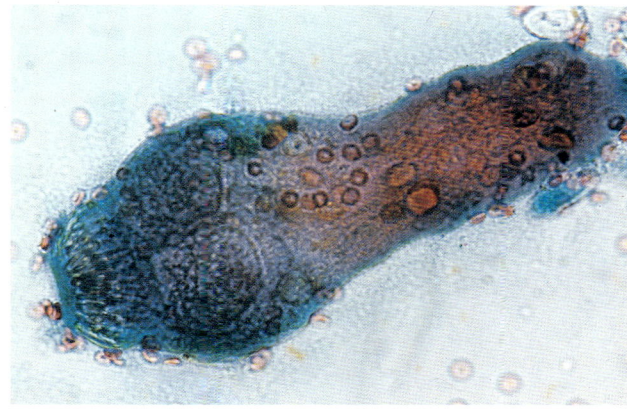

FIGURE 6.29 Hydatid cyst from a liver abscess that emptied into the peritoneum. The aspirate yielded a chocolate-colored fluid containing a few scolices of *Echinococcus granulosus.* (Pap × 400) (Courtesy M. Melamed, MD)

tions and the popularity of air travel, parasitic infestations are expected to occur more often in nonendemic areas. Hydatid disease is the most common helminthic infection spreading to the serosal spaces (Fig. 6.29). The scolices of *echinococcus* are very prone to degeneration, but its characteristic shape allows recognition. In rare instances the hooklets may be intact with good appreciation of cytologic detail (Fig. 6.30). *Microfilaria* are frequent invaders of effusions in tropical climates. The parasite inhabits dilated lymphatics of the soft tissues but may gain access to submesothelial layers of

the serosal cavities because of blockage and retrograde migration. In addition to effusions the parasite has been identified in pulmonary cytologic specimens, nipple discharges, gynecologic smears, and aspirates of lymphedematous extremities. *Microfilaria* stain either palely or rather vividly with Papanicolaou's stain and are identifiable by their slender elongated shape (Figs. 6.31 and 6.32).

Strongyloides stercoralis only seldom appears in effusions but may do so in hyperinfections of the immunosuppressed host. There are cytologic differences be-

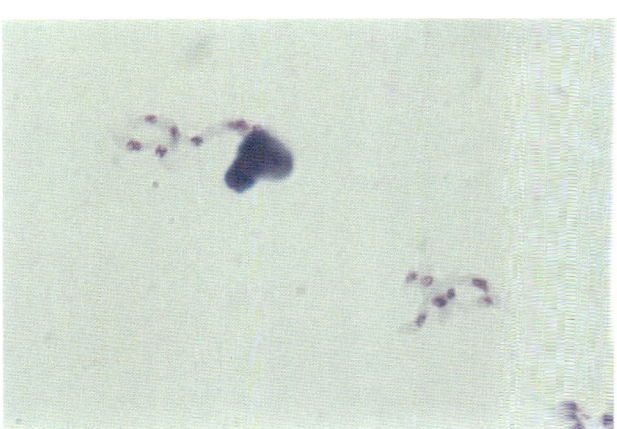

FIGURE 6.28 *Toxoplasma gondii* tachyzoite in ascitic fluid from a patient with AIDS. This patient also had a rare case of ulcerative colitis and bowel perforation, noted at autopsy. (MGG × 240) (Courtesy of Dr. L. Ash)

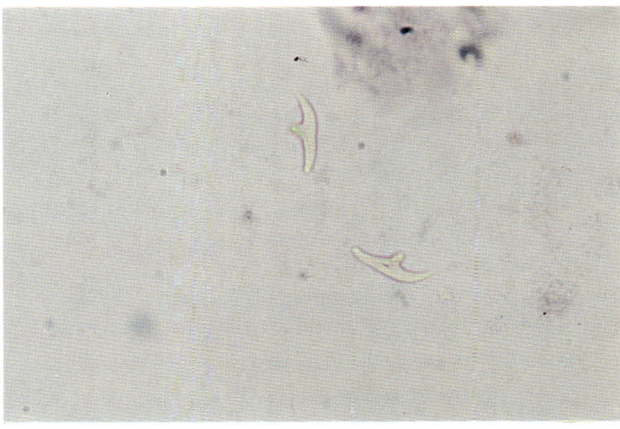

FIGURE 6.30 Free-floating hooklets from a hydatid cyst. Even without staining, these structures can be identified because of their birefringence. (Phase × 40) (Courtesy of Dr. L. Ash)

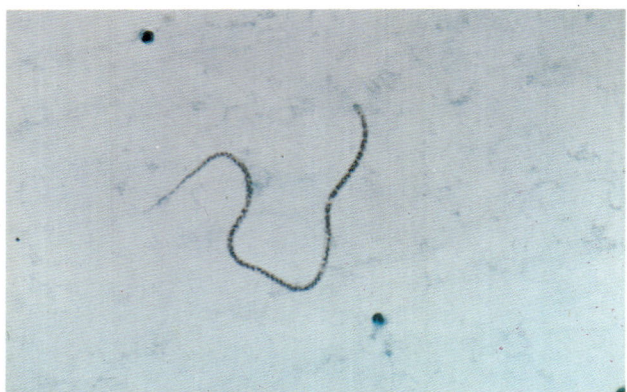

FIGURE 6.31   Filariasis in pleural fluid of an Asian Pacific immigrant. (Pap × 40) (Courtesy M. Melamed, MD)

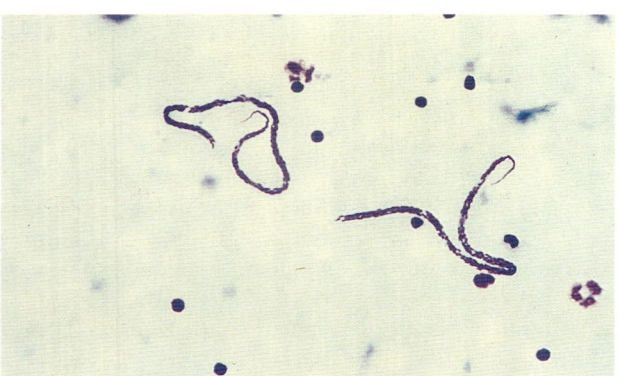

FIGURE 6.32   Pleural fluid with filarial form. This example was identified as *Mansonella ozzardi,* but *Wuchereria bancrofti* may also block lymphatics and gain access to a serosal cavity by retrograde movement. (Diff-Quik × 40)

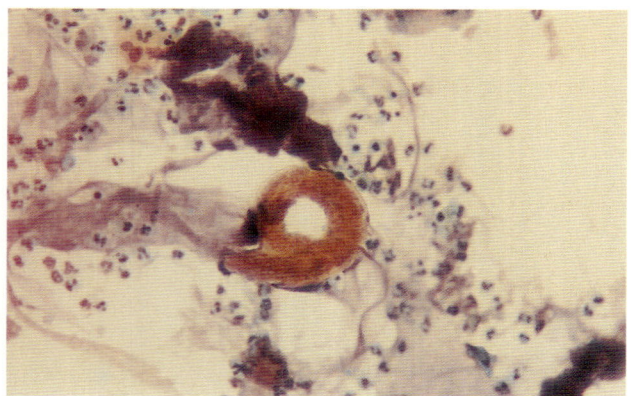

FIGURE 6.33   *Strongyloides stercoralis* in a patient with disseminated strongyloidiasis. A coiled, partially degenerated organism is seen, but it is impossible to appreciate its internal structure. (Pap × 60)

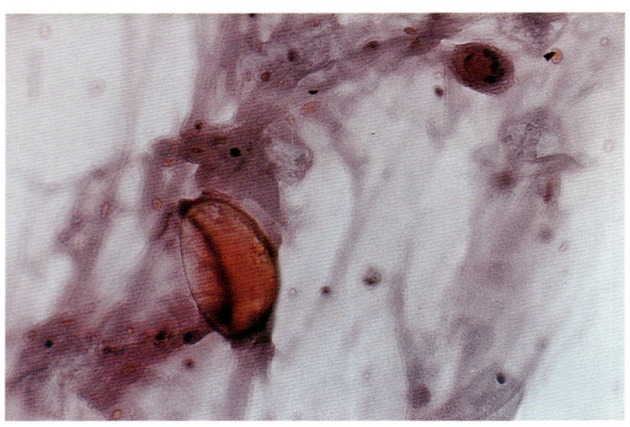

FIGURE 6.34   Single ovum of *Paragonimus* in serous fluid. (Pap × 90) (Courtesy M. Melamed, MD)

tween the male and the female adult worms, but they are difficult to appreciate in Papanicolaou-stained preparations (Fig. 6.33). Paragonimiasis affects primarily the lungs and has been documented in the sputum. However, in malnourished hosts the process may disseminate into the pleural space (Fig. 6.34). The organism stains brownish-yellow by Papanicolaou's method and can be recognized by its characteristic operculum. In the northeastern portion of Brazil, *Schistosoma mansoni* is a rather prevalent infestation. Ova may travel to the lung and are even occasionally observed in effusions in malnourished hosts suffering from anasarca (Fig. 6.35).

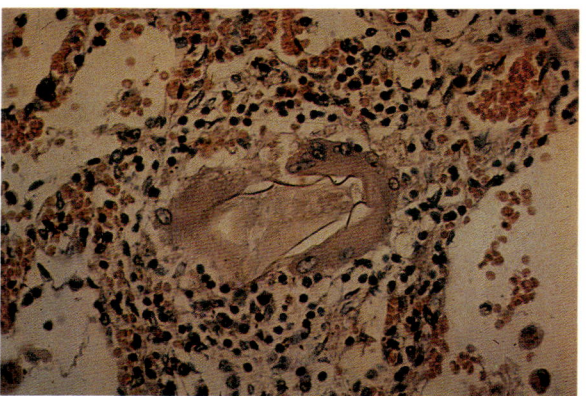

FIGURE 6.35   *Schistosoma mansoni* in a native of northeastern Brazil. A heavy infestation with *Schistosoma* coupled with malnutrition may result in anasarca. Transudates from the peritoneum and, rarely, the pleura may harbor the parasite. (H&E × 60)

BIBLIOGRAPHY

Viral Infections

Bedrossian U, Lozano E, Bedrossian C. Immunoperoxidase method to detect herpes simplex virus in cytologic specimens. *Lab Med.* 1984;15:673–676.

Fine NL, Smith LR, Sheedy PF. Frequency of pleural effusions in mycoplasma and viral pneumonia. *N Engl J Med.* 1970;283:790–793.

Fermaglich DR. Pulmonary involvement in infectious mononucleosis. *J Pedr.* 1975;86:93–95.

Goodman LD, Gupta PK, Frost JK, et al. Cytodiagnosis of viral infections in body cavity fluids. *Acta Cytol.* 1979;23:204–208.

Grix A, Giammona SJ. Pneumonitis with pleural effusion in children due to mycoplasma pneumonia. *Am Rev Respir Dis.* 1974;109:665–671.

Gross PA, Gerding DN. Pleural effusion associated with viral hepatitis. *Gastroenterology.* 1971;60:898–902.

Milder JE, McDearmon SL, Walzer PD. Presumed respiratory syncytial virus pneumonia in an adolescent compromised host. *South Med J.* 1979;72:1195–1198.

Sarkar TH. Infectious mononucleosis with pleural effusion. 1969;56:359–360.

Speer ME, Schaeffer RL, Barrett FF. Adenovirus type 7 pneumonia associated with large pleural effusion. *South Med J.* 1977;70:119–120.

Bacterial Infections

Bartlett JG, Finegold SM. Anaerobic infections of the lung and pleural space. *Am Rev Respir Dis.* 1974;110:56–77.

Bartlett JG, Gorbach SL, Thadepalli H, et al. Bacteriology of empyema. *Lancet.* 1974;1(853):338–340.

Campbell RA. Pneumococcal peritonitis in cirrhosis. *N Eng J Med.* 1968;278:743.

Epstein M, Calia FM, Gabuzda GJ. Pneumococcal peritonitis in patients with postnecrotic cirrhosis. *N Engl J Med.* 1968;278:69–73.

Taryle DA, Potts DE, Sahn SA. The incidence and clinical correlates of parapneumonic effusions in pneumococcal pneumonias. *Chest.* 1978;74:170–173.

Walker A, Walker G, Feldman P. Diagnosis of *Legionella micdadei* pneumonia from cytologic specimens. *Acta Cytol.* 1983;27(3):252–254.

Funguslike Bacteria

Frazier AR, Rosenow ED III, Roberts GD. Nocardiosis: A review of 25 cases occurring during 24 months. *Mayo Clin Proc.* 1975;50:657–663.

Karetzky MS, Garvey JW. Empyema due to *Actinoncycosis naeslundi. Chest.* 1974;65:229–230.

Neu HC, Silva M, Hazen E, et al. Necrotizing nocardial pneumonitis. *Ann Int Med.* 1967;66:274–284.

Varkey B, Landis FB, Tang TT, et al. Thoracic actinomycosis: Dissemination to skin, subcutaneous tissue, and muscle. *Arch Intern Med.* 1974;134:689–693.

Acid Fast Bacteria

Epstein DM, Kline LR, Albelda SM. Tuberculous pleural effusion. *Chest.* 1987;91(1):106–109.

Spieler P. The cytologic diagnosis of tuberculosis in pleural effusions. *Acta Cytol.* 1979;23:374–379.

Tani E, Schmitt F, Oliveira M, et al. Pulmonary cytology in tuberculosis. *Acta Cytol.* 1987;31(4):460–463.

Fungal Infections

Brewer PL, Himmelwright JP. Pleural effusion due to infection with *Histoplasma capsulatum. Chest.* 1970;58:76–79.

Covell JL, Lowry EH, Feldman PS. Cytologic diagnosis of blastomycosis in pleural fluid. *Acta Cytol.* 1982;26:833–837.

Epstein R, Cole R, Hunt KK Jr. Pleural effusion secondary to pulmonary cryptococcosis. *Chest.* 1972;61:296–298.

Ericsson CD, Pickering LK, Salmon GW. Pleural effusion in histoplasmons. *J Pediatr.* 1977;90:326–327.

Hargis JL, Bone RC, Miller FC, et al. Pulmonary blastomycosis diagnosed by thoracentesis. *Chest.* 1980;77:455–460.

Jay SJ, O'Neill RP, Goodman N, et al. Pleural effusion a rare manifestation of acute pulmonary blastomycosis *Am J Med Sci.* 1974;274:325–328.

Jay SJ, O'Neill RP, Goodman N, et al. Pleural effusion: A rare manifestation of acute pulmonary blastomycosis. *Am J Med Sci.* 1977;274 325–328.

Lonky SA, Catarzaro A, Moser KM, et al. Acute coccidioidal pleural effusion. *Am Rev Respir Dis.* 1976;114:681–688.

Pinckney L, Parker BR. Primary coccidioidomycosis in children presenting with massive pleural effusion. *AJR.* 1978; 130:247–249.

Tani E, Franco M. Pulmonary cytology in paracoccidioidomycosis. *Acta Cytol.* 1984;28(5):571–575.

Opportunistic Fungi

Hillerdal G. Pulmonary aspergillus infection invading the pleura. *Thorax.* 1981;36:745–751.

Reyes CV, Kathuria S, MacGlashan A. Diagnostic value of calcium oxalate crystals in respiratory and pleural fluid cytology. *Acta Cytol.* 1979;23:65–68.

Shapiro BS. *Candida* peritonitis. *Conn Med.* 1966;30:727–728.

Walsh TJ, Bulkley BH. Aspergillus pericarditis—clinical and

pathologic features in the immunocompromised patient. *Cancer* 1982;49:48–54.

Protozoal Infections

Bedrossian CWM, Mason MR, Gupta PK. Rapid cytologic diagnosis of pneumocystis: A comparison of effective techniques. *Sem in Diagn Pathol.* 1989;6:245–261.

Bloch T, Davis TE, Schwenk CR. *Giardia lamblia* in peritoneal fluid. *Acta Cytol.* 1987;31:785–790.

Drew PA, Krauss JS. Identification of *Giardia lamblia* in peritoneal fluid of trauma patients. *Acta Cytol.* 1989;33:283–284.

Ibarra-Perey C. Thoracic complications of amebic abscess of the liver. *Chest.* 1981;79:672–676.

Markowitz S, Leiman G. Cytologic detection of *Pneumocystis carinii* by ultraviolet light examination of Papanicolaou-stained sputum specimens. *Acta Cytol.* 1986;30(1):79–80.

Memik F. Trichomonads in pleural effusion. *JAMA* 1968; 204:1145–1146.

Miller MJ, Leith DE, Brooks JR, et al. Trichomonas empyema. *Thorax.* 1982;37:384–385.

Rasaretnam R, Paul AS, Yoganotham M. Pleural empyema due to ruptured amoebic liver abscess. *Br J Surg.* 1974; 61:713–715.

Walsh T, Berkman W, Brown N, et al. Cytopathologic diagnosis of extracolonic amebiasis. *Acta Cytol.* 1983;27(6): 671–675.

Walzer PD, Rutherford I, East R. Empyema with *Trichomonas* species. *Am Rev Respir Dis.* 1978;118:415–418.

Helminthic Infections

Aragnina MA, Esner B, Jotti RM, Re R. *Strongyloides stercoralis* in Papanicolaou-stained smears of ascitic fluid. *Acta Cytol.* 1980;24:36–39.

Balikian JP, Mudarris FF. Hydatid disease of the lungs: A roentgenologic study of 50 cases. *AJR.* 1974;122:692–707.

Figueroa JM. Presence of microfilariae of *Mansonella ozzardi* in ascitic fluid. *Acta Cytol.* 1973;17:73–75.

Hira P, Lindberg LG, Ryd W, et al. Cytologic diagnosis of Bancroftian filariasis in a non-endemic area. *Acta Cytol.* 1988; 32:267–269.

Jacobson ES. A case of secondary echinococcosis diagnosed by cytologic examination of pleural fluid and needle biopsy of pleura. *Acta Cytol.* 1973;17:76–79.

Johnson JR, Falk A, Iber C, et al. Paragonimiasis in the United States. A report of nine cases in immigrants. *Chest.* 1982; 82:168–171.

Kapila K, Verma K. Cytologic detection of parasitic disorders. *Acta Cytol.* 1982;26:359–362.

Liepman M. Disseminated *Strongyloides stercoralis:* A complication of immunosuppression. *JAMA.* 1975;231:387–389.

Lintermans JP. Fatal peritonitis, an unusual clinical complication of *Strongyloides stercoralis* infestation. *Clin Pediatr.* 1975;14:974–978.

Naylor B. Pleural, peritoneal and pericardial fluids. In: Bibbo M, ed. *Comprehensive Cytopathology.* W.B. Saunders; Philadelphia: 1991:chap 22, 541–614.

Okuyama T, Imai S, Tsubura Y. Egg of *Schistosoma japonicum* in ascitic fluid. *Acta Cytol.* 1985;29:651–652.

Pollock TW, Perenvich EN. Hyperinfection with *Strongyloides stercoralis* in a patient with Hodgkin's disease. *J Am Osteopath Assoc.* 1976;76:171–175.

Walter A, Krishmaswami H, Cariappa A. Microfilarial of *Wuchereria bancrofti* in cytologic smears. *Acta Cytol.* 1983; 27(4):432–436.

Xanthakis DS. Hydatid cyst of the liver with intrathoracic rupture. *Thorax.* 1981;36:497–501.

Yacoubian HD. Thoracic problems associated with hydatid cyst of the dome of the liver. *Surgery.* 1976;79:544–548.

Yokogawa M. IGE raised levels in sera and pleural exudates of patients with paragonimus. *Am J Trop Med Hyg.* 1976; 25:581–586.

CHAPTER SEVEN

Iatrogenic, Organ-related, and Systemic Processes

As previously noted, mesothelial cells are extremely reactive to physical, chemical, and biologic injury. Cellular response is florid but varies little among the various insults. However, careful correlation between the clinical history and the cytomorphologic alterations makes it possible to recognize some of the causative factors involved. It is extremely important to be familiar with the different causes so as not to misinterpret the cytologic changes. Particularly costly is to misdiagnose these changes as malignant.

Some reactive, nonneoplastic changes have an obscure, poorly understood pathogenesis, to the point that to attach too great a significance to terms such as "atypical" mesothelial cells or "suspicious" mesothelial cells serves little purpose. Others are traceable to a specific organ, particularly with the assistance of good clinical data. Still other nonmalignant alterations relate to metabolic and poorly understood systemic conditions which may be first manifested by effusion. In these cases a precise cytologic diagnosis will make an extensive evaluation unnecessary. The major difficulty in identifying the etiology of the mesothelial injury is that mesothelial cells are normally extremely reactive and may exhibit a number of morphologic changes, many of which are nonspecific (Table 7.1).

NON-SPECIFIC "REACTIVE" CHANGES

The boundary between normal and hyperplastic mesothelial cells is imprecise and these two cell populations are usually represented in reactive, non-malignant conditions. "Reactive" changes of some degree seem to affect mesothelial cells in any kind of effusion. In fact,

the mere presence of excessive fluid causes the mesothelium to react to its accumulation. This natural phenomenon is frequently cited in cytologic reports to the annoyance of some authors, who argue validly that such a pervasive response may be totally meaningless to the clinician. It is important, however, that the cytopathologist recognize reactive changes as part of normalcy, so that they are not overinterpreted. We refer to them as "the many faces of mesothelial cells" to stress the concept that mesothelial cells cannot be stereotyped and that despite the variation of appearances, one can still recognize them as a single cell population in the cytologic specimens. This is an extremely useful concept because malignant cells tend to stand out in such a milieu of quiescent and reactive mesothelial cells, identifiable quite obviously as a group quite different from their mesothelial neighbors. In contrast, reactive mesothelial cells seem to belong next to one another even when their nuclei denote hyperplasia (Fig. 7.1).

If a group of enlarged cells cannot be readily recognized as alien chances are it is not malignant. The features enabling the recognition of reactive cells as mesothelial in origin can be as subtle as their clasping articulations or a clear ecto-endoplasmic demarcation (Fig. 7.2). Variation of the nuclear size and shape, per se, should not be cause for alarm (Fig. 7.3). As mesothelial cells react to their environment they may acquire unusual granulations in the cytoplasm, the cause of which remains obscure (Fig. 7.4). Long-standing reactive pleurisies may also lead to altered shapes of the cell cytoplasm (Fig. 7.5).

Hyperchromasia without a change of other nuclear parameters such as size and shape, distribution of the chromatic granules, and evenness of the nuclear envelope, is one of the most common nonspecific changes

TABLE 7.1 The Many Faces of Mesothelial Cells

Cell Group- ings	Intercellular Relationships	Cellular Morphology
Single cells	Pinching	Enlargement
Doublets	Clasping	Elongation
Triplets	Windows	Hyperchromasia
Flat groups	Side-by-side	Chromatin clearing
Rosettes	Molding	Multinucleation
Cells in a row	Syncytia	Increased nuclear:
Tight cell balls	Cell-in-cell	cytoplasmic ratio
Pseudoacini		Granulation
		Blebbing
		Signet-rings
		Mitosis

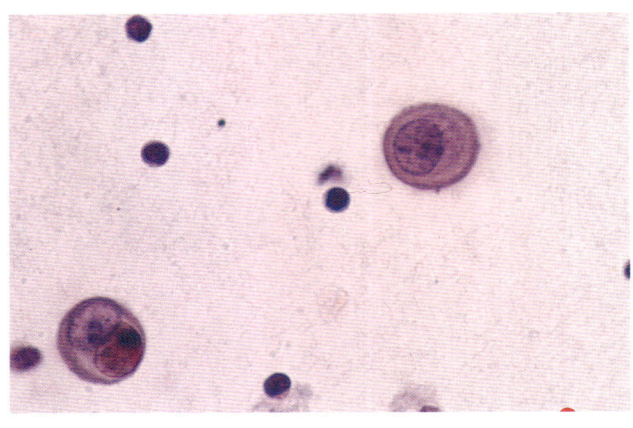

FIGURE 7.2 Hyperplastic mesothelial cells with apparent ecto-endoplasmic demarcation. Another mesothelial cell clasps a degenerating neighbor, simulating binucleation. (Pap × 90)

demonstrated by "reactive" mesothelial cells. Accentuation of cytoplasmic vacuolization is another common finding, often leading to rounded or, sausage-shaped semilunar vacuoles at the periphery of the cytoplasm (Fig. 7.6). These are shown to contain glycogen, digestible by diastases. Not infrequently, the vacuolization acquires the signet ring–like appearance or may appear between cells, but the absence of malignant changes in the nuclei prevents one from misdiagnosing them as adenocarcinoma (Fig. 7.7). Macrophages may also undergo this signet-ring–like transformation, and they may be impossible to distinguish from mesothelial cells by routine stains alone.

Florid alterations of mesothelial cells may be caused simply by increased fluid pressure related to accumula-tion of the effusion and its resulting irritation of the mesothelium. This phenomenon is particularly common in pericardial fluid (Fig. 7.8). As such, they may appear in transudates due to congestive heart failure and numerous other processes where it is not possible for the pathologist to make a specific diagnosis. These cells may appear cytologically "atypical" but invariably one still appreciates their mesothelial derivation (Fig. 7.9). Other instances exist, in which a combination of microscopic examination and clinical correlation allows the recognition or the suggestion of possible causes of serous fluid accumulation (Table 7.2).

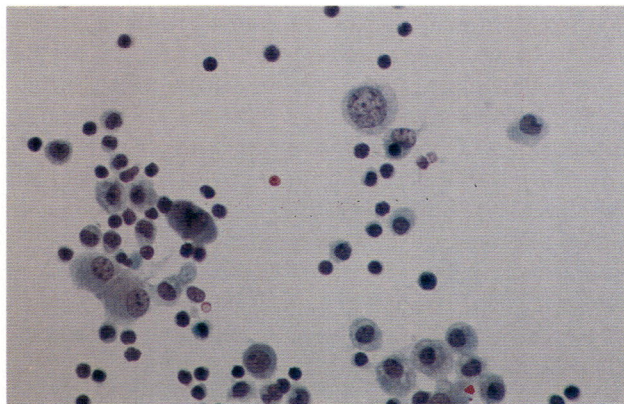

FIGURE 7.1 Reactive mesothelial hyperplasia with cells occurring singly, and as doublets. Note the variation in size and in the tinctorial properties of the nuclei. Numerous lymphocytes are noted in the background. (Pap × 40)

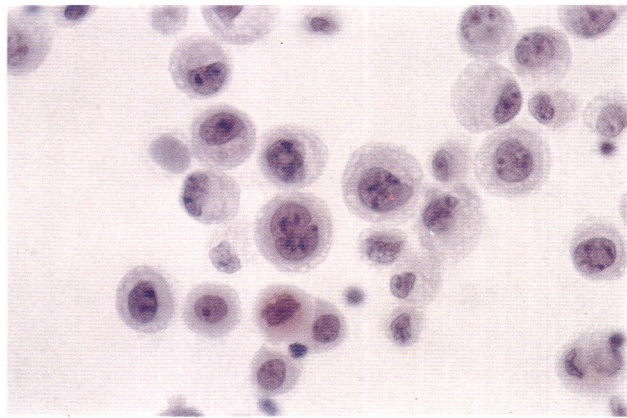

FIGURE 7.3 Mesothelial cells with variation of their nuclei. Note the prominent nucleoli and dense cytoplasm in some but not all reactive cells. (Pap × 120)

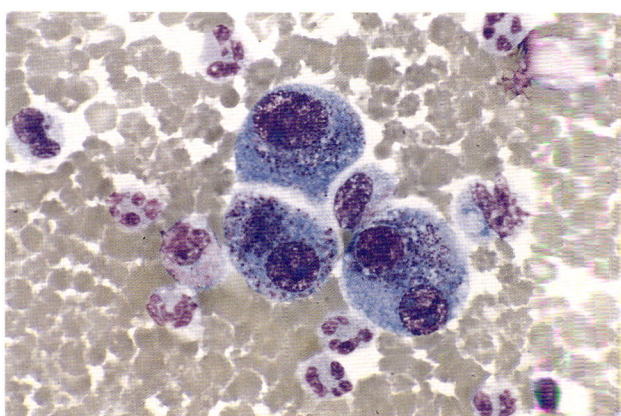

FIGURE 7.4 Cytoplasmic granulation in hyperplastic mesothelial cells. This poorly understood reactive process may be similar to the toxic granulation of inflammatory cells. (MGG× 120) (Courtesy of S. Zaleski, CT)

A   B

FIGURE 7.6 Altered pattern of vacuolization in reactive mesothelial cells. (A) Large, coalesced vacuole (Pap× 120); (B) Semilunar, perinuclear vacuole. (DQ× 120)

Radiation Effect

Radiation pneumonitis is a rare but significant complication of radiotherapy to the chest and mediastinum. The process may occur immediately after radiation but more often presents as asymptomatic pericarditis and pleuritis, discovered by chest x-ray. The onset of the process may be delayed by months, even several years. In 20 to 30% of these cases effusion will form in either of the pleural cavities or the pericardial sac and may be diagnosed cytologically. Persistent postradiation pleural and pericardial effusions are high in protein and contain lymphocytes in elevated proportion.

Mesothelial cells increase in number when exposed to radiation and show nonspecific reactive changes including nuclear enlargement and slight hyperchromasia. The presence of vacuoles in both the cytoplasm and the nucleus, however, is a rather suggestive evidence of radiation effect as is the finding of blebs in macrophage (Fig. 7.10) Another finding suggestive of radiation is elongation of mesothelial cells, which may also appear misshapen by cytoplasmic extensions or frag-

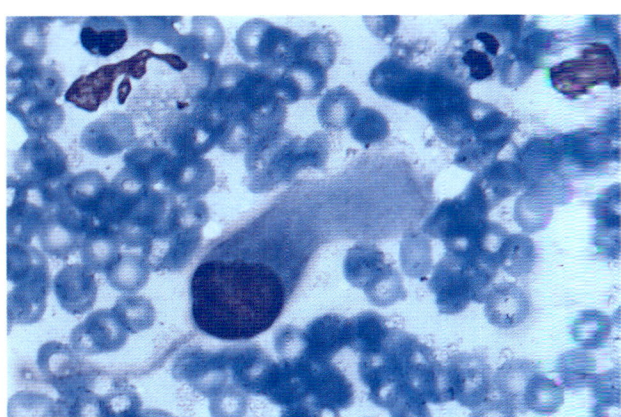

FIGURE 7.5 Cytoplasmic elongation in reactive pleuritis. The corresponding biopsy specimen showed mesothelial cells flattened out over an area of infarction. (MGG× 120)

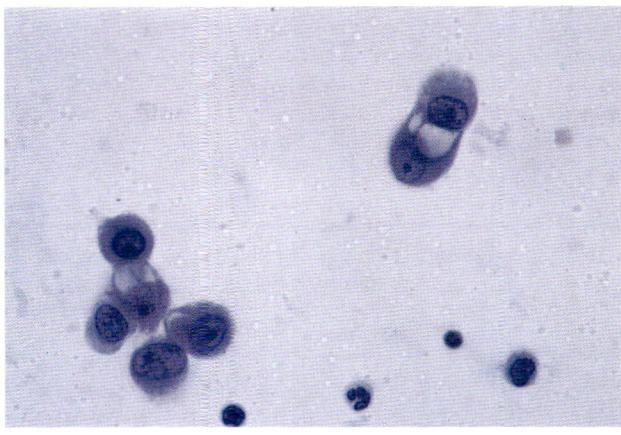

FIGURE 7.7 Intercellular vacuolization of reactive mesothelial cells. Cells also show articulations and "windows" between one another. (Pap× 60)

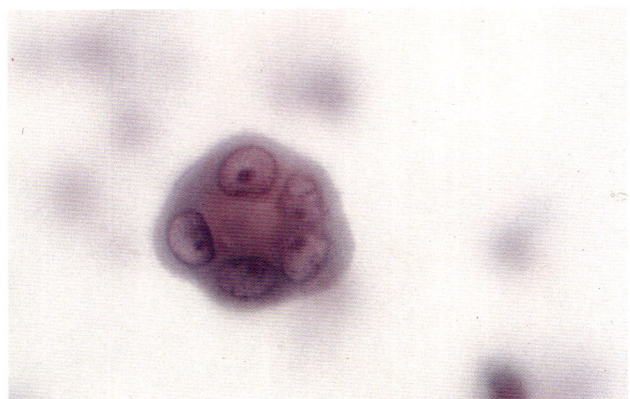

FIGURE 7.8 Pseudoacinar arrangement of mesothelial cells from pericardial fluid. Crowded microvilli in the center simulate an inspissated secretion. Refocusing elucidates the intercellular relationships and demonstrates the cell borders better. (Pap × 90)

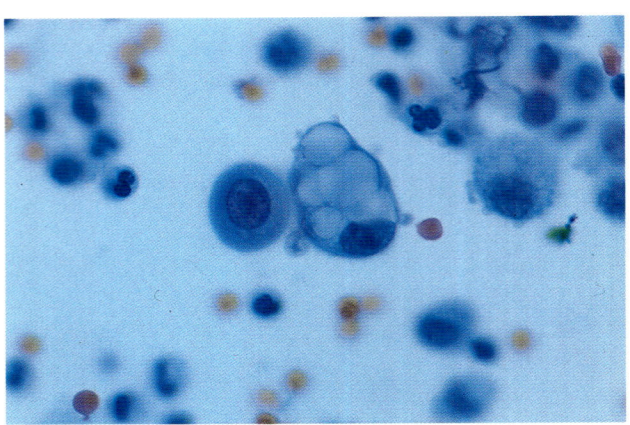

FIGURE 7.10 Radiation effect in a pleural effusion. Marked vacuolization of mesothelial cells and bleb formation are common outcomes of irradiation. (Pap × 90)

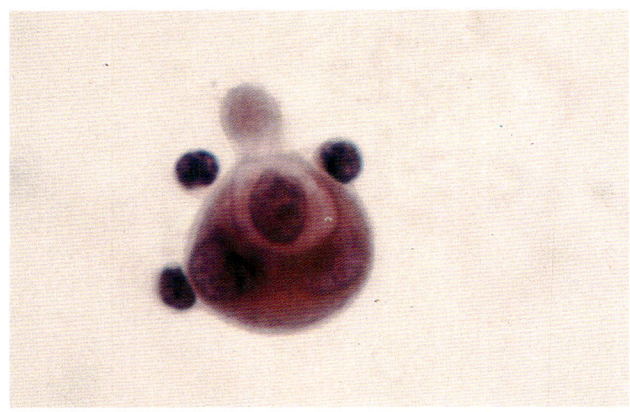

FIGURE 7.9 Clasping among reactive mesothelial cells, creating the ilusion of engulfment. The clasped cell actually lies in a concavity of the embracing cells. Note the cytoplasmic knob protruding from the clasped cell, a characteristic feature of mesothelial cells. (Pap × 90)

mentation. Multinucleation of elongated cells and prominent nucleoli are noted less frequently, but proliferative changes and cell ball formation are not a prominent feature of radiation effect. The cytoplasmic vacuoles may be filled with smudged condensations of protoplasmic material or appear as empty blebs.

In acute radiation effect, necrotic debris is present in the background, and dead cells may contain hyaline inclusions in the cytoplasm. The serous fluids contain numerous RBCs, a large number of leukocytes including neutrophils and lymphocytes, and reactive mesothelial cells. These cells may be multinucleated and may form rosettes but rarely form cell balls. Individual cells exhibit florid vacuolization. The combination of nuclear and cytoplasmic vacuolization and a bizarre shape of the mesothelial cells is suggestive of radiation injury in the proper clinical setting, but a specific diagnosis is difficult in the absence of a supportive history.

Chemotherapeutic Effect

Any treatment may affect human epithelia in an untoward fashion, resulting in toxic effects. Particularly prone to this type of complication are the lung and the bladder, which are frequently the target of drug reactions. By comparison, the serosal membranes are less seriously affected but they too may develop alterations as a result of drug therapy. Drug toxicity in the serous cavities can be the result of a direct, chemically mediated effect or may be related to immunologic phenomena. An example of the latter is nitrofurantoin,

TABLE 7.2 Iatrogenic Conditions, Organ Related and Systemic Processes, Affecting the Serous Membranes

Iatrogenic	Organ-related	Systemic	Extraneous
Radiation	Infarction	Sarcoidosis	Talcum
Chemotherapy	Cirrhosis	Amyloidosis	powder
Hemodialysis	Uremia	Sickle-cell	Asbestos
Washings	Pancreatitis	anemia	Pigmentation
Pleurodesis	Endometriosis	Collagen	Other foreign
Endoscopy	Pneumothorax	diseases	matter

which causes allergic pleuro-pneumonitis and occasionally, serofibrinous effusion. Cytologically, it is not possible to distinguish drug-related from other causes of serofibrinous effusions. In allergic reactions the degree of atypia in the mesothelial cells is generally rather low and the process tends to disappear when the drug is discontinued. Lymphocytes and occasionally eosinophils are noted in the effusion, which is generally a transudate or an exudate of relatively low specific gravity. Quite often, these transient effusions are diagnosed radiologically and too small to warrant drainage and cytologic evaluation.

The effusion resulting from direct toxic effect of drugs such as procarbezine and methotrexate is exudative in nature and contains many lymphocytes and reactive mesothelial cells. If the patient had a pleural effusion at the beginning of chemotherapy for breast and other carcinomas, the proportion of leukocyte and macrophages has some prognostic value. Good therapeutic response is accompanied by a decrease in the number of tumor cells, a reduction in the number of macrophages, and an increase in the number of lymphocytes. In contrast, an increase in the number of macrophages usually accompanies a poor response. The chemotherapeutic effect extends to the cancerous cells, which undergo marked atypia followed by degeneration and disappearance from the effusion.

Mesothelial cells also reflect the chemotherapy effect in the absence of a malignant effusion. The most common alteration is vacuolization of the cytoplasm and lesser involvement of the nuclei. The mesothelial cells may appear hyperplastic and hypertrophic and a few may mimic malignant cell groups with nuclear enlargement and hyperchromasia (Fig. 7.11). There is minimal inflammatory reaction and the process appears to be dose related. Procarbazine-related exudative pleural effusions tend to persist for a period of months and clear slowly after interruption of the drug administration (Fig. 7.12).

A very characteristic reaction of mesothelial cells is elicited by amiodarone, an antiarrhythmic drug effective in intractable arrhythmias. The major changes occur in the lung and have been described as a phospholipidosis, responsible for clear vacuolization of alveolar macrophages. In a small proportion of patients receiving the drug, an effusion will develop that contains foamy mesothelial cells and macrophages. By electron microscopy, not only alveolar macrophages but also epithelial and endothelial cells of the lung are seen to be engorged with lamellated phospholipid inclusions that are pathognomonic of amiodarone toxicity (Fig. 7.13). The vacuolization induced by amiodarone is finer and more

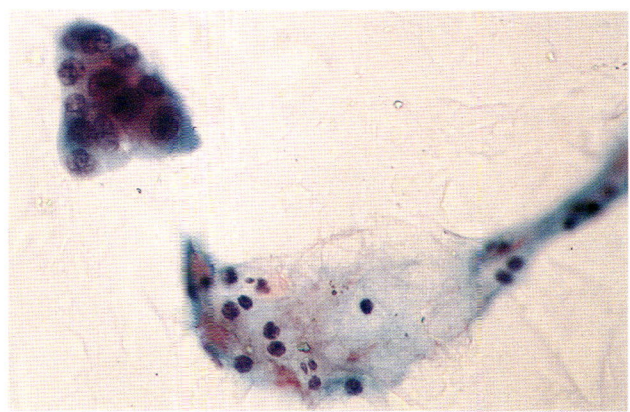

FIGURE 7.11 Pleural fluid from patient on multidrug chemotherapy. Fragmentation of cells, hyperchromasia of nuclei, and amphophilia of the cytoplasm are all features of chemotherapy effect. (Pap × 60)

homogeneous than in lipoid granulomas that result from the instillation of lipid into a serosal cavity. As noted above, drugs other than amiodarone may cause a nonspecific vacuolization change of mesothelial cells. These vacuoles are coarser than the ones induced by amiodarone toxicity and as seen by electron microscopy they represent degenerative vacuoles rather than lamellated phospholipid-laden vesicles. Some drugs cause a lupuslike phenomenon which may manifest itself by pleural effusion. This type of reaction is indistin-

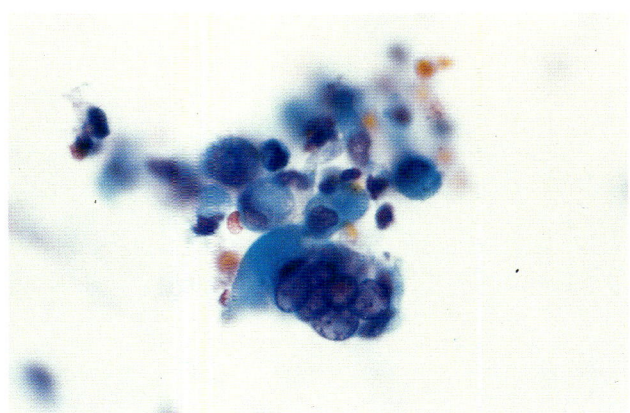

FIGURE 7.12 Multinucleated mesothelial cell from a patient receiving procarbazine. Without a proper clinical history, both chemotherapy and radiation effects are difficult to interpret. (Pap × 90)

guishable from naturally occurring lupus-related effusions.

Instillation of chemotherapeutic agents in a serosal cavity has been tried as a local treatment of malignant effusion. Cytology is very useful in the followup of these cases, where it may detect the presence of malignant cells, demonstrate their viability, and disclose any cytologic alterations induced by the chemotherapy in malignant as well as in mesothelial cells. Just as in systemic chemotherapy, cytology may be used to monitor immunologic response to the treatment in the form of a predominant lymphocytic or histiocytic response to the instillation of the drug. A predominantly lymphocytic response is associated with a good prognosis whereas an increased number of macrophages occur in patients whose clinical course is deteriorating.

Solid tumors may evolve from a low level of anaplasia to a very bizarre multinucleated stage following the administration of chemotherapeutic agent into a serous cavity. Lymphomas and leukemias in effusion may present with a nuclear fragmentation pattern due to karyorrhexis induced by systemic chemotherapy or radiation. The most dramatic changes in the cytologic appearance of neoplastic cells occur when a radiomimetic drug is associated with radiation. In intrapleural chemotherapy with alkylating agents, extreme vacuolization of nucleus and cytoplasm and frank ballooning or death of the tumor cells are practically indistinguishable from radiation effect.

Dialysis Effect

Patients in renal failure may develop effusions affecting the pleura, pericardium, and peritoneum. Chronic peritoneal dialysis may cause severe atypical hyperplasia of mesothelial cells occurring in association with hemorrhagic ascites. The effect is most dramatic in the peritoneum but may also affect the pleural spaces. Mesothelial cells mechanically dislodged by the dialysis catheters attain unusual groupings and may appear atypical (Fig. 7.14). Repeated dialysis sessions increase the danger of infection, and both bacterial and fungal peritonitis have been recorded in dialysis patients. In noninfectious processes, the dominant feature is the presence of fresh and old RBCs, macrophages exhibiting erythrophagocytosis or a hemosiderin-laden cytoplasm, and reactive mesothelial cells. With chronicity, both lymphocytosis and eosinophilia may occur in the ascitic fluid and, by mechanisms unknown, be accompanied by recurrent pleural effusions.

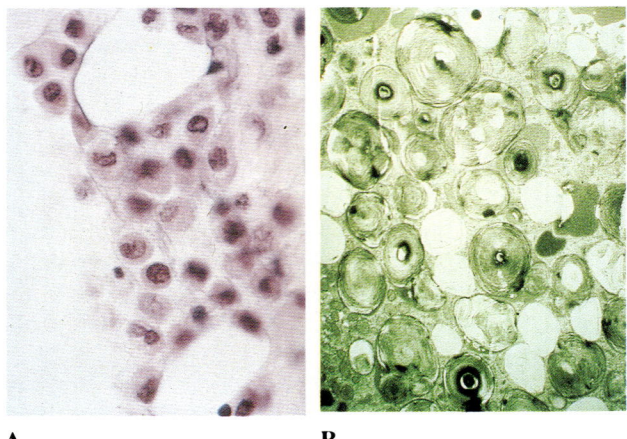

A   **B**

FIGURE 7.13 Effect of amiodarone on a pleural effusion. (*A*) Foamy histiocytes with bean-shaped nuclei and a hypervacuolated cytoplasm. (Pap × 90) (*B*) By electron microscopy, lamellated, osmophilic inclusion bodies are noted in the cytoplasm. (EM × 6,000)

Peritoneal Washings

The pouch of Douglas, also known as the cul-de-sac, accumulates up to 10 to 20 mL of peritoneal fluid in symptomless women. For a time, aspiration of this material—culdocentesis—held the hope for a screening modality capable of detecting early neoplasia of the ovaries and fallopian tubes. This practice has been mostly abandoned, but peritoneal fluids and cells are still harvested in an attempt to diagnose ovarian neoplasis either in its primary site or as metastatic implants throughout the peritoneal cavity.

As first mentioned in Chapter 2, the procedure of obtaining cells from the peritoneum is not without its traumatic consequences. Depending on the vigor of the aspirator, normal mesothelial cells are scraped forcibly and appear either as small or large sheets of cells. The sheets are mosaiclike, with monotonous nuclei, abundant cytoplasm, and laterally apposed cell surfaces. In these cases, evenly spaced nuclei, the absence of nuclear atypia, and the very low nuclear:cytoplasmic ratios are all deterrents to overdiagnosis. The problems occur in women who have had previous gynecologic surgeries and have therefore developed a chronically inflamed and reactive mesothelial lining of the pelvic peritoneum and its vicinity. The cells exfoliating from these areas or being scraped during peritoneal washings may present considerable diagnostic difficulty. The use of cell blocks may alleviate the diagnostic difficulties in

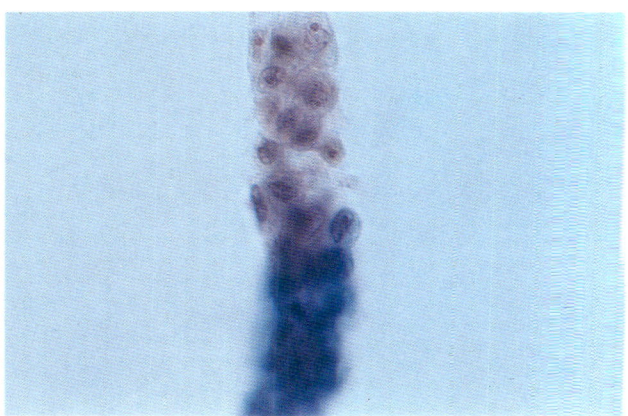

FIGURE 7.14 Tubular group of mesothelial cells freed from a dialysis catheter. Note the prominent nucleoli of the reactive mesothelial cells. (Pap × 90)

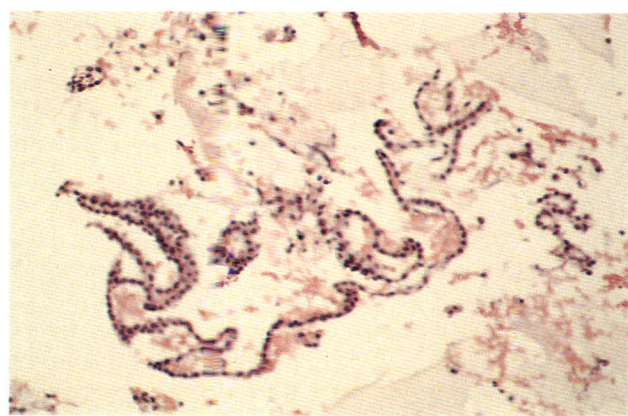

FIGURE 7.15 Typical effect of pelvic washings. The cell block shows monolayers of stripped mesothelial cells with regularly shaped and spaced nuclei. (H&E × 120)

these cases by demonstrating typical monolayers of mesothelial cells (Fig. 7.15). Poorly preserved and ineptly handled specimens result in cellular material of difficult interpretation. Not only do they contain clusters of atypical cells, but individually their nuclei may be hyperchromatic owing to pyknosis secondary to degeneration.

To avoid the pitfalls of misdiagnosing benign washings as malignant, one has to keep in mind that only viable cells should form the basis of a solid interpretation. The rule of identifying cell groups that stand out from the background mesothelial cells is not easily applicable in peritoneal washes because these specimens are extremely cellular and contain, in addition to the groups of atypical mesothelial cells, a large number of normal mesothelial cells in the benign appearing sheet-like arrangement. Large numbers of RBCs are common in peritoneal lavages. Treating the specimen first by a lysing agent and filtering it through a millipore membrane filter reduces the negative effect of RBC contamination. If surgery has been performed within months of the second-look operation, it is not uncommon for the macrophages to "tell the story" of the events taking place during and after surgery. Macrophages may contain hemosiderin, fragmented or intact RBC, cellular debris, carbon, starch granules, talcum powder, or other foreign matter (Fig. 7.16). Talcum powder is frequently overlooked in the examination of peritoneal lavage fluid, despite its characteristic appearance (Fig. 7.17). The presence of a talcum powder, may considerably alter the cell shape and mimic signet rings Fig. 7.18). Polarization microscopy helps characterize the

contaminants particularly in the case of talcum powder and starch granules (Fig. 7.19).

Rows of mesothelial cells that break off and coil upon themselves are generally easy to recognize as benign in cell blocks from peritoneal washings. These preparations can be the target of special stains and immunocytochemistry if a suspicion of malignancy exists. Another element sometimes found in these specimens are psammoma bodies, which should not cause alarm in the absence of obviously malignant cells. If the preparations are poor and diagnosis is based on only a few degenerated cells, the likelihood of a false-positive diagnosis is greater.

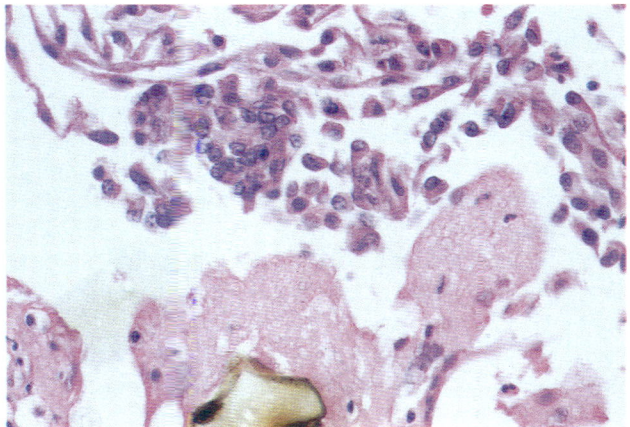

FIGURE 7.16 Cell block from peritoneal washing. Reactive rows of mesothelial cells are noted in the vicinity of fibrin-coated suture material. (H&E × 180)

Pleurodesis

Spontaneous, repeated pneumothoraces occur somewhat infrequently, either idiopathically or as a consequence of eosinophilic granuloma in the young and COPD in the elderly. Traumatic pneumothoraces may also become recurrent and necessitate treatment by obliteration, known as pleurodesis. The success rate of this treatment is variable, and persistent small effusions need to be aspirated repeatedly to avoid secondary infection. These fluids reflect the chronicity of the process in the form of a predominantly lymphocytic effusion accompanied by a few eosinophils. Very often, particularly in chemical pleurodesis induced by tetracycline, the mesothelial cells appear reactive with the spectrum of changes common in chronic irritative processes. Pleurodesis may be attempted by instillation of talcum powder, starch or leucite beads. The particles of talc are irregular in size and shape, depending on the purity of the product, in contrast to the rounded, more regular appearance of starch granules. Pleurodesis may also be accomplished by olive oil instillation and the use of liquid glue, but we are yet to see a pleural fluid following these therapeutic procedures.

ORGAN-RELATED PROCESSES

Infarction

The serosal membranes reflect upon themselves to constitute the visceral layer covering every major organ of the thoracic and intraabdominal compartments. When the blood supply to these organs is suddenly and severely curtailed, infarction takes place, accompanied by an inflammatory response of the overlying mesothelium. Serous effusions become progressively hemorrhagic so that a period of serosanguinous fluid accumulation is typical of the early stages of ischemia. This is followed by exudation of inflammatory cells and reactive hyperplasia of mesothelial cells. In the presence of blood, mesothelial cells develop nuclear hyperchromasia and prominent nuclei. Together with a sheetlike exfoliation and degeneration of the mesothelial cells, this picture can lead to interpretational difficulties (Fig. 7.20). In the late stages of infarction, multinucleated mesothelial cells and histiocytic cells make their appearance, and the latter are prone to hemosiderin accumulation.

Gradually, the hemorrhagic fluid is reabsorbed only to be replaced by a fibrinous layer—provided there is

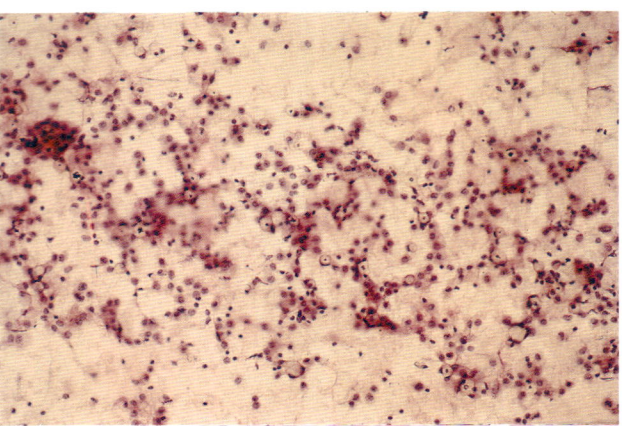

FIGURE 7.17   Reactive mesothelial cells in a specimen from a second-look operation. The peritoneal wash contains many spherical structures with dots in their centers. (Pap × 40)

no secondary infection. Not uncommonly, the underlying dead tissue becomes an excellent culture medium for bacteria and fungi, and the exudate becomes overtly purulent and foul-smelling. In infarctions of the gut, bacteria may seep through a boggy, leaky bowel wall and cause peritonitis. When healing finally occurs, the surface of the involved organ is filled with a crust that includes a bottom layer of proliferating fibroblastlike submesothelial cells and a top layer of hyperplastic and hypertrophic mesothelial cells. Microinfarctions of the subpleural area are not unusual in eosinophilic granuloma of the lung, leading to air leakage and hemothoraces. In severe emphysema, small ruptured subpleural blebs may also rupture and cause small serosanguinous effusions containing lymphocytes, eosinophils, and histiocytes filled with either fresh RBCs or hemosiderin. Because these patients are elderly smokers, not infrequently one also sees pigmented macrophages laden with carbon particles in the effusion.

Uremia

Uremic hemopericarditis and, less frequently, uremic pleuritis and nephrogenic ascites are consequences of advanced renal failure. The pleural effusion in these instances is bloody and may reveal lysed and fragmented RBCs in the form of Heinz bodies. The mesothelial cells are extremely reactive and may appear atypical because of the chronic presence of blood and the high urea content of the accumulated fluid (Fig. 7.21). With correction of the renal failure, the effusion

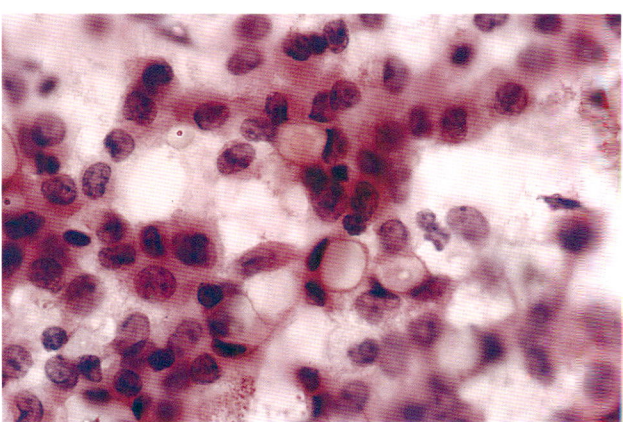

FIGURE 7.18   Signet ring-like appearance of mesothelial cells due to the presence of starch granules in the cytoplasm. Note the variation in the nuclear size, shape, texture, and tinctorial properties of the surrounding mesothelial cells. (Pap × 120)

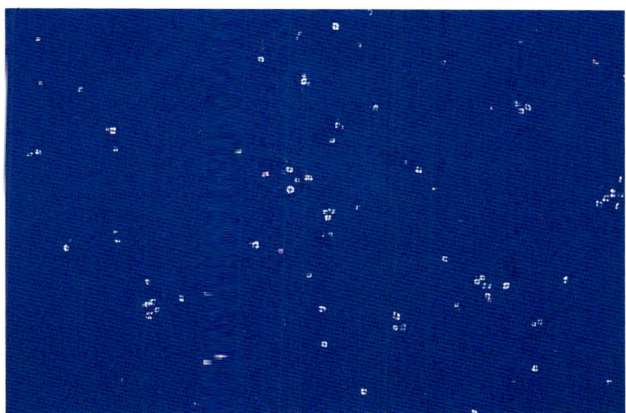

FIGURE 7.19   Same specimen as figure 7.18 examined by polarization microscopy. Starch granules, a common contaminant of talcum powder, demonstrate their typical "maltese cross" birefringence. (Polarized light × 40)

may subside and appear only as a serofibrinous transudate, poor in cells except for the presence of hemosiderin-laden macrophages, lymphocytes, and a rare eosinophil. Koss documented a case in which the abnormalities of mesothelial cells mimicked malignancy even in histologic sections of the pleura at autopsy.

Pancreatitis

Pancreatitis may be accompanied by chronic ascites and may also cause recurrent episodes of hemorrhagic pleural effusions. The cytologic picture of pancreatic ascitis is similar to that of uremic effusions with numerous, often degenerated RBCs, lymphocytes, eosinophils, and reactive mesothelial cells (Fig. 7.22). In full-blown cases, pancreatic enzymes leak into the peritoneal cavity, causing fat necrosis and hemorrhagic effusions. We have seen such cases only at autopsy. They are characterized by low cellularity and considerable autolysis with only rare, degenerated mesothelial cells present. As should be expected, amylase determination is a more reliable diagnostic method for pancreatic ascitis than cytologic examination of the fluid.

Cirrhosis

The presence of atypical clusters of mesothelial cells in ascitic and pleural fluids of patients with liver disease

ranks among the most challenging and neglected aspects of effusion cytology. The extent to which these cells may mimic adenocarcinoma may be astonishing, and, in fact, ploidy studies have shown that these cells may lead to a false-positive diagnosis even by flow cytometric examination. To the clinician, hepatogenic ascites constitutes a difficult dilemma because it is difficult to distinguish between infected and noninfected cirrhotics by examination of the ascitic fluid. Often the ascitic fluid of cirrhotic patients will reveal an increased WBC count, elevated protein content and specific gravity, and no evidence of spontaneous bacterial peritonitis. In general, the accumulated fluid has the characteristics of an exudate, but in extreme cases, hypoproteinemia causes a transudate. Sometimes the fluid may show jaundice. In exudates, the salient feature is hypercellularity due to the presence of proliferating and atypical mesothelial cells.

Virtually all features described previously under "reactive" and "atypical" mesothelial cells can be induced by alcoholic cirrhosis or hepatitis. The most common presentation is in the form of large numbers of cell balls, some attaining up to one hundred individual cells. Only the fact that no alien cell population stands out from the background of mesothelial hyperplasia stops the experienced cytopathologist from rendering a positive diagnosis of metastatic adenocarcinoma. Mesothelioma is ruled out by the clinical history and the lesser number of mesothelial cells in cirrhosis-related hyperplasia. Pleural fluids in patients with cirrhosis, contain considerably fewer cell balls than ascitic fluid. The major problem with cirrhosis occurs when the ascitic fluid is not promptly brought to the laboratory or is left unrefrigerated for a prolonged period. In these cases, the more viable clusters of cells acquire unusual hyperchromasia owing to pyknosis of the nuclei and may stand out from their degenerated neighbors. A good clinical history is essential in these instances if a false-positive diagnosis is to be avoided.

Ancillary procedures have not been extensively explored in the investigation of cirrhosis-related ascites. In a study of pleural effusion by pulse cytophotometry we were puzzled by a "false positive" aneuploidy induced by cirrhosis. Subsequent users of flow cytometry and image analysis observed the same phenomenon, so an increased DNA content cannot be perceived as a sign of malignancy in cirrhotic patients.

SYSTEMIC PROCESSES

Sarcoidosis

The etiology of sarcoidosis, a multisystem disease, remains an enigma even though a poorly understood immunologic mechanism appears the basis of its pathogenesis. The intrathoracic manifestations of sarcoidosis are commonly restricted to the lungs and the hilar lymph nodes, but pleural involvement has been observed in fatal sarcoidosis. Although not a frequent complication of sarcoidosis, both pericardial and pleural effusions secondary to it have been documented in the literature. All reported cases have had in common lymphocytosis, slight eosinophilia, and a slight to moderate reactive hyperplasia of the mesothelial cells. In most cases, T cells are the predominant lymphocyte population, a feature also observed in the bronchoalveolar fluid of patients with active sarcoidosis. In a few cases, giant cells identical to those noted in the lung and hilar lymph nodes were present in the pleural effusion.

Amyloidosis

Koss documented a case of amyloidosis in which rather atypical hyperchromatic cells were noted in the ascitic fluid. We have seen a similar case, characterized by the presence of lymphocytes, plasma cells, and giant cells in a hypocellular serous fluid from the pleural cavities. Of note was the presence of small chunks of amyloid, probably derived from a large, solitary, plaquelike lesion of the lung and pleura, noted at pneumonectomy. Only a few reactive mesothelial cells were present, some of which displayed enlarged and hyperchromatic nuclei.

EXTRANEOUS ELEMENTS

Noncellular Structures

Effusions may demonstrate a number of noncellular elements which may nevertheless reflect underlying pathologic processes. Some of these represent extraneous material introduced into the pleural and peritoneal space for diagnostic and therapeutic purposes. Talc, lipid contrast medium, and latex beads all fall in this category. Talcum powder was formerly discussed in relation to pleurodesis in patients with persistent pleurisy due to tuberculosis and other chronic pulmonary diseases. Talc may also enter the pleural and peritoneal spaces during surgery, accumulating and becoming the source of effusions. The mesothelium is extremely reactive to foreign substances, and the resulting mesothelial hyperplasia may be quite intense. Talc crystals are approximately the size of a mesothelial cell and give, as noted previously, the characteristic maltese cross appearance under polarized light. In cases of extreme obesity, excessive fat accumulates in the submesothelial layer where it excites a foreign body granuloma containing histiocytes, epithelial cells, and multinucleated giant cells.

Certain structures can be formed by the degradation of cellular products: corpora amylacea, calcific concretions, and psammoma bodies. They too are unwelcome elements in a serous cavity and may result in mesothelial hyperplasia. Psammoma bodies are the most conspicuous because of their unique concentric laminations and association with neoplasia. It should be remembered, however, that the mesothelium is prone to form these structures in nonmalignant conditions such as postsurgical status, particularly of the pericardium and pelvic peritoneum.

Products of cellular metabolism may accumulate in effusions in the form of crystals with typical morphology that makes them easy to identify. Charcot–Leyden crystals form as a degradation product of eosinophilic granules, acquiring an eosinophilic color and an angular lozenge shape as illustrated in chapter 5. They are quite variable in size and as such may occur either intracellu-

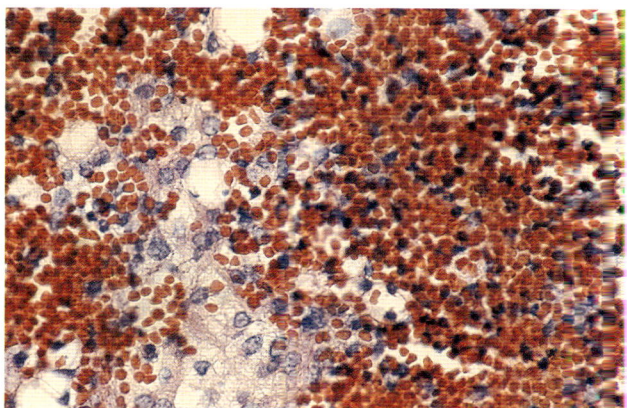

FIGURE 7.20 Sheet-like reactive mesothelial cells in a pulmonary infarct. Even though RBCs and fibrin may later be resorbed, these reactive cells persist for months after the acute episode. (H&E × 40)

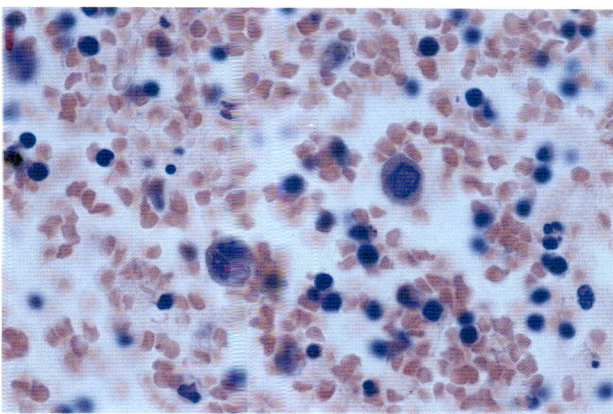

FIGURE 7.22 Reactive mesothelial cells in pancreatic ascites. Pyknosis has set in and these cells can be easily mistaken for malignant cells. The smudged RBCs, however, are indicative of degeneration. (H&E × 60)

larly or in a free state. Cholesterol crystals are typical of pseudochylous effusions of long duration. They are formed endogenously by the breakdown of cellular products, and their accumulation imparts a glistening appearance to the effusions. Old fibrinopurulent pleuritis, the pleurisy of rheumatoid arthritis, and tuberculous empyema are prone to the development of cholesterol-containing effusions. Stacked, rectangular, and angulated cholesterol crystals fail to stain with Papanicolaou's and Romanowsky's methods, but reflect and

refract the light under polarization. The resulting effect leads to a multicolored kaleidoscope, worthy of abstract art status (Figs. 7.23 and 7.24).

In old hemorrhagic effusions, hemoglobin crystals resembling Heinz bodies may be formed, but the most common outcome is accumulation of hemosiderin. The resulting effusion is chronic, with lymphocytsis and macrophages showing erythrophagocytosis (Fig. 7.25). If the effusion is left standing without prompt fixation, hematoidin, an oxidized product of hemoglobin, is formed instead. Lymphoplasmacytic effusions may on occasion display a few cells with Russell bodies or fully formed immunoglobulin crystals (Mott cells). We have not seen such an example, but the phenomenon is beautifully illustrated by Spriggs and Bodington in their monograph.

Asbestos Bodies and Other Foreign Substances

With asbestiform minerals preferring the pleura and peritoneum as their target, it is a wonder that asbestos bodies are not found more frequently in effusions. Asbestos fibers may be uncoated or coated by a mixture of protein and iron, in which case some authors refer to them as ferruginous bodies. Uncoated asbestos fibers are not readily visible under light microscopy, and because they are extremely thin, they polarize the light only faintly or do not polarize it at all. Despite a diligent search, including chlorine bleach digestion and iron

FIGURE 7.21 Hyperplastic mesothelial cells secondary to uremia. Despite the bizarre shape of their cytoplasm, the cells leave windows between one another. Also note the degenerative changes of the nuclei. (H&E × 90)

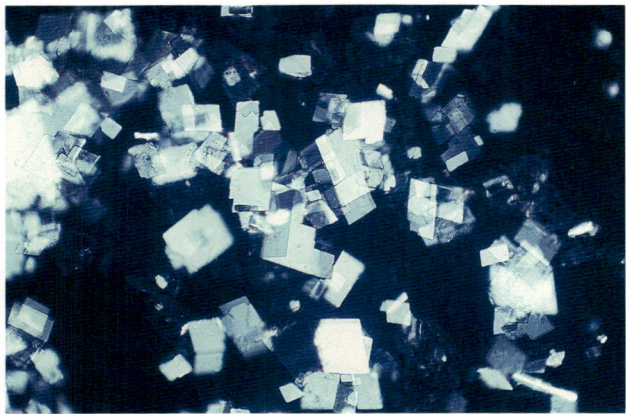

FIGURE 7.23   Cholesterol crystals in long-standing effusion. Notice squared off crystalline structures against a dark background. (Courtesy of P. Gupta, MD)

TABLE 7.3   Cytologic Pitfalls in Reactive Mesothelial Hyperplasia

Papillary cluster with collaginous core
Psammoma bodies
Degeneration of cytoplasm
Hyperchromatic nuclei
High nuclear : cytoplasmic ratio
Prominent nucleoli
Signet-ring change
High mitotic rate

staining of pleural tissues from asbestos workers, only a rare case will show asbestos bodies (Figs. 7.26 and 7.27). The most likely explanation is that fibers break down once they reach the pleura and the peritoneum, their fragments being too small to fully form asbestos bodies.

Despite being invisible, air is the most ubiquitous substance in the universe. A welcome guest in the alveoli of the lung, air is inhospitable in the body cavities. Both pneumothorax and pneumoperitoneum act as irritants to the mesothelial surfaces, causing reactive eosinophilic pleuritis and peritonitis (Fig. 7.28). No one knows what mediates the eosinophilotactic effect of the air, but eosinophils release their granules in the submesothelial layer, leading to fibrosis overlaid by reactive mesothelial hyperplasia.

Diagnostic Pitfalls

Effusions often constitute a difficult facet of cytology for anyone to master. The florid and variegated appearance of mesothelial hyperplasia may lead to a false-positive diagnosis, particularly if the cytopathologist is not aware of the underlying causes of the effusion (Table 7.3). This occurs because many of the cytologic alterations noted in reactive mesothelial cells mimic certain aspects of malignancy. These include: nuclear hyperchromasia, high nuclear : cytoplasmic ratio, slight thickening of the nuclear membranes, high mitotic rate and prominent nucleoli. Occasionally, medium to moderately sized papillary groups display a definite collagenous core. Groups such as these may be mistaken for carcinoma, particularly if one pays no attention to the clinical history and ignores clues to nonmalignancy such as the absence of more than one cell type in the effusion. It is anecdotally believed that mesothelial spherules with a collagenous core are more common in the pericardium because of the beating of the heart (Fig. 7.29). Even though no statistical study exists to support such a contention, small mesothelial excrescencies are often encountered in the pericardium at autopsy (Fig. 7.30). Recognition of the collagenous core in cytologic specimens can be accomplished by refocusing the microscope or the use of Masson's (Fig. 7.31) stain. The pericardium is also the site of mesothelial proliferations lacking a collagenous core and displaying a scalloped contour (Fig. 7.32). The resulting proliferative spheres may be hollow or solid and show considerable complexity but do not show features of malignancy (Fig. 7.33).

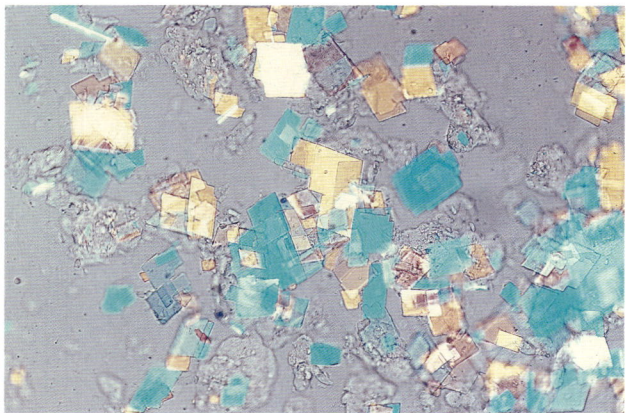

FIGURE 7-24   Same case as figure 7.24 depending on the filter utilized, the crystalline particles acquire different discoloration. (Polarized light × 80) (Courtesy of P. Gupta, MD)

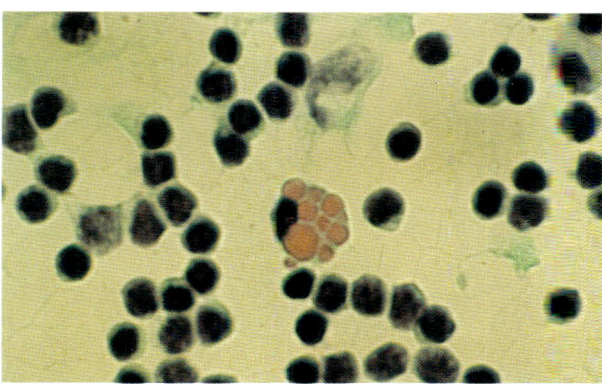

FIGURE 7.25 Erythrophagocytosis in hemorrhagic ascites secondary to peritoneal dialysis. Note the lymphocytosis indicative of the chronic reactive process. (Pap × 60) (Courtesy D. Hidvegi, MD)

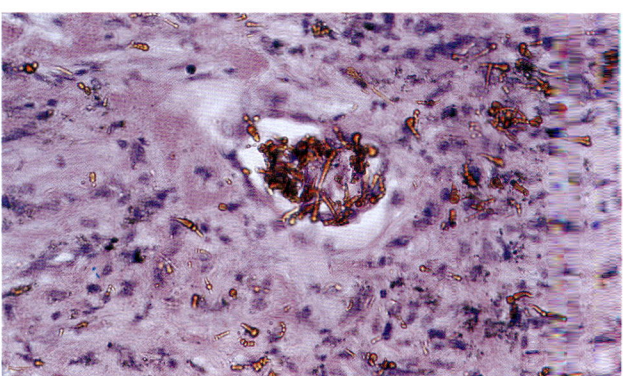

FIGURE 7.26 Pleural strippings from an asbestos worker digested and concentrated as a cell block. Note asbestos bodies near the center surrounded by fragmented ferruginous structures. (H&E × 40)

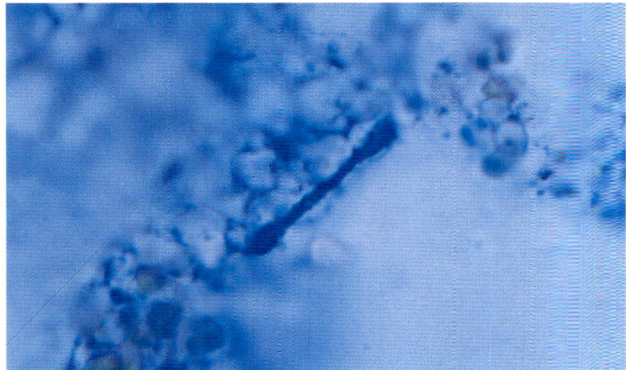

FIGURE 7.27 Same case as Fig 7.26. Filter preparation digested by chlorine bleach and stained by Prussian blue. Note the typical asbestos body among the liquefied cellular debris. (MGG × 60)

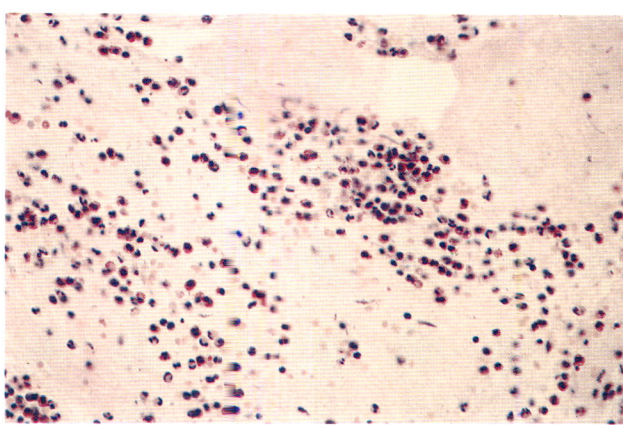

FIGURE 7.28 Effusion from a patient recovering from pneumothorax. Leukocytes show binucleation and faint granularity of the cytoplasm, typical of eosinophils stained by Papanicolaou's method. (Pap × 40)

Dark cells, with high N/C ratio are typical of endometriosis and may be misinterpreted as malignant. A great deal of caution should be exercised where dark, small cells appear in sheets and the possibility of endometriosis should be entertained (Fig 7.34). Another cause of concern that might develop into false-positive diagnosis is the presence of psammoma bodies in a degenerated specimen. As the cytoplasm is partially lost, the nuclear:cytoplasmic ratio is artificially increased in cells undergoing degeneration. Pyknosis sets in and nuclei may appear enlarged, compounding the interpretational dilemma. A peculiar form of degeneration leads to the formation of detached ciliary tufts (DCTs) without

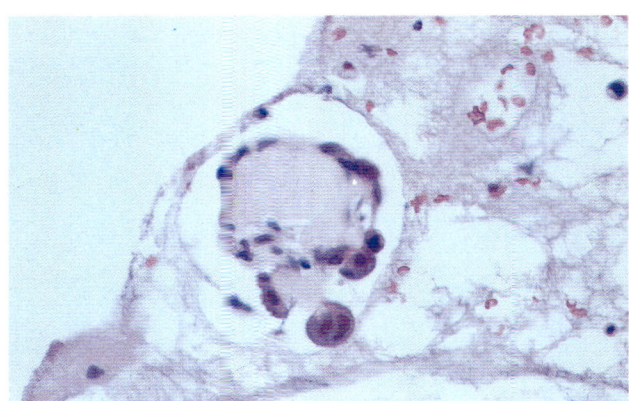

FIGURE 7.29 Cell block from hyperplastic pericardial mesothelium. Note the papillary proliferation reactive mesothelial cells showing a collagenous core. (H&E × 40)

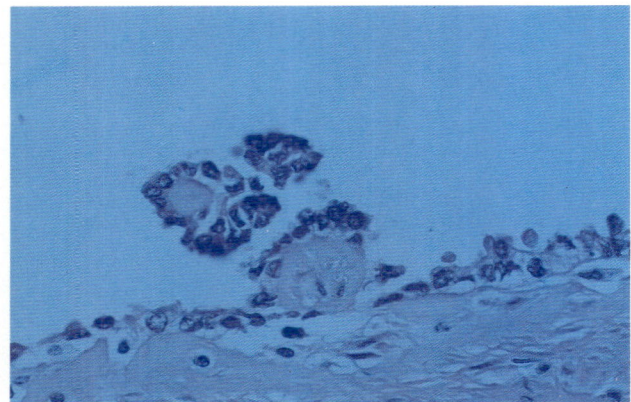

FIGURE 7.30 Autopsy section from hyperplastic pericardial mesothelium. The papillary excrecencies display a collagenous core. (H&E × 40)

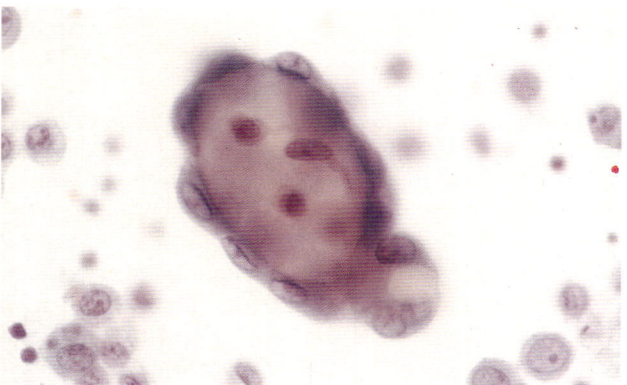

FIGURE 7.31 Cytologic specimen from pericardial fluid. Note the fibrous core containing elongated, fibroblast-like cells, surrounded by mesothelial cells. (Pap × 240)

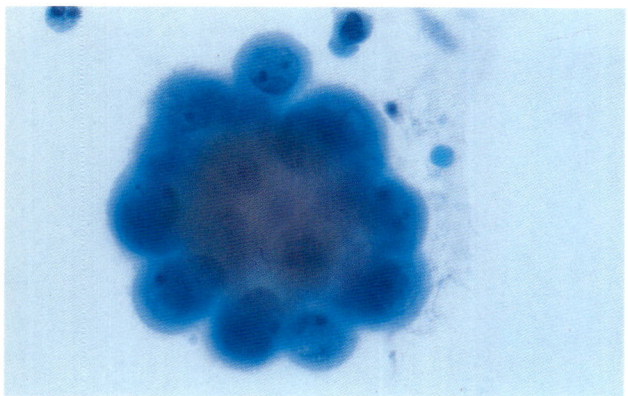

FIGURE 7.32 Proliferative sphere of mesothelial cells with typical scalloped contour. Even after refocusing the microscope, no collagenous core was identified. (Pap × 240)

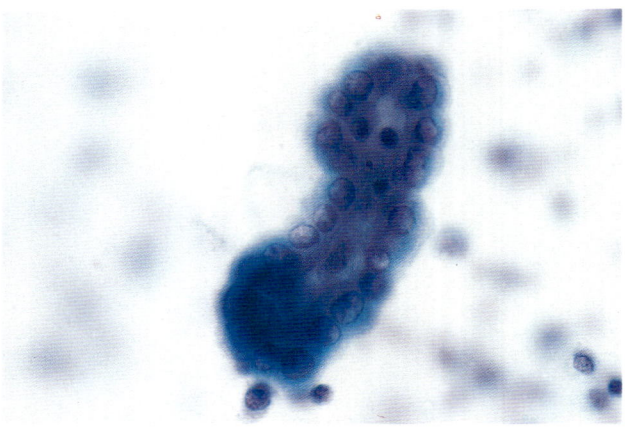

FIGURE 7.33 Proliferative mesothelial sphere of greater complexity. Notice fibrovascular core surrounded by hyperplastic mesothelial cells (Pap × 180).

attachment of cytoplasm or another cell component. However, these are seldom confusible with malignancy. Mesothelial cells may also degenerate in the form of signet-ring—like elements, and set the stage for undue worry. One should also ignore other causes of false alarm such as a high mitotic rate and multinucleation. Both mesothelial cells and macrophages benefit from the excellent nourishment provided by the natural "culture medium" that the effusion represents these cells continue to proliferate even after the specimen is collected until fixative is added. Koss emphasizes that a great insurance against false-positive interpretation of

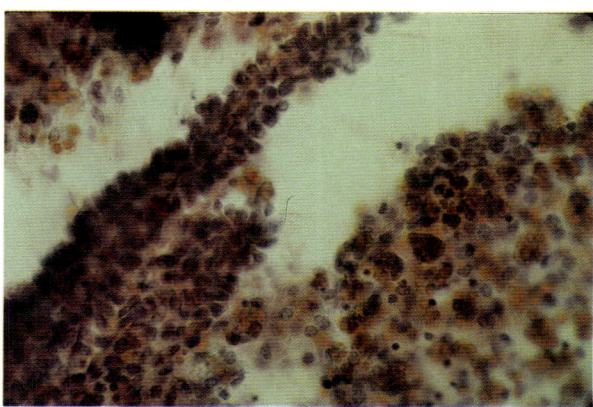

FIGURE 7.34 Ascites from a patient with endometriosis of the peritoneum. Sheets of endometrial cells are darker and larger than the individual mesothelial cells. The background contains hemosiderin. (Courtesy D. Hidvegi, MD)

effusions is not to venture a diagnosis of malignancy unless technically adequate preparations are available for examination.

BIBLIOGRAPHY

Radiation

Ariel IM, Oropeza R, Pack GT. Intracavitary administration of radioactive isotopes in the control of effusions due to cancer. Results in 267 patients. *Cancer.* 1966;19:1906–1112.

Martin RG, Ruckdeschel J, Chang P, et al. Radiation-related pericarditis. *Am J Cardiol.* 1975;35:216–220.

Masland DS, Rotz CT, Harris JH Jr. Postradiation pericarditis with chronic pericardial effusion. *Ann Intern Med* 1968;68:97–102.

Cham WC, Freiman AH, Carstens PHB et al. Radiation therapy of cardiac and pericardial metastases. *Radiology.* 1975;114:701–704.

Torres E, Guevara E. Pleuritis by radiation: Report of two cases. *Acta Cytol.* 1981;25:427–429.

Chemotherapy

Bedrossian CWM. Iatrogenic and toxic injury. In: Dail D, Hammar S, eds. *Pulmonary Pathology.* New York: Springer-Verlag; 1988: chap 14.

Cava E, Marsan C, Accard JL, et al. Modifications cytologiques des epanchements pleuraux malins traites par chimiotherapie locale. *Arch Anat Cytol Pathol.* 1980;28:350–354.

Ecker MD, Jay B, Keohane MF. Procarbezine lung. *AJR.* 1978;131:527–528.

Hailey FJ, Glascock HW Jr, Hewitt WF. Pleuropneumonic reactions to nitrofurantoin. *N Engl J Med.* 1969;281:1087–1090.

Kok-Jensen A, Lindeneg O. Pleurisy and fibrosis of the pleura during methysergide treatment of hemicrania. *Scand J Respir Dis.* 1970;51:218–222.

LeWitt PA, Calne DB. Pleuropulmonary changes during long-term bromocriptine treatment for Parkinson's disease. *Lancet.* 1981;1:44–45.

Walden PAM et al: Pleurisy and methotrexate treatment. *BMJ.* 1977;2:867.

Dialysis

Berger HW, Rammohan G, Neff MS, et al. Uremic pleural effusion: A study of 14 patients on chronic dialysis. *Ann Intern Med.* 1975;82:362–364.

Cardon G, dellaGiustina D. Atypical mesothelial cells in peritoneal dialysis fluid. *Acta Cytol* 1983;27:706–708.

Galen MA, Stinberg SM, Lowrie EG, et al. Hemorrhagic pleural effusion in patients undergoing chronic hemodialysis. *Ann Intern Med.* 1975;82:359–361.

Johnson R, Ramsey P, Gallagher N, et al. Fungal peritonitis in patients on peritoneal dialysis: Incidence, clinical features, and prognosis. *Am J Nephrol.* 1985;5:169–175.

Peritoneal Washings

Barbee CL, Gilsdorf RB Diagnostic peritoneal lavage in evaluating acute abdominal pain. *Ann Surg.* 1975;181:853–856.

Evans C, Rashid A, Rosenberg IL, et al. An appraisal of peritoneal lavage in the diagnosis of the acute abdomen. *Br J Surg.* 1975;62:119–120

Zuna RE, Mitchell ML. Cytologic findings in peritoneal washings associated with benign gynecologic disease. *Acta Cytol.* 1988;139–142.

Pleurodesis

Adler RH. A talc powder aerosol method for the prevention of recurrent spontaneous pneumothorax. *Ann Thorac Surg.* 1968;5:474–477.

Jackson JW, Bennett MH. Chest wall tumor following iodized talc pleurodesis. *Thorax.* 1969;28:788–793.

Goldszer RC, Bennett J, VanCampen J, et al. Intrapleural tetracycline for spontaneous pneumothorax. *JAMA* 1979;241:724–725.

Ofoegbu RO. Pleurodesis for spontaneous pneumothorax: Experience with intrapleural olive oil in high risk patients. *Am J Surg.* 1980;140:673–681.

Infarction

Holt S, Kirkman N, Myerscough E. Hemothorax after subclavian vein cannulation. *Thorax.* 1977;32:101–103.

Kossowsky WA, Epstein PJ, Levine RS. Post–myocardial infarction syndrome: An early complication of acute myocardial infarction. *Chest.* 1973;63:35–40.

Stelzner TJ, King TE, Antony VB, et al. Post–cardiac injury syndrome (PCIS): Pleuropulmonary manifestations. *Am Rev Respir Dis.* 1982;125:81A.

Urschel HC Jr, Razzuk MA, Gardner M. Coronary artery bypass occlusion secondary to post-cardiotomy syndrome. *Ann Thorac Surg.* 1976;22:528–531.

Cirrhosis

Darnis F. Cirrhosis edema-ascites syndrome. The role of hormonal abnormalities in the pathogenesis. *Minn Med.* 1971;54:143–150. Review.

Cline MM, McCallum RW, Guth PH. The clinical value of ascitic fluid in alcoholic liver disease. *Gastroenterology.* 1976;70:408–412.

Pearlman DM. Hepatogenic ascites: Pathogenesis and management. *NY State J Med.* 1968;68:1837–1842.

Wilson JAP, Suguitan EA, Cassidy WA. Characteristics of ascitic fluid in the alcoholic cirrhotic. *Dig Dis Sci.* 1979;24:645–648.

Uremia

Alfrey AC, Goss JE, Ogden DA: Uremic hemopericardium. *Am J Med.* 1968;45:391–400.

Berger HW, Rammohan G, Neff MS, et al. Uremic pleural effusion: A study in 14 patients on chronic dialysis. *Ann Intern Med.* 1975;82:362–364.

Buja LM. Friedman CA, Roberts WC. Hemorrhagic pericarditis in uremia. Clinicopathologic studies in six patients. *Arch Pathol.* 1966;90:325–330.

Craig R, Sparberg M, Ivanovich P, et al. Nephrogenic ascites. *Arch Intern Med.* 1974;134:276–279.

Gilbert L. Fibrinous uremic pleuritis: A surgical entity. *Chest.* 1975;67:53–56.

Lindsay J Jr, Crawley IS, Callaway GM Jr. Chronic constrictive pericarditis following uremic hemopericardium. *Am Heart J.* 1970;79:390–395.

Nidus BD, Matalon R, Cantacuzino D, et al. Uremic pleuritis—a clinicopathological entity. *N Engl J Med.* 1969;281:255–256.

Pancreatitis

Anderson WJ, Skinner DB, Zuidema GD, et al. Chronic pancreatic pleural effusions. *Surg Gynecol Obstet.* 1973;137:827–830.

Chochran JW. Pancreatic pseudocyst presenting as massive hemothorax. *Am J Gastroenterol.* 1978;69:84–87.

Coupland G. Pancreatic ascites in childhood. *J Pediatr Surg.* 1970;5:570.

Donowitz M, Kerstein MD, Spiro HM. Pancreatic ascites. *Medicine.* 1974;53:183–195.

Kirianoff T, Strauch GO, Rogers JF. The nature of pancreatic ascites. *Conn Med.* 1969;33:573–575.

Miridjanian A, Ambruoso VN, Derby BM, et al. Massive bilateral hemorrhagic pleural effusions in chronic relapsing pancreatitis. *Arch Surg.* 1969;98:62–66.

Schindler SC, Schaefer JW, Hull D, et al. Chronic pancreatic ascites. *Gastroenterology.* 1970;59:453–459.

Shetty AN. Pseudocysts of the pancreas: An overview. *South Med J.* 1980;73:1239–1242.

Svane S. Recurrent, hemorrhagic pleural effusion and eosinophilia accompanying pancreatitis. *Acta Chir Scand.* 1966;131:352–356.

Noncellular Structures

Martin A, Carstens P, Yam L. Crystalline deposits in ascites in a case of cryoglobulinemia. *Acta Cytol.* 1987;31(5):631–636.

Naylor B, Novak PM. Charcot-Leyden crystals in pleural fluids. *Acta Cytol.* 1985;29:781–784.

Pfitzer P. Eosinophil pleural effusion with Charcot-Leyden Crystals. *Acta Cytol.* 1985;29:906–907.

Reyes CV, Katchuria S, MacGlashan A. Diagnostic value of sodium oxalate crystals in respiratory and pleural cytology: A case report. *Acta Cytol.* 1979;23:65–68.

Asbestosis

Bedrossian CWM, Landas S, Schwartz D. Significance and follow-up of asbestos bodies in cytologic specimens. (In preparation)

Epler GR, McLoud TC, Gaensler EA. Prevalence and incidence of benign asbestos pleural effusion in a working population. *JAMA* 1982;247:617–622.

Gaensler EA, Kaplan AI. Asbestos pleural effusion. *Ann Intern Med.* 1971;74:178–191.

Hillerdai G, Ozesmi M. Benign asbestos pleural effusion: 73 exudates in 60 patients. *Eur J Respir Dis.* 1987;71(2):113–121.

Mattson SB. Monosymptomatic exudative pleuresy in persons exposed to asbestos dust. *Scand J Respir Dis.* 1975;56:263–272.

Sarcoidosis

Chusid EL, Viera LOBD, Siltzbach LE. Sarcoidosis of the pleura. In: Iwai K, Hoseda Y, eds. *Proceedings of the Sixth International Conference on Sarcoidosis.* Tokyo: University Park Press; 1974:373–378.

Greman GS, Castele RJ, Altose MD, et al. Lymphocyte subpopulations in sarcoid pleural effusion. *Ann Intern Med.* 1984;100:75–79.

Kinney E, Murthy R, Ascunce G, et al. Pericardial effusions in sarcoidosis. *Chest.* 1979;76:476–478.

Papowitz AJ, Jk LI. Abdominal sarcoidosis with ascites. *Chest.* 1971;59:692–695.

Sharma OP, Gordonson J. Pleural effusion in sarcoidosis: A report of six cases. *Thorax.* 1975;30:95–101.

Shiff AD, Blatt CJ, Colp C. Recurrent pericardial effusion secondary to sarcoidosis of the pericardium. *N Engl J Med.* 1969;281:141–143.

Stork WJ, Greenberg SD, Bedrossian CWM. Fatal sarcoidosis. In: Iwai K, Hoseda Y, eds. *Proceeding of the Sixth International Conference on Sarcoidosis.* Tokyo: University Park Press; 1974:462–472.

CHAPTER EIGHT

Mesothelioma

Mesothelioma has gained a lot of attention because of the medico-legal implications of asbestos exposure. Whether or not there is a true increase in the incidence of mesothelioma is the subject of ongoing epidemiologic studies. Nevertheless, the cytopathologist should be familiar with the cytologic appearance of this neoplasm and should suspect mesothelioma in the correct clinical setting. This includes a history of asbestos exposure, appropriate radiologic findings, a bloody effusion lacking plausible explanation and clinico-radiologic data excluding a primary tumor elsewhere. A bloody effusion is an almost universal mode of presentation of mesothelioma. Approximately 90% of mesotheliomas are pleural in origin, the remainder appearing in the peritoneum either alone or in combination with pleural ones. Only rarely does one see a pericardial mesothelioma without involvement of the adjacent pleura and lung. One of the most striking features of mesothelioma is the high number of cells noted in the effusion. Even when the mesothelial cells are relatively bland, their excessive number raises the suspicion of mesothelioma. Another cardinal feature: cells in mesothelioma resemble one another unlike carcinomatous cells that stand out from their mesothelial neighbors.

The diffuse type of epithelial mesothelioma is the prototype of malignant mesothelioma, arising most frequently in the pleura and less commonly in the peritoneal and the pericardial sacs (Fig. 8.1). The tumor is related to asbestos exposure anywhere from ten to thirty years prior to the onset of symptoms. Chest pain and weight loss are followed by pleural effusion which is detected by the chest X ray. The diagnosis may be established by pleural biopsy or by cytologic examination of the effusion—malignant mesothelial cells are very numerous and they may attain a solid acinar or papillary configuration and any combination thereof. Mesotheliomas may cover an extensive area which comes into contact with the serosal cavity. This explains the very large number of cells present in cytologic speci-

mens showing mesothelioma (Fig. 8.2). Mesotheliomas may closely mimic adenocarcinoma in cytologic and tissue biopsy specimens. In biopsy specimens mesotheliomas have a variegated histologic appearance ranging from solid, to acinar; from tubulo-papillary to anaplastic. In cytologic specimens the cells are larger than both normal mesothelial cells and carcinoma cells. They occur either singly or as cell balls ranging from few to literally thousands of cells. Despite the extreme variety in the size and shape of the groups, the nuclei of the tumor cells are monotonous in appearance and there is never a distinct impression of more than one cell population (Fig. 8.3). The chromatin distribution is finely to coarsely granular and nucleoli are not so prominent as those seen in adenocarcinoma. The greatest diagnostic difficulty is to distinguish mesothelioma from mesothelial hyperplasia because of the similarities of their nuclei. Clinical history and the number and size of the clusters are crucial in establishing the correct diagnosis. Ancillary procedures capable of establishing the intermediate filament content of the cells do not solve this dilemma because both nonmalignant and malignant mesothelial cells share the same intermediate filaments. Ploidy determination, however, is of assistance by demonstrating aneuploidy in mesothelioma, whereas a diploid population is the rule in hyperplasia. Measurement of proliferative activity also holds some promise in the distinction between mesothelial hyperplasia and mesothelioma.

MESOTHELIAL PROCESSES DETECTED BY CYTOLOGY

Nonmalignant Mesothelial Proliferations

The peritoneal mesothelium shares many characteristics with the cells covering the surface of the gonads. No

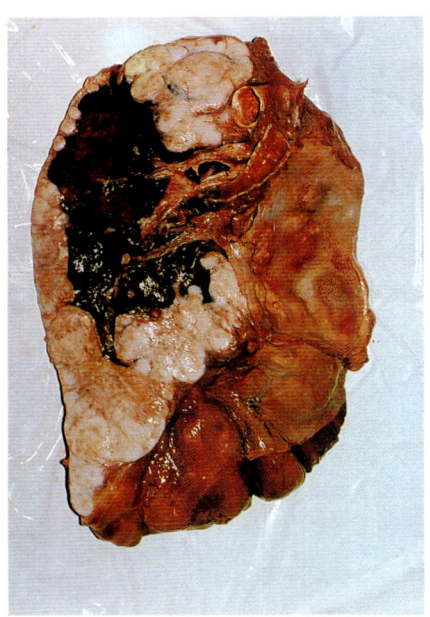

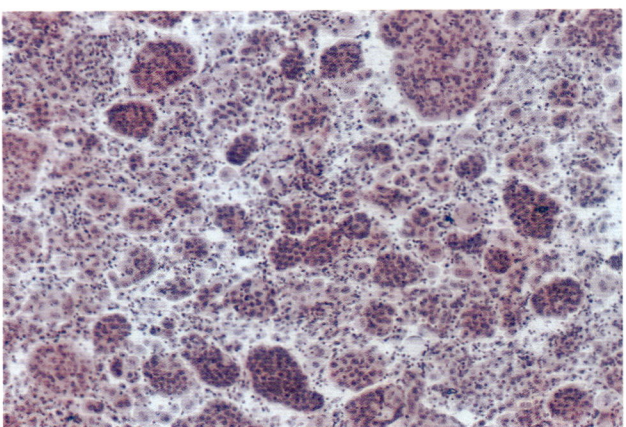

FIGURE 8.3 Cytologic specimen from mesothelioma. The pleural fluid contains thousands of tumor cells resembling one another. Note the enormous size of the cell balls. (Pap × 60)

FIGURE 8.1 Gross appearance of the lungs in malignant mesothelioma. The neoplasm involves the visceral pleura, extends along the subpleural space and penetrates the right lung parenchyma at several points. (Courtesy M. Melamed, MD)

wonder the pelvic peritoneum may be the site of benign tumors that resemble those of testicular and ovarian origin. In the testes these are known as adenomatoid tumors but in the ovaries the tendency is to classify them as papillary serous tumors of the ovary. This is

significant because papillary excrecencies arising from the surface of the ovary may represent a localized form of mesothelioma. The converse may also occur, with papillary tumors affecting the abdominal peritoneum in a multifocal fashion, and both ovaries being spared. The problem is compounded by the fact that the peritoneal mesothelium is apparently related to tissues of müllerian origin and is subject to the same influences that act upon structures of müllerian origin. This relationship is attested by endometriosis, which usually affects the pelvic mesothelium, and by decidual reaction of the peritoneum, which may occur extensively during pregnancy. When evaluated by immunocytochemistry some peritoneal papillary tumors share certain antigens, such as placental lactogen and CA-125, with papillary serous tumors of the ovary and with other müllerian-derived tissues which include the normal fallopian tube, the endometrium and the endocervix. Both sexes may also show benign proliferative groups of mesothelial cells unrelated to the gonads as discussed in the previous chapter.

Benign Papillary Mesothelioma

The presence of papillary clusters in peritoneal fluid or pelvic washings is a common problem facing the cytopathologist. Sometimes these have either a very well differentiated or a deceptively benign-appearing cytologic configuration. Psammoma bodies are frequently noted in association with the papillary tufts. The first

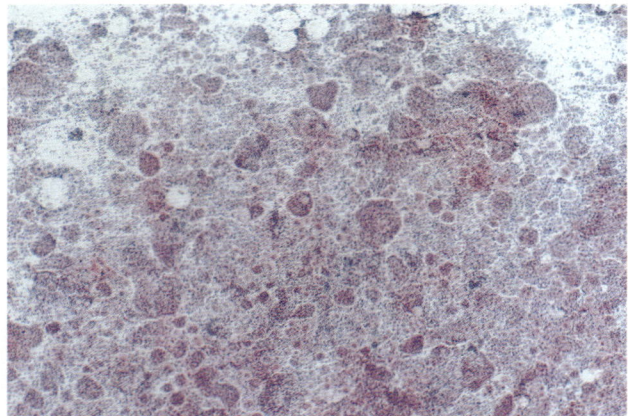

FIGURE 8.2 Low power view of malignant mesothelioma. The wall-to-wall cellularity is typical of this neoplasm and not attained by mesothelial hyperplasia (Pap × 40)

differential diagnosis to be considered is ovarian neoplasm, most commonly a papillary serous cystadenocarcinoma or a borderline serous tumor. If ovarian involvement is ruled out by CT scan or laparoscopy, some nonmalignant conditions that should be considered are benign inclusion cysts of the peritoneum, chronic salpingitis, and chronic peritonitis. If these pelvic conditions are eliminated, the diagnosis of benign papillary mesothelioma of the peritoneum should be entertained in contradistinction to that of diffuse malignant mesothelioma. In the latter, the nuclei are considerably more bizarre, the number of cells is extremely high, and the psammoma bodies are a minor component of the cellular sample. Differentiation between benign papillary mesothelioma and papillary serous carcinoma of the ovary may be moot, since the specialized ovarian epithelium could well be the origin of both papillary serous carcinoma and mesothelioma. In addition, benign-appearing mesothelial proliferations may behave in a malignant fashion and affect a considerable area of mesothelial surfaces to which it extends by implantation.

MALIGNANT EPITHELIAL MESOTHELIOMA

Epithelioid mesotheliomas are more often accompanied by effusion than any other type. Mesotheliomatous effusions are characterized by a bloody but not necessarily necrotic background. The dominant feature is the monotony exhibited by exceedingly numerous mesothelial cells (Fig. 8.4). Most of them are clustered or arranged

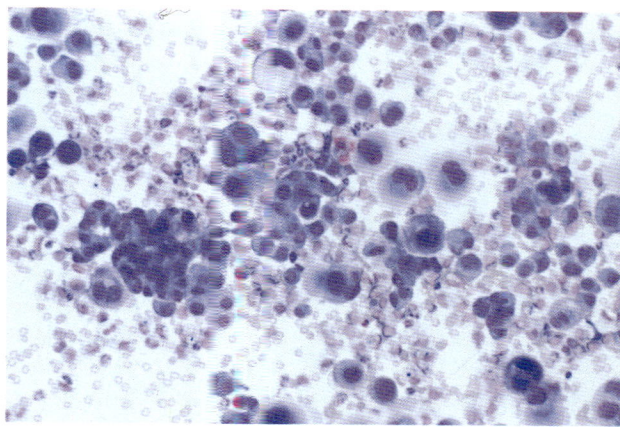

FIGURE 8.5 Malignant mesothelioma by Romanovskis stain. The cells are enlarged but the N/C ratio is not markedly elevated. Notice high cellularity and degeneration of tumor cells. (Pap × 90)

in cell balls, but smaller groups, as well as doublets and isolated mesothelial cells are also present (Fig. 8.5). Individual cells resemble their normal counterparts and they are related to other cells in a mesothelial-like fashion (Fig. 8.6). Malignant cells may also display multinucleation, but their nuclei are not nearly as bizarre as the cells of a sarcoma. The most common cellular feature, however, is for mesotheliomatous cells to appear as cellular aggregates (Fig. 8.7). Some of the cell aggregates have smooth outlines, but scalloped borders often result from protruding single cells or small groups of cells. In the tight cell groups the articulation between cells may be very intimate, but in the looser cell aggregates the

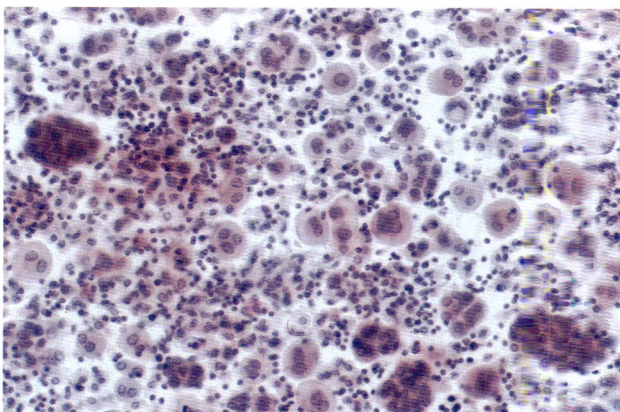

FIGURE 8.4 Pap stained appearance of malignant mesothelioma. Notice spectrum from hyperplastic to neoplastic mesothelial cells. (Pap × 90)

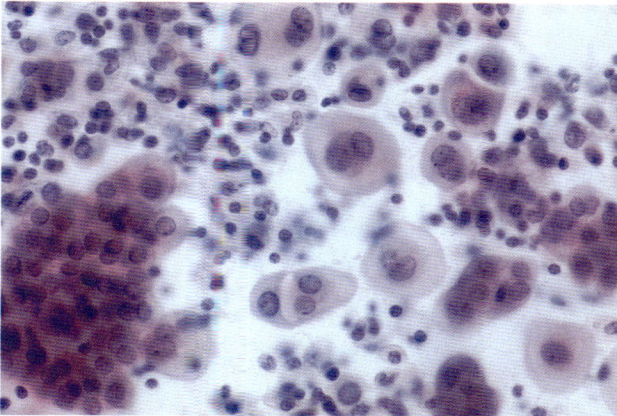

FIGURE 8.6 Medium power view of malignant mesothelioma. The tumor cells show the same intercellular arrangements of ordinary mesothelial cells (Pap × 120)

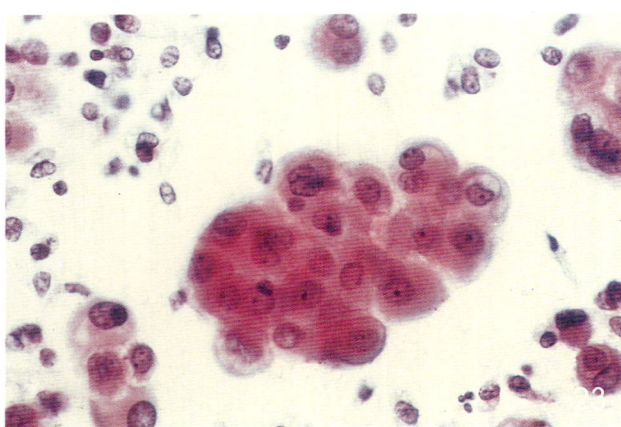

FIGURE 8.7 Group of malignant mesothelial cells showing articulations between themselves similar to those of their nonmalignant counterparts. The cytoplasm is dense and eosinophilic. Note the lymphocytes dwarfed in the background. (Pap × 120)

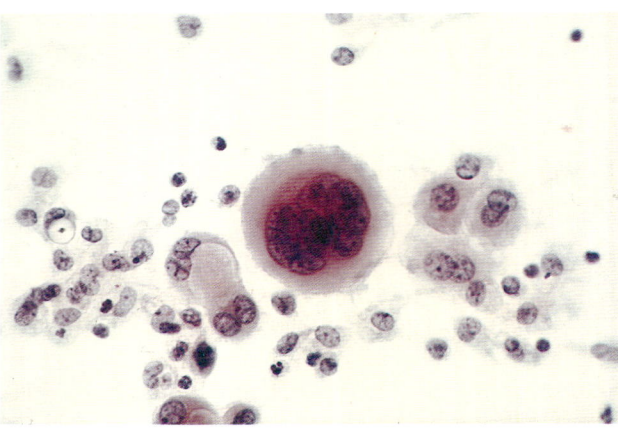

FIGURE 8.9 Multinucleated mesothelial cells in malignant mesothelioma. Several bizzare hyperchromatic nuclei overlie one another. (Pap × 120) (Courtesy of S-B. Buckner CT)

characteristic crescent-shaped window can be observed between the cells. Mesotheliomatous cells appear to extend clawlike prongs in an attempt to engulf their smaller neighbors but without quite succeeding. The result may be a simulation of a cell-in-cell arrangement when in reality the smaller cell lies in a dimple of the other (Fig. 8.8). The empty spaces thus created may require refocusing for their full appreciation, but they may be enhanced by the EMA immunostain. Mesotheliomatous cells may form intracytoplasmic lumina but they never do so to the extent that carcinomas may do. In contrast with carcinoma mesothelioma seldom sheds

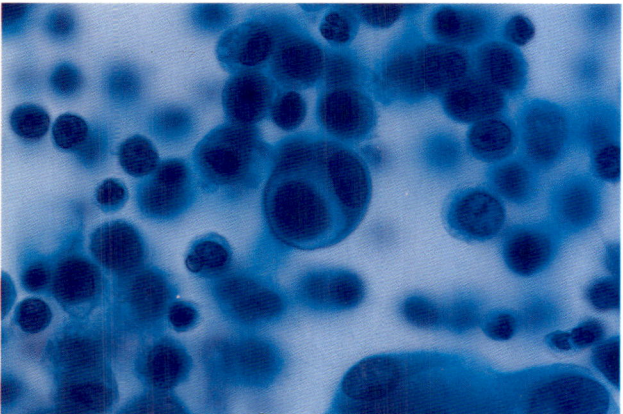

FIGURE 8.8 Cell-in-cell arrangement, simulated by one mesothelial cell engulfing another in the classic clasplike arrangement. The smaller cell is pyknotic, indicative of degeneration. (Pap × 120)

large pleomorphic cells. Even when malignant mesothelial cells are very large they still resemble their benign counterpart (Fig. 8.9). The cytoplasm of malignant mesothelial cells bears striking resemblance to that of their nonmalignant counterpart. Preserved are (1) the two-tone quality of the cytoplasmic texture, (2) the amphophilia represented by dark-maroon perinuclear zones and paler periphery, (3) the ruffled cellular borders in an irregular fashion, (4) peripheral vacuolization, and (5) an occasional cell pinching another, causing a protrusion of the cytoplasm of the pinched member of the pair. Because of the stickiness of the slender microvilli or bleb formation within these, pseudovacuolization is very common at the edge of malignant mesothelial cells. These and other less common cytologic features of mesothelioma are summarized in Table 8.1. The cytologic monotony of mesothelioma extends to the nuclei, mostly medium sized and rounded to oval in shape. They are larger than normal and reactive mesothelial cells, but the chromatin distribution and the appearance of the nucleoli may be deceptively bland. Irregular chromatin distribution and bright eosinophilic nucleoli as noted in adenocarcinoma are not the rule in malignant mesothelioma. Intranuclear inclusions are also rare in mesothelioma, even though they are common in certain types of adenocarcinoma. Although mesotheliomas may attain a biphasic epithelial and spindle pattern, the epithelial pattern predominates and the cells tend to ball up in the effusion. Thus, the lack of a biphasic pattern in cytologic specimens is not a reason to rule out mesothelioma. Cell clusters with scalloped borders and variable sizes, composed of thousands of tumor cells, are the most helpful feature in differentiating mesothelioma from carcinoma. In mesothelioma all

TABLE 8.1 Cytologic Features that Enable One to Recognize Malignant Cells as Deriving from Mesothelioma

Groupings of Cells:
Excessive number of malignant cells
No evidence of a two-cell population
High number of cells in the cell balls
Doublets and triplets still recognizable
Rare acinar groups with extracellular lumina
Individual cells betray their mesothelial origin
Individual Cells:
Ecto–endoplasmic demarcation
Fuzzy border around entire perimeter
Clasplike articulation between two cells
Protrusion from pinched member of the pair
Window-like spaces between the cells
Peripheral revacuolization of bleb formation
Bland nuclei, resembling one another

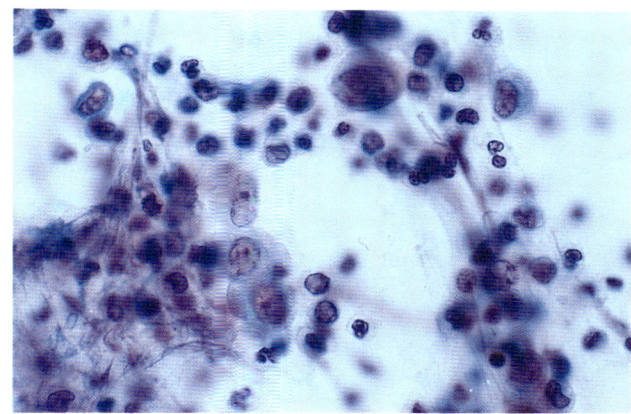

FIGURE 8.10 Malignant cells from biphasic mesothelioma. Note the prominent nucleoli and clear-appearing cytoplasm. (Pap × 90)

cells in the effusion bear a resemblance to one another, even though they may vary in their degree of atypia. In carcinoma, on the other hand, a distinct two-cell population can be identified because the alien malignant cells bear little resemblance to the mesothelial cells in the background.

Another important differential is between mesothelioma and mesothelial hyperplasia, a difficult task in cytologic specimens. A helpful but often ignored cue is the number of cells, rather excessive in mesothelioma, and small in hyperplasia. Repeat taps are also helpful in the distinction between mesothelioma and hyperplasia. The large number of cells is stable in mesothelioma while it waxes and wanes in mesothelial hyperplasia. Upon close inspection mesothelial cells in mesothelioma are severalfold larger than their normal and reactive counterparts. If the two-tone cytoplasmic features are still recognizable, their identification is easier once. In hyperplasia, tumor cells may show bizarre cytoplasmic shapes, nuclear pleomorphism, coarse chromatin clumping, enlarged nucleoli, and abnormal mitoses. These cells may stand out from their neighbors and appear alien to the observer. As such, they may necessitate ancillary procedures to distinguish them from carcinoma.

Biphasic Mesothelioma

In biphasic mesothelioma, the dual nature of the mesothelial cells is easily discernible in histologic sections. The surface of the serosal membrane is lined by cuboidal cells supported by a fibrovascular layer containing

plump spindle cells. These spindle cells are believed to be capable of transformation into cuboidal cells as they divide and migrate upward toward the surface. During the process of division and differentiation, these cells are subject to carcinogenic stimuli giving rise to mesotheliomas with two cell populations. The spindle-cell component resembles sarcomatous mesothelioma but blends imperceptibly with the epithelial component. These epithelioid cells may occur singly or as solid sheets of plump cells, or it may attain full organization into rows of cells that line slits, small acinar spaces, and large glandlike luminas. They may be further organized in papillary groups identical to the ones seen in tubulopapillary variants of malignant epithelial mesothelioma. The epithelioid component of biphasic mesothelioma is much more likely to exfoliate than the sarcomatous one, and consequently the effusion often contains cell balls, rosettes or papillary groups. Cytologically, the cells are indistinguishable from those of ordinary epithelial mesotheliomas. Nuclei are enlarged and display prominent nucleoli. The cytoplasm is lacy and clear-appearing or disfigured peripherally vacuolated by strongly PAS-positive material, with the ultrastructural appearance of glycogen (Fig. 8.10). Hyaluronic acid is elevated in the effusion and can also be demonstrated in the intercellular spaces of both the epithelial and sarcomatous components as noted in histologic sections.

Biphasic mesotheliomas may be poorly differentiated and need to be distinguished from renal cell carcinomas, which also contain glycogen and lipid and may mimic both the sarcomatous element and the epithelial component with all of its variations in cell arrangement (Fig. 8.11). Mesotheliomas may accumulate intracytoplasmic inclusions that should not be confused with the

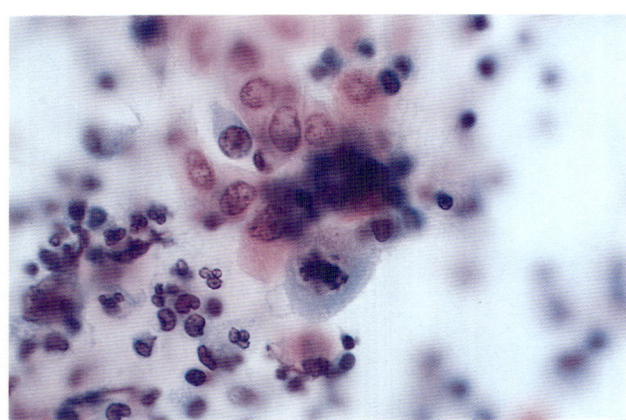

FIGURE 8.11 Poorly differentiated mesothelioma with malignant mesothelial group of cells, one of which is undergoing mitosis. Note the PMNs in the background. (Pap × 90)

hyaline droplets of renal cell carcinoma (Fig. 8.12). The lipid content of renal cell carcinomas is much greater than that of mesothelioma, their microvilli are much shorter as seen by electron microscopy, and they lack hyaluronic acid. Both mesothelioma and renal cell carcinoma may be positive for keratins and negative for CEA, but only renal cell carcinoma expresses antigens of the uroseries. Seminomas may bear some resemblance to the epithelial component of biphasic mesothelioma, but they occur in a different age group and express the placental variant of alkaline phosphatase and occasionally, alpha$_1$ antitrypsin, seldom, if ever expressed by malignant mesothelial cells.

Sarcomatous Mesothelioma

The diffuse sarcomatous variant is much less common than either the epithelial or the biphasic variant of mesothelioma. It is characterized by spindle cells that lay down a considerable amount of collagen, making them, at times, difficult to differentiate from fibrosarcomas and other sarcomas of the pleura. The tumor, however, also secretes hyaluronic acid, and the individual cells coexpress keratin and vimentin whereas they are negative for CEA and the other semispecific markers of spindle cell sarcomas. Cytologically, the effusions tend to be small because the aggressive behavior of these neoplasms kills the patient before large amounts of fluid have accumulated. Cellularity is sparse, with plump and spindle cells showing some variation in size and shape (Fig. 8.13). Cytologically, one of the elements, more frequently the plump cells, tend to predominate (Fig. 8.14). In cell blocks, a myxoid component can be noted in the intercellular spaces, corresponding to the areas of strongest positivity for hyaluronic acid with the alcian blue stain. The tumor, however, may lack a significant amount of intercellular substance and appear epithelioid. By electron microscopy at least a few of the cells conserve their florid microvillous surface, and the finding of these microvilli in direct juxtaposition with intervening collagen is a feature not seen in any other neoplasm except mesothelioma. This tumor is difficult if not impossible to separate cytologically from fibrosarcoma of the pleura, but its positivity for keratin of various molecular weights allows such a distinction to be made (Fig. 8.15).

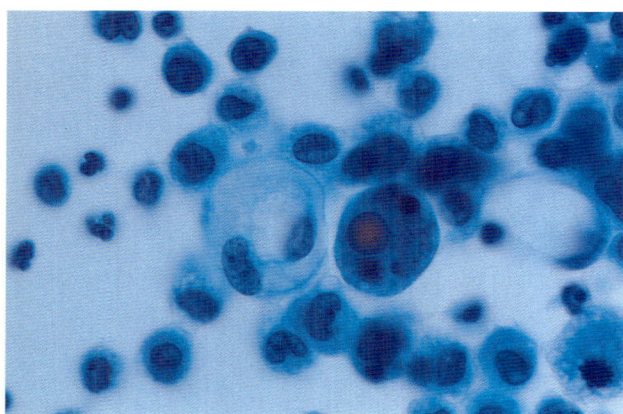

FIGURE 8.12 Biphasic malignant mesothelioma. Note the contrast between one cell with abundant clear cytoplasm and another cell with a discrete eosinophilic inclusion. (Pap × 120)

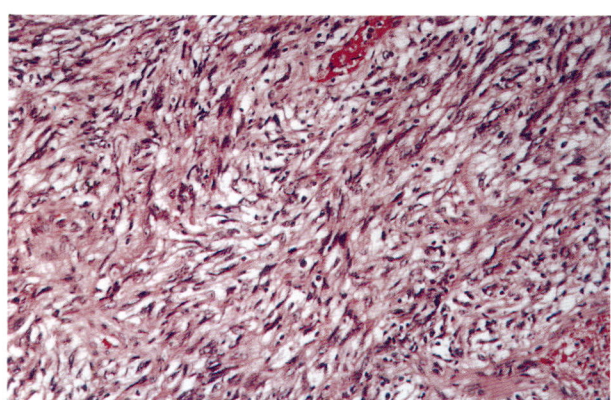

FIGURE 8.13 Sarcomatous mesothelioma. Note the plump and spindle cells with elongated nuclei, amidst cells with clear cytoplasm. (H&E × 40)

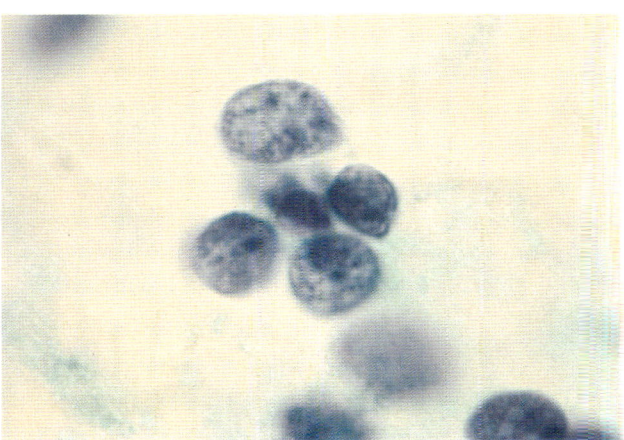

FIGURE 8.14 Scant cellular specimen from FNA of a sarcomatous mesothelioma. These tumors shed scant cellular material in comparison to epithelial mesothelioma. Notice plump, rather than spindle-shaped tumor cells. (Pap × 200)

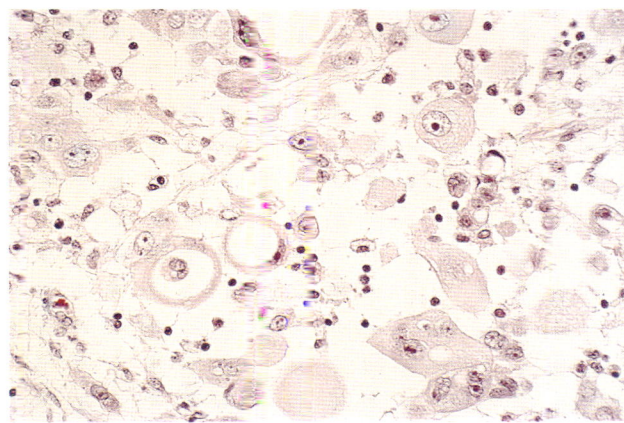

FIGURE 8.16 Anaplastic mesothelioma with large single cells, groups of cells, giant cells, and cells with large intracytoplasmic lumina. Note also the rare spindle cells near the top. (H&E × 40)

As opposed to localized fibrous tumor of the pleura, diffuse sarcomatous mesothelioma extends over a large surface and penetrates to a great depth into the chest wall or the lung. The tumor resembles fibrosarcoma, from which it can be differentiated by its production of hyaluronic acid and its lesser tendency to form collagen. Coexpression of vimentin and keratin and florid microvilli over the cell surface set this tumor apart from other sarcomas. The close apposition of the microvilli against collagen is rather characteristic of sarcomatous mesothelioma. As with localized fibrous tumors, only rarely

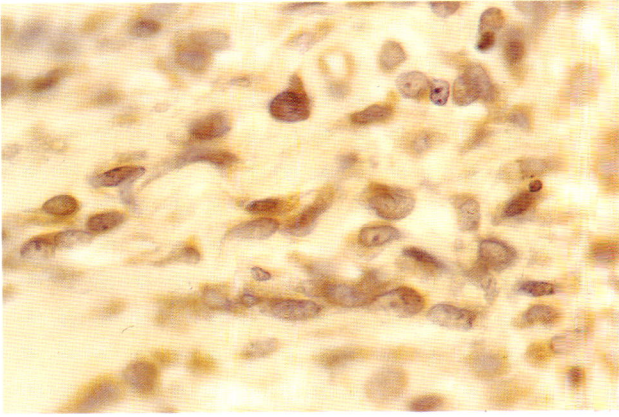

FIGURE 8.15 Weak keratin positivity in sarcomatous mesothelioma. This immunostain highlights plump cells not easily discernible by routine stains alone. (P.A.P. × 90)

will a diffuse sarcomatous mesothelioma lead to effusion. When it does, hyperplastic mesothelial cells are the dominant cytologic feature. In needle aspirates the spindle malignant cells are frequently disassociated. The cytologic features are those of a sarcoma with bizarre elongated cells, dark hyperchromatic nuclei, and frequent mitosis.

Anaplastic Mesothelioma

Anaplastic mesotheliomas run a rampant course with extreme morbidity and a high mortality. The tumors are composed of a mixture of spindle cells, plump cells, and bizarre cells so that the differential diagnosis is often with malignant fibrous histiocytoma (MFH) and other pleomorphic sarcomas (Fig. 8.16). However, these tumors are negative for histiocytic markers such as α_1AT/α_1ACT and muramidase whereas they are weakly positive for keratin and vimentin. Some anaplastic mesotheliomas may contain foci of heterologous sarcomatous elements. There are also pleural-based sarcomas that may show the production of myxomatous, chondroid, and even osteoid material, and yet they bear some resemblance to mesothelioma. When these tumors occur in asbestos workers, it is tempting to view the mesothelium as a totipotential tissue, capable of a greater repertoire of malignant transformation, rather than the narrow pathway of mesothelioma. As a rule, asbestos exposure should be ruled out whenever a malignant effusion is documented and there is diffuse pleural

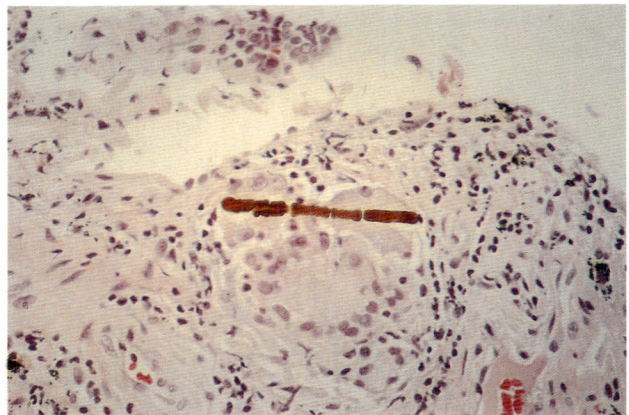

FIGURE 8.17 Asbestos body surrounded by giant cell reaction. Impregnation by proteinecous material containing iron is responsible for the rusty color of the coated fiber. (H&E × 40)

CONDITIONS CONFUSIBLE WITH MALIGNANT MESOTHELIOMA

Two conditions have been clinically and pathologically confused with mesothelioma: localized fibrous tumor and sarcomas of the pleura. Their differentiation from diffuse malignant mesothelioma is important for medicolegal purposes but their true pathogenesis and cell of origin is still controversial. If one considers their origin to be from the mesothelial fibroblastlike cells of the submesothelial layer, then they would belong in the mesotheliomatous categories. However, some cases occur in the absence of documented asbestos exposure, and we presently consider these separately from asbestos-related mesotheliomas, even though their etiology is not completely understood.

involvement in the absence of an extra-pleural primary site for the neoplasm. Objective link between mesothelioma and asbestos exposure is attained by demonstrating excessive numbers of asbestos bodies. These are seldom seen in effusions but are demonstrable in tissue sections of the lung and pleura and in cytologic specimens such as sputum and BAL. Asbestos bodies are formed by interaction with the host and appear golden brown by the impregnation of an iron-containing proteinaceous coat (Fig. 8.17). In its natural state, uncoated asbestos fibers are thin and brittle and cannot be detected in routine cytologic and histologic preparations (Fig. 8.18).

Localized Fibrous Tumor (Pleural Fibroma)

Benign, localized "mesotheliomas" are in reality bulky, pedunculated fibrous tumors that arise from the parietal pleura, compress the lung and may appear intrapulmonary on the chest roentgenogram (Fig. 8.19). Localized fibrous tumors are well circumscribed and surrounded by a capsule. Invariably, there is no history of asbestos exposure, no asbestos-associated lesions such as asbestosis or pleural plaques are present, and the process is localized to one area of one lung, the other being unaffected. These fleshy tumors may give rise to

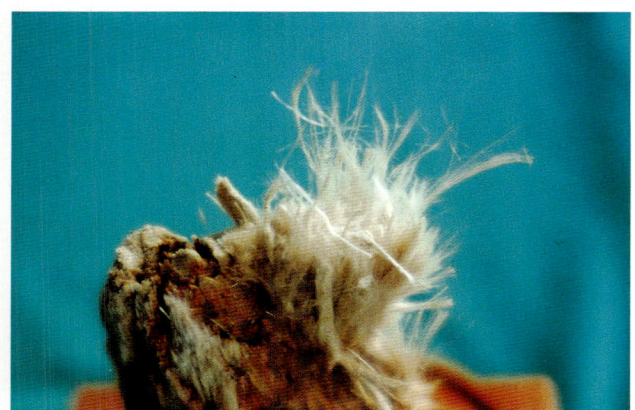

FIGURE 8.18 Asbestos fibers in natural state. Uncoated fibers split and fragment into rather delicate segments undetectable by ordinary light microscopy. (Courtesy of Richard Bedrossian)

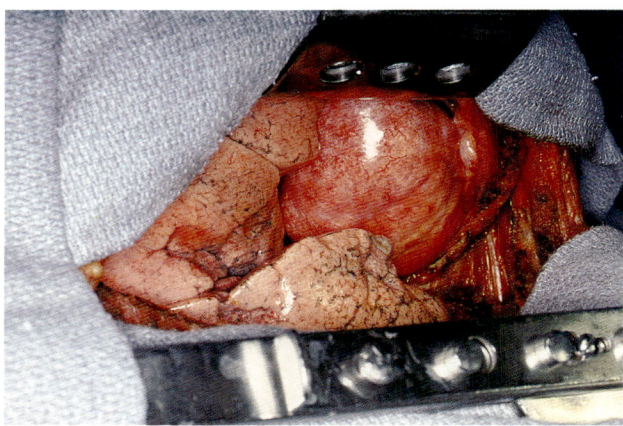

FIGURE 8.19 Benign localized mesothelioma from a woman never exposed to asbestos. Note the well-circumscribed lesion, compressing lung parenchyma. (Courtesy of K. Naunheim, MD)

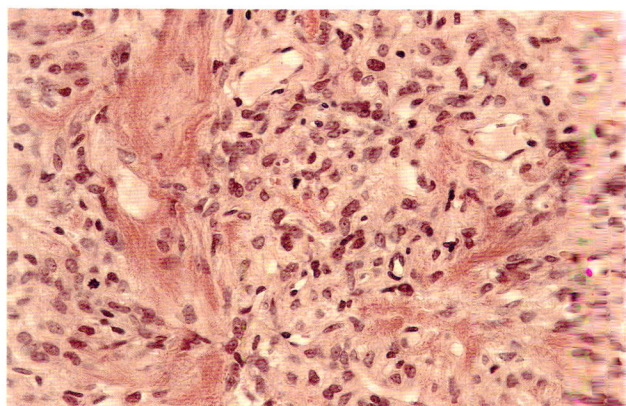

FIGURE 8.20 Histologic section of the tumor shown in Figure 8.19. Note the spindle cells separated by bundles of collagen and the bland appearance of the tumor cells. (H&E × 60)

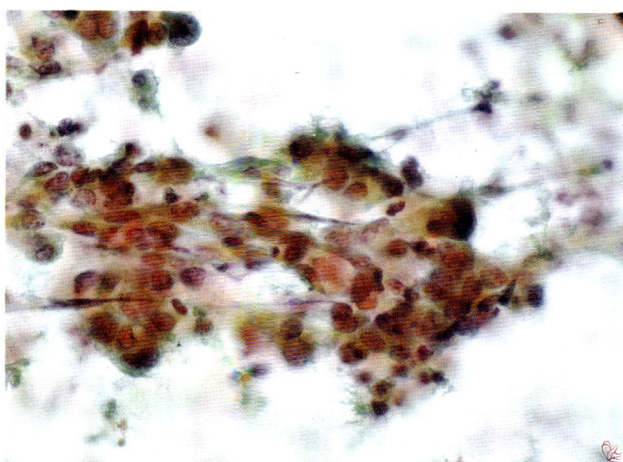

FIGURE 8.21 Cytologic specimen from a malignant spindle cell tumor of the pleura sampled by FNA. Spindle cells in fluid specimens tend to appear plumper than in biopsy specimens. (Pap × 180)

only a small amount of pleural effusion, so they are more often diagnosed by fine-needle aspiration of a pleural-based mass. Cellularity is sparse, and only a single cell population of bland spindle cells is observed with ovoid or cigar-shaped nuclei and tapered cytoplasmic extremities (Fig. 8.20). These keratin-negative cells are positive for vimentin but negative for other mesenchymal markers so that they are best classified as a localized fibroma of the pleura. Cytologic specimens are seldom seen in this condition since the cells do not exfoliate into the pleural effusion. In FNA specimens the cells from pleural fibroma are plump but do not form groupings as in epithelial mesothelioma. The tumor is difficult to distinguish from leiomyoma, synovial sarcoma, and neurofibroma on cytologic grounds alone, but these lesions are rare in the pleura. Pleural fibromas may be asymptomatic for many years, and local excision is usually curative.

Pleural Sarcomas

Fibrosarcoma of the pleura is a tumor segregated by Carter from the sarcomatous mesothelioma group on the basis of its negativity for keratin. Not only do these tumors fail to coexpress keratin and vimentin, but in one case we recently examined, vimentin positivity was weak and focally distributed. It is possible that this tumor is a neoplasm of primitive submesothelial cells without full mesotheliomatous differentiation. In our opinion, the most important measure when faced with this entity is to obtain a good clinical history to exclude

asbestos exposure. We have seen one case without asbestos exposure and one case with asbestos exposure and the cytologic and histopathologic features of the two cases were practically identical (Fig. 8.21). The answer to the medicolegal questions in cases of fibrosarcomas in patients exposed to asbestos is a difficult one. If this tumor occurs with (1) other clinicopathologic evidence of asbestos-related diseases such as asbestosis and pleural plaques, (2) a large number of asbestos bodies in sputum or broncheoalveolar lavage specimens or (3) an elevated asbestos fiber count in a digested specimen or under especialized ultrastructural examination we tend to conclude that the fibrosarcoma of the pleura is probably related to occupational exposure to asbestos-containing dust.

DISTINCTION OF MESOTHELIOMA FROM ADENOCARCINOMA

Nowhere is the difficulty in distinguishing mesothelioma from adenocarcinoma more pungent than in small biopsies. The proximity between the pleura—the site of mesotheliomas—and the lung parenchyma—the site of adenocarcinoma—is so close that the tumors could easily be confusible or actually run into one another (Fig. 8.22). Both mesothelioma and adenocarcinoma may invade the loose connective tissue of the serosal membrane and manifest themselves as neoplastic cell balls

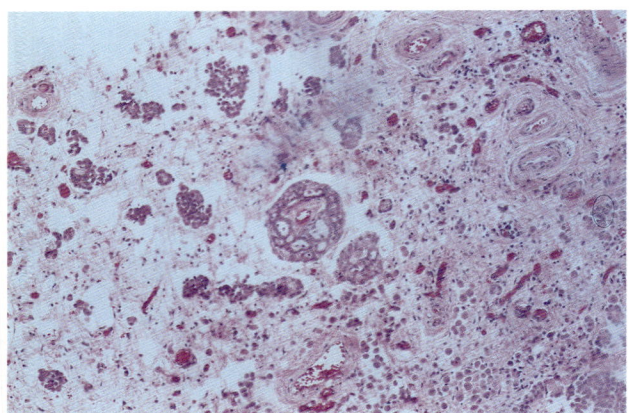

FIGURE 8.22   Edge between mesothelioma and the pleural surface from tumor that presented as a subpleural mass. Cell balls float in viscid proteoglycans. Note the cribriform group with a vascular core near the center. (H&E × 40)

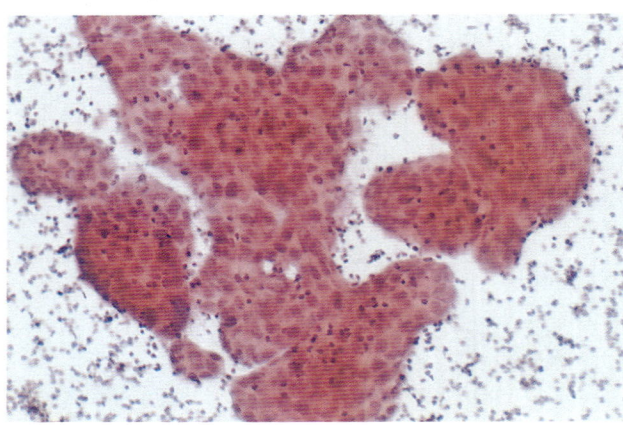

FIGURE 8.24   Malignant mesothelioma sampled by FNA. Notice enormous tissue fragments dwarfing the individual cells in the background (Pap × 60)

or free floating acini (Fig. 8.23). Mesotheliomas may invade vertically and present as a subpleural mass. Conversely adenocarcinomas may spread horizontally along the pleural surfaces in a psuedomesotheliomatous pattern. Depending on the size and the doubling time of the neoplasm, mesotheliomas may be rather necrotic and hemorrhagic. This tends to confuse the clinical picture and make the distinction between mesothelioma and adenocarcinoma even more difficult.

The significant medicolegal implication resulting from the recognition of mesothelioma dictates extreme caution at arriving at this diagnosis. At times, in histologic preparations and cell blocks, the tumor will betray

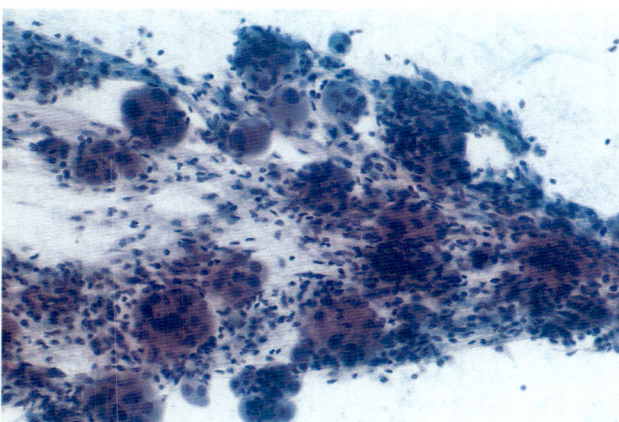

FIGURE 8.23   FNA specimen from subpleural mass. The mesothelioma shows both spindle cells and epithelial like cell groups. (Pap × 60)

its mesothelial origin; for instance, the finding of classical articulations between malignant mesothelial cells (Fig. 8.24). The cell block may also contain the architectural features of mesothelioma including papillary fronds of mesothelial cells supported by a fibrovascular core (Fig. 8.25). The cytopathologist, however, should, if at all possible, back up cytomorphologic impressions with specialized techniques of greater accuracy and precision. Because metastatic adenocarcinoma is such a common affliction of serous fluid, this diagnosis must be excluded prior to accessing the diagnosis of mesothelioma. Several staining methods have been tried in attempts to distinguish adenocarcinoma from mesothelioma (Table 8.2). However, if at all possible, electron microscopy should be obtained because ultrastructural features constitute the gold standard for the diagnosis of mesothelioma. By electron microscopy, glycogen appears either as discrete granules or in the form of clear spaces secondary to glycogen removal during processing. Glycogen may also be visualized by light microscopy. The amount of glycogen in mesothelioma may be rather small, represented by regular aggregates, peripherally located, at times overlapping the nuclei. Glycogen can be highlighted by special stains, in the form of punctate areas which are positive with PAS in appropriately fixed preparations. Diastase digestion removes the positivity.

Mesotheliomas may display small peripheral vacuoles that are easily demonstrated with the MGG stain but not as neatly appreciated with Papanicolaou's method. Mesotheliomas may also form larger vacuoles that appear as beaded area of PAS-positivity immedi-

TABLE 8.2 Staining Characteristics of Mesothelioma and Adenocarcinoma

	Mesothelioma	Adenocarcinoma
Routine Stains	Two-tone appearance with Papanicolaou Peripheral blebs with Romanowsky's stain	Homogeneously distributed stain No peripheral blebs noted
Special Stains	Cytoplasm contains PAS (+), digestible material Coalesced vacuoles may appear sausage-shaped Extracellular space contains alcian blue (+) material removable by hyaluronidase	Glycogen content is small PAS (+) vacuoles not removed by digestion No hyaluronic acid present in extracellular space
Immunostains	CEA consistently negative EMA variably positive with frequently "thick" membrane pattern Both low and high molecular weight keratin positive Leu M$_1$ invariably negative	CEA consistently positive EMA frequently positive in cytoplasm and cell periphery Positive only with low molecular weight keratin Leu M$_1$ occasionally positive

Modified from: Bedrossian CWM. Immunocytochemistry. In: Astarita RW, ed. *Practical Cytopathology.* New York: Churchill Livingstone 1990: chap 14, 403–457. With permission.

ately beneath the cell border. These vacuoles may coalesce in the form of crescent-shaped areas at the periphery of the cells. With the PAS stain these spaces appear as a sausage-shaped rim of positivity. The slender microvilli may also trap the PAS stain in the absence of true vacuolization. The microvilli are responsible for the lacunae between tumor cells and the surrounding stroma (Fig. 8.26). With electron microscopy not only the lacunae but the spaces between mesothelial cells are occupied by their profuse microvilli (Fig. 8.27). By immunoperoxidase staining the thick membrane positivity of EMA appears double-decked because part of the immunostain lines up along the tips of the microvilli and part is deposited along the cell membrane (Fig. 8.28). This phenomenon is also observed in cytologic

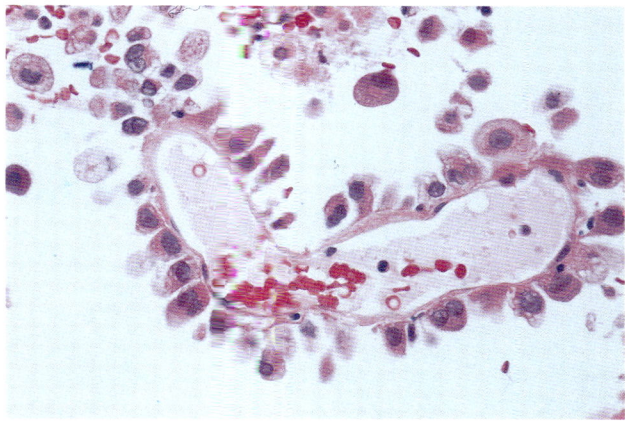

FIGURE 8.25 Cell block from mesothelioma sampled by FNA. Tumor cells supported by fibrovascular core display mesothelial characteristics (H&E × 120)

specimens that show a thick rim of EMA positivity at the periphery of cell groupings (Fig. 8.29). The shorter microvilli of malignant epithelial cells do not lead to this phenomenon, so a single-layer linearity is the rule in carcinoma. A crownlike pattern of staining similar to that of EMA can be seen with alcian blue. The alcian blue positivity, however, is removable by hyaluronidase digestion, whereas in adenocarcinoma it is not. In metastatic carcinoma the secretory vacuoles are irregular in size and shape. They may be scattered in location or, when coalesced and of sufficient size, they may push the nucleus aside. They are negative for fat, except in renal cell carcinoma, positive for PAS, even after diastase digestion, and visible both with MGG and Papani-

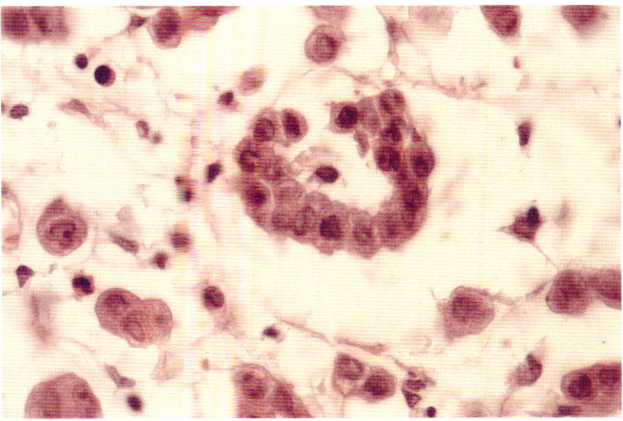

FIGURE 8.26 Loose connective tissue of pleura involved by mesothelioma. Note acinar groups, doublets, and single malignant mesothelial cells surrounded by ample clear spaces. (H&E × 120)

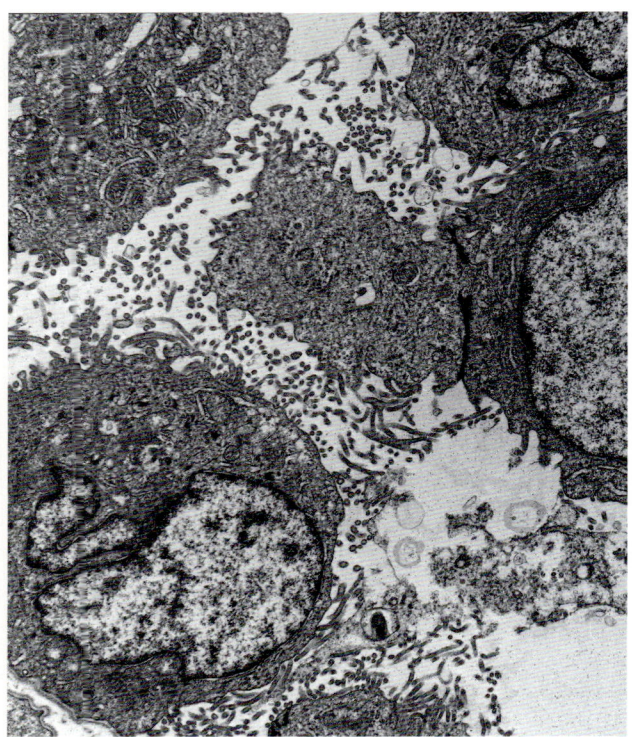

FIGURE 8.27   Ultrastructure of mesothelioma. The interface between cells is occupied by microvilli. (EM × 12,000) (From Eedrossian et al. *Sem Diagn Pathol* 9:124–140, 1992 with permission)

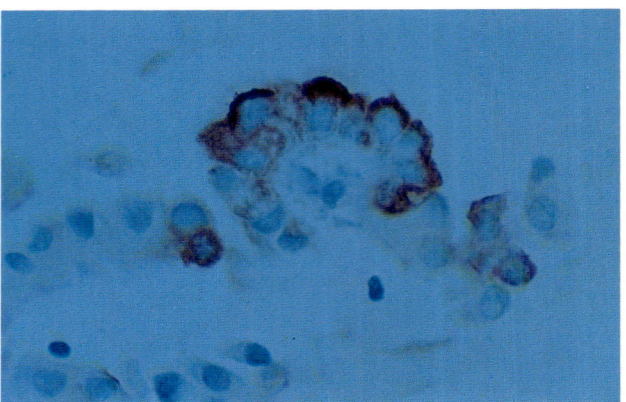

FIGURE 8.29   Cytologic smear from same specimen shown in Figure 8.28 stained by EMA. The thick membrane pattern delimits the group of neoplastic mesothelial cells, while benign mesothelial cells in the background are negative. (P.A.P. × 60)

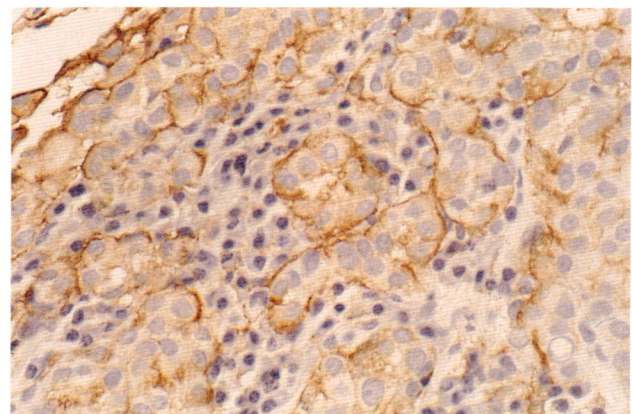

FIGURE 8.28   Thick membrane pattern with EMA. Immunostaining clearly separates cords of neoplastic mesothelial cells from the surrounding stroma. (P.A.P. × 90) (Courtesy of HS-Y Leong, MD)

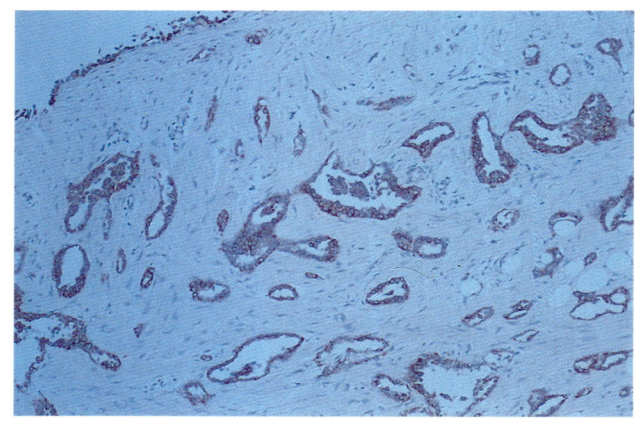

FIGURE 8.30   Mesothelioma stained for keratin. The immunostain delineates cells lining luminal spaces but shows no thick membrane pattern. (P.A.P. × 100)

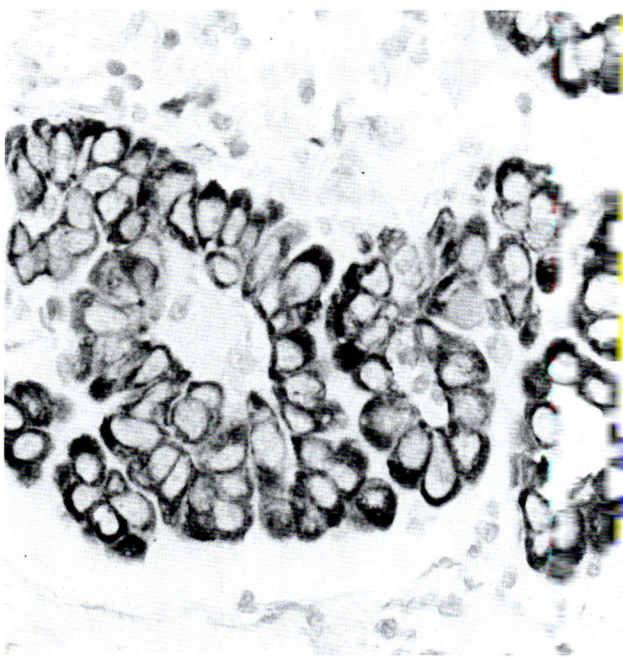

FIGURE 8.31 Cell block of mesothelioma stained for keratin. Note the strong staining of cytoplasm, delimiting the tubulopapillary arrangement of the tumor cells. (P.A.P. × 120)

TABLE 8.3 Ultrastructural Distinction between Mesothelioma and Adenocarcinoma

	Mesothelioma	Adenocarcinoma
Cell Surface	Microvilli evenly distributed around entire cell	Microvilli concentrated at poles
	Slender, bushy microvilli	Short, stubby microvilli
	No glycocalyceal bodies	Glycocalyceal bodies noted
Cell Junctions	Apical tight junctions	Terminal bars near lumen
	Well developed desmosomes	Poorly developed junctions
	Rare elongated desmosomes	Desmosomes, if noted, are normal length
Cytoplasm	Tonofilaments surround the nucleus	Irregularly distributed intermediate filaments
	Abundant glycogen	Variable amount of glycogen
	No secretory granules	Numerous secretory granules

Modified from: Bedrossian CWM. Immunocytochemistry. In: Astarita RW, ed. *Practical Cytopathology*. Churchill Livingstone 1990: chap 14, 403–457. With permission.

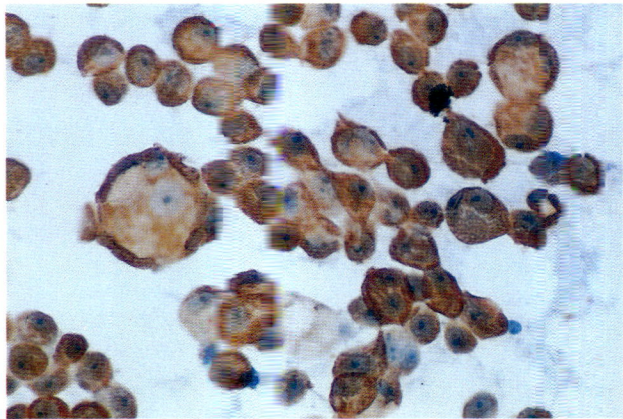

FIGURE 8.32 Cytospin of pleural fluid stained for keratin. The neoplastic cells show a perinuclear pattern of immunopositivity, typical of mesothelioma (P.A.P. × 120)

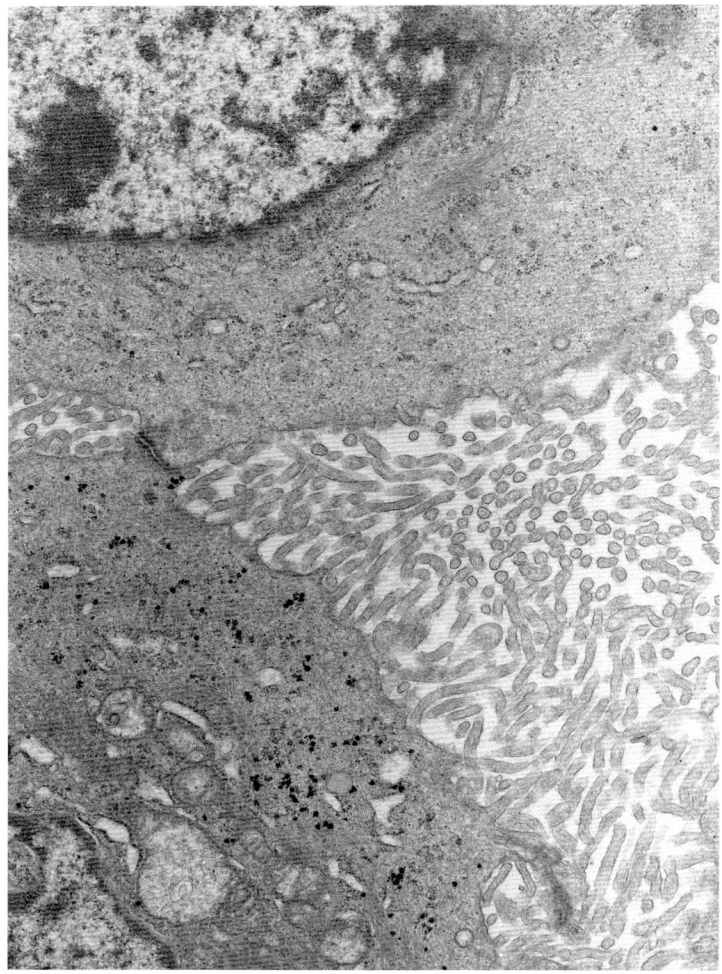

FIGURE 8.33 Mesothelial cells by TEM. Notice slender, bushy microvilli along the free surfaces of the cells and absence of secretory products in the cytoplasm. (EM × 8,000) (Courtesy of S. Bonsib, MD)

colaou's stains. A strongly positive mucin stain is powerful evidence against mesothelioma. CEA positivity and keratin negativity favor carcinoma whereas the reverse suggests mesothelioma (Fig. 8.30). The keratin positivity in mesothelioma is stronger around the nucleus as opposed to the diffuse and weak positivity of carcinoma (Fig. 8.31 and 8.32). Vimentin has been negative in the majority of cytologic samples of mesotheliomas we examined, even though it has been variably reported in the literature pertaining to histologic sections of mesothelioma. Other markers that are useful in the diagnosis of mesothelioma are discussed in more detail in Chapter 15.

In our experience electron microscopy is the most reliable method of diagnosing mesothelioma by the demonstration of these three ultrastructural features: (1) long and slender microvilli, often bushy and multibranched (Fig. 8.33), (2) tightly woven perinuclear intermediate filaments which are practically absent near the periphery of the cell (Fig. 8.34) and (3) no mucin-secreting apparatus in the cytoplasm, even though it may contain a well developed rough endoplasmic reticulum. Other ultrastructural features play a supportive role in the distinction between adenocarcinoma (Table 8.3). SEM is helpful in demonstrating slender as opposed to blunt microvilli in mesothelioma, in sharp contrast with adenocarcinoma (Fig. 8.35). However, as discussed in chapter 14, SEM plays more of a supportive rather than a primary role in the ultrastructural diagnosis of mesothelioma.

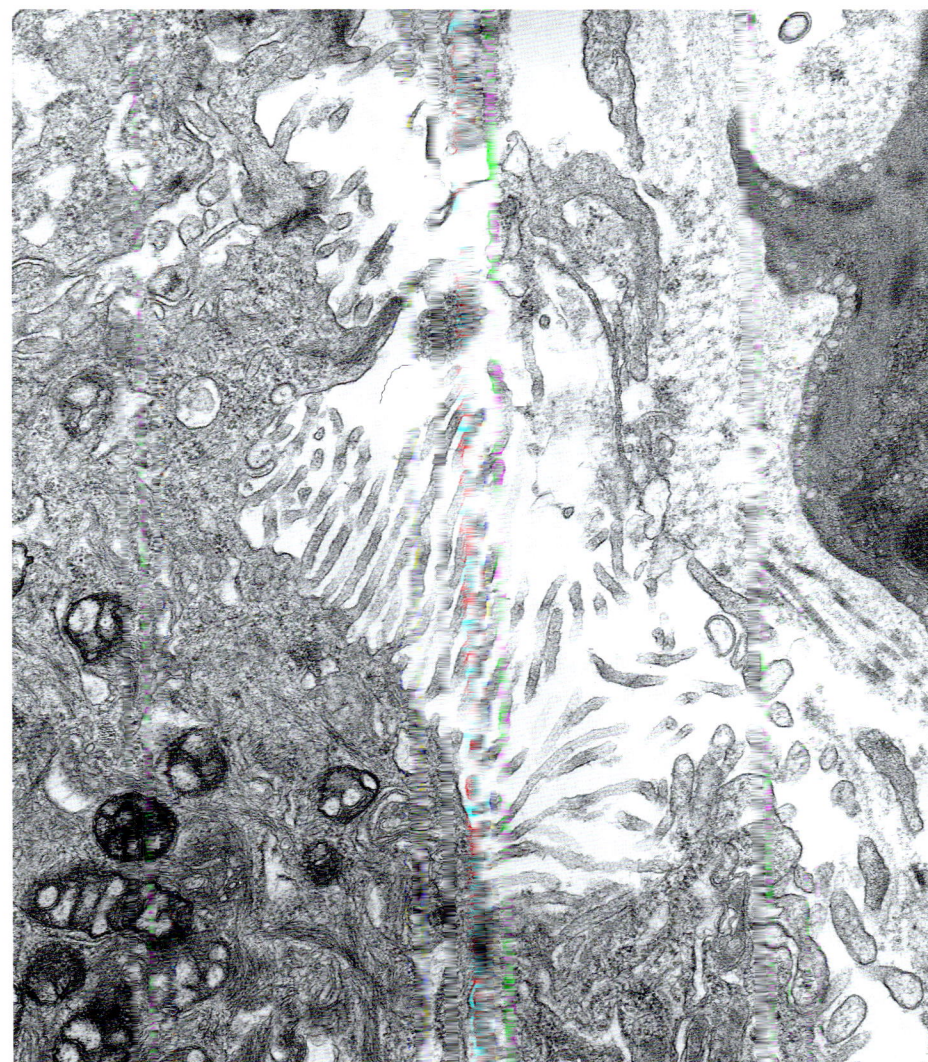

FIGURE 8.34 Microvillous-stromal contact in malignant mesothelioma. The microvilli are rather long and the cytoplasm is rich in intermediate filaments. (EM × 7,500)

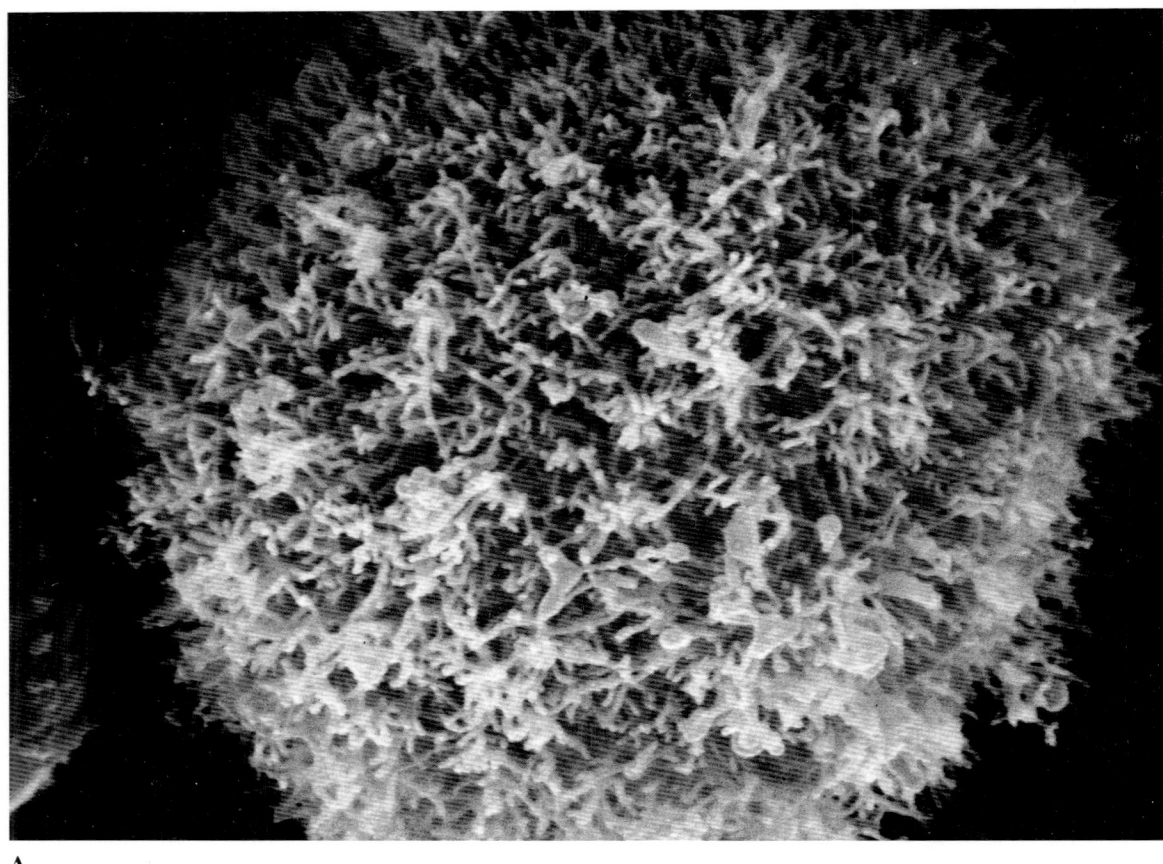

A

FIGURE 8.35   Contrast between mesothelioma and adenocarcinoma. (*A*) Mesothelioma cells are covered by numerous slender microvilli and display a scalloped contour. (SEM× 4,000)

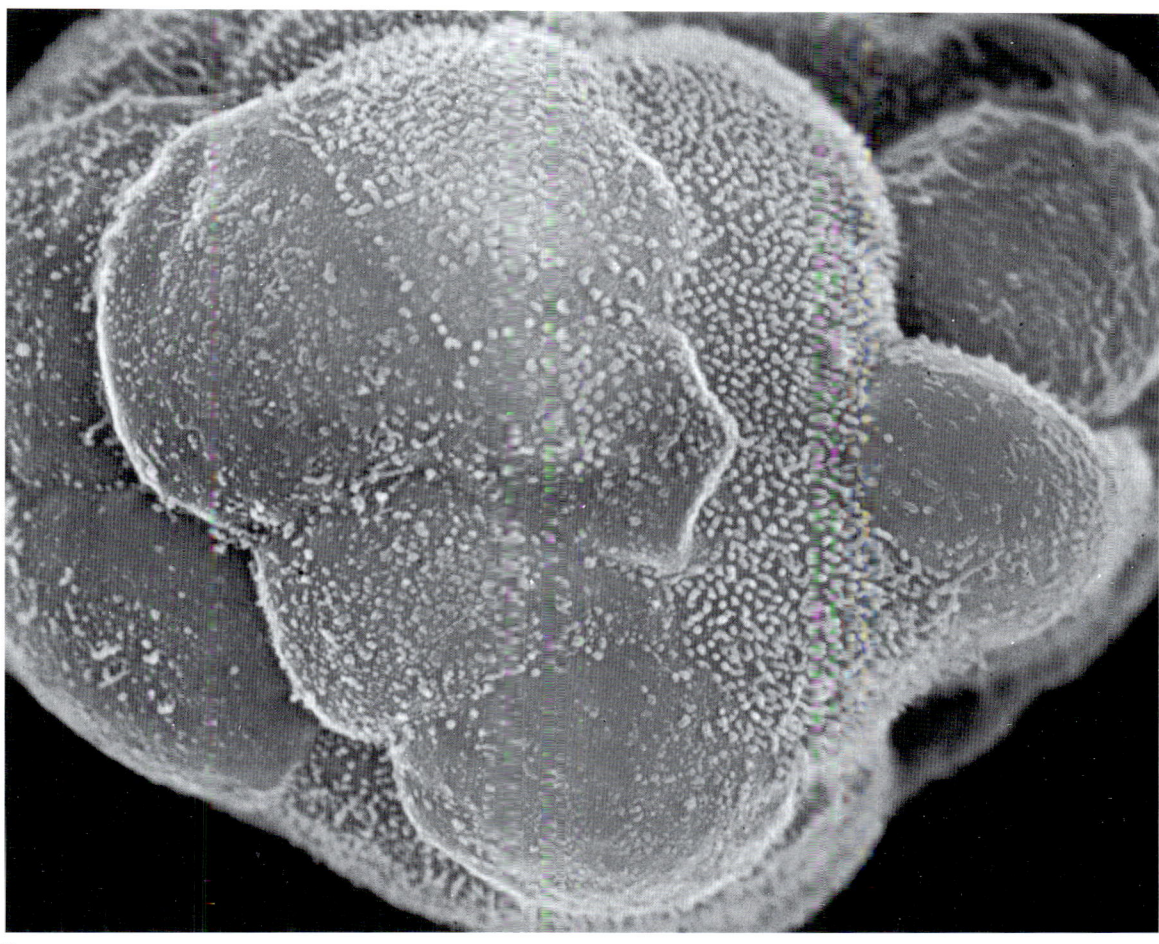

B

FIGURE 8.35 (B) Stubbly and sparse microvilli are noted in this adenocarcinoma. Notice the flat community border shared by several tumor cells (SEM × 4,000) (Courtesy of T. Mukerjee, MD)

BIBLIOGRAPHY

Malignant Mesothelioma

Antman KH. Clinical presentation and natural history of benign and malignant mesothelioma. *Semin Oncol.* 1981; 8:313–320.

Oels HC, Harrison EG Jr, Carr DT, et al. Diffuse malignant mesothelioma of the pleura: A review of 37 cases. *Chest.* 1971;60:564–570.

Roberts GH. Diffuse pleural mesothelioma. A clinical and pathological study. *Br J Dis Chest.* 1970;64:201–211.

Roggli V, Johnston W, Kaminsky D. Asbestos bodies in fine needle aspirates of the lung. *Acta Cytol.* 1984;28(4): 493–498.

Wagner J. Mesothelioma and mineral fibers. *Cancer.* 1986; 57(10):1905–1911.

Whitwell F, Rawcliffe RM. Diffuse malignant pleural mesothelioma and asbestos exposure. *Thorax.* 1971;26:6–22.

Cytologic Diagnosis

Berge T, Grontoff O. Cytologic diagnosis of malignant pleural mesothelioma. *Acta Cytol.* 1965;9:207–212.

Boon ME, Veldhuizen RW, Ruinaard C, et al. Qualitative distinctive differences between the vacuoles of mesothelioma cells and of cells from metastatic carcinoma exfoliated in pleural fluid. *Acta Cytol.* 1984;28:443–449.

Butler EB, Berry AV. Diffuse mesothelioma diagnostic criteria using exfoliative cytology. In: *Biological Effect of Asbestos.* Delahaye M, deJong AAW, Versnel MA, et al.: *Cytopathology of malignant mesothelioma: Reappraisal of the diagnostic value of collagen cores.* 1990;1:137–145. Lyon: WHO International Agency for Research on Cancer; 1972.

Klemprran S. The exfoliative cytology of diffuse pleural mesothelioma. *Cancer.* 1962;15:691–704.

Kobayashi Y, Takeda S. Yamamoto T, et al. Cytologic detection of malignant mesothelioma of the pericardium. *Acta Cytol.* 1978;22:344–349.

Naylor B. The exfoliative cytology of diffuse malignant mesothelioma. *J Pathol Bacteriol.* 1963;86:293–298.

Roberts GH, Campbell GM. Exfoliative cytology of diffuse mesothelioma. *J Clin Pathol.* 1972;25:577–582.

Tao LC. The cytopathology of mesothelioma. *Acta Cytol.* 1979;23:209–213.

Triol JH, Conston AS, Chandler SVD. Malignant mesothelioma cytopathology of 75 cases seen in a New Jersey community hospital. *Acta Cytol.* 1984;28:37–45.

Whitaker D, Shilkin KB. The cytology of malignant mesothelioma in Western Australia. *Acta Cytol.* 1978;22:67–70.

Benign Mesothelial Proliferation

Becker S, Pepin D, Rosenthal D. Mesothelial papilloma: A case of mistaken identity in a pericardial effusion. *Acta Cytol.* 1976;20(3):266–268.

Ehya H. Cytology of mesothelioma of the tunica vaginalis metastatic to the lung. *Acta Cytol.* 1985;29(1):79–84.

Guffanti MC, Faleri ML. Benign-appearing mesothelioma cells in a serous effusion. *Acta Cytol.* 1985;29:90–92.

Klima M, Gyorkey F. Benign pleural lesions and malignant mesothelioma. *Virchows Arch [A].* 1977;376:181–193.

Klima M, Spjut HJ, Seybold WD. Diffuse malignant mesothelioma. *Am J Clin Pathol.* 1976;65:583–600.

Rosai L, Denner LP. Nodular mesothelial hyperplasia in hernia sacs: A benign reactive conditioning stimulating a neoplastic process. *Cancer.* 1975;35:165–175.

Ryan G, Groberty J, Majno G. Mesothelial injury and recovery. *Am Lab Pathol.* 1973;71:93–112.

Yazdi HM, Hajdu SI, Melamed MR. Cytopathology of pericardial effusions. *Acta Cytol.* 1980;24:401.

Benign Papillary Mesothelioma

Kannerstein M, Churg J, McCaughey W, et al. Papillary tumors of the peritoneum in women: Mesothelioma or papillary carcinoma. *Am J Obstet Gynecol.* 1977;127(3):306–313.

Moore JH, Crum CP, Chandler JG, et al. Benign cystic mesothelioma. *Cancer.* 1980;45(9):2395–2399.

Epithelial Mesothelioma

Chahinian AP, Pajak TF, Holland JF, et al. Diffuse malignant mesothelioma. *Ann Intern Med.* 1982;96(6):746–755.

Dionne GP, Wang N. A scanning electron microscopic study of diffuse mesothelioma and some lung carcinomas. *Cancer.* 1977;40:707–715.

Biphasic Mesothelioma

Lewis R, Sisler G, Mackenzie J. Diffuse, mixed malignant pleural mesothelioma. *Ann Thorac Surg.* 1981;31(1):53–60.

McCaukey WTE: Criteria for diagnosis of diffuse mesothelial tumors. *Ann NY Acad Sci.* 1985;132:603–613.

Sarcomatous Mesothelioma

Arai H, Kang K, Sato H, et al. Significance of the quantification and demonstration of hyaluronic acid in tissue specimens for the diagnosis of pleural mesothelioma. *Am Rev Respir Dis.* 1979;120:529–532.

Sterrett G, Whitaker D, Shilkin K, et al. Fine needle aspiration cytology of malignant mesothelioma. *Acta Cytol.* 1987; 31(2):185–193.

Anaplastic Mesothelioma

Kjellevold K, Nesland J, Holm R, et al. *Pathol Res Pract.* 1986;181:767–771.

Spriggs A, Grunge H. An unusual cytologic presentation of mesothelioma in serous fluids. *Acta Cytol.* 1983;27(3):288–292.

Conditions Confusible with Malignant Mesothelioma

Benisch B, Peison B, Sobel H, et al. Fibrous mesotheliomas (pseudofibroma) of the scrotal sac. *Cancer.* 1981;47(4):731–735.

Carter D, Otis CN. Three types of spindle cell tumors of the pleura: fibroma sarcoma and sarcomatoid mesothelioma. *Am J Surg Pathol* 1988;12:747–753.

Dervan PA, Tobin B, O'Connor M. Solitary (localized) fibrous mesothelioma: Evidence against mesothelial cell origin. *Histopathology.* 1986;10:867–875.

Foster E, Ackerman L. Localized mesotheliomas of the pleura. *Am J Clin Pathol.* 1960;34(4):349–364.

Gondos B. Electron microscopic study of papillary serous tumors of the ovary. *Cancer.* 1971;27(6):1455–1464.

Moran CA, Suster S, Koss MN. The spectrum of histologic growth patterns in benign and malignant fibrous tumors of the pleura. *Semin Diagn Pathol* 1992;9:169–180.

Distinction From Adenocarcinoma

Battifora H, Kopinski ML. Distinction of mesothelioma from adenocarcinoma: An immunohistochemical approach. *Cancer.* 1985;55:1697

Bedrossian CWM, Bonsib B, Moran C: Differential diagnosis between mesothelioma and adenocarcinoma: A multimodal approach based on ultrastructure and immunocytochemistry. *Sem Diagn Pathol.* 1992;9:124–140.

Boon M, Kwee H, Alons C, et al. Discrimination between primary peritoneal mesotheliomas by morphometry and analysis of vacuolization pattern of the exfoliated mesothelial cells. *Acta Cytol.* 1982;26(2):103–108.

Cibas ES, Corson JM, Pinkus GS. The distinction of adenocarcinoma from malignant mesothelioma in cell blocks of effusions. *Hum Pathol.* 1987;18:67–74.

Kobzik L, Antman K, Warhol M. The distinction of mesothelioma from adenocarcinoma in malignant effusions by electron microscopy. *Acta Cytol.* 1985;29:219–225.

Kwee WS, Veldhuizen RW, Along CA, et al. Quantitative and qualitative differences between benign and malignant mesothelial cells in pleural fluid. *Acta Cytol.* 1982;26:401–406.

Legrand M, Pariente R. Ultrastructural study of pleural fluid in mesothelioma. *Thorax.* 1974;29:164–171.

Naylor B. The exfoliative cytology of diffuse malignant mesothelioma. *J Pathol Bacteriol.* 1963;86:293–298.

Suzuki Y, Churg J, Hammerstein M. Ultrastructure of human malignant diffuse mesothelioma. *Am J Pathol.* 1976;85:241–262.

Van der Kwast TH, Versrel MA, Delahaye M, et al. Expression of EMA on malignant mesothelioma cells: An immunocytochemical and immunoelectron microscopic study. *Acta Cytol.* 1988;32:169–174.

Wange NS. Electron microscopy in the diagnosis of pleural mesotheliomas. *Cancer.* 1973;31:1046–1053.

Warhol MJ, Hickey WF, Corson JM. Malignant mesothelioma: Ultrastructural distinction from adenocarcinoma. *Am J Surg Pathol.* 1982;16:307–314.

Waxler B, Eisenstein R, Battifora H. Electrophoresis of tissue glycosaminoglycans as an aid in the diagnosis of mesotheliomas. *Cancer.* 1979;44:221–227.

CHAPTER NINE

Epithelial Malignancies

Carcinomas metastasize widely via the lymphatics, reaching first the regional lymph nodes and subsequently distant sites. The serosal membranes with their rich plexuses of lymphatic channels are frequent sites of seeding, but a malignant effusion may also occur in the absence of serosal metastasis. This occurs when circulating cells simply gain access to a serosal cavity without implanting the serosal membrane. A negative serosal biopsy is meaningless in the face of a positive cytologic result in a malignant effusion. It may in fact indicate that the serosa is not involved by metastasis, but if there is radiologic evidence of metastasis, the biopsy comes from a negative "skip-area" of the serosa. Correlative studies between pleural biopsy and cytologic examination of pleural effusion suggest that metastases tend to be patchy, thus explaining the higher yield of cytology as opposed to biopsy of the pleura. The reverse situation is extremely rare; that is, one very seldom sees a positive biopsy without the presence of malignant cells in the pleural effusion. Barring a difficulty in the collection or cytopreparation of the specimen such an event should not be seen, and if it occurs, the tap should be repeated to ensure the good technical quality of the cytologic sample.

COMMON AND UNCOMMON CARCINOMAS

Adenocarcinomas are by far the most common malignancies affecting effusions of the serous cavities. These tumors may be poorly differentiated or may exhibit full adenocarcinomatous differentiation, which aids enormously in their correct diagnosis and classification (Table 9.1).

If the adenocarcinomatous nature of the process is established, mesothelioma and other types of neoplasm are excluded. Establishing the primary site is the next important step since some adenocarcinomas may respond to therapy applied to the primary site, even in the presence of malignant effusion and distant metastasis. Cytomorphologic examination may offer some clues regarding the primary site of the neoplasm, and it helps to know the frequency of the primary sources of epithelial malignancies. These range from common (lung, breast, ovary, uterus, stomach, colon, pancreas) to a number of progressively less frequent sources of origin (esophagus, kidney, bladder, liver, prostate, thyroid, adrenal), which will be discussed later on.

In general, adenocarcinomas share certain cytologic features expressed in the manner the cells interrelate and in the texture of the cytoplasm, which reflects their secretory status (Table 9.2). It is therefore a relatively easy task to make the diagnosis of adenocarcinoma in a malignant effusion. Such a finding is clinically important in patients whose primary lesion is known, but occasionally the malignant effusion may arise from a second primary site. In patients whose primary neoplasm is not known, clinicians often ask the cytopathologist for a possible source of the malignant cells. In this chapter we describe and illustrate the most common cytologic features of the several carcinomas that occur in malignant effusions. In Chapter 13 we analyze the different presentations of carcinoma in effusions and present our approach to the search for the primary site. It pays dividends to be familiar with the statistical odds for the various primary sites represented in effusions, particularly in one's own institution. The accuracy of "predicting" or "confirming" the primary site by cytology is surprisingly high in some primary sites (Table 9.3).

TABLE 9.1 Expressions of Adenocarcinomatous Differentiation

Morphologic	Histochemical	Immunocytochemical	Ultrastructural
Gland or acinar formation	PAS with diastase digestion	CEA	Surface microvilli
Tridimensional cell groups	Mucicarmine (neutral mucin)	EMA	Intracytoplasmic lumina
Signet-ring configuration	Alcian blue pH 1.5 (acid mucin)	Secretory piece	Terminal bars
Mucosubstance accumulation	Colloidal iron (Mowry's)	Leu M$_1$	Secretory granules
		B72.3	
		HMFG-1	

Modified from: Bedrossian CWM. Immunocytochemistry. In Astarita RW, ed. *Practical Cytopathology.* New York: Churchill Livingstone; 1990: chap 14, 403–457. With permission.

TABLE 9.2 Cytologic Features of Adenocarcinoma in Effusions

Cell Groups	Individual Cells
Solid cell balls	Signet-ring appearance
Papillary formations	Intracytoplasmic umira
Free-floating acini	Clear cell change
Columnar cell fronds	Intracytoplasmic "dot"
Single-file rows	Multinucleated giant cells
	Granular cell change

COMMON EPITHELIAL NEOPLASMS

Breast

Breast carcinoma is the most frequent source of malignant pleural effusion in the female. Prevalence of the breast as the primary site ranges from 40 to 50% and the effusion has a high risk of recurrence. The most common subtype represented is infiltrative duct adenocarcinoma, which accounts for over 90% of the cases. The malignant effusion in these cases contains a large

TABLE 9.3 Frequency of Metastasis in Effusions

Primary Site	Number of Cases (%) Frequency	Accuracy in Cytologic Sample, %	Accuracy in Small Biopsy, %
Breast	155 (40)	79	72
Ovary	84 (22)	70	83
Pancreatic bile ducts	24 (7)	44	75
Lung	23 (6)	50	29
Stomach	23 (6)	52	40
Mesothelioma	19 (5)	53	80
Colon	16 (4)	50	100
Melanoma	9 (2)	50	100
Uterus	9 (2)	0	0
Urothelial	7 (2)	29	50
Prostate	5 (1)	20	0
Rare primaries	9 (< 2)	0	0
Total	387 (100)		

Adapted from: Spieler P. Gloor F. Identification of types and primary sites of malignant tumors by examination of exfoliated tumor cells in serous fluids. *Acta Cytol* 1985;29:753–767. With permission.

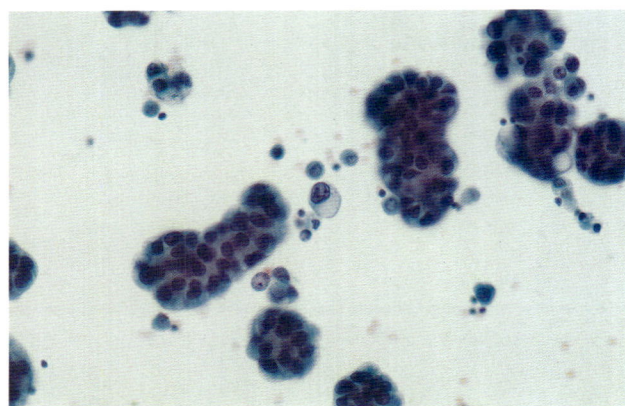

FIGURE 9.1   Cells from ductal adenocarcinoma of the breast. They share a common border, and the nuclei are at different planes of focus. Some of the cells show evidence of secretion, but the majority are nonvacuolated. (Pap×60)

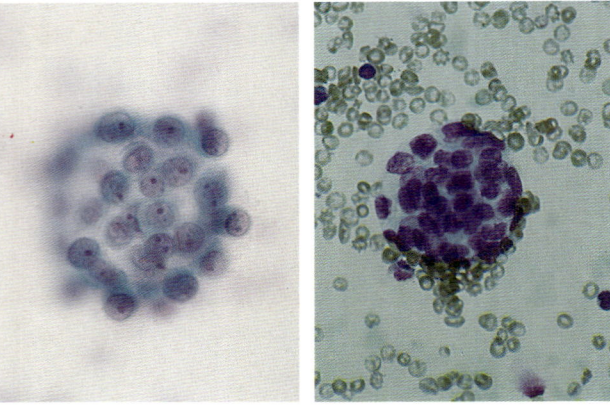

A   B

FIGURE 9.3   (*A*) Cell ball stained by Papanicolaou's method. Fine distribution of the chromatin and conspicuous nucleoli are noted, giving the impression of tridimensionality, a feature best appreciated by refocusing the microscope. (Pap× 90) (*B*) Cell ball stained by Diff-Quik. Apart from their abundant cytoplasm, the nuclei vary in size and shape but display less detail of the chromatin distribution than is seen with the Papanicolaou stain. (D.Q. × 90)

number of malignant cells arranged in cohesive groups (Fig. 9.1). The malignant cells tend to ball up in the effusion and form spheres which may reach enormous proportions (Fig. 9.2). The interior of the cell balls may be entirely made up of tumor cells, appear hollow, or contain a small amount of collaginous stroma. Nuclear features are first appreciated with the Pap stain than with Diff-Quik (Fig. 9.3). Special stains show the secretory pole in the outer rather than the inner aspect of the cell groups in breast carcinoma. Occasionally, the original shape of the infiltrating tumor cords is preserved

in the effusion with elongated or stellate groups of cells being shed from the neoplasm. Rarely, single-file arrangement is observed, particularly in lobular carcinoma of the breast.

The cytoplasm of mammary adenocarcinomatous cells is usually lacy, with routine stains (Fig. 9.4). The texture of the cytoplasm can be highlighted by immuno-

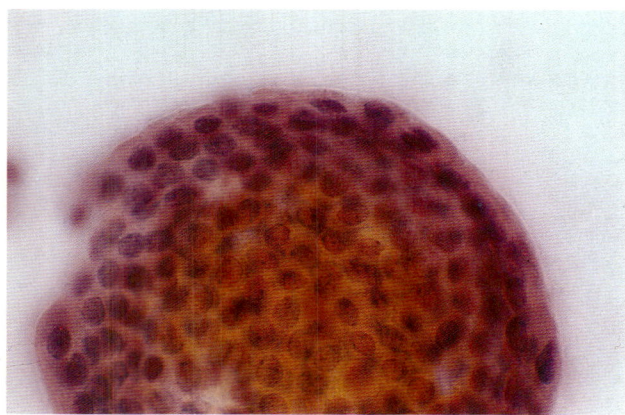

FIGURE 9.2   Large, nearly spherical cell ball. Some of the nuclei are seen en face, some sideways; most are relatively bland. However, the enormous size of the group is typical of ductal adenocarcinoma of the breast. (Pap× 90)

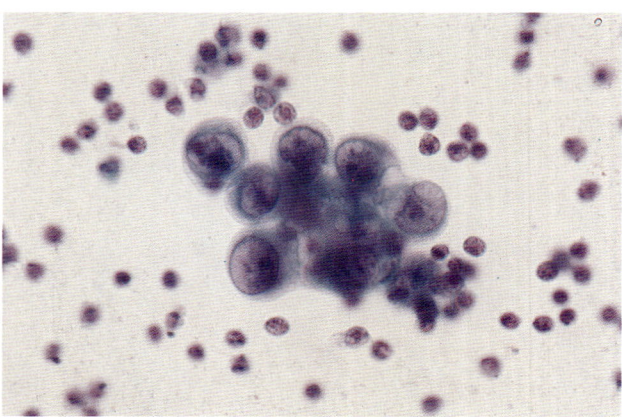

FIGURE 9.4   Cell group from breast carcinoma stained by Papanicolaou's method. Note the high nuclear: cytoplasmic ratio, chromatin clearing, and vacuolization of the cytoplasm. (Pap× 180)

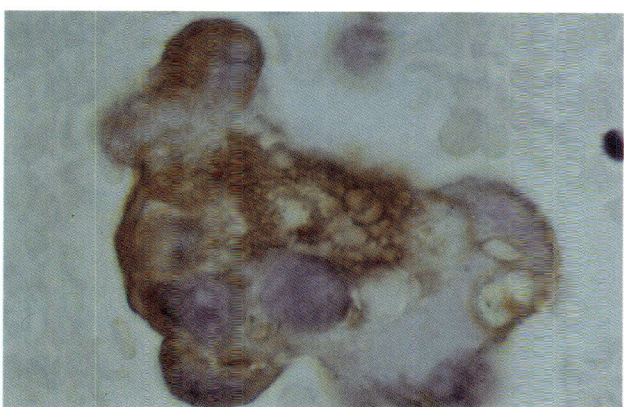

FIGURE 9.5 Cell group from same case shown in Figure 9.4, stained for CEA. Vacuoles and intracytoplasmic lumina are clearly delineated by the immunostain. Note the negative inflammatory and mesothelial cells in the background. (P.A.P. × 180)

cytochemistry, giving a positive reaction for CEA (Fig. 9.5). Cells of breast carcinoma may appear signet-ring in shape and be positive for mucicarmine or the combined alcian blue–CEA stain. In cells with intracytoplasmic lumina this feature may be highlighted by the demonstration of actin using appropriate antibodies. The anti-EMA antibody enhances the outer border of the cell groups with the thick cell membrane pattern shown by mesothelioma. The degree of anaplasia of the tumor cells ranges from very bland elements, difficult to distinguish from mesothelial cells, to anaplastic cells with bizarre sizes and shapes. The most difficult form to recognize is a carcinoma of the breast that sheds mainly single cells (Fig. 9.6). This type may be virtually impossible to identify because of its morphologic similarities with mesothelial cells. The most helpful criterion to recognize their malignant nature is the large size of the tumor cells, sometimes two to three times that of mesothelial cells. Occasionally these malignant cells have intracytoplasm lumina, typical of breast carcinoma (Fig. 9.7). This feature corresponds to the magenta dot of MGG-stained preparations but may also be visible with H&E or the Pap stain (Fig. 9.8). DNA ploidy abnormalities may not always assist in the recognition of malignancy, whereas determination of the percentage of cells in the S-phase is a good prognostic indicator. The greater the aneuploidy and the percentage of cells in the S-phase, the more aggressive the breast carcinoma is expected to be. Estrogen receptor analysis may be performed in FNAs of the breast and have also been used in malignant effusions. Other types of breast carcinoma in the effusion such as small duct carcinoma and lobular carcinoma are recognized by the small size of their cells and their lesser tendency toward cell ball formation. However, cytologic recognition of these and of comedocarcinoma and tubular carcinoma in effusions cannot be made with certainty without prior knowledge of the histologic type in the primary site. Cystosarcoma phyllodes is characterized by large sheets of tumor cells and occasional spindle cell elements, but we are yet to see an example of this tumor in an effusion specimen.

Lung

Carcinoma of the lung is not a single entity and four major types are recognized: adenocarcinoma, squamous cell carcinoma, large cell carcinoma, and small cell carcinoma. Carcinomas of the lung frequently cause pleural effusion by obstructing the hilar lymph nodes or the pleural lymphatics by direct seeding (Fig. 9.9). The effusion may present initially as a transudate but soon an exudate will form, either by an inflammatory response or by the presence of malignant cells in the effusion. The frequency of the various histologic types of lung cancer resulting in pleural effusion is different than their frequency in the primary site. By far adenocarcinoma is the most common type. This is due to the propensity of these tumors to arise in peripheral air spaces and spread to the overlying pleura either directly or via the lymphatics. Acinar, glandular, solid, and papillary areas may sometimes be found in a single histologic section of the tumor. In the effusion, however, the predominant appearance is that of cohesive cell groups

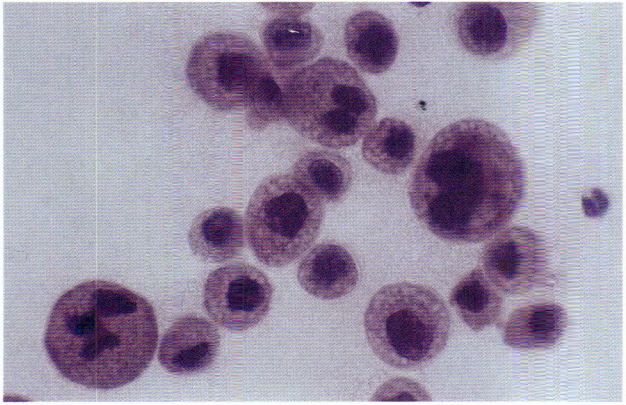

FIGURE 9.6 Single cells of ductal adenocarcinoma of the breast. The cytoplasm is vacuolated, and the nuclei assume bizarre pleomorphic shapes. (H&E × 800)

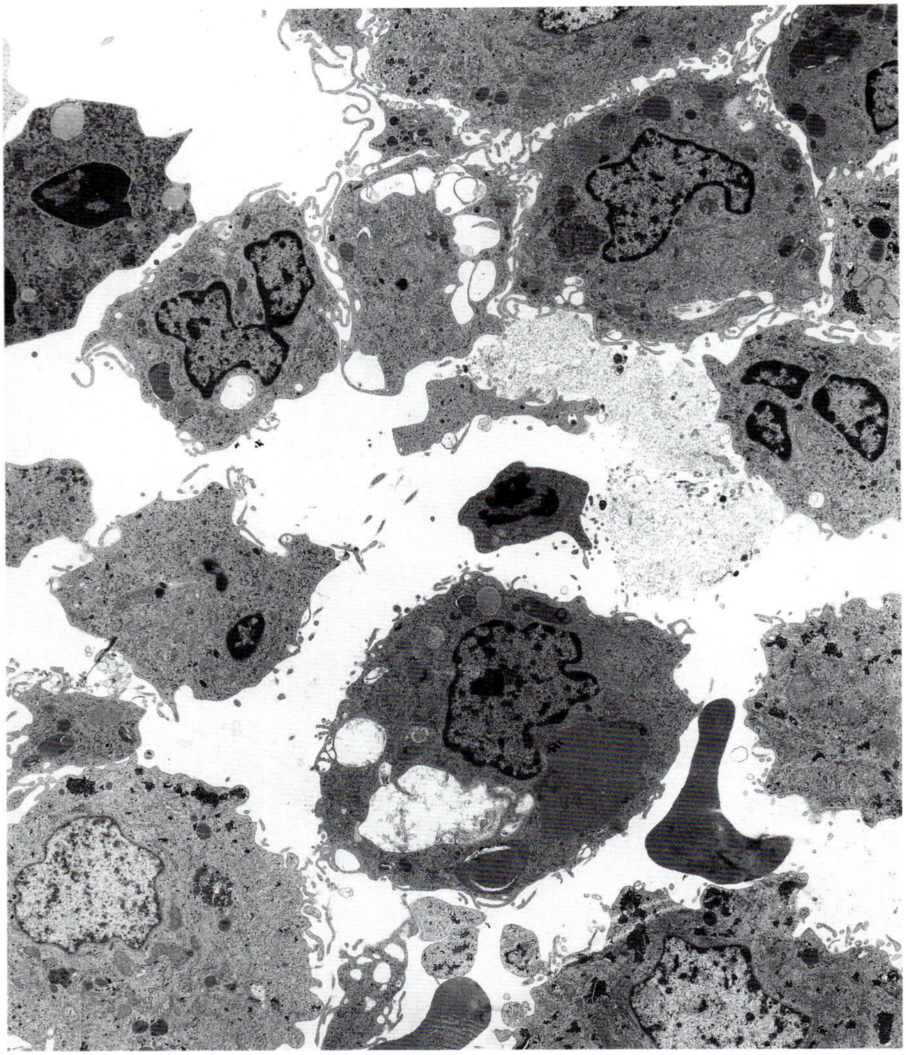

FIGURE 9.7 Single malignant cells in breast carcinoma. Notice vacuoles in the cytoplasm and intracytoplasmic lumen in dark cell near center. (EM × 6,000)

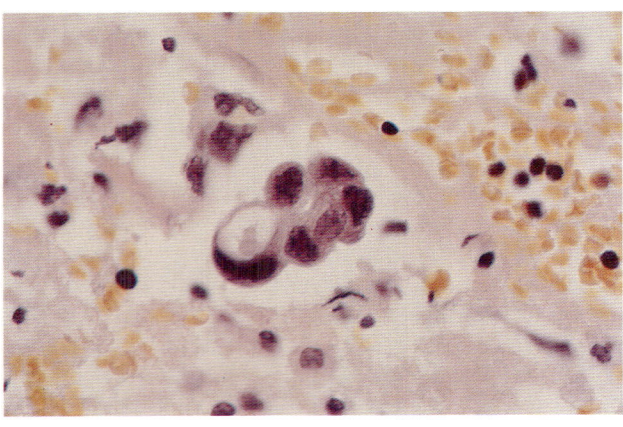

FIGURE 9.8 Neoplastic ductal cells of the breast with intracytoplasmic lumina. Note the pink appearance of the secretory material, corresponding to the purplish ''magenta dot'' in Diff-Quick-stained material. (H&E × 120)

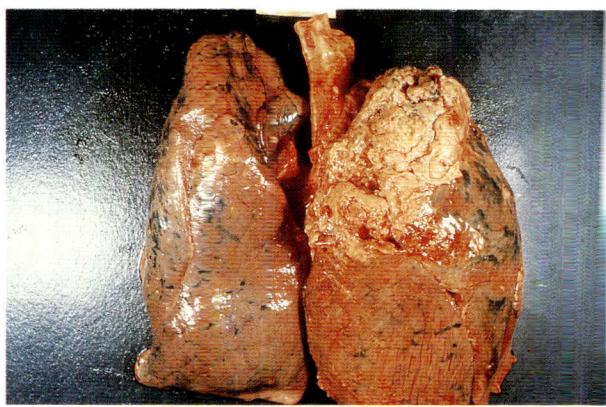

FIGURE 9.9 Gross specimen of a lung affected by adenocarcinoma. The tumor occupies most of the posteroapical region of the right lung over a vast surface in direct contact with the pleural space.

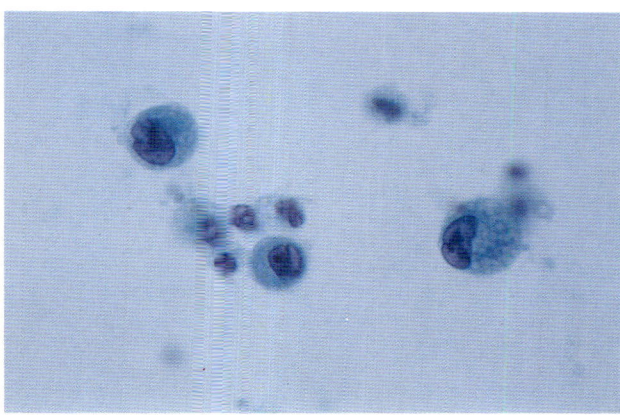

FIGURE 9.11 Adenocarcinoma of the lung presenting as single cells. Note the irregularities of the nuclear envelope and the moderately abundant, lacy cytoplasm. (Pap × 120)

with individual cells tightly woven around each other (Fig. 9.10). The cells may share a smooth common border or may alter the boundaries of the group in the form of scalloping. When compared with groups of mesothelial cells, malignant cells do not leave a window between each other, and their nuclear shapes are molded by their neighboring elements. The cells in adenocarcinomatous groups are moderately sized, but individual tumor cells may appear rather large and multinucleated, mimicking the histologic appearance of the

neoplasm. Occasionally the tumors may shed single cells or very small acinar or glandular structures which may be difficult to distinguish from breast or gastrointestinal carcinoma (Fig. 9.11). Poorly differentiated malignant cells may be difficult to recognize even in small pleural biopsies (Fig 9.12). This same difficulty is carried over to effusions containing poorly differentiated malignancies that give little clue as to their source of origin. Single malignant cells, or tumor cells in doublets, or small groups may be difficult to distinguish from meso-

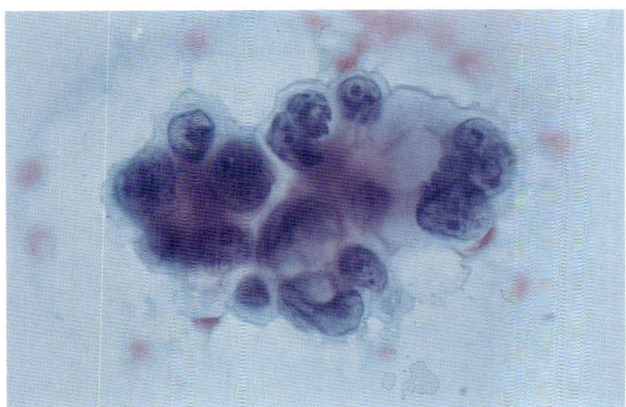

FIGURE 9.10 Adenocarcinoma of the lung in a pleural effusion. Cohesive groups of tumor cells with irregular, overlapping nuclei attest to the tridimensional growth pattern of this neoplasm. (Pap × 240)

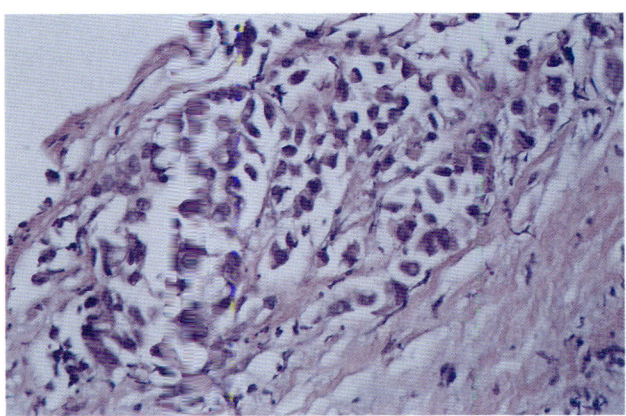

FIGURE 9.12 Permeation of pleura by adenocarcinoma of the lung. In contrast to mesothelioma, the cells stand out as alien to the area and fail to form cohesive cellular groupings (H&E × 90)

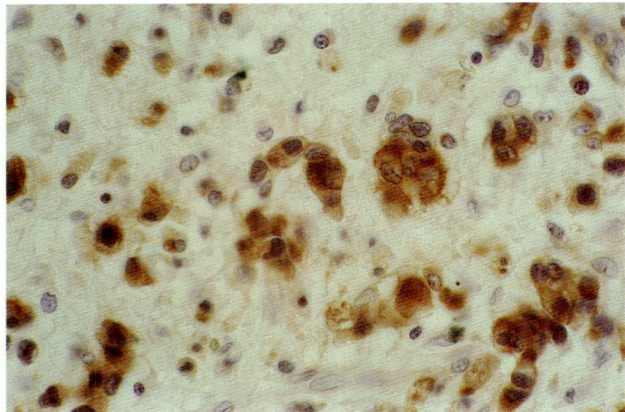

FIGURE 9.13   Lung adenocarcinoma with individual malignant cells, positive for CEA. The CEA-positive cells are easily distinguishable from the smaller negative cells in the background. (P.A.P. × 100)

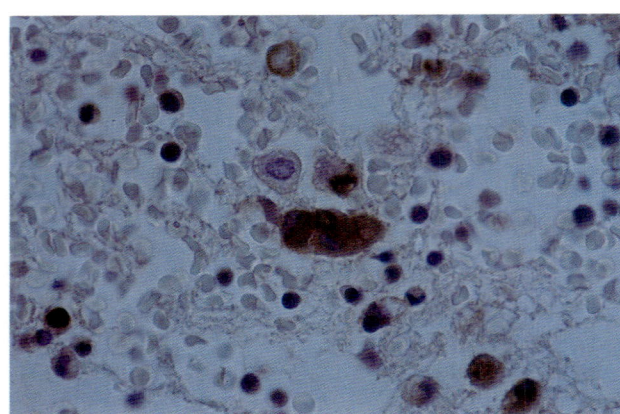

FIGURE 9.15   Cell block from the sample shown in Figure 9.14. Large malignant cells are positive for Leu-M1, while mesothelial cells are negative. Note the macrophages showing positivity unrelated to adenocarcinoma. (P.A.P. × 100)

thelial cells. When all the cells in an effusion appear malignant they may be difficult to recognize due to the absence of mesothelial cells against which they could be contrasted. Immunostains may be of value in these cases (Fig. 9.13). Ideally, cell blocks should be submitted to a panel of stains to confirm the adenocarcinomatous nature of the neoplasm (Figs. 9.14 and 9.15). Not uncommonly the cell-in-cell appearance will occur either by cannibalism among bizarre tumor cells or by

superimposition of a smaller cell upon the soft underbelly of a larger cell. At least one member of the pair is vacuolated, thus betraying their true adenocarcinomatous nature.

The bronchioalveolar variety of adenocarcinoma often presents with true papillary formations dominating the histologic picture (Fig. 9.16). Cytologically the cell groups are characterized by a central vascular core and disposition of the tumor cells petal-like and resembling

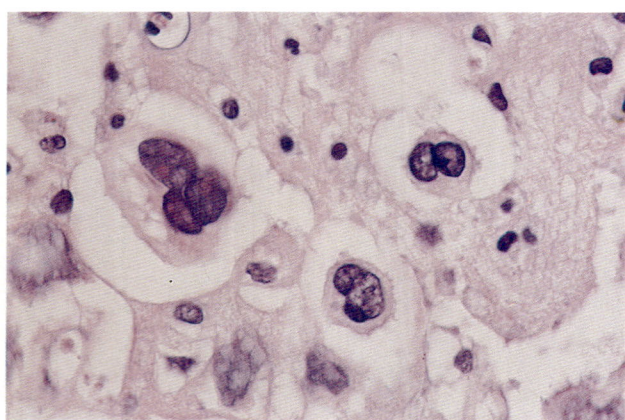

FIGURE 9.14   Adenocarcinoma of the lung in cell block. Large malignant cells occur in doublets or triplets, without spaces between one another. Notice the clear halo separating the tumor cells from their proteinaceous background. (H&E × 240)

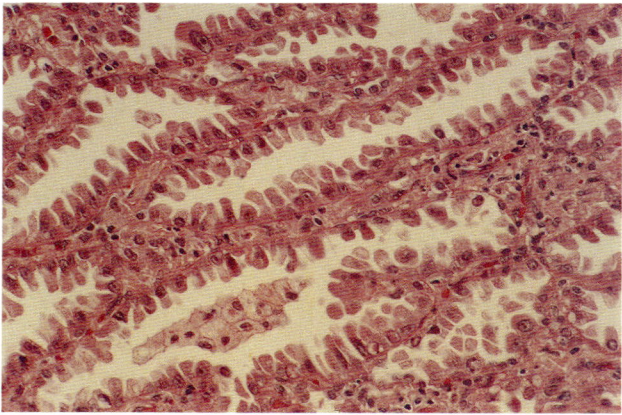

FIGURE 9.16   Histologic section of bronchioloalveolar carcinoma. In this well-differentiated region, the tumor cells are bland and grow along alveolar septa. (H&E × 140)

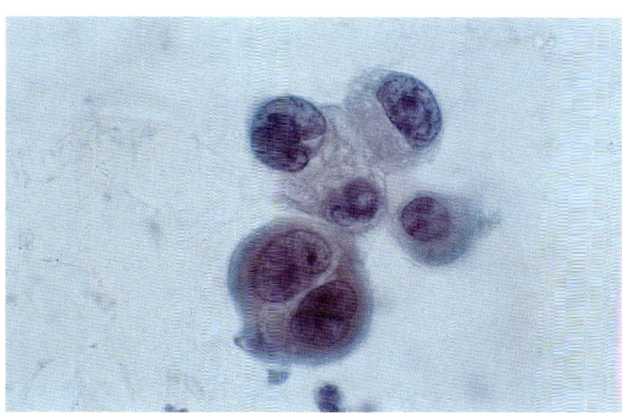

FIGURE 9.17 Bronchioloalveolar carcinoma in pericardial effusion. Note the tumor cells in petal-like arrangements, as in a flower. The nuclei are irregular in shape and the chromatin distribution is rather variable; the nucleoli are very prominent. (Pap × 240)

a floret (Fig. 9.17). Psammoma bodies may occur in these tumors, raising other diagnostic possibilities which should be considered in light of the clinical data. Ultrastructurally, some bronchioalveolar carcinomas are recognized by lamellated inclusion bodies (Fig. 9.18). Other examples of bronchioloalveolar carcinoma show mucosubstance or clara cell-type granules. In the giant cell variety of adenocarcinoma, multinucleated or rather enormous mononucleated cells occur against a background that resembles adenocarcinoma. Unless the number of giant cells is overwhelming, this diagnosis is not possible in a cytologic specimen because the appreciation of medium-sized tumor cells may be grossly obscured by the presence of mesothelial cells.

Squamous cell carcinoma of the lung has a slower pattern of spread, remaining in the primary site for a longer time. This tumor extends mainly to the hilar lymph nodes. Near-hilar tumors, however, may break the serosal planes and extend into the pleural cavities and pericardial sac. In contrast to adenocarcinoma, which is more frequent among women, squamous cell carcinoma predominates in cigarette-smoking emphysematous males. These patients are usually elderly, and the effusion may be a terminal event in the course of a cavitating neoplasm. In squamous cell carcinoma most tumor cells occur as single elements. If groups are formed, they appear as small sheets (Fig. 9.19). None of the helpful features such as overt keratinization, sharp angular nuclear borders, or frequent elongated or tadpole shapes noted in sputum are clearly evident in

an effusion. Instead the predominant feature is the presence of rounded or oval cells with abundant transparent cytoplasm or, depending on the fixation, multilayered sheets of condensation. These correspond to the degree of keratinization, which is seldom fully noticeable in effusions. The nuclei are sharply bordered, large, and hyperchromatic, and nucleoli are often obscured by coarse chromatin granules. Histologically solid sheets of tumor cells are the rule, thus explaining the paucity of tumor cells in effusions (Fig. 9.20). If the tumor cells are numerous they may form angulated clusters but the groups lack the tightly woven character of the tridimensional clusters of adenocarcinoma (Fig. 9.21). When true groupings are formed they are more sheetlike in configuration and their nuclei exhibit a parallel rather than a haphazard orientation. Despite the lack of orangeophilia, the cells often express keratin (Fig. 9.22). When bizarre squamous cells attain a cell-in-cell arrangement, the possibility of an esophageal primary tumor should be considered, since this is a common feature of squamous cell carcinoma of the esophagus. Another feature that is common in squamous cell carcinoma of the esophagus but may be also seen in primary tumors of the lung is cavitation. These tumors are characterized by the presence of neutrophils burrowing into degenerative holes in the cytoplasm of tumor cells. Not uncommonly, infection supervenes and the tumor cells have to be diligently sought in a purulent exudate (Fig. 9.23). Certain tumors of the lung are poorly differentiated, showing neither squamous nor adenocarcinomatous full blown differentiation. Some of these may fulfill the criteria of large cell undifferentiated carcinoma (Fig. 9.24). The majority of these tumors share features with adenocarcinoma (Fig. 9.25). A minority of large cell carcinomas of the lung demonstrate attempts at squamous differentiation (Fig. 9.26).

Small cell carcinoma differs from the other types of lung cancers by requiring chemotherapy rather than surgical treatment. The neoplasm spreads early to mediastinal lymph nodes and may also involve the pleura and the pericardium (Fig. 9.27). The small metastatic cells tend to degenerate rapidly, but they retain their positivity to neuroendocrine markers (Fig. 9.28). However, it is infrequent for the oat cell variety of cell carcinoma of the lung to appear in malignant effusions. The cells in the serous fluid acquire a characteristic aspect of capping one another in two-cell to three-cell groupings (Fig. 9.29). However, if specimens are not properly processed, degenerating cells may form artifactually large clumps (Fig. 9.30). Occasionally, larger groups are formed, within which curved nuclei are noted in an on-

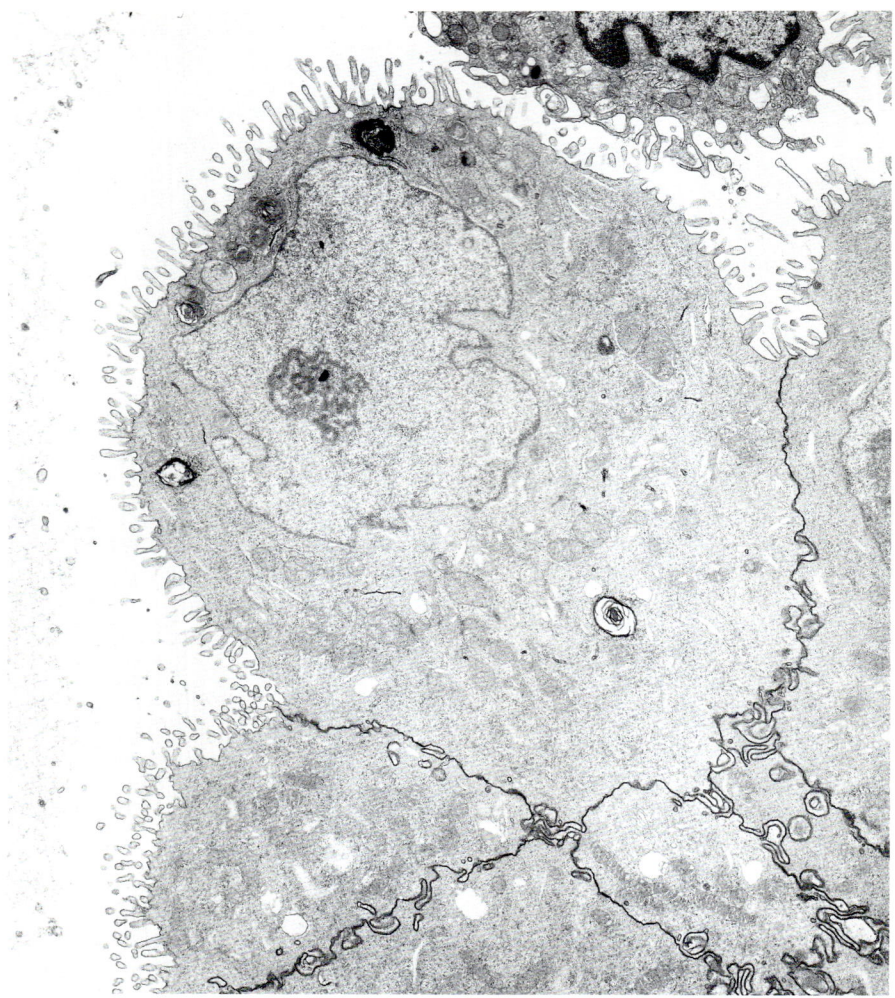

FIGURE 9.18 Ultrastructural appearance of bronchiolealveolar carcinoma. Note complex interdigitation among the cells. Abundant cytoplasm and lamellated inclusions are typical of Type II derived neoplasms. (TEM× 8,000)

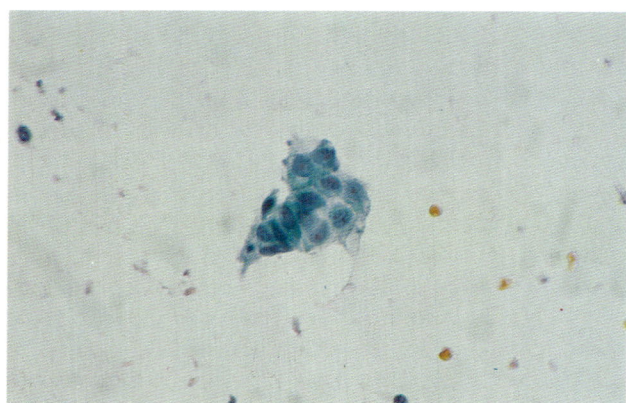

FIGURE 9.19 Poorly differentiated squamous cell carcinoma of the lung that extended to pleural space. The malignant squamous cells are loosely arranged as a flat sheet with angulated borders. (Pap× 60)

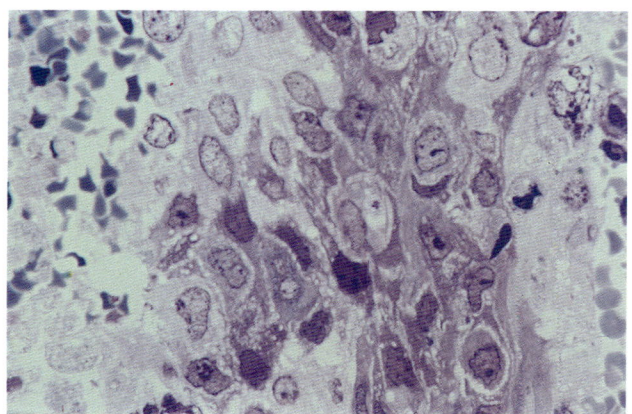

FIGURE 9.20 Semi-thin section of squamous cell carcinoma from plastic embedded cell block. Notice intercellular bridges and marked variation of chromatin pattern within the nuclei. (Toluidine Blue× 240)

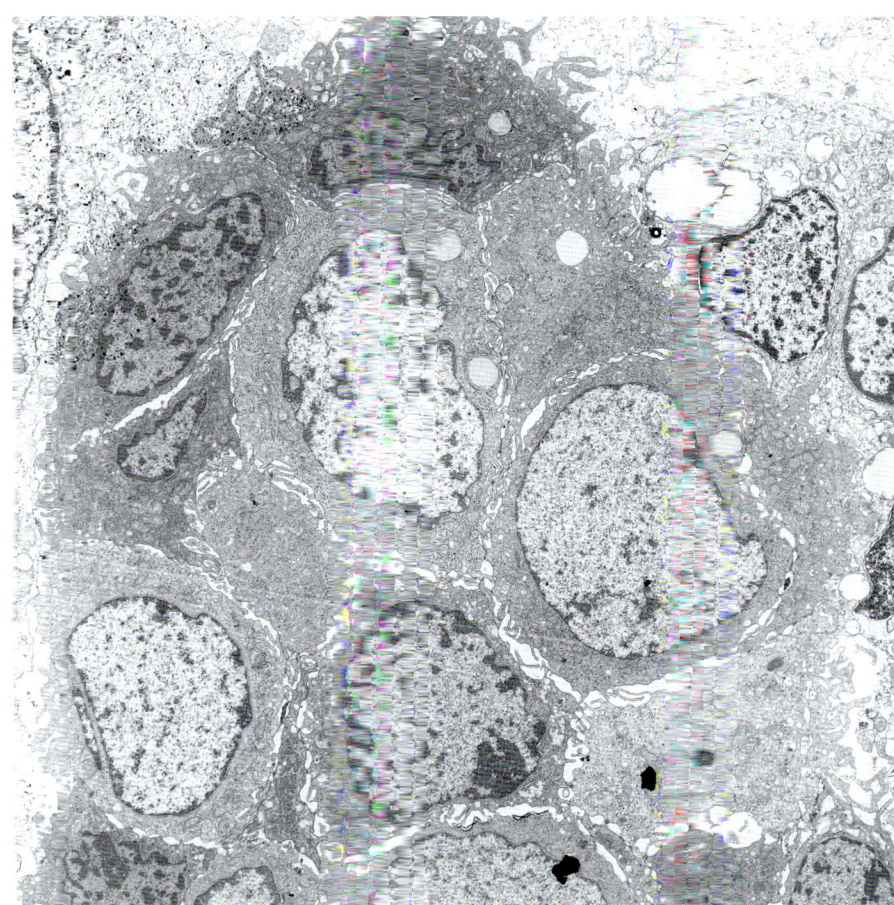

FIGURE 9.21 Squamous cell carcinoma of the lung examined ultrastructurally. The angulated sheet of tumor cells appears cohesive, but not to the extent noted in adenocarcinoma. (EM × 6,000)

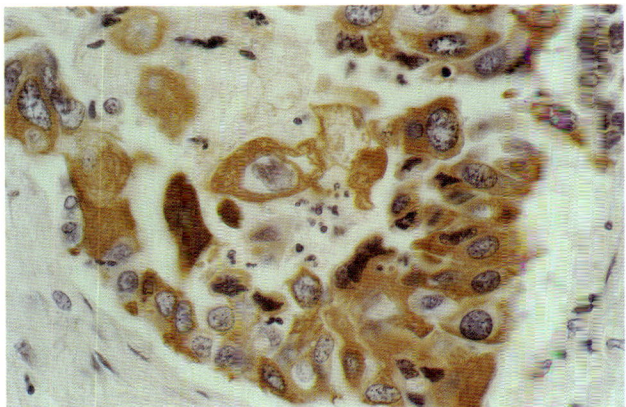

FIGURE 9.22 Keratin positivity in sheet of cells showing angulated edges. The antibody is against low molecular weight cytokeratin, thus explaining the lack of overt keratinization as seen by the Papanicolaou stain. (P.A.P. × 120)

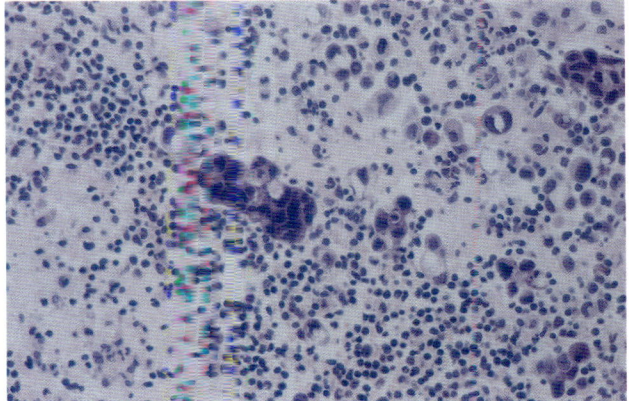

FIGURE 9.23 Cavitary squamous cell carcinoma with superinfection. Notice small groups of malignant cells against a purulent background. (Pap × 40)

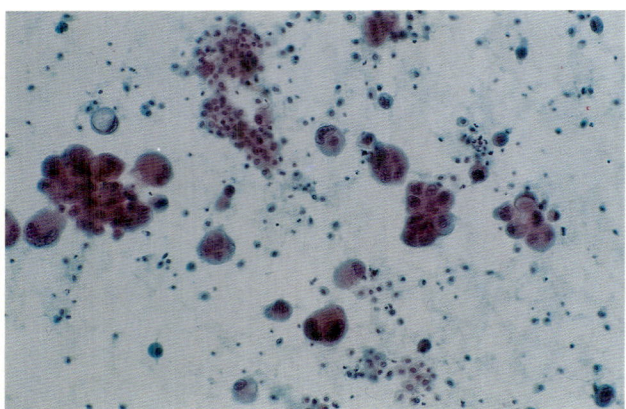

FIGURE 9.24   Large cell carcinoma of the lung in pleural effusion. Very large cells, singly and in groups, resemble oversized adenocarcinomatous cells and dwarf the mesothelial cells in the background. (Pap × 40)

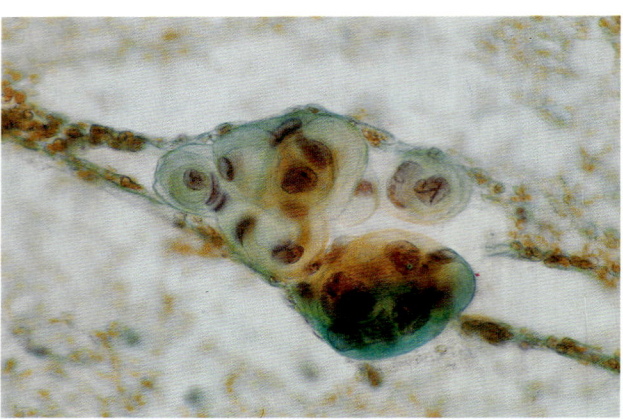

FIGURE 9.26   Large cell carcinoma with partial squamous differentiation. Cells arranged as squamous pearls display dense whorls of cytoplasm wrapped around neighboring cells. (Pap × 240)

ion-ring arrangement. Another characteristic feature of oat cell carcinoma is the absence of nucleoli (Fig. 9.31). Because the effusion is not an inhospitable environment, such as the bronchial lumen, small cell carcinomas of the lung may show a large amount of cytoplasm. We have seen oat cell carcinomas that were positive for CEA and could easily be misdiagnosed as adenocarcinoma in pleural fluid. The pathognomonic criterion of oat cell carcinoma is the demonstration of neuroendo-

crine differentiation, either by electron microscopy or immunocytochemistry.

Ovary

Ovarian carcinoma is the most common cause of ascites in women. A combination of papillary clusters of malignant cells and psammoma bodies is virtually pathogno-

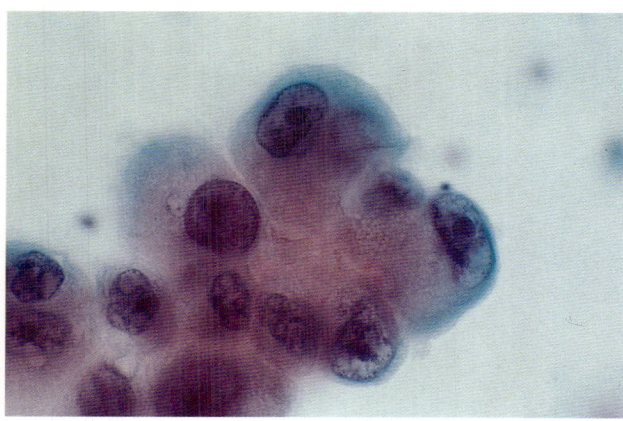

FIGURE 9.25   High-power view of a cell group from specimen shown in Figure 9.24. Large expanses of undifferentiated cytoplasm are shared by nuclei showing enormous nucleoli. (Pap × 240)

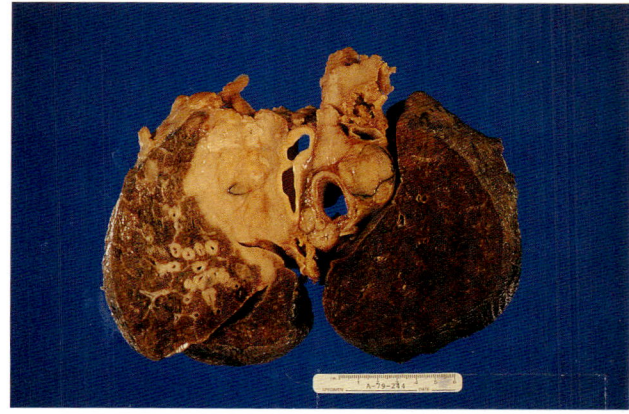

FIGURE 9.27   Small cell carcinoma extending to the medial aspect of the pleura. This tumor also contributes to pleural effusion by obstructing lymph nodes or permeating lymphatics of the lungs.

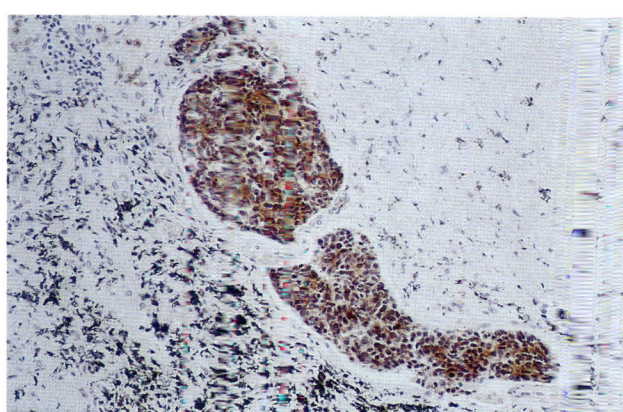

FIGURE 9.28   Metastatic deposit in a hilar lymph node showing hyperpigmentation. The neuroendocrine nature of this small cell carcinoma is confirmed by its positivity for neuron-specific enolase (NSE). (P.A.P. × 90)

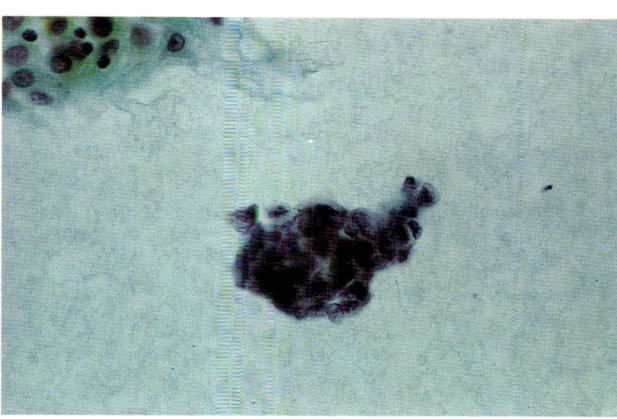

FIGURE 9.30   Small cell carcinoma, long-standing specimen. The cells appear degenerated and form groups mimicking acinar spaces. The correct diagnosis is made by paying particular attention to individual single cells. (Pap × 120)

monic for ovarian carcinoma (Fig. 9.32). Less frequently mucinous tumor cells are noted in association with papillary clusters (Fig. 9.33). The cells may be pulled off from the stroma and appear as hollow ringlets; or they may exfoliate still attached to a fibrovascular core. If the mucinous component predominates, the ovarian tumor is difficult to differentiate from neoplasms arising in the gastrointestinal tract or the lung (Fig. 9.34). Tumors that spread readily into the peritoneal cavity tend to be poorly differentiated and may be impossible to distinguish from pancreatic carcinomas despite their positivity with the mucin stains (Fig. 9.35). Neoplasms of borderline or low malignant potential may occasionally spread into the ascitic fluid where the cells are deceptively bland (Fig. 9.36). Papillary serous adenocarcinomas lack evidence of mucus secretion and display florid papillary formations (Fig. 9.37). These tumors are frequently diagnosed in washings during sec-

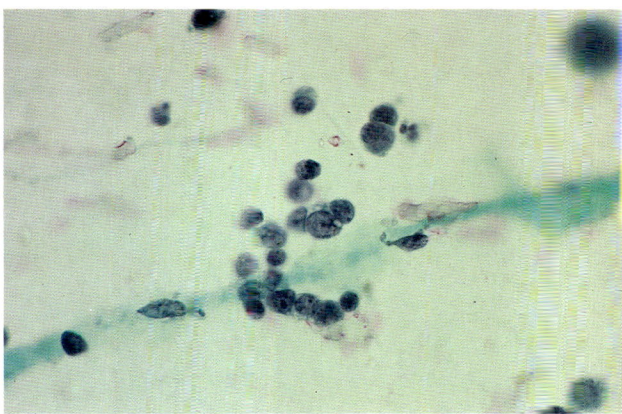

FIGURE 9.29   Small cell carcinoma, promptly processed specimen. The single cells appear crisp, with a slight tendency to mold. Note few cells lined up as a tandem (Pap × 120)

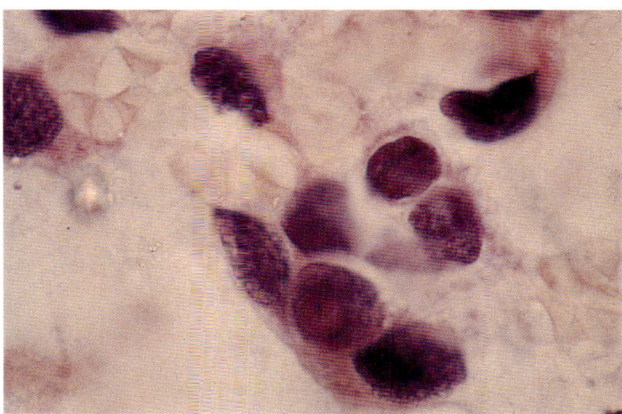

FIGURE 9.31   Molding of nuclei in small cell carcinoma. The neuroendocrine features are well appreciated: 1) negligible, wispy cytoplasm; 2) hyperchromatic, evenly distributed nuclear chromatin and 3) inconspicuous or absent nucleoli. (Pap × 400)

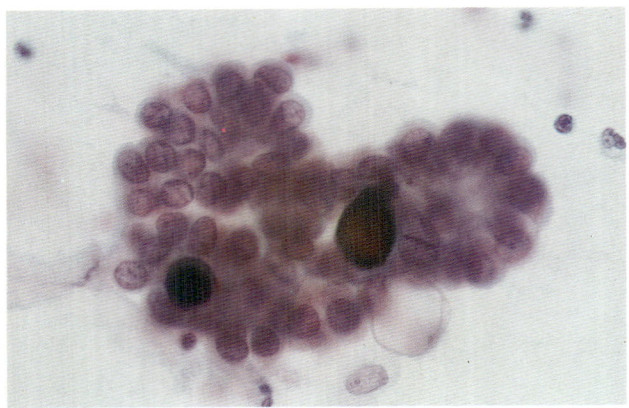

FIGURE 9.32 Papillary carcinoma of the ovary arranged around psammoma bodies. Only a rare cell shows evidence of mucinous differentiation. (Pap × 120)

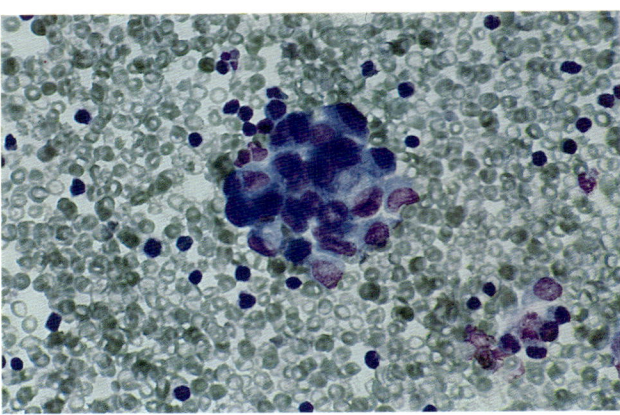

FIGURE 9.34 Papillary mucinous cystadenocarcinoma of the ovary. The cell group shows clustering of cells with abundant cytoplasm. (MGG × 100)

ond-look operations. Cytologically, papillary serous adenocarcinomas range from rather cohesive groups of cells to cells that shed individually (Fig. 9.38). Few of these tumors, however, may be positive for CEA (Fig. 9.39). Ovarian tumors that shed individual cells can be confused with breast carcinomas, but the tumor cells tend to be larger than those of breast origin and display more prominent nucleoli. The presence of psammoma bodies alone is not sufficient for a malignant diagnosis or for establishing an ovarian origin for a neoplasm (Fig. 9.40). If only degenerating atypical cells accompany a psammoma body, repeat taps are indicated in an at-

tempt to confirm or reject the diagnosis of carcinoma. Ultimately, by cytomorphology only it is not possible to pinpoint an ovarian origin except in cases where the history and other clinical data suggest the ovary as the primary site.

Uterus

Uterine carcinomas, particularly those tumors arising in the cervix, metastasize frequently to the retroperitoneal space. The tumor cells form irregular groups with at-

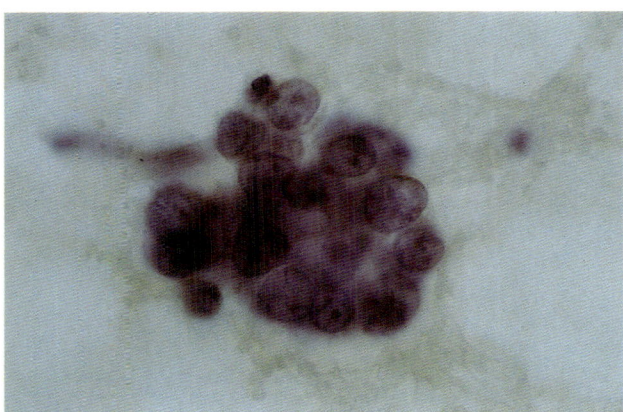

FIGURE 9.33 Pap-stained appearance of papillary carcinoma of the ovary. Evidence of secretion is not as as readily apparent as with the MGG stain. (Pap × 120)

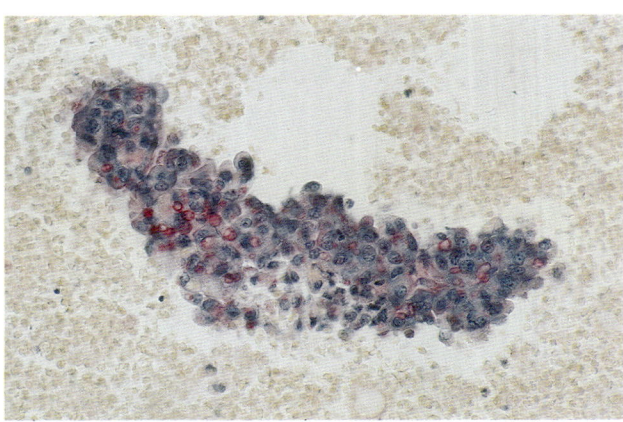

FIGURE 9.35 The mucicarmine stain clearly outlines the secretory products of numerous cells in the group. (Mucicarmine × 120)

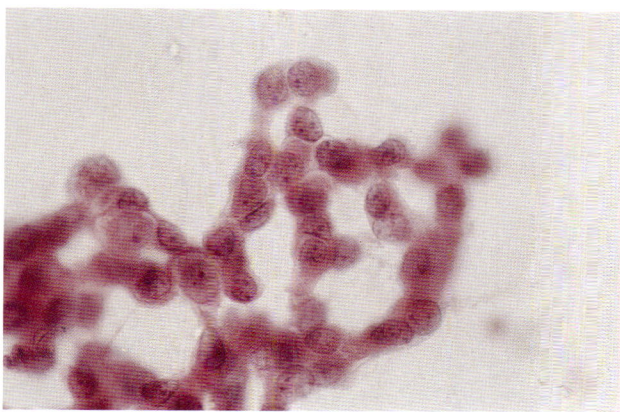

FIGURE 9.36   Peritoneal wash showing low grade papil-lary serous cystadenocarcinoma of the ovary. In this in-stance, the cells are less cohesive and show attempts at rudi-mentary gland formation. (Pap × 120)

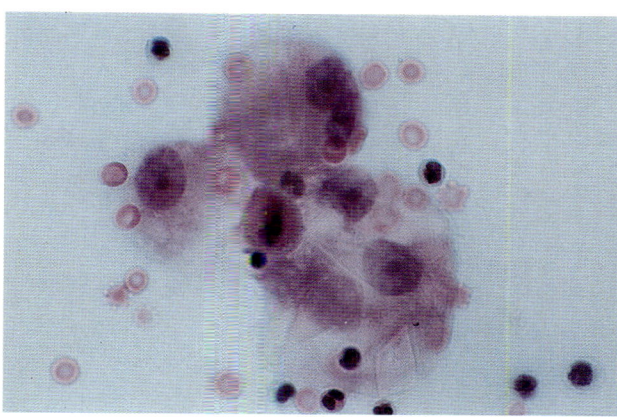

FIGURE 9.38   Small group of malignant serous ovarian cells. The cytoplasm is nearly transparent and shows no evi-dence of secretion. Nuclei display evenly distributed, pow-dery chromatin and prominent nucleoli. (Pap × 120)

tempts to mold around one another (Fig. 9.41). These tumors may spread into the ascitic fluid and present as tumor cells either singly or arranged in small cell groups (Fig. 9.42). Cytologically, squamous cell carcinomas of the cervix may display both a glassy-cell and a clear-cell appearance (Fig. 9.43). They may also form psammo-mabodies and as such, enter the differential diagnosis with renal-cell carcinoma (Fig. 9.44). Ascites caused by endometrial adenocarcinomas are rare, presenting as nonmucinous, slightly elongated tumor cells (Fig. 9.45). Carcinosarcomas and mixed müllerian neoplasms are relatively uncommon, but because of their aggressive nature they frequently lead to ascites (Fig. 9.46). The tumor cells are bizarre and in the case of mixed mülle-rian neoplasms they may exhibit a prominent epithelial component. Not infrequently, only the epithelial com-ponent is manifested and shows mucinous differentia-tion (Fig. 9.47). These cases are impossible to distin-guish from ordinary adenocarcinoma. As with other primary sites, diagnosis is facilitated by clinical data and comparison with sections from the original tumor.

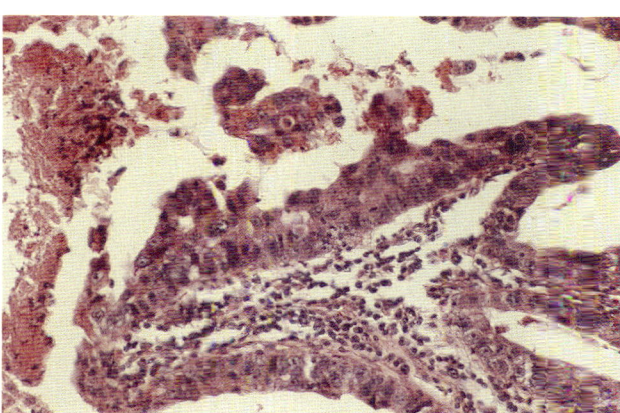

FIGURE 9.37   Cell block from papillary serous ovarian carcinoma. Neoplastic cells separated by a loose core pro-ject above the surface at different heights. (H&E × 120)

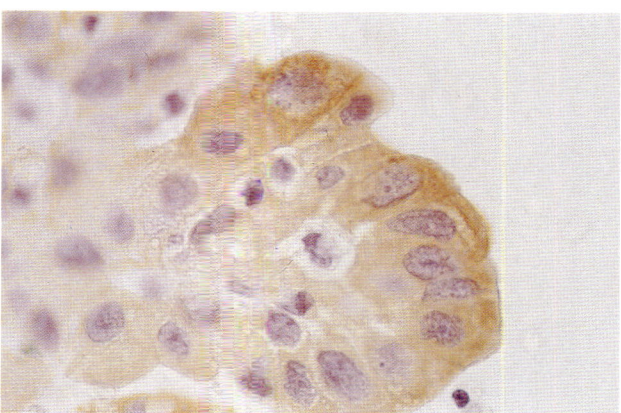

FIGURE 9.39   CEA staining of papillary mucinous ovar-ian cystadenocarcinoma. The immunostain outlines the fluffy secretory apparatus of the tumor cells. (P.A.P. × 90)

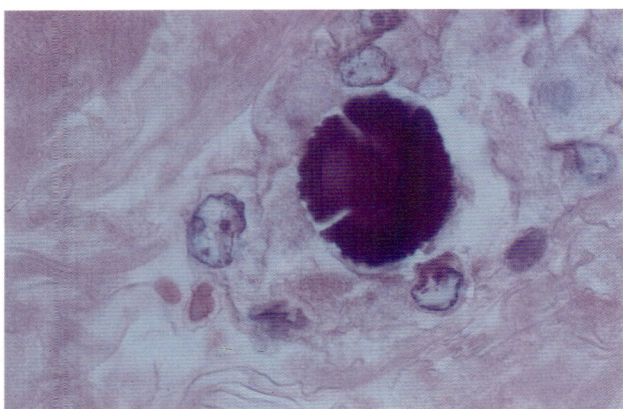

FIGURE 9.40 Psammoma body in papillary carcinoma of the ovary. The presence of such structures warrants a search for malignant cells but is not sufficient per se for a diagnosis of malignancy. (H&E × 400)

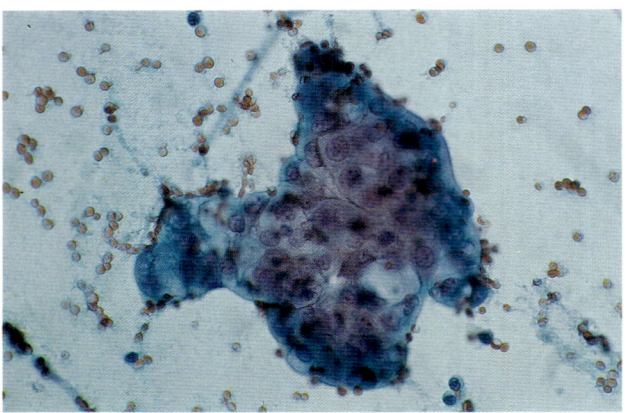

FIGURE 9.42 Sheet of polygonal cells from nonkeratinizing squamous cell carcinoma arising in the cervix. Even though the group is cohesive, it lacks the tightly woven appearance of adenocarcinoma. (Pap × 120)

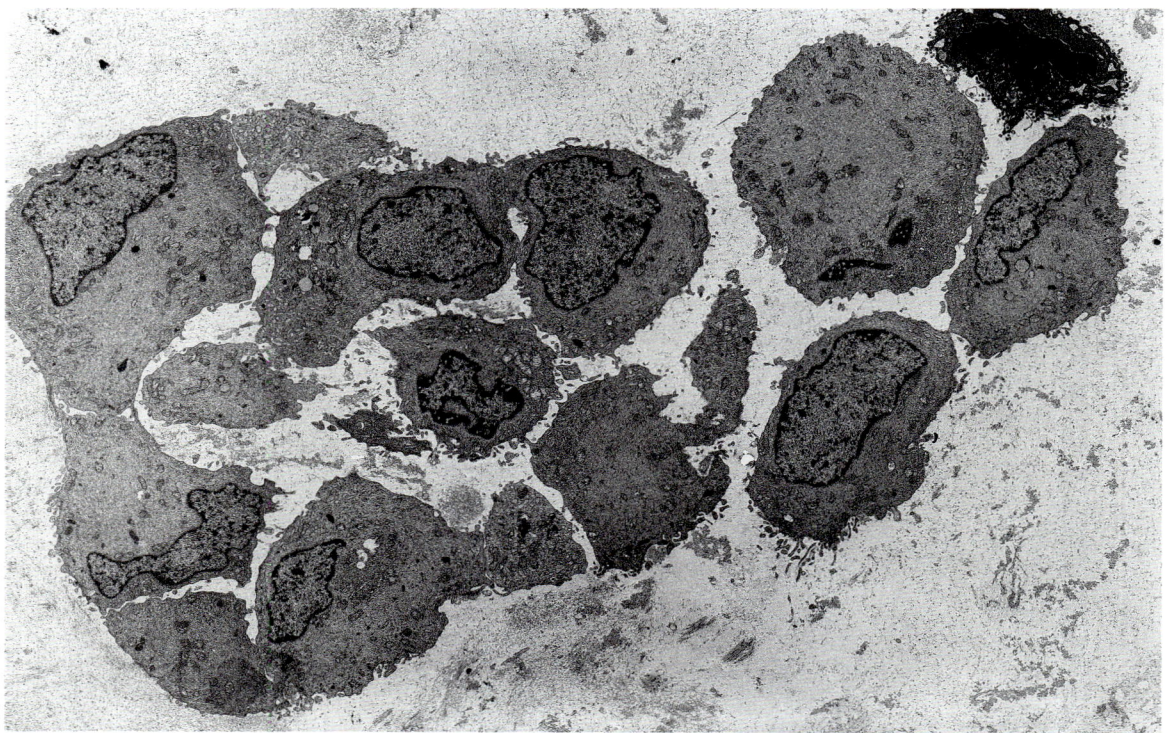

FIGURE 9.41 Loosely cohesive group of cells in adenocarcinoma. Microvilli and scalloped edges are typical of adenocarcinomatous differentiation. (EM × 7,800)

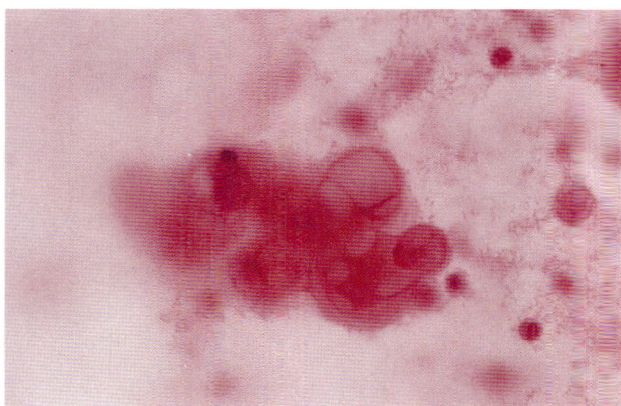

FIGURE 9.43   Clear cell variant of cervical adenocarcinoma. Note the large, clear cells arranged around small fragmented psammoma bodies. (H&E × 180)

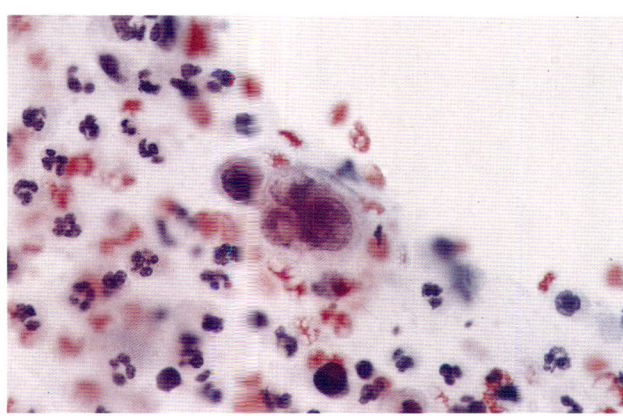

FIGURE 9.45   Cul-de-sac aspirate of endometrial adenocarcinoma showing bizarre malignant cells. The markedly inflammatory background accounts for the degeneration noted in the tumor cells. (Pap × 240)

Stomach

Gastric carcinomas constitute from 20 to 30% of primary sites in some series of malignant effusions. The tumors are not restricted to the ascitic fluid but may metastasize above the diaphragm and present as or pleural effusions and more rarely pericardial effusions. Large, single tumor cells are the rule but occasionally they may shed in small clusters (Fig. 9.48). Individual cells are difficult to distinguish from breast carcinoma except in the signet-ring variety where the mucin positivity makes the stomach a more likely source. These signet-ring cells display large mucus droplets which push the nucleus to one side of the cytoplasm (Fig. 9.49).

The intestinal type of gastric carcinoma sheds slightly elongated cells, but their columnar shape may be lost in effusions because of the rounding-up tendency of cells in fluid media. Anaplastic carcinoma, as

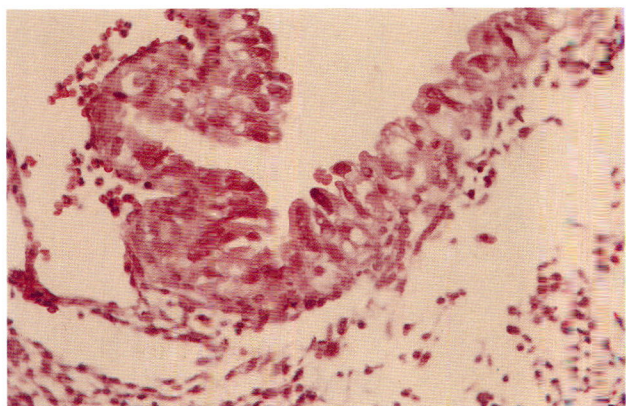

FIGURE 9.44   Portion of a cell block with clear cell carcinoma of the uterine cervix. Note the large, vacuolated cells supported in part by smaller, spindle-shaped mesenchymal cells. (H&E × 120)

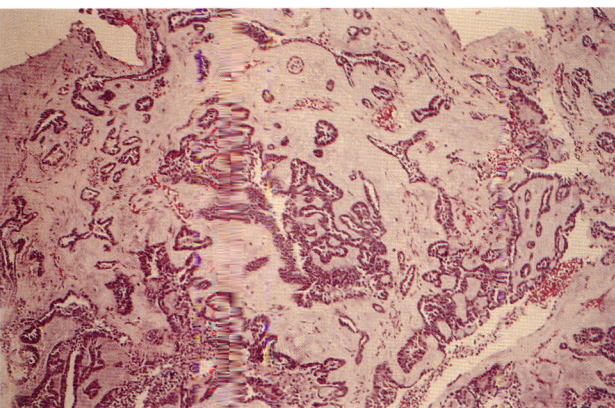

FIGURE 9.46   Tissue section of malignant mixed mesodermal tumor. The epithelial and myxomatous mesenchymal components form an intricate array of slit-like spaces infiltrating the retroperitoneum. (H&E × 90)

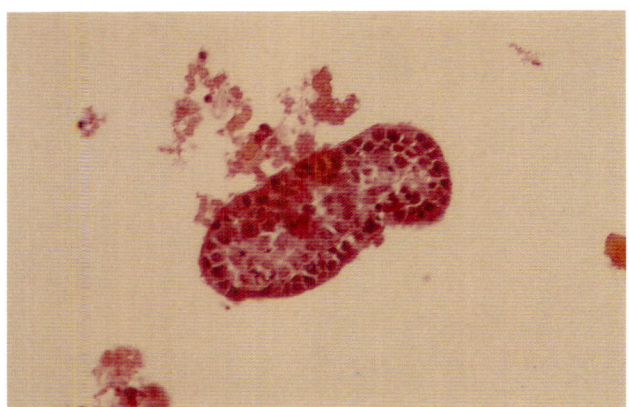

FIGURE 9.47   Detached group of cells from malignant mixed mesodermal tumor. Very often, only epithelial-like elements such as these are represented in the effusion. (H&E × 120)

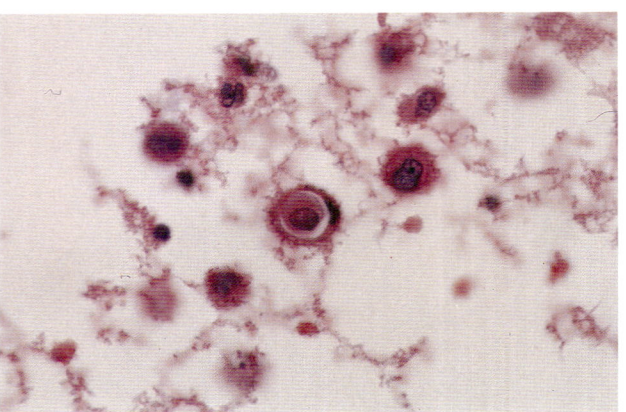

FIGURE 9.48   Single cells of gastric carcinoma. Notice the cell-in-cell phenomenon created when a tumor cell sits on top of the concavity of another tumor cell. (Pap × 240)

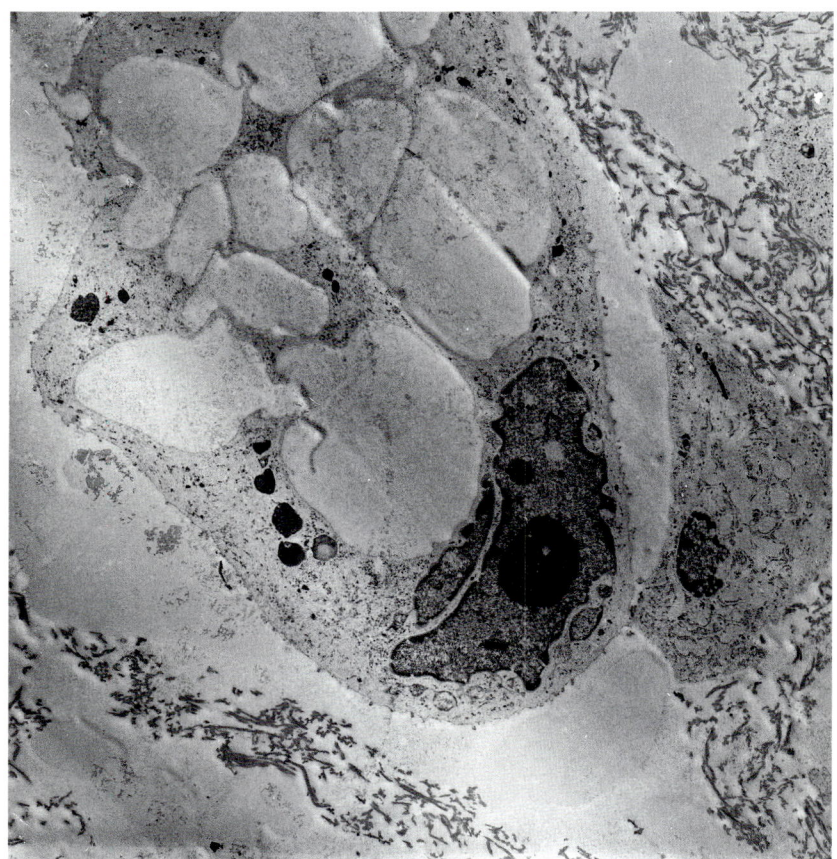

FIGURE 9.49   Degenerating single cell in carcinoma of the stomach. The clear vacuoles in the cytoplasm are responsible for the signet-ring appearance of the cell. (EM × 9,000)

the name indicates, exfoliates bizarre cells with foamy vacuolated cytoplasm and, occasionally, single cells with a large secretory vacuole and stripped nuclei secondary to tumor necrosis. We have yet to see an example of adenosquamous carcinoma arising in the stomach and presenting as a malignant effusion.

Colon

Colonic carcinomas comprise less than 5% of the primary source of malignant effusions. The vast majority present as clusters of elongated or rounded tumor cells some of which exhibit vacuolization (Fig. 9.50). Considerable molding may lead to the formation of cell balls but the tumor cells are considerably bigger than those seen in breast carcinoma. Even in instances where the cells retain their columnar shape the cytoplasm ranges from scant and granular to abundant and signet-ring—like. The chromatin distribution is coarse and nucleoli are usually very prominent. Poorly differentiated adenocarcinomas present with loosely arranged tumor cells with high nuclear:cytoplasmic ratio (Fig. 9.51). The nuclei are crowded in the clusters, but careful search reveals tumor cells still retaining their full columnar shape even though mucin-containing elements are found only with difficulty (Fig. 9.52). Lack of differentiation results in tumors composed of undifferentiated small true round cells resembling a neuroendocrine neoplasm.

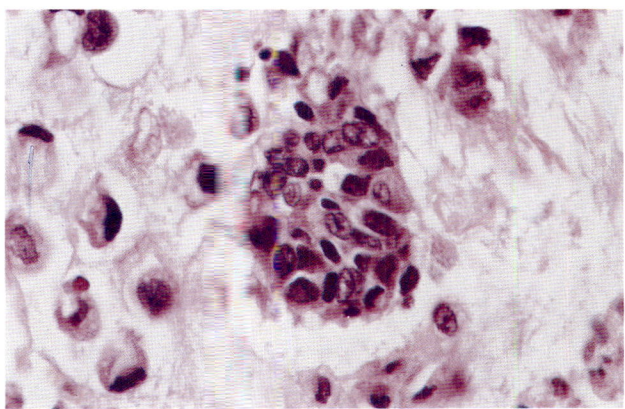

FIGURE 9.51 Cell block with degenerating cells of colonic adenocarcinoma. Note the irregularity of the nuclear envelope and the marked variation in nuclear size and shape. (H&E × 120)

Pancreas

Pancreatic neoplasms rank lower in frequency to gastric tumors as the source of malignant effusions (5–10% of the cases). The majority of these tumors are adenocarcinomas that shed small tumor cells arranged in papillary formations. The nuclei vary considerably in shape but

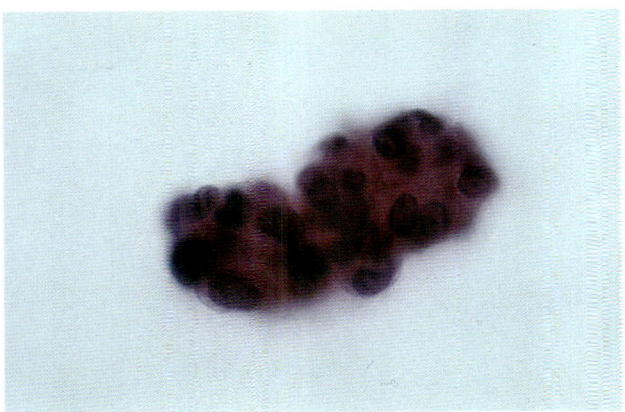

FIGURE 9.50 Colonic carcinoma. Cluster of tumor cells showing some elongation of the nuclei. In fluids, all cells tend to "ball up"; consequently, the tall columnar shape at the primary site is not always reflected in effusions. (Pap × 120)

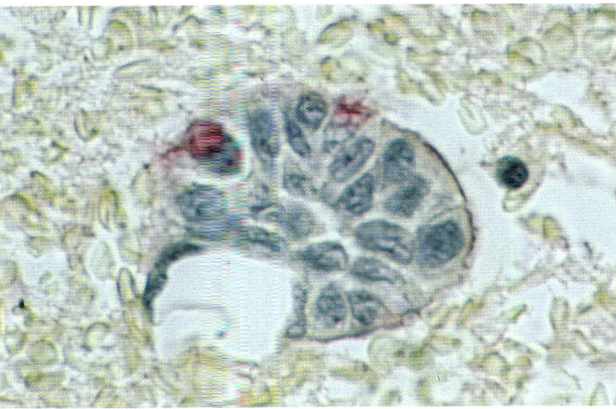

FIGURE 9.52 Focal mucicarmine positivity noted in colonic adenocarcinoma. The group shares a common border, but the nuclei overlap and are oriented in different directions. (Mucicarmine × 120)

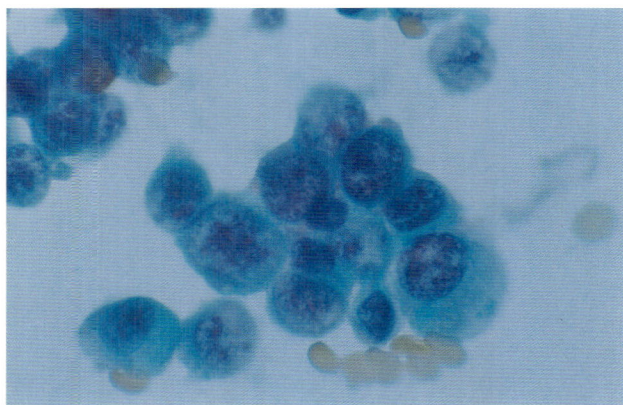

FIGURE 9.53 Poorly differentiated adenocarcinoma of the pancreas. The prominent nucleoli require differentiation form lymphoma, a task made easier by the tight groups of tumor cells. (Pap × 140)

not so much in size. The nuclear contour is crinkled with irregular distribution of chromatin granules beneath the nuclear envelope. The scant granular cytoplasm is rather cyanophilic with occasional vacuolization (Fig. 9.53). By electron microscopy the cells are closely apposed to one another and show evidence of glandular differentiation (Fig. 9.54). By immunocytochemistry the cells are frequently positive for CEA (Fig. 9.55). Mucin-producing adenocarcinomas of the pancreas are indistinguishable from their counterparts in the colon and in the stomach (Fig. 9.56). A high degree of cohesiveness characterizes the tumor cells, but in poorly differentiated carcinomas single large tumor cells may appear in the effusion (Fig. 9.57). Islet-cell tumors cannot be distinguished from a carcinoid tumor in cytologic samples (Fig. 9.58). Another tumor difficult to separate from other primary sources is anaplastic carcinoma of the pancreas.

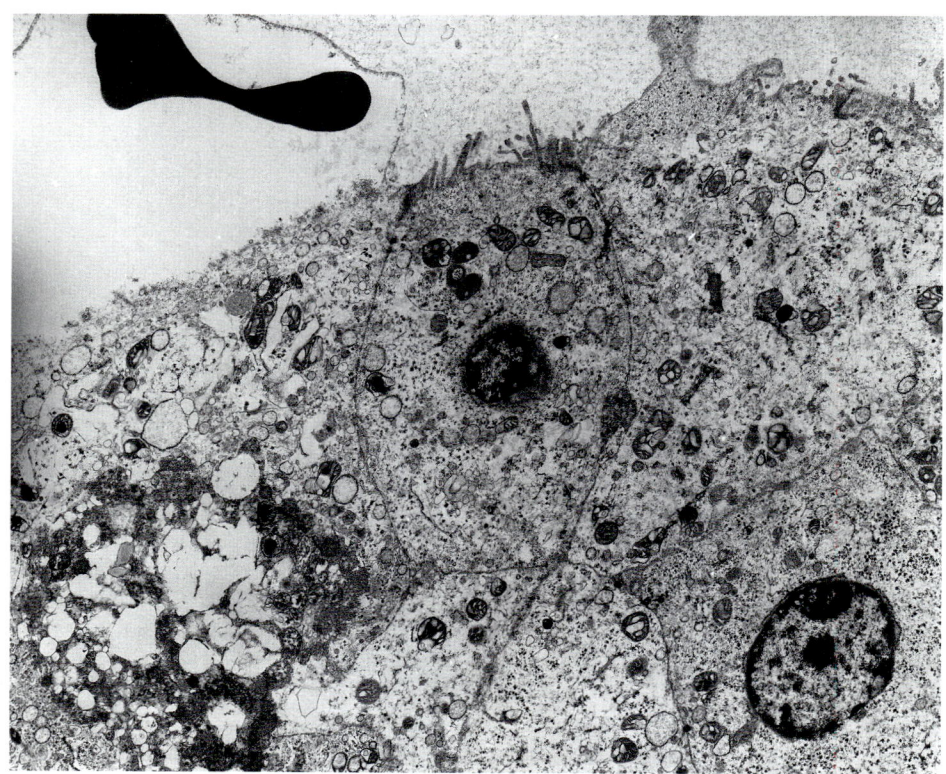

FIGURE 9.54 Poorly differentiated adenocarcinoma of the pancreas. Notice short microvilli, secretory vacuoles and confluence of cell borders off center. (EM × 7,800)

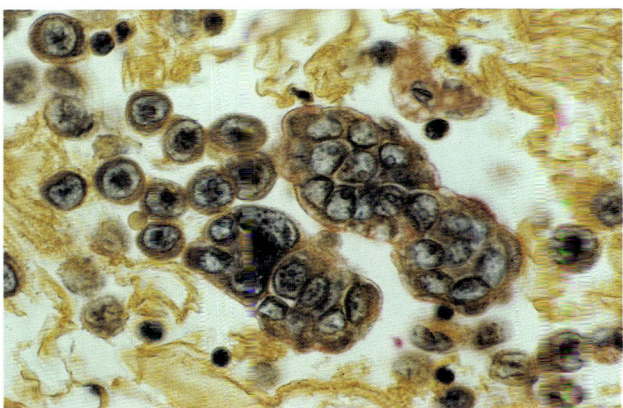

FIGURE 9.55 Pancreatic adenocarcinoma positive for CEA. Both single cells and clusters show prominent nucleoli (P.A.P. × 120)

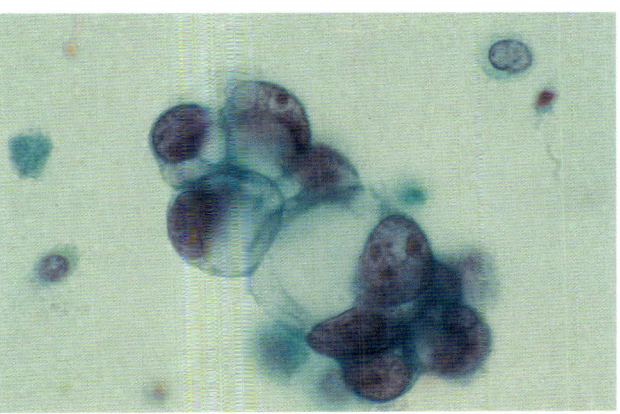

FIGURE 9.56 Vacuolated cells from carcinoma of the pancreas. The primary site of such a tumor cannot be accurately predicted without clinical information. (Pap × 120)

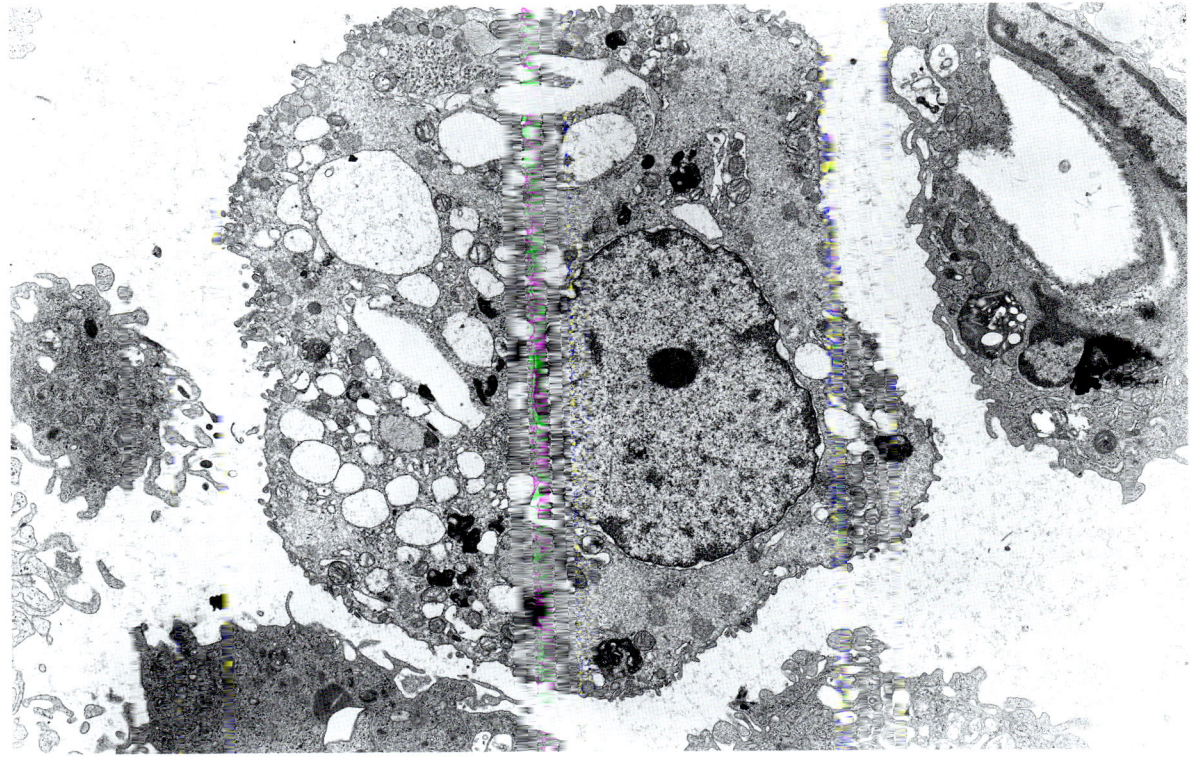

FIGURE 9.57 Mucus-secreting cell from adenocarcinoma of the pancreas. Microvilli are short and sparse; the cytoplasm contains secretory products and dilated vacuoles (EM × 8500)

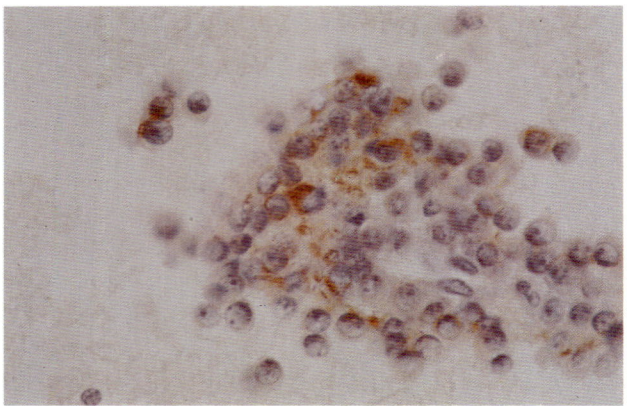

FIGURE 9.58   Islet cell tumor in ascites, probably secondary to extensive liver invasion. The cells are small, tightly packed, and positive for chromogranin. (P.A.P. × 120)

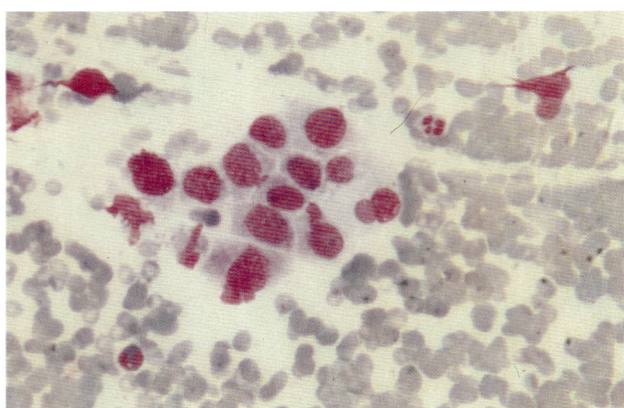

FIGURE 9.60   With the Diff-Quik stain, squamous cell carcinoma forms a geometric design. The cells are polygonal, but the nuclear features cannot be readily appreciated. (Pap × 120)

LESS COMMON EPITHELIAL NEOPLASMS

Esophagus

Squamous cell carcinoma of the esophagus is one of the rarest neoplasms to give origin to malignant effusions. The malignant squamous cells tend to be more bizarre than those originating in the lung, with frequent multinucleation and cell in cell pattern. The cytoplasm ranges from deep orangophilic in keratinizing neoplasms to cyanophilic in less well differentiated tumors (Fig. 9.59). The number of cells tends to be small, and degenerated cells may appear rather bland. In Diff-Quik preparations the cytoplasm stains light blue (Fig. 9.60). Based on cytology alone it is not possible to discern the esophageal origin particularly if another source such as the lung cannot be discarded on clinical grounds (Fig. 9.61). Other, albeit uncommon, sources of squamous cell carcinoma in effusions include the larynx and the uterine cervix in the female. Mature squamous cells may also appear in pleural effusions originating from ruptured cystic teratomas of the mediastinum.

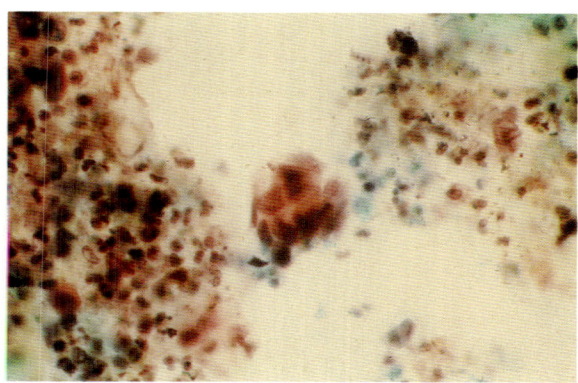

FIGURE 9.59   Moderately well-differentiated squamous cell carcinoma of the esophagus with a few keratinized cells. A fistulous tract between the esophagus and pericardium accounts for the dirty background. (Pap × 90)

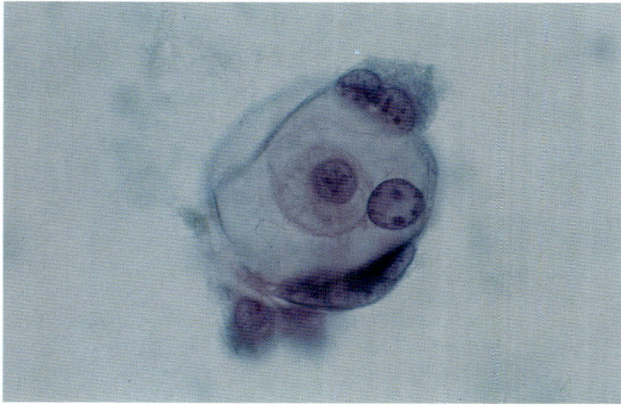

FIGURE 9.61   Cell-in-cell phenomenon in a keratinized pearl from esophageal carcinoma. In effusions these cells have a tendency to balloon up and it is not possible to establish their primary source. (Pap × 400)

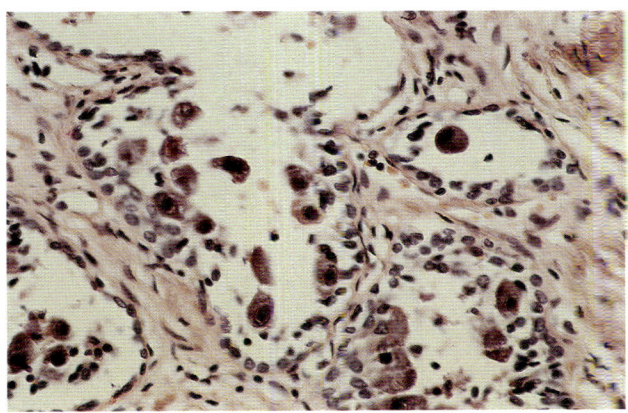

FIGURE 9.62 Mixture of cells in retroperitoneal implant from renal cell carcinoma. Cuboidal, rounded, and slightly elongated, cells show nuclei oriented in many directions. Notice also spindled elements with marked anisocytosis and anisonucleosis. (H&E × 120)

Kidney

Renal cell carcinomas comprise less than 2% of tumors noted in malignant effusions. The cells are large, with abundant pale granular cytoplasm and rounded nuclei but they may be rather pleomorphic, recapitulating their appearance in the primary site (Fig. 9.62). Most often renal cell carcinomas occur as single cells, though they may be artificially clustered in cell blocks and cytospin preparations (Fig. 9.63). If available, previously ob-

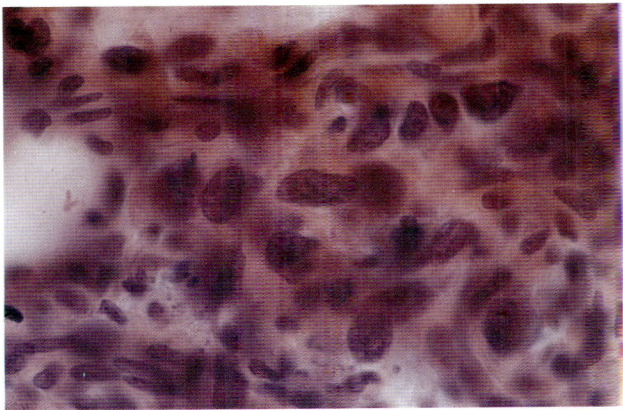

FIGURE 9.63 Cell block from renal cell carcinoma shown in figure 9.62. Note pleomorphic nuclear features and variation in size and shape of the cells. (H&E × 240)

tained histologic sections of the primary tumor are useful when compared to the effusion material. If alerted to this, prior to receiving the cytologic specimen, a simple oil-red-O stain of air-dried smear may obviate a more expensive workup. By E.M., not only lipid, but lakes of glycogen are typical of renal cell carcinoma (Fig. 9.64). The tumors may be rich in intermediate filaments which account for the eosinophilic appearance of the cells in cytologic preparations (Fig. 9.65). Nuclei of renal cell carcinomas are oval shaped and display prominent nucleoli. When these cells appear in sheets, they must be differentiated from mesothelial cells.

Urinary Bladder

Urothelial neoplasms of high grade malignancy may spread to the ascitic fluid but only rarely do they give rise to pleural effusions. The cells are arranged in syncytia, but as part of the generalized balling-up phenomenon they may appear as papillary clusters (Fig. 9.66). The nuclei are crisp, irregular in size and shape, and packed with finely dispersed chromatin granules that largely obscure small, sometimes multiple nucleoli. The cytoplasm is moderately dense with minimal vacuolization and slight cyanophilia. These tumors may be difficult to distinguish from other poorly differentiated carcinomas because they are commonly positive for CEA, and display only a small amount of nondescript cytoplasm (Fig. 9.67).

Liver

A primary tumor that very rarely presents as a malignant effusion is hepatocellular carcinoma. The tumor cells tend to occur in isolation without forming clusters or cell balls. Groupings, if they do occur, are irregular in size and appear as though attempting to form cords, as in histologic sections. The tumor cells are large with unusual shapes often encompassing intracytoplasmic lumina and with bizarre nuclei which may lead to their misinterpretation as choriocarcinoma. Nucleoli are enormous, often spiculated and brightly red. Cholangiocarcinomas, on the other hand, resemble adenocarcinomas of the colon or ovary. The tumor cells are tall and tightly molded, with basally placed nuclei and finely vacuolated cytoplasm. Pseudoacinar and floret arrangements are also identified or the cells may be rich in mucin, even attaining a signet ring–like configuration. Without clinical data, cholangiocarcinomas cannot be easily identified in effusions or metastatic sites.

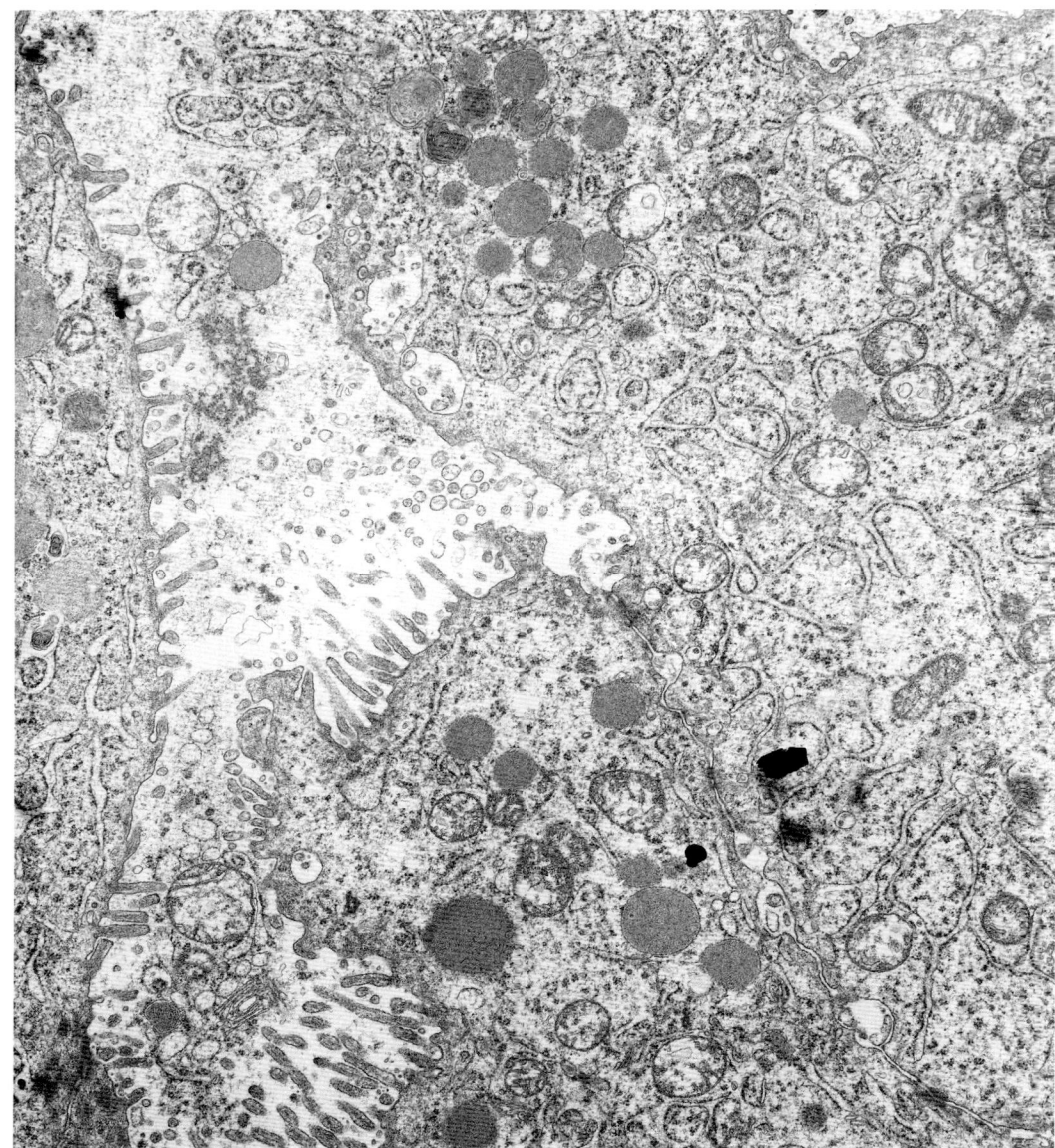

FIGURE 9.64 Ultrastructure of renal cell carcinoma. The combination of glycogen, lipid, and medium-length microvilli is typical of origin from the kidney. (EM × 7,800)

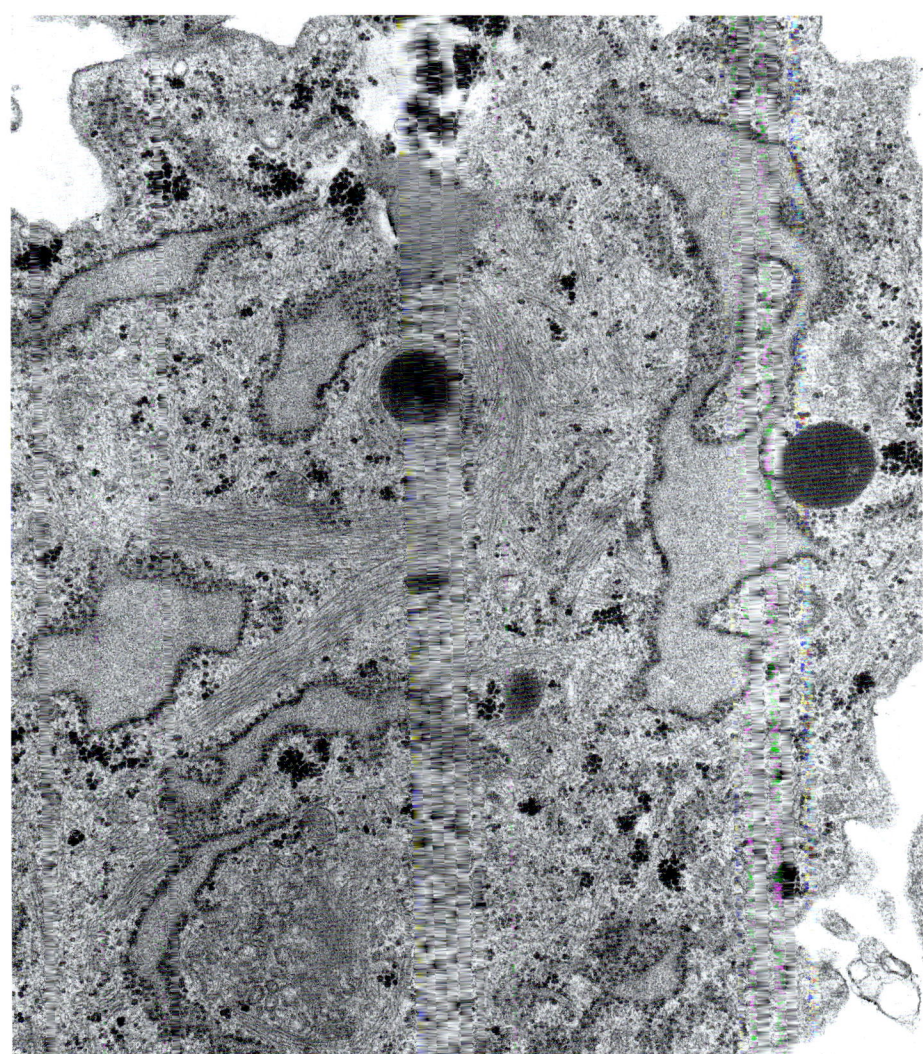

FIGURE 9.65 Another appearance of renal cell carcinoma. Dilated E.R. vesicles, occasional lipid droplet and abundant intermediate filaments would result in granular appearance of the tumor cells. (EM × 7,800)

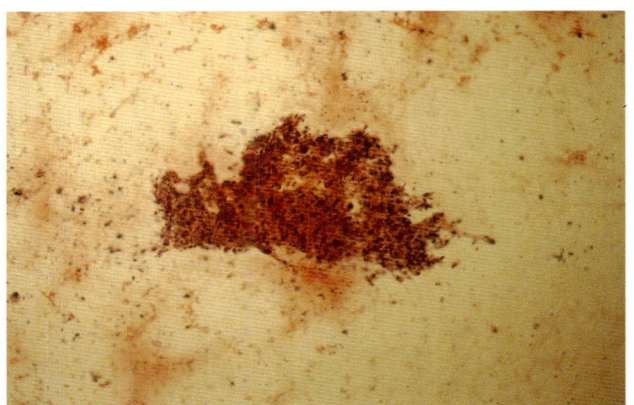

FIGURE 9.66   Large fragment of malignant urothelial cells in transitional cell carcinoma that extends into the peritoneal cavity. The cells are large, but the abundant cytoplasm lacks secretory vacuoles. (Pap× 90)

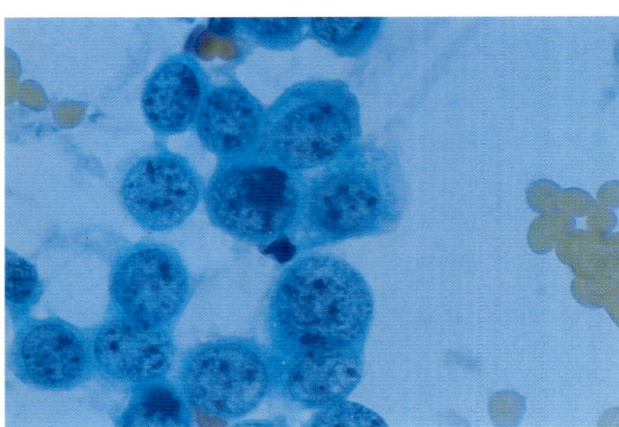

FIGURE 9.67   Group of urothelial cells in ascite fluid. There is no attempt at acinar, glandular or papillary formation (Pap× 240)

Prostate

Except for its small cell variant, prostatic carcinoma seldom presents as a peritoneal effusion. In this aggressive form of prostatic cancer, tumor cells may be recovered in pelvic washes. The cells tend to recapitulate their cytologic appearance in the primary site, in which they are small and may form microacini. Nucleoli are small and the finely dispersed chromatin granules are evenly distributed. Wide dissemination to bone, soft tissues, and retroperitoneum may lead to peritoneal effusion. The tumor may also affect the lungs, where it can be confused with a primary bronchogenic carcinoma. In conventional prostatic carcinoma, pleural effusion may follow from lymphatic obstruction caused by metastasis of the tumor onto the pleura. These tumors resemble nonmucinous carcinomas from other sites but tend to form rather compact masses of small, bland-appearing tumor cells.

Thyroid

Well-differentiated thyroid neoplasms follow a protracted course and only rarely give rise to malignant effusions. In these rare instances, the follicular and papillary nature of the neoplasm is reflected in the cytologic appearance of the effusion. Papillary tumors with psammoma bodies need to be differentiated mainly from

ovarian carcinoma, and this can be easily accomplished by the absence of mucin in the thyroid neoplasm. Follicular tumors may be nondescript and necessitate markers for their recognition. Poorly differentiated thyroid neoplasms, in particular the undifferentiated spindle and giant cell variant, may disseminate widely with malignant effusions in pleural, pericardial, and peritoneal spaces. The cells are large with bizarre shapes of the cytoplasm, multinucleation, and extremely prominent macronucleoli. The differential diagnosis is with a sarcoma or an undifferentiated large cell carcinoma of nonthyroid origin.

Adrenal

These clear cell neoplasms are rarely diagnosed cytologically, even in the primary site. They are often difficult to differentiate from renal cell tumors, with which they share the cytologic features of abundant, finely vacuolated cytoplasm, large nuclei with prominent nucleoli, and the presence of lipid in the tumor cells. If all of these features are noted in a malignant effusion, either the kidney or the adrenal should be considered as possible primary sites. The distinction between these two sites is difficult, however, even with the use of electron microscopy and immunocytochemistry. The differentiation between origin in the kidney or the adrenal is seldom accomplished without a thorough clinical and radiologic investigation.

TABLE 9.4   Differential Diagnosis of Malignant Effusions Caused by Epithelial Neoplasms

Primary Neoplasm	Cytologic Findings	Immunodiagnostic Markers	Ultrastructural Features
COMMON			
Lung	Cell balls, vacuolated cells	Surfactant apoprotein, CEA	Lamellar bodies, fluffy granules
Breast	Cell balls, single cells	Lactalbumin, estrogen receptor	Intracytoplasmic lumina
Ovary	Papillary clusters, psammoma bodies	OC-125	Microvilli, cilia
Uterus	Cell balls, vacuolated cells	CEA, EMA	Small secretory granules, short microvilli
Stomach	Single cells, signet-ring	CEA, EMA	Filamentous cores, deep rootlets
Colon	Tall columnar cells	CEA, EMA	Filamentous cores, deep rootlets
Pancreas	Cell balls, giant cells	DU-Pan 2	Small secretory granules, short microvilli
UNCOMMON			
Esophagus	Keratinization, cannibalism	Keratin (HMW)	Desmosomes, tonofilaments
Kidney	Single cells, granular cytoplasm	Secretory piece, URO series	Glycogen particles, lipid droplets
Bladder	Fluffy cell groups	Keratin, CEA	Intercellular junctions, no secretory granules
Liver	Single large cells, cords of cells	Alpha-fetoprotein, hBsAg, α_1ACT, keratin (LMW)	Bile canaliculi, bizarre mitochondria
Prostate	Microacini, cell balls	PSA, PSAP	Short microvilli, abundant organelles
Thyroid	Cell balls, vacuolated cells	Thyroglobulin, calcitonin, CEA	Complex nuclear contour, amorphous colloid/NE granules
Neuroendocrine carcinoma	Small cells, onion skin	NSE, chromogranin, hormones	Neuroendocrine granules, paranuclear tufts

DISTINCTION OF CARCINOMAS FROM OTHER NEOPLASMS

At times the diagnosis of malignant effusion is easily established but its carcinomatous nature is in doubt. In these cases, it is useful to ascribe the tumor cells to a given cytologic category such as small cell, large cell, spindle cell, or pleomorphic cell and then to proceed with the differential diagnosis by correlating clinical data to the site of the effusion. A simple special stain or a panel of immunostains may resolve the dilemma and place the tumor in a narrower diagnostic category such as carcinoma, lymphoma, sarcoma, or melanoma, or it

may simply categorize the malignant effusion as being of either epithelial or nonepithelial origin. The use of ancillary methods, especially electron microscopy and immunocytochemistry together with cytomorphology and clinical data may assist in ascertaining the primary source of the epithelial neoplasms (Table 9.4).

By comparison, nonepithelial tumors often resist all efforts at identification and subclassification. The number of special stains and immunocytochemical markers is considerably smaller in nonepithelial as compared with epithelial neoplasms. They also seem to derive and differentiate little from a totipotential mesenchymal cell. The difficulties in recognizing and classifying nonepithelial are considered in the next chapter. A more thorough discussion of ways to identify the primary souce of malignant effusions is contained in chapter 13.

BIBLIOGRAPHY

Lung

Sahn SA. Pleural effusion in lung cancer. *Clin Chest Med.* 1982;3(2):443–452.

Salhadin A, Nasiell M, Nasiell K, et al. The unique cytologic picture of oat cell carcinoma in effusions. *Acta Cytol.* 1976; 20:298–302.

Takenaga A, Matsuda M, Horai T, et al. Scanning electron microscopy in the study of lung cancer. *Acta Cytol.* 1977;21(1):90–95.

Tsumuraya M, Kodama T, Kameya T, et al. Light and electron microscopic analysis of intranuclear inclusions in apillary adenocarcinoma of the lung. *Acta Cytol.* 1981;25(5):523–532.

Yam LT, Winkler CF. Immunocytochemical diagnosis of oat cell carcinoma in pleural effusion. *Acta Cytol.* 1984;28: 425–430.

Breast

Ashton, PR, Hollingsworth AS, Johnston WW. The cytopathology of metastatic breast cancer. *Acta Cytol.* 1975;19:1–6.

Danner D, Gmelich J. A comparative study of tumor cells from metastatic carcinoma of the breast in effusions. *Acta Cytol.* 1975;19(6):509–518.

McCarty K, Worlman J, Moore J, et al. Malignant effusions in recurrent breast cancer. *Cancer.* 1980;45:1609–1614.

Mallonee MM, Lin F, Hassanein R. A morphologic analysis of the cells of ductal carcinoma of the breast and of adenocarcinoma of the ovary in pleural and abdominal effusions. *Acta Cytol.* 1987;31:441–447.

Spriggs A, Jerrome DW. Intracellular mucous inclusions. *J Clin Pathol.* 1975;28:929–936.

Ovary

Covell J, Carry J. Feldman P. Peritoneal washings in ovarian tumors. *Acta Cytol.* 1985;29:310–316.

Ehya H, Lang WR. Cytology of granulosa cell tumour of the ovary. *Am J Clin Pathol.* 1986;85:402–406.

Graham J, Burstein P, Graham R. Prognostic significance of pleural effusion in ovarian cancer. *Am J Obstet Gynecol.* 1970;106:312–313.

Gupta PK, Albritton N, Erozan YS, et al. Occurrence of cilia in exfoliated ovarian adenocarcinoma cells. *Diagn Cytopathol.* 1985;1:228–231.

Kannerstein M, Churg J, McCaughey W, et al. Papillary tumors of the peritoneum in women: Mesothelioma or papillary carcinoma. *Am J Obstet Gynecol.* 1977;127(3):306–313.

Kashimura M, Matsukusma K, Kamura T, et al. Cytologic findings in peritoneal fluids from patients with ovarian serous adenocarcinoma. *Acta Cytol.* 1986;2(1):13–16.

Kashimura M, Tsukamoto N, Matsuyama T, et al. Cytologic findings of ascites from patients with ovarian dysgerminoma. *Acta Cytol.* 1983;27(1):59–62.

Kobayashi T, Teraoka S, Tsujioka T, et al. Ciliated ovarian adenocarcinoma cells in ascitic fluid cytology. *Diagn Cytopathol.* 1988;4(3):234–238.

McGowan L, Bunnag B, Arias LB. Peritoneal fluid cytology associated with benign neoplastic ovarian tumors in women. *Am J Obstet Gynecol.* 1972;11:961–966.

Uterus

Bewtra C, Greer K. Ultrastructural studies of cells in body cavity effusions. *Acta Cytol.* 1985;29(3):226–238.

Hidvegi D, Demay R, Sorensen K. Uterine Müllerian adenosarcoma with psammoma bodies: Cytologic, histologic and ultrastructural studies of a case. *Acta Cytol.* 1982;26: 323–326.

Hirai Y, Chen J, Hamada T, et al. Clinical and cytologic aspects of primary fallopian tube carcinoma. A report of ten cases. *Acta Cytol.* 1987;31(6):834–840.

Labay GR, Feiner FS. Malignant pleural endometriosis. *Am J Obstet Gynecol.* 1971;110:478–480.

Ziselman E, Harkavy S, Hogan M, et al. Peritoneal washing cytology. *Acta Cytol.* 1984;28(2):105–110.

Zura R, Mitchell M. Cytologic findings in peritoneal washings associated with benign gynecologic disease. *Acta Cytol.* 1988;32(2):139–147.

Stomach

Duane GB, Kanter MH: Light and electron microscopic characteristics of signet-ring adenocarcinoma cells in serous effusions and their distinction from mesothelial cells. *Acta Cytol.* 1985;29:211–218.

Kobayashi T, Gotah T, Kamachi M, et al. Immunocytochemical presentation of α-fetoprotein–producing gastric cancer in ascitic fluid. *Diagn Cytopathol.* 1988;4:116–120.

Colon

Legrand M, Pariente R. Electron microscopy in the cytological examination of metastatic pleural effusions. *Thorax.* 1976; 31:443–449.

Polsalaky Z, McGinley D, Polsalaky I. Electron microscopic identification of the colorectal origins of tumor cells in pleural fluid. *Acta Cytol.* 1983;27(1):45–48.

Pancreas

Goodale R, Gajl-Peczdska K, Dressel T, et al. Cytologic studies for the diagnosis of pancreatic cancer. *Cancer.* 1981; 47:1652–1655.

Combs G, Hidvegi DF, Ma Y, et al. Pleomorphic carcinoma of the pancreas: a rare case report of combined histologic features of pleomorphic adenocarcinoma and giant cell tumor of the pancreas. *Diagn Cytopathol.* 1988;4:316–322.

Esophagus

Cobb CJ, Wynn J, Cobb SR, et al. Cytologic findings in an effusion caused by rupture of a benign cystic teratoma of the mediastinum. *Acta Cytol.* 1985;29:1015–1020.

Smith-Purslow MJ, Kini SR, Naylor B. Cells of squamous-cell carcinoma in pleural, peritoneal and pericardial fluids: Origin and morphology. *Acta Cytol.* 1989;33:245–253.

Kidney/Bladder

Johnston W. The malignant pleural effusion. *Cancer.* 1985; 56:905–909.

Sears D, Hajdu S. The cytologic diagnosis of malignant neoplasms in pleural and peritoneal effusions. *Acta Cytol.* 1987; 31:85–97.

Liver

Woyke S, Domagala W, Olszewski W. Ultrastructure of hepatoma cells detected in peritoneal fluid. *Acta Cytol.* 1974;18: 130–136.

Yazdi H. Cytopathology of clear cell hepatocellular carcinoma in ascitic fluid. *Acta Cytol.* 1985;29:911–913.

Prostate

Broghamer W, Richardson R, Faurest S, et al. Prostate and phosphatase immunoperoxidase staining of cytologically positive effusions associated with adenocarcinomas of the prostate and neoplasms of uncertained origin. *Acta Cytol.* 1985; 29(3):274–278.

Thyroid

Yazdi HM, Hajdu SI, Melamed MR. Cytopathology of pericardial effusions. *Acta Cytol.* 1980;24:401–406.

Adrenal

Walts AE, Said JW. Specific tumor markers in diagnostic cytology: Immunoperoxidase studies of carcinoembryonic antigen, lysozyme and other tissue antigens in effusions, washes and aspirates. *Acta Cytol.* 1983;27:408–413.

CHAPTER TEN

Nonepithelial Neoplasms

Nonepithelial neoplasms constitute a heterogeneous group of primary sources of malignant effusion. When these lesions occur as a terminal event the diagnosis is simple, with the help of the clinical history and comparison of the cells in the effusion with those of the parent neoplasm. In effusions where the primary lesion is occult, as for example in amelanotic melanoma, the challenge to disclose the primary site is considerable. Perhaps of all categories of neoplasms, nonepithelial malignancies benefit the most from the use of a multimodal approach to cytologic examination. (Table 10.1) Immunocytochemistry plays a significant role in distinguishing non-epithelial tumors from the more common carcinomas.

MELANOMA

Not infrequently, malignant melanoma will metastasize widely and reach one of the serosal cavities. The cells of melanoma may occur singly or may form occasional loose cell groups. They may stand out as an alien cell population with abundant cytoplasm and eccentric nuclei which tends to overshadow the mesothelial cells. The individual cells are pleomorphic, frequently multinucleated with a considerable number of binucleated cells (Fig. 10.1). The cytoplasm is amphophilic, and nuclei display prominant nucleoli. Large round intranuclear inclusions are frequently observed and may completely obscure the nucleus. The chromatin granules are coarse but evenly distributed within the nuclear envelope.

Cytoplasmic pigment may be totally absent in melanoma or, rarely, it may form coarse granules that obscure cytologic detail. Melanoma cells without pigment may be difficult to distinguish from mesothelial cells. Most frequently, however, the pigment appears as a fine dust in the cytoplasm in contrast with the large clumps seen in macrophages that phagocytize melanin

(Fig. 10.2). Phagocytosis of melanin is more likely to occur in necrotic tumors which also show nuclear debris in the background. When cohesive groups are present in melanoma, they are composed of cells tightly wrapped around one another. However, the nuclei of the individual cells fail to mold to the same extent as in adenocarcinoma. As the cells in effusion tend to conform their dimensions to the surrounding fluid medium, rounding up of tumor cells is commonplace. However, melanomas may present rather bizarre cells. For these reasons melanomas often have to be differentiated from other large cell neoplasms (Table 10.2).

With the Diff-Quik stain, the cells of melanoma are considerably larger and paler than the surrounding mesothelial cells. Occasionally, melanoma cell variants such as anaplastic, bland, epithelioid, and clear-celled types may metastasize and give rise to a malignant effusion. In these cases, melanin may be demonstrated histochemically by the Fontana–Mason stain or immunocytochemically with anti S-100 or the HMB 45 antibody. By electron microscopy it is necessary to find premelanosomes and melanosomes to confirm the diagnosis of melanoma. These ancillary techniques are particularly useful when the least common variants of melanoma—the spindle cell and the small cell variants—need to be differentiated from poorly differentiated epithelial or mesenchymal neoplasms. Not infrequently, the precise classification of these tumors is impossible without clinical data suggesting the primary site.

SARCOMAS

Sarcomas constitute fewer than 2% of the tumors recognized in effusions. It is useful, when suspecting a nonepithelial neoplasm, to classify it in a general broad category from which special studies may further subclassify the tumor in question. Spindle cells, undifferentiated

TABLE 10.1 Antibodies Useful in the Study of Nonepithelial Neoplasms

Antibody	Applicable Neoplasm
Vimentin	Mesenchymal tumors (general)
Keratin	Synovial sarcoma, epithelioid sarcoma
Desmin	Myogenous tumors (smooth muscle, striated muscle)
Myoglobin	Rhabdomyoma, rhabdomyosarcoma
Factor VIII–related antigen, *Ulex europaeus* agglutinin	Vasoformative tumors (excluding Kaposi's sarcoma)
α_1-AT, lysozyme, α_1-ACT	Malignant fibrous histiocytoma
S-100 protein	Granular cell tumor, neurofibroma, schwannoma, clear cell sarcoma, malignant schwannoma, chondrosarcoma

From: Bedrossian CWM. Immunocytochemistry. In: Astarita RW, ed. *Practical Cytopathology.* New York: Churchill Livingstone; 1990: 403–457. With permission.

small round cells and pleomorphic tumor cells including multinucleated elements may be noted in the effusion generated by a sarcoma. They are distinguishable from carcinoma by their characteristic loose cell arrangement and unique cytologic features. In comparison to carcinoma, sarcomas fail to form cell balls, papillary groups, gland lumina, and acinar structures but appear in a rather noncohesive dispersed fashion in a malignant effusion. Occasionally, the malignant cells may form large tissue fragments, particularly in neoplasms that extend to rather than metastasize into a serosal cavity.

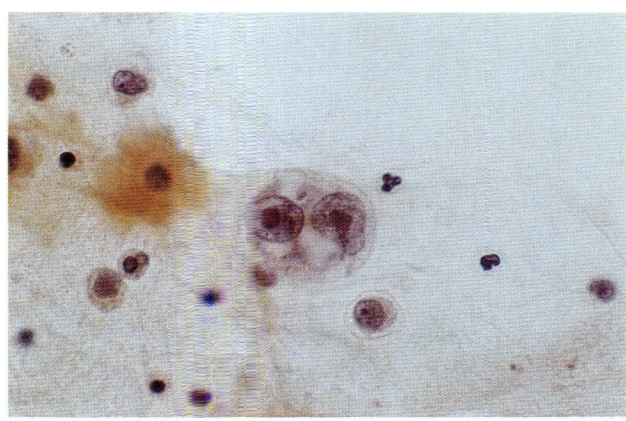

FIGURE 10.1 Malignant melanoma with clear vacuolization. The large binucleate element and smaller cells with a high nuclear:cytoplasmic ratio attest to the protean morphology of this neoplasm. (Pap × 400)

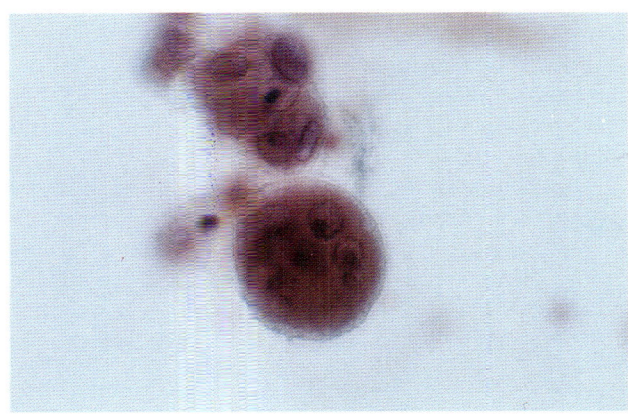

FIGURE 10.2 Large bizarre neoplastic cell in malignant melanoma. Note dusty cytoplasm without pigment or vacuolization. The diagnosis was made by comparing the appearance of the cells at the primary site. (Pap × 400)

TABLE 10.2 Differential Diagnosis of Large Cell Neoplasms

Tumor Type	Special Stain	Electron Microscopy	Immunocytochemistry
Melanoma	Fontana–Masson	Premelanosomes	S-100, monoclonals
Carcinoma	PAS, mucicarmine	Desmosomes, microvilli	CEA, EMA, keratin
Lymphoma	MGP	Nuclear protrusions, nucleoli	LCA, LN 1 & 2 monoclonals
Histiocytic tumor	Leder's	Lysosomes, branching cisternae	α_1-AT/α_1ACT, muramidase
Germ cell tumor	PAS	Secretory granules, glycogen	BaCG, AFP, PL, ALPase
Plasma cell myeloma	MGP	Stacks of RER	IgG, IgM

TABLE 10.3 Diagnosis of Spindle Cell Neoplasms

Tumor Type	Special Stain	Electron Microscopy	Immunocytochemistry
Fibrosarcoma	Masson's (blue)	Extracellular collagen	Vimentin
Leiomyosarcoma	Masson's (red)	Pinocytotic vesicles, dense bodies	Desmin
Schwannoma	Picrosirius	Crystals, cytoplasmic extensions	S-100
Kaposi's sarcoma	Elastic	Pericytes, tight junctions	Factor VIII–negative
Carcinoma	Kreyberg	Desmosomes, microvilli	Keratin

Spindle Cell Tumors (Table 10.3)

As compared with aspirates or histologic sections of the parent neoplasm, metastatic spindle cell sarcomas tend to exhibit plumper and rounder cells in malignant effusions. The cells may either appear smaller than originally expected, or larger than the sarcoma in its native site. Examples of fibrosarcoma, leiomyosarcoma, hemangioendothelioma, synovial sarcoma, and malignant schwannoma have all been illustrated in textbooks and case reports of malignant effusion. The AIDS epidemic has enabled us to document widely disseminated vascular neoplasms that we have seen recently in pleural effusions.

The retroperitoneal space may be the site of fibrosarcomas that extend to the ascitic fluid. *Fibrosarcomas* often present as single spindle cells or as small groups of tumor cells interwoven with intercellular collagen. Cells range from plump to fiber-like. Nuclei are elongated and with pointed ends (Fig. 10.3). Anisokaryosis is rather common, and nuclei exhibit irregular chromatin granules. Occasional multinucleated giant cells are present and indistinguishable from those of other sarcomas (Fig. 10.4).

In *leiomyosarcoma,* single spindle-shaped cells predominate but they may be plump or arranged in loose clusters forming parallel bundles. Cells have indistinct cell borders or may form syncytia, sharing cytoplasmic material with neighboring elements (Fig. 10.5). Abundant eosinophilic cytoplasm is the rule, and nuclei are either cigar-shaped or rounded (Fig. 10.6). As with other sarcomas, pleomorphism may occur. Chromatin is finely distributed, with multiple distinct nucleoli identified within it. In the primary site, mitoses are frequent, and they may be present occasionally in malignant effusions.

In *malignant schwannoma* (neurofibrosarcoma) a large number of cells are usually present in the effusion. Elongated spindle nuclei predominate. The chromatin distribution is obviously malignant with coarse clumping

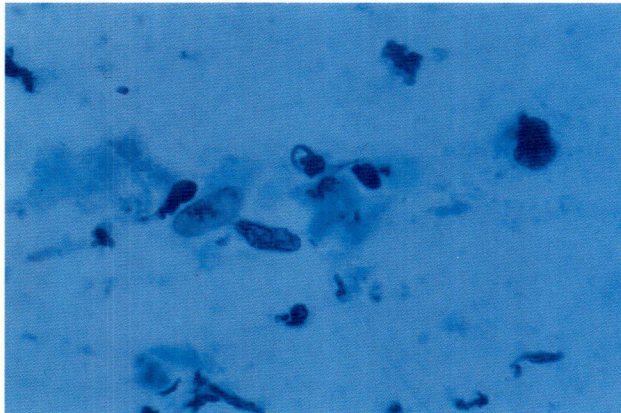

FIGURE 10.3 High-grade fibrosarcoma in the retroperitoneal space. Tumor cells are sparse and demonstrate a mixture of plump and elongated nuclei. (Pap × 240)

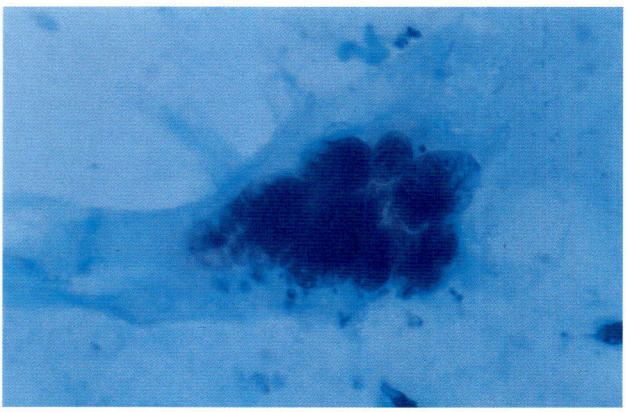

FIGURE 10.4 Giant cell in high-grade fibrosarcoma. Short of ancillary studies, only a previous diagnosis allows classification of a high-grade sarcoma in cytologic material. (Pap × 240)

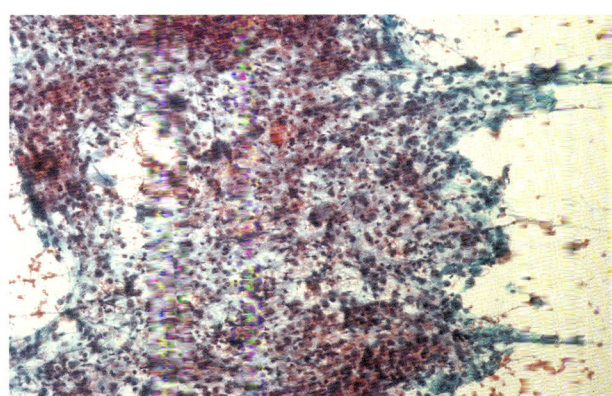

FIGURE 10.5 Peritoneal washing in uterine leiomyosarcoma. The large sheets of tumor cells demonstrates eosinophilia of the cytoplasm. (Pap × 120)

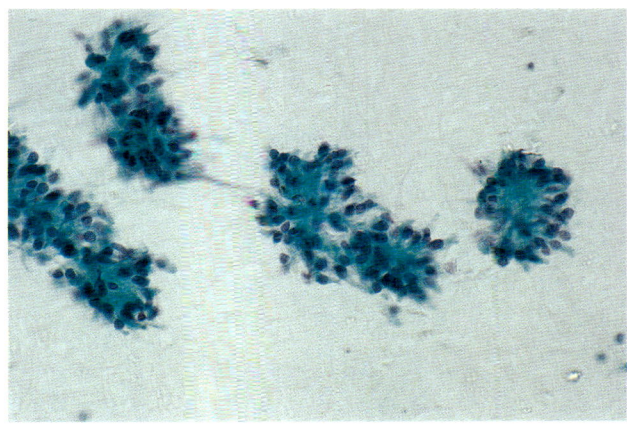

FIGURE 10.7 Omental ependymoma in peritoneal fluid. Note the spindle cells held together by a fibrous intercellular matrix. (Pap × 120)

and crowding beneath the nuclear membrane. Wispy, fragile cytoplasm may lead to frequent bare nuclei showing pointed rather than blunt ends. Malignant schwannomas may be rather pleomorphic with frequent multinucleated giant cells, difficult to differentiate from other soft tissue sarcomas.

One example of omental ependymoma has been documented in ascitis. Spindle cells held together by intercellular matrix resemble malignant cells of other types of sarcoma (Fig. 10.7). These tumors may be rich in blood vessels rendering their distinction from vascular tumors extremely difficult on cytologic grounds alone (Fig. 10.8). Both *synovial sarcoma* and *hemangiopericytoma* may present with a predominance of spindle

cells difficult to differentiate from the other spindle cell sarcomas. Knowledge of the primary diagnosis and the use of special stains, immunocytochemistry and electron microscopy make it possible to recognize these neoplasms.

An angioendothelioma and a hemangioendothelial sarcoma have been documented in malignant effusions. The angiosarcoma in our AIDS patient was composed of plump spindle cells with a moderate degree of pleomorphism. RBCs and fragmented vessel walls were noted within the tumor nests (Fig. 10.9). Tumor giant cells, plump cells, and accompanying vascularity were identified in keeping with direct extension of the tumor into the pleural cavity. The cell blocks revealed small

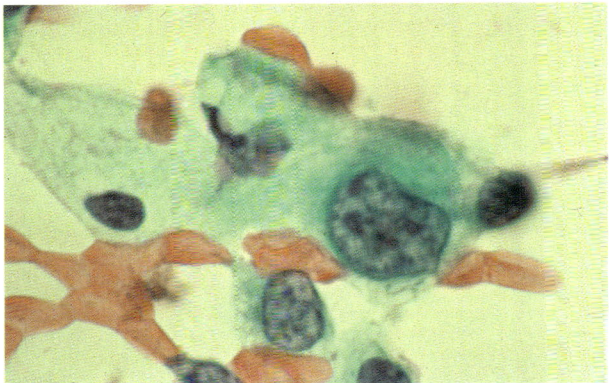

FIGURE 10.6 Large neoplastic cell from leiomyosarcoma. Note the marked variation in size and shape of the nuclei, with irregular distribution of chromatin and aberrant nucleoli. (Pap × 800)

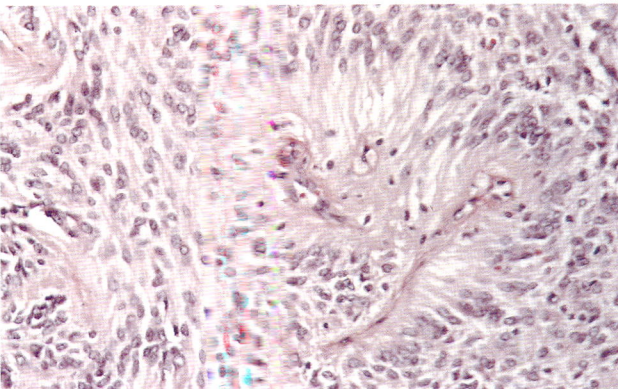

FIGURE 10.8 Tissue fragment from the case in Figure 10.12. The fibrillary intercellular matrix is traversed by delicate blood vessels. (H&E × 130) (Figs. 10.7 and 10.8 courtesy of N. Sneige, MD)

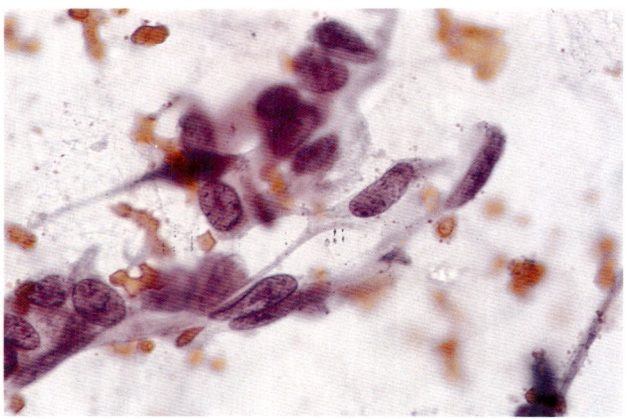

FIGURE 10.9   Angiosarcoma in a cul-de-sac aspirate. Note the spindle cells within a vascular matrix containing RBCs. (Pap × 240)

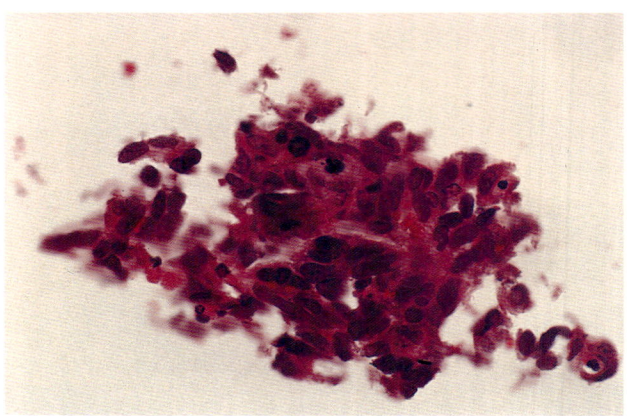

FIGURE 10.10   Kaposi's sarcoma from the pleura of a patient with AIDS. A rather anaplastic group of tumor cells displays pink eosinophilic cytoplasm. (Pap × 180)

tissue fragments allowing for immunocytochemical confirmation of the nature of the tumor. Kaposi's sarcoma has exploded in frequency among the AIDS population. Kaposi's tumor cells are rather pleomorphic with spindle, plump, and multinucleated elements forming irregular vascular channels (Fig. 10.10). In effusions, the tendency toward cell balling may mimic an epithelial neoplasm particularly in cell blocks (Fig. 10.11). The diagnosis can be confirmed by the use of immunocytochemistry which is positive for vimentin but not for Factor VIII or *Ulex europeans* antigens.

Pleomorphic Cell Tumors (Table 10.4)

Pleomorphic tumor cells tend to occur frequently in malignant fibrous histiocytoma, pleomorphic rhabdomyosarcoma, pleomorphic liposarcoma, osteosarcoma, chondrosarcoma, and malignant melanoma. However, a few of these giant cells are present in virtually all sarcomas. It is not possible to distinguish the bizarre giant

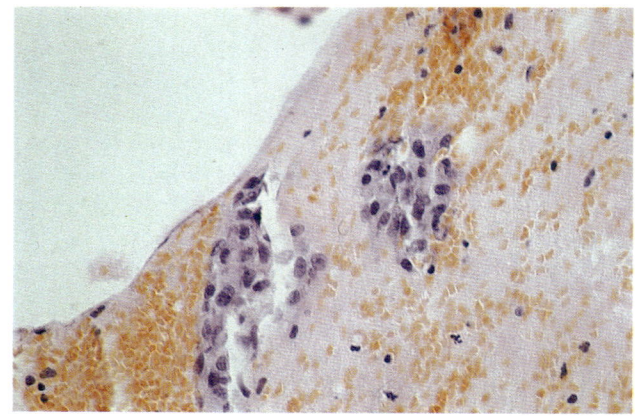

FIGURE 10.11   Cell block from Kaposi's sarcoma, same patient as in Figure 10.10. Note the groups of tumor cells against a fibrinous background. (H&E × 120) (Figs. 10.10 and 10.11, courtesy of D. Solomon, MD)

TABLE 10.4   Differential Diagnosis of Pleomorphic Cell Neoplasms

Tumor Type	Special Stain	Electron Microscopy	Immunocytochemistry
Anaplastic carcinoma	PAS, mucin, bile	Sparse organelles, nuclear whorls	CEA, EMA, BhCG
MFH		Rough ER, no filaments	α_1AT/α_1ACT, lysozyme
Liposarcoma	Oil–red O	Clear vacuoles, nuclear indentation	Vimentin, S-100
Rhabdomyosarcoma	Trichrome	Actin, myosin	Myoglobin, creatine kinase, Z-band protein, vimentin
Chordoma	Mucicarmine	MER complexes, glycogen	EMA, S-100

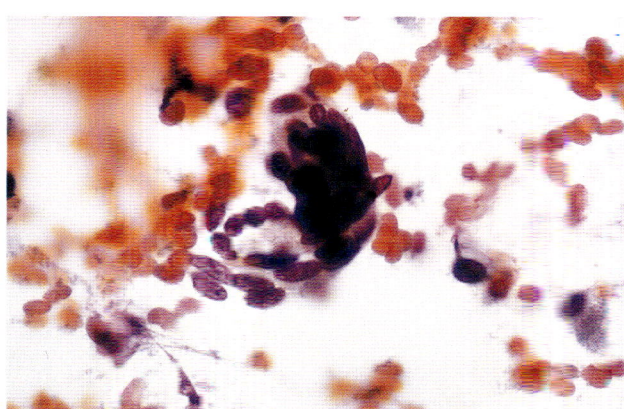

FIGURE 10.12 High-grade sarcoma impossible to classify cytologically. Despite the use of special stains, no primary site could be identified. (Pap × 160)

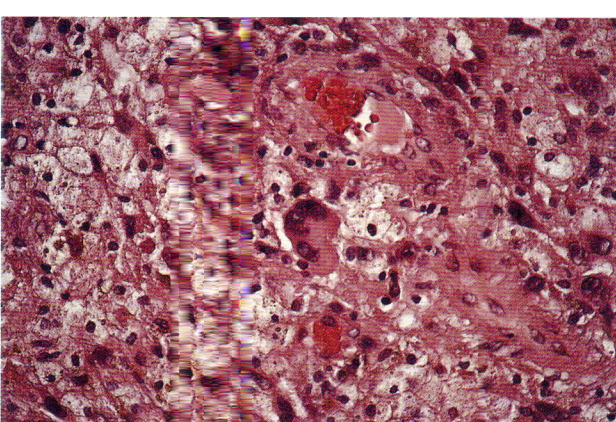

FIGURE 10.13 Cell block from liposarcoma. Large giant cells side by side with lipid-filled tumor cells are typical of this neoplasm. (H&E × 120)

cells of one sarcoma from those of another except with the help of ancillary studies.

In *malignant fibrous histiocytoma* (MFH), the neoplastic cell population is rather pleomorphic. Spindled, fibroblastlike cells are noted and the background is usually necrotic. Plump cells with pale cytoplasm intermixed with clear cells with abundant vacuolated cytoplasm are usually observed. Invariably, there is marked nuclear pleomorphism with frequent bizarre multinucleated tumor cells (Fig. 10.12). Nucleoli vary but may be extremely prominent and mitoses are frequent. Tumor cells may show bizarre shapes of the cytoplasm suggesting a rhabdosarcomatous differentiation. Many lesions diagnosed as pleomorphic rhabdomyosarcomas in the past are now believed to represent malignant fibrous histiocytoma. Distinction between these two types of sarcoma can be accomplished by immunocytochemistry or electron microscopy. Malignant fibrous histiocytoma is positive for vimentin and at least one of the histiocytic markers: α_1-antitrypsin, α_1-antichimotrypsin, or lysozyme. Pleomorphic rhabdomyosarcoma is positive for vimentin but negative for the histiocytic markers. Rhabdomyosarcomas are positive for desmin and at least one of the markers of striated muscle differentiation: myoglobin, creatine kinase or Z-band protein.

The frequency of *pleomorphic liposarcoma* is on the rise, and these tumors have been documented in effusions both in Von Ham's monograph and Takahashi's atlas. The cytologic presentation is indistinguishable from other pleomorphic cell sarcomas, but careful scrutiny may identify dispersed cells exhibiting lipoblastic differentiation. Clear vacuoles that slightly indent the

nuclei are characteristic of this neoplasm (Fig. 10.13). These tumors are positive for S-100 and vimentin and by electron microscopy reveal large lipid vacuoles indenting upon the nuclei. Pleomorphic liposarcomas resemble malignant fibrous histiocytoma cytologically. As in other sarcomas the neoplastic tissue becomes necrotic and may yield small tissue fragments (Fig. 10.14). If the tumor has been previously suspected, a portion of the effusion may be prepared for air-dried smears that can be stained for fat with oil–red O. In the MGG or Diff-Quik stained smears, fat vacuoles are more easily identified than in wet (alcohol) fixed smears. The cells appear loosely cohesive, and multivacuolated li-

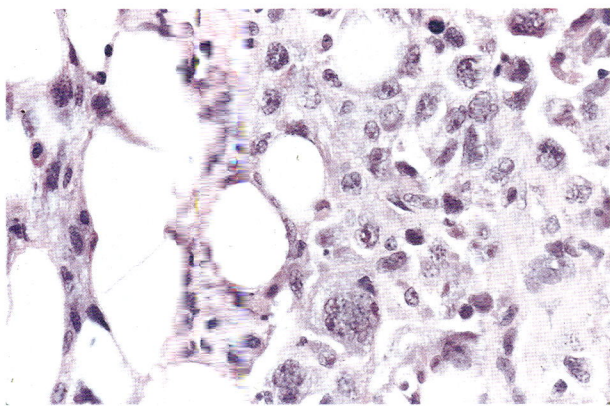

FIGURE 10.14 Tissue fragment from pleomorphic liposarcoma. Note the bizarre giant cells intermingled with tumor cells displaying abundant clear cytoplasm. (H&E × 90)

poblasts may appear in clusters. In the mixoid variant of liposarcoma, small tissue fragments are noted floating in the effusion. These may reveal the classic plexiform vascular pattern of this neoplasm.

Skeletal sarcomas such as osteosarcoma and chondrosarcoma may invade locally or metastasize into one of the serosal cavities. A pleomorphic cytologic picture with spindled and round cells is characteristic of osteosarcoma. In the primary site, the presence of osteoid is crucial for the diagnosis. In metastatic sites the tumor is usually rather undifferentiated and can be seldom separated from the other sarcomas. Intense alkaline phosphatase positivity is characteristic of osteosarcoma. In chondrosarcoma the cells are intimately meshed in a mixoid fibrillary chondroid background. Binucleated cells are typical of these neoplasms. They are positive for S-100 and vimentin, and a few examples have been positive for keratin.

In *chordoma* the characteristically enormous physaliphorous cells exhibit abundant, pale hypervacuolated cytoplasm with sharply demarcated cell boundaries. These cells may have one, two, or (often) many nuclei with finely distributed chromatin and small nucleoli. The background contains the same mixoid ground substance as that of other cartilaginous tumors. These neoplasms may also present with epithelial-like cells which may be rather deceptive. These tumors are frequent in the sacrococcygeal area and may be diagnosed by aspirating the cul-de-sac contents. Chordomas are positive for vimentin, S-100, keratin, and even the neural endocrine markers. By electron microscopy these cells show short, microvilli-like cell processes, desmosomes, and microchondria–RER complexes, the latter being rather characteristic for chordoma. A lesser number of pleomorphic cells than those of chordoma characterize clear cell sarcomas that start in the soft tissues and may extend to the serous cavities. These nonpigmented tumors give the same immunocytochemical profile as cutaneous melanoma and have been considered to represent melanomas of the soft parts.

Round Cell Tumors

In addition to sarcomas, small blue round cell tumors (SBRCT) include lymphomas and neuroendocrine tumors. Sarcomas composed of round cells include Ewing's sarcoma of bone and soft tissues, embryonal rhabdomyosarcoma, stromal sarcoma of the uterus, and nephroblastoma of the kidney. With a clinical history suggesting the primary site, cytologic examination of the malignant effusion may allow the recognition of these neoplasms. If the primary tumor is unknown, however, the differential diagnosis often depends on special stains, immunocytochemistry, or electron microscopy. Ewing's sarcoma and embryonal rhabdomyosarcoma are discussed in detail in Chapter 11. Only one example of uterine stromal sarcoma has been illustrated in the literature. The tumor demonstrated small to medium-sized rounded cells with a high nuclear:cytoplasmic ratio. These cells must be differentiated from lymphoma and the other blue round cell tumors. Examples of nephroblastoma have been described by Hajdu in his monograph and include not only small blue round tumor cells but rudimentary organoid groups of cells, cigar-shaped spindle cells, and occasionally multinucleated elements. Other mesenchymal neoplasms containing small blue round cells include small cell osteosarcoma, mesenchymal chondrosarcoma, and small cell malignant melanoma. These tumors are difficult to distinguish from one another, and immunocytochemistry is often needed to discriminate among them (Table 10.5).

Mesenchymal chondrosarcoma and small cell osteosarcomas are positive for vimentin, but only chondrosarcoma is positive for cytokeratin. Small cell malignant melanoma is also positive for vimentin but negative for keratin and positive for S-100 or HMB-45. Positivity for antidesmin will identify embryonal rhabdomyosarcomas, whereas in Ewing's sarcoma positivity extends to vimentin and neuron-specific enolase (NSE) but not to neurofilament.

TABLE 10.5   Diagnosis of Small Cell Neoplasms

Tumor Type	Special Stain	Electron Microscopy	Immunocytochemistry
Ewing's sarcoma	PAS +, PTAH −	Glycogen, perinuclear space	NSE −, vimentin +
Neuroblastoma	Churukian's, Pascual's	Microtubules, NE granules	NSE +, NF −
Rhabdomyosarcoma	PAS −, PTAH +	Z-bands, contractile nuclei	Vimentin +, myoglobin +
Lymphoma	Reticulum around individual cells	No junctions, nuclear protrusions	Pan-B, Pan-T, LCA, UCHL 1
Oat cell carcinoma	Fontana–Masson, Grimelius	No axons, NE granules	NF −, NSE +

TABLE 10.6 Ultrastructural and Immunocytochemical Features of Various Sarcomas

Sarcoma	Ultrastructure	Immunocytochemistry
SPINDLE		
Fibrosarcoma	Long spindle cells interweaving collagen, dilated cysternae of RER	Vimentin
Leiomyosarcoma	Myofilaments, dense bodies, basal lamina, plaquelike junctions, subplasmalemmal densities	Vimentin, desmin, smooth muscle actin
Schwannoma	Interdigitating cell processes, long-spaced collagen, longitudinal microtubules, irregular crystals	Vimentin, S-100
PLEOMORPHIC		
Rhabdomyosarcoma	Thick and thin filaments, microtubules, glycogen, Z-bands	Vimentin, desmin, HHF-35, myoglobin
Liposarcoma	Lipid droplets, indented nuclei	Vimentin, S-100
Angiosarcoma	Slender intercellular clefts, Weibel–Palade bodies (rare)	Vimentin, Factor VIII, ACE, *Ulex europaeus* -glutamin
EPITHELIOID		
Epithelioid sarcoma	Abundant intermediate filaments, desmosomelike junctions, filopodia	Vimentin, keratin
Granular cell sarcoma	Aggregates of lysosomes, microtubules, redundant membranes	Vimentin, S-100
Alveolar soft part sarcoma	Rhomboid crystals, prominent Golgi complexes, dense core granules	Vimentin
Synovial sarcoma	Short, nonbranching spindle cells, closely apposed cells, no collagen	Vimentin, keratin

From: Bedrossian CWM. Electron microscopy and immunocytochemistry as adjuncts to cytopathology. In: Proceedings of WHO National Training Course on the Application of Electron Microscopy in Biomedical Research and Diagnosis of Human Diseases, Beijing, 1990. World Health Organization. With permission.

It should be obvious from the foregoing discussion that classification of sarcomas is usually a difficult if not futile exercise. Many surgeons rely on grading rather than on classifications based on histogenesis and differentiation. Nevertheless, pathologists still use morphologic subdivisions to identify these neoplasms (Table 10.6).

GERM CELL NEOPLASMS

Germ cell tumors may arise in gonadal and extragonadal sites, invade locally, or metastasize widely, and give rise to malignant effusions.

Embryonal carcinomas arising in the testicle or in the midline are composed of large polygonal cells intermixed with primitive mesenchymal spindle elements. In malignant effusions, however, the tendency to arrange in cell balls is frequently manifested (Fig. 10.15). The cells may form microglandular aggregates within which cell borders are indistinct. Pale, pleomorphic nuclei exhibit a clear cell chromatin pattern and prominent nucleoli. The nucleus may be eccentric because of the presence of PAS-positive large glycogen vacuoles. Embryonal cell carcinomas are positive for placental alkaline phosphatase (PLAP) and alpha fetoprotein (AFP) but negative for beta human chorionic gonadotropin (β-HCG).

Endodermal sinus tumors are related histogenetically to embryonal cell carcinomas but arise in the pediatric age group. These tumors present with a predominance of tightly packed uniform cells which may form tubulo papillary cell clusters. As in embryonal cell carcinoma, the chromatin pattern is clear and nucleoli are prominent. These tumors show prominent cytoplasmic vacuolization because of the presence of glycogen and are positive for AFP and PLAP.

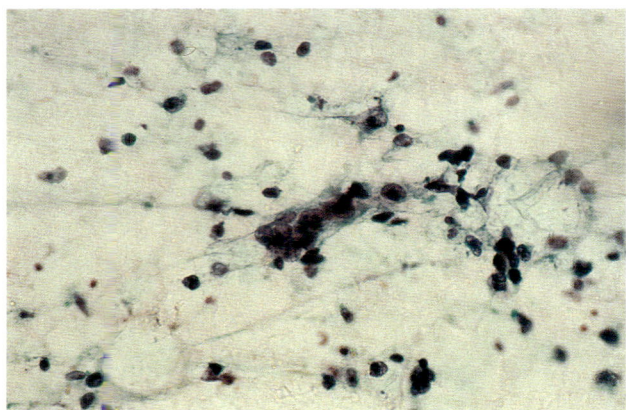

FIGURE 10.15   Germ cell neoplasm with features of embryonal cell carcinoma. The small cells attempt form acinus-like clumps. (Pap × 90)

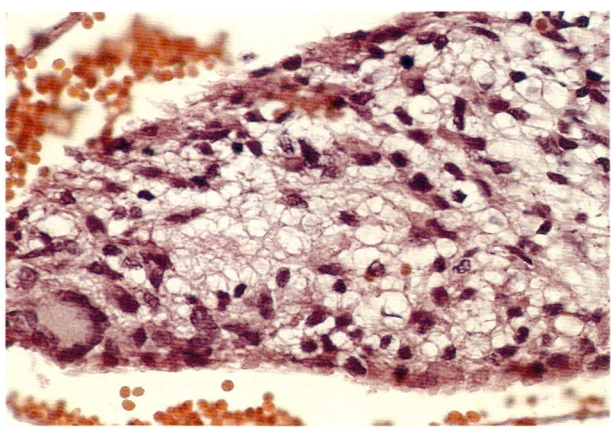

FIGURE 10.16   Tissue fragment of teratoma. Note the immature tumor cells held together by a fibrillary matrix. (H&E × 180)

Choriocarcinomas may present as the predominant pattern of the germ cell tumor or as a minor component in the other cell types. They are characterized by the presence of disassociated or clustered cytotrophoblastic cells with abundant amphophilic cytoplasm. Multinucleated syncytiocytotrophoblasts are also present, with a large number of bizarre hyperchromatic nuclei with irregular chromatin clumping. These tumors may form implants within the serosal cavities and present as floating tissue fragments with a prominent vascular network. Cell blocks from these preparations are very useful for the β-HCG reaction that characterizes choriocarcinoma. AFP and PLAP are usually negative in choriocarcinoma but positive in embryonal carcinoma and endodermal sinus tumor.

Teratomas contain several epithelial and mesenchymal elements which may be mature and immature and display different propensities to metastasis. Common mature elements include sheets of squamous cells, ciliated or intestinal-type epithelium with numerous goblet cells, and structures mimicking skin adnexa. The immature elements resemble those of embryonal carcinoma or may contain partially differentiated mesenchymal tissues such as glia (Fig. 10.16). The metastasizing element present in the effusion may be either an adenocarcinoma, a squamous cell carcinoma, or an undifferentiated small cell neoplasm without obvious epithelial or mesenchymal derivation. Primitive neural rosettes have been described in pleural effusions, and occasionally more mature neural elements may be identified. Seminomas rarely extend to the pelvic cavity where they can be recognized by a mixture of medium-sized germ cells and lymphocytes (Fig. 10.17).

CARCINOSARCOMAS

There is a group of neoplasms that show both epithelial and mesenchymal differentiation. These tumors arise in embryonic rests within certain parenchymal organs (uterus, ovaries, lungs, kidney) or in nonparenchymal structures (soft tissues) of the midline, retroperitoneum or notochord, metastasizing early and widely. They are relatively rare neoplasms, but authors in large cancer centers have accumulated some experience. Steven Hajdu has written extensively on this subject, and Bernard Naylor has shown examples of these neoplasms in his workshop. We have seen a few cases, mainly in

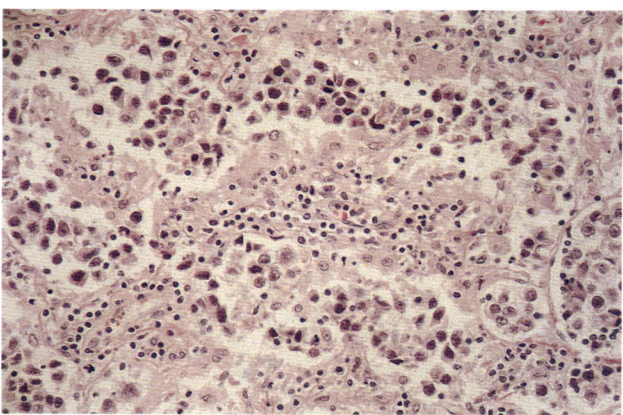

FIGURE 10.17   Seminoma in peritoneal fluid. The cell block demonstrates tumor cells with a moderate amount of cytoplasm against a background containing lymphocytes. (H&E × 40)

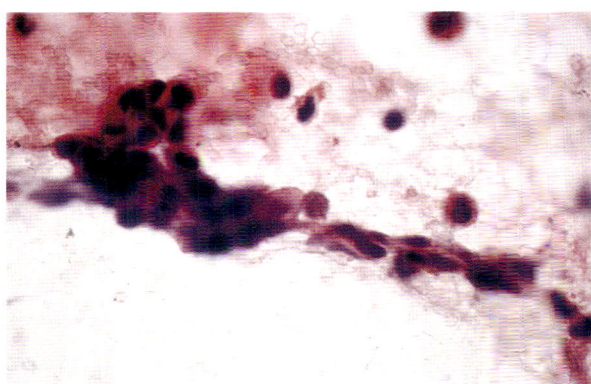

FIGURE 10.18 Cul-de-sac aspirate in malignant mixed mullerian tumor (MMMT). Note the large bundles of spindle cells intermixed with isolated elements. (Pap × 120)

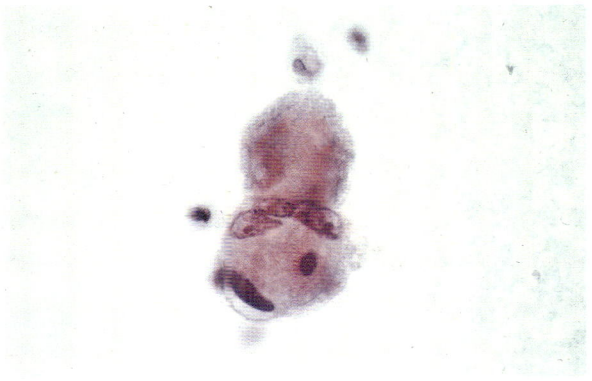

FIGURE 10.19 Bizarre giant cell in MMMT. Note the peripheral location of the nuclei and the myoid appearance of the abundant cytoplasm (Pap × 180)

the form of outside consultation. The prototype of these unique neoplasms is the so-called malignant mixed müllerian tumor (MMMT) that may originate in the uterus or in the ovaries. The neoplasm is characterized by a dual population of tumor cells that blend in one another in the primary site but tend to metastasize as a single element. MMMTs usually reach the malignant effusion as poorly differentiated or well differentiated adenocarcinoma. In the case described by Hidvegi the epithelial element was admixed with psammoma bodies. For this reason, diagnosis is difficult if one overlooks the smaller population of single bizarre cells indicative of its mesenchymal inclinations.

Less frequently, a great degree of pleomorphism may be exhibited by MMMT in effusions. In such cases, epithelial-like cells appear admixed with spindle-shaped cells. The sarcomatous element may show a tendency toward chondrosarcomatous differentiation. In turn the epithelial cells may appear endometrioid or even undifferentiated (Fig. 10.18). Occasionally, the tumor cells may contain hyaline globules in the cytoplasm corresponding to accumulations of alpha-one antitrypsin. A variety of multinucleated cells are identified in association with ordinary cell groups representing adenocarcinomatous and undifferentiated areas of the neoplasm (Fig. 10.19). The pleomorphic sarcomatous elements may show differentiation toward a variety of directions including that of rhabdomyoblasts with distinct cross striations, or they may resemble the cells of leiomyosarcoma (Fig. 10.20). In the example described by Silverman, epithelial-like cells mimicked adenocarcinoma. Epithelial-like cells tend to form loose aggregates with amphophilic cytoplasm but obvious vacuolization may

occasionally be evident. The bizarre tumor giant cells are indistinguishable from those of other sarcomas.

Both the lung and the kidney may be the source of tumors variously called "blastomas" or "carcinosarcomas," the most common of which is nephroblastoma (Wilm's tumor). The small round cell mesenchymal component is rather ubiquitous, but the tumor attempts to form rudimentary organoid structures and occasionally such tubular groupings are noted in malignant effusions. In pulmonary blastomas, the cells can be rather vacuolated and resemble germ cell tumors of the ovary. In Wilm's tumor the tubular structures are formed by very tall nonsecreting cells that form a very small lumen, devoid of secretory materials. These neoplasms resemble embryonic attempts at reproducing the lungs and

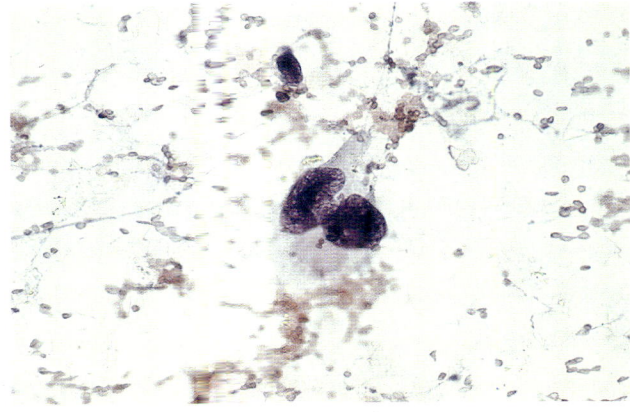

FIGURE 10.20 Malignant cells from MMMT. Nuclei are obviously malignant, but cytoplasm yields no clues as to the differentiation of the neoplasm. (Pap × 180)

the kidney, respectively, but they are not true germ cell neoplasms. Accordingly, they do not express the onco-fetal markers expressed by tumors derived from germ cells.

BIBLIOGRAPHY

Melanoma

Freidman M, Rao U, Fox S. The cytology of metastatic balloon cell melanoma. *Acta Cytol.* 1982;26(1):39–43.

Hajdu S, Savino A. Cytologic diagnosis of malignant melanoma. *Acta Cytol.* 1973;17(4):320–327.

Walts AE. Malignant melanoma in effusions: A source of false negative diagnosis. *Diagn Cytopathol.* 1986;2:150–153.

Sarcomas

Hajdu SI, Hajdu EO. *Cytopathology of Sarcomas and Other Nonepithecial Malignant Tumors.* Philadelphia: WB Saunders; 1976.

Hajdu SI, Koss LG. Cytologic diagnosis of metastatic myosarcomas. *Acta Cytol.* 1969;13:545–551.

Massoni E, Hajdu S. Cytology of primary and metastatic uterine sarcomas. *Acta Cytol.* 1984;28(2):93–100.

Nguyen G, Jeannot A. Cytology of synovial sarcoma in pleural fluid. *Acta Cytol.* 1982;26(4):517–520.

Nguyen GK, Shnitra TK, Jewell LD, et al. Exfoliative cytology of clear cell sarcoma metastasis in pleural fluid. *Diagn Cytopathol.* 1986;2:144–149.

Spindle cell tumors

Dekmezian RH, Sneige N, Ordonez NG. Ovarian and omental ependymomas in peritoneal washings. *Diagn Cytopathol.* 1986;2:62–68.

Gaba AR, tine G, Raju UB. Malignant angioendothelioma. Cytologic, histologic and ultrastructural findings. *Acta Cytol.* 1983;27:76–80.

Lopes Cardozo P. Atlas of Clinical Cytology. Leiden's Hertogenbosch, Targa bv, 1976.

Spriggs A, Boddington MM. Atlas of serous fluid cytopathology. A guide to the cells of pleural, pericardial, peritoneal and hydrocele fluids. In: Gresham GA, ed. *Current Histopathology Series,* vol 14. Dordrecht: Kluwer Academic; 1989.

Young JA, Crocker J. *Colour Atlas of Pulmonary Cytopathology.* Oxford: Harvey Miller; 1985.

Pleomorphic cell tumors

Geisinger KR, Naylor B, Beals TF, et al. Cytopathology including transmission electron microscopy, of pleomorphic liposarcoma in pleural fluids. *Acta Cytol.* 1980;24:435–441.

Koss LG. *Diagnostic Cytology and Its Histopathologic Bases,* 3rd ed. Philadelphia: JB Lippincott; 1979.

Satake T, Matsuyama M. Cytologic features of ascites in malignant fibrous histiocytoma of the colon. *Acta Pathol. Jpn.* 1988;38:921–928.

Takahashi M. *Color Atlas of Cancer Cytology,* 2nd ed. New York, Igaku-Shoin; 1981.

von Haam E. Cytology of transudates and exudates, vol 5. In: Wied GL, ed. *Monographs in Clinical Cytology.* Basel: S Karger; 1977.

Yang H-Y, Weaver LL, Foti PR. Primary malignant fibrous histiocytoma of the pleura. A case report. *Acta Cytol.* 1983;27:683–687.

Round cell tumors

Akhtar M, Bedrossian CWM, Ali MA, et al. FNA biopsy of pediatric neoplasm. *Diagn. Cytopathol.* 1992;8:258–265.

Farr GH, Hajdu SI. Exfoliative cytology of metastatic neuroblastoma. *Acta Cytol.* 1971;16:203–206.

Jobst SB, Ljung B-M, Gilkey FN, et al. Cytologic diagnosis of olfactory neuroblastoma. Report of a case with multiple diagnostic parameters. *Acta Cytol.* 1983;27:299–305.

Venegas RJ, Sun NC. Cardiac tamponade as a presentation of malignant thymoma. *Acta Cytol.* 1988;32:257–262.

Zirkin HJ. Pleural fluid cytology of invasive thymoma. *Acta Cytol.* 1985;29:1011–1014.

Carcinosarcomas

Hidvegi DF, DeMay R, Sorensen K. Uterine Müllerian adenosarcoma with psammoma bodies. *Acta Cytol.* 1982;26:323–326

Motoyama T, Watanabe H. Ascitic fluid cytologic features of a malignant mixed mesodermal tumor of the ovary. *Acta Cytol.* 1987;31(1):63–67.

Silverman JF, Gardner J, Larkin EW, et al. Ascitic fluid cytology in a case of metastatic malignant mixed mesodermal tumor of the ovary. *Acta Cytol.* 1986;30:173–176.

Tsukamoto N, Matsukuma K, Daimaru Y, et al. Cytologic presentation of ovarian adenosquamous carcinoma in ascitic fluid: A case report. *Acta Cytol.* 1984;28:703–705.

von Haam E. Cytology of transudates and exudates. In: Wied G, ed. *Monographs in Clinical Cytology.* Basel: Karger; 1977:10–83.

Germ cell tumors

Cobb CJ, Wynn J, Cobb SR, et al. Cytologic findings in an effusion caused by rupture of a benign cystic teratoma of the mediastinum into a serous cavity. *Acta Cytol.* 1985;29:1015–1020.

Grunze H. The comparative diagnostic accuracy, efficiency and specificity of cytologic techniques used in the diagnosis of malignant neoplasms in serous effusions of pleural and pericardial cavities. *Acta Cytol.* 1964;8:150–153.

Kashimura M. Tsukamoto N, Matsuyama T. et al. Cytologic findings of ascites from patients with ovarian dysgerminoma. *Acta Cytol.* 1983;27:59–62.

Kimura N, Namiki T. Wada T, et al. Peritoneal implantation of endodermal sinus tumor of the pineal region via a ventriculoperitoneal shunt. *Acta Cytol.* 1984;28:143–147.

Morimoto N, Ozawa M. Diagnostic value of hyaline globules in endodermal sinus tumor: Report of two cases. *Acta Cytol.* 1981;25(4):417–420

Pagès A, Marsan C. Cytopathologie des épanchements des sereuses. In: Sicard A, Marsan C, eds. *Atlas de Cytologie,* vol 3. Paris: Varia; 196

Roncalli M, Gribaudi E, Simoncelli D, et al. Cytology of yolk-sac tumor of the ovary in ascitic fluid. *Acta Cytol.* 1988; 32(1):113–116.

CHAPTER ELEVEN

Leukemia and Lymphoma

Both leukemia and lymphoma may spread to the serosal spaces, particularly in the pediatric age group. In the adult, lymphoma may lead to effusion as part of an aggressive biologic behavior of the neoplastic process. Effusions may also develop late as part of the indolent but relentless course of low grade lymphomas. Without the clinical history it is impossible to tell leukemia apart from lymphoma on the basis of cytomorphology alone. Another difficulty is to distinguish a florid lymphocytosis from lymphomatous involvement. Even with surface markers and other sophisticated tools, this distinction is difficult. However, flow cytometry and immunophenotyping have greatly facilitated the classification of lymphoma once this diagnosis has been established.

NORMAL LYMPHOCYTES

Lymphocytes are unique in that they derive from a central replenishable source, populate their own lymphoid organs, and are also a major contributor to the function of every other organ of the body. If this were not enough, lymphocytes are also capable of circulation and migration and play an important role in immune modulation and other important regulatory mechanisms. It is not surprising, therefore, that lymphocytes are present in effusions triggered by a variety of mechanisms including inflammation, infection, adverse reactions to drugs, and neoplastic processes, both within and outside the lymphoid system. In fact, lymphocytes are also capable of significant interactions with other neoplastic cells. This versatile and prolific participation in a variety of disease processes implies great adaptability on the part of lymphocytes which, in turn, is reflected in their assumption of great morphologic diversity.

Lymphocytes originate from bone marrow–derived pluripotent stem cells that later differentiate under the influence of the thymus and the bone marrow. The resulting cells, T lymphocytes and B lymphocytes respectively, proliferate and mature in lymph nodes and other lymphoid organs, but in this process, they become susceptible to hyperplasia and malignant transformation.

LYMPHOID HYPERPLASIA

Tuberculosis, viral infections, chronic nonspecific pleuritis, collagen diseases, and carcinomatosis may all be accompanied by effusions with a high number of lymphocytes. The lymphocytes are stimulated but they are not transformed, even though their cytologic appearance may cause considerable difficulty in interpretation. Of all the conditions capable of inducing lymphoid hyperplasia, tuberculosis is most consistently associated with effusions showing lymphocytosis and a scarcity of mesothelial cells (Fig. 11.1). In pulmonary tuberculosis the number of T lymphocytes is increased in the pleural effusion, whereas the number of B lymphocytes is considerably lower than in the serum. These cells are polyclonal in contrast to the monoclonal cell population of malignant lymphoma. If surface immunoglobulins are studied, IgG and both kappa and lambda light chains are demonstrated.

Often one is not able to suspect the etiology of the lymphoid hyperplasia, but lymphoma is not an obvious possibility. These cases are characterized by an increased number of lymphocytes some of which appear activated (Fig. 11.2). When polys and histiocytes are admixed, a reactive process is more likely, particularly if the histiocytes appear as macrophages with phagocytosed debris in their cytoplasm (Fig. 11.3). These so-called tingible-body macrophages, however, are not iron-clad evidence of benignancy: necrotizing infections may also be accompanied by these cells. In lymphoid hyperplasia, the plasma cell count is elevated, whereas

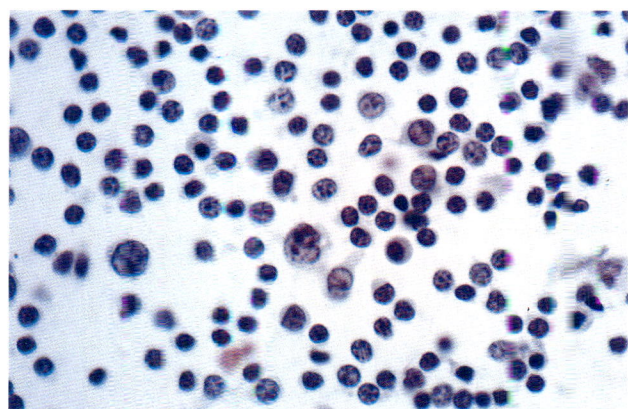

FIGURE 11.1 Tuberculous effusion. Note the absence of mesothelial cells and the monotonous population of lymphocytes, some of which are atypical. By flow cytometry and marker studies, the majority of these cells are T lymphocytes. (Pap × 120)

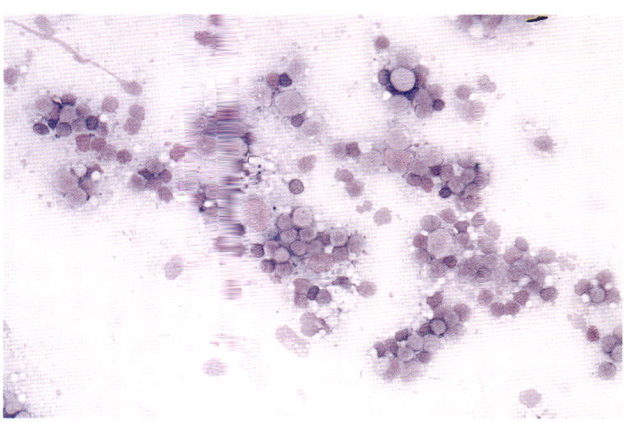

FIGURE 11.3 Same case as in Figure 11.2. With Wright's stain, the heterogeneity of the lymphocytic population is better appreciated. The large, pale cell with debris in the cytoplasm is a tingible body macrophage. (Wright × 100)

in lymphomas few plasma cells are present. Lymphocytosis with a significant number of plasma cells is common in rheumatoid arthritis, malignant diseases, and syphilis. Another condition causing lymphoplasmacytic proliferation is AIDS, but only infrequently is this disease accompanied by effusion. The lymphocytoses of AIDS may occasionally be accompanied by lymphoid elements known as polykarions with abundant cytoplasm shared by lymphohistiocytic nuclei.

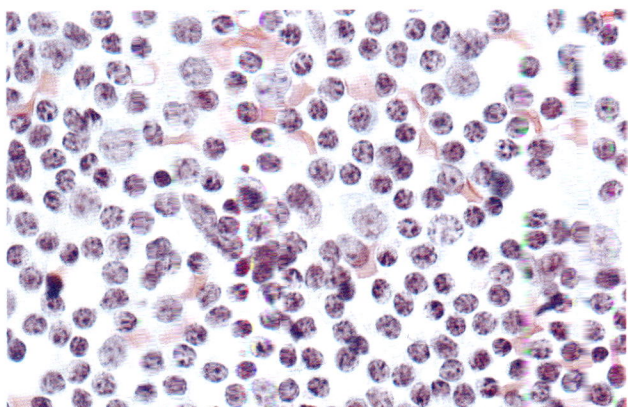

FIGURE 11.2 Reactive lymphocytosis. There is increased cellularity due mainly to lymphocytes, mostly small and mature. Note also the larger pale cells corresponding to histiocyte-like activated lymphocytes. (Pap × 120)

NON-HODGKIN'S LYMPHOMA

In contrast to inflammatory conditions, lymphomas are less frequently accompanied by effusion. However, leukemias that escape remission and lymphomas that fail to respond to chemotherapy may spread to any of the serosal cavities. If the diagnosis has been previously established, very little difficulty exists in recognizing lymphoma in the effusion. If the diagnosis is to be established for the first time by cytologic examination of the effusion, certain criteria have to be met. First of all, most if not all cells encountered in the specimen must be lymphocytes even though occasionally they may exhibit different stages of maturation. Frequently, however, most lymphocytes exhibit the same degree of maturation so that a monotonous population of lymphoid cells is considered the salient cytologic feature of lymphoma. Second, the lymphocytes must appear in large numbers so that the cell count is extremely elevated, at the expense of mesothelial cells which are overwhelmed by the excessive number of lymphoid elements. Third, the lymphocytes must show a degree of cytologic atypia that distinguishes them from normal lymphocytes.

In small cell lymphomas, particularly those of low grade malignancy the cells are mature, small and do not appear atypical but it is possible to suggest the diagnosis of lymphoma on the basis of the clinical history and the monotony of the cell population. In large cell lymphomas, particularly those of high grade malignancy, less difficulty exists in recognizing the lympho-

TABLE 11.1   A Comparison Between Cytologic and Histologic Classifications of Lymphoma

Cytologic Classification	Working Formulation	Rappaport Equivalent	Markers Expressed
Small Size:			
Small (mature) lymphocyte	Low grade, small lymphocytic	WDL (CLL)	Mostly B cell
Small (plasmacytoid) cell	Low grade, Lymphoplasmacytoid	WDL (CLL)	Blast B cell
Small (cleaved) cell	Low grade, follicular, small cleaved	PDL (nodular)	Monoclonal B cell
Small (non-cleaved) cell	High grade, small non-cleaved cell	Diffuse undifferentiated (Burkitt's, Non-Burkitt's)	Blast B cell
Medium Size:			
Convoluted cell	Intermediate grade medium-size non-cleaved cells	N/A[a]	Peripheral T cell
Intermediate, (cleaved) cell	Intermediate grade "small" cleaved cells	PDL (diffuse)	Variable
Lymphoblastic cell	High grade, lymphoblastic	Lymphoblastic	Thymic T cell
Large Size:			
Large (cleaved) cell	Intermediate grade, large cleaved cell	Diffuse histiocytic	Mostly B cell
Large (immunoblastic) cell	High grade, large cell immunoblastic	Diffuse histiocytic	Blast B cell
Large (non-cleaved) cell	Intermediate grade, large non-cleaved	Diffuse histiocytic	Mostly B cell
True histiocyte	Histiocytic	Diffuse histiocytes	Tissue macrophage

[a]N/A = not applicable.

matous process. However, there are no definitive cytologic criteria of malignancy applicable to individual lymphocytes in a body fluid. A sign that received considerable attention in the cytology literature is irregularity of the nuclear contour, with sharp protrusions abutting from the nuclear envelope. This same phenomenon, however, is noted in atypical lymphocytosis, so it cannot be considered a reliable sign of lymphoma. In tuberculosis and mononucleosis the problem is compounded by rather numerous lymphocytes in the effusion in the presence of variable numbers of non-lymphoid cells. In inflammatory and infectious conditions, the atypical lymphocytes display several stages of maturation and are accompanied by a mixture of tingible body macrophages, plasma cells, and polymorphonuclear leukocytes. The mere presence of tingible body macrophages does not guarantee a diagnosis of nonmalignancy per se, because high grade lymphomas may be accompanied by necrosis followed by phagocytosis of necrotic debris.

Classification of Lymphomas in Effusions

It is possible to classify lymphomas cytologically and histologically into the two broad categories of large cell and small cell lymphoma. There also remains a less obvious third group of lymphomas of medium sized cells, intermediate between small cell and large cell lymphomas (Table 11.1). The cytologic classification of lymphoma benefits from the utilization of multiple staining methods such as Papanicolaou's, MGG, Wright's stain, Diff-Quik and H&E. The latter provides good definition of nuclear features in histologic sections and can also be applied to effusions.

By combining cytomorphologic features in Papanicolaou- and Diff-Quik stained preparations with the knowledge of the clinical course, further insight can be gained. Once the diagnosis of lymphoma has been established, subclassification of the lymphoma is best accomplished by flow cytometry or surface markers. Certain antibodies are capable of classifying the lymphomas

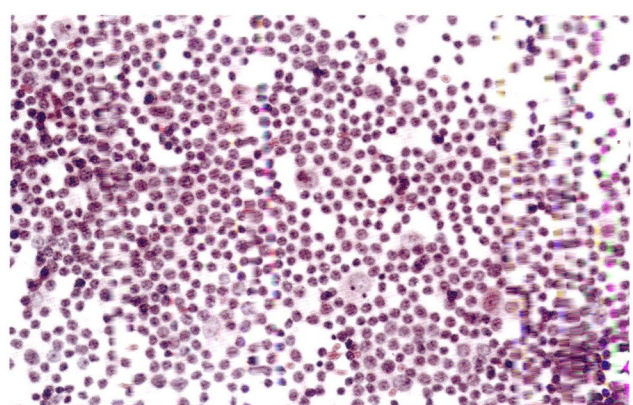

FIGURE 11.4 Highly cellular small cell lymphocytic lymphoma of the WDL subtype. The small lymphocytes are mature, with only an occasional well-preserved large cell. Without a clinical history, one would be hard pressed to render a positive diagnosis in this case. (Pap × 90)

FIGURE 11.5 Monotonous population of mature lymphocytes in the same case as Figure 11.4. There is minimal variation in size and shape of the small lymphocytes. (Pap × 180)

into broad B-cell and T cell categories and work well in B5-formalin fixed cell blocks. Marker studies may also be performed in cytospin preparations with reliable results.

SMALL CELL LYMPHOMAS

This group includes small cell lymphoma of the chronic lymphocytic leukemia/well differentiated lymphoma (CLL/WDL) variety, small cleaved lymphoma and lymphoplasmacytoid lymphomas, all of which may be recognized by cytologic criteria and correspond to well defined clinicopathologic entities. The cells of CLL are considerably smaller than large lymphocytes and are characterized by monotonous nuclei with coarse chromatin distribution. The absence of other lymphoid and nonlymphoid inflammatory cells is very important to excluding a reactive process. A clue to the CLL diagnosis is offered by the presence of occasional lymphoid cells with very coarse large chromatin clumps that set them apart from the other lymphoid elements ("cellules grumelees"). CLL is predominantly a clonal B-cell condition, a fact easily verifiable in the cell block, whereas reactive processes are usually T-cell positive and polyclonal. It is not possible to distinguish cells deriving from CLL from those of WDL by cytologic means alone. A monotonous population of mature lymphocytes derived from WDL may also be difficult to distinguish from a reactive process (Fig. 11.4) The condition, however,

may be accompanied by hyperplastic mesothelial cells, thus making the diagnosis of tuberculosis less likely (Fig. 11.5).

In small cleaved cell lymphoma and lymphoplasmacytoid lymphoma, the number of cells and the monotony of the cell population are more reliable indicators of malignancy than cytologic atypia (Fig. 11.6). Appreciation of plasmacytoid features is best accomplished in Wright-stained preparations (Fig. 11.7). Poorly differentiated lymphomas (PDL) composed

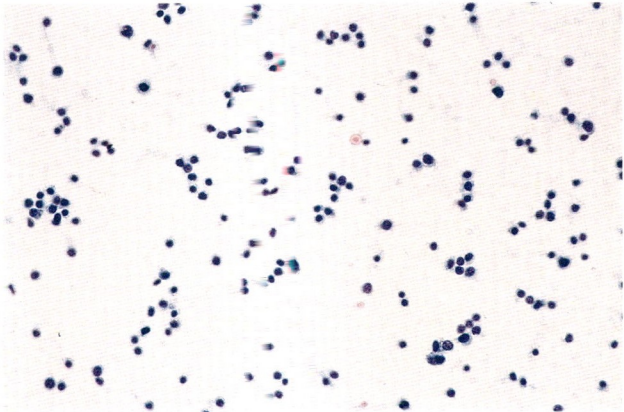

FIGURE 11.6 Small cell lymphoma with plasmacytoid differentiation. The number of cells is small, and only a rare mesothelial cell and a few RBCs are noted in the background. (Pap × 40)

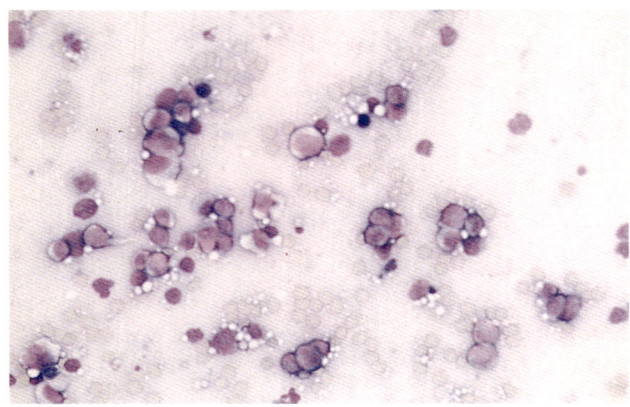

FIGURE 11.7 Same case as in Figure 11.6. With the Wright stain, the plasmacytoid features of this lymphoma are better appreciated. Note the eccentric nuclei and the abundant bluish cytoplasm with clear vacuoles. (Wright× 100)

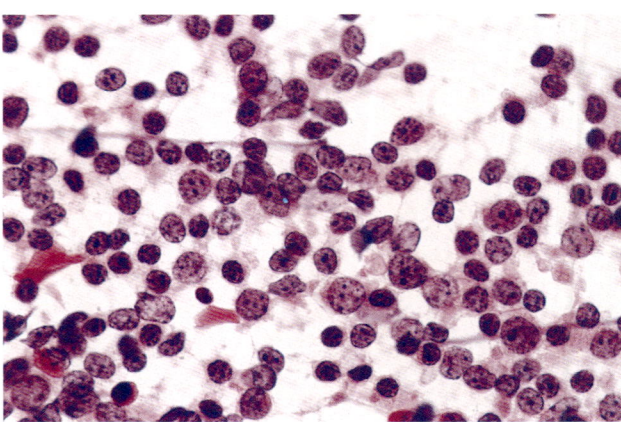

FIGURE 11.9 Same specimen as that shown in Figure 11.8. Lymphocytes show irregularities of the nuclear contour, variation in size and shape, and multiple small nucleoli. (Pap× 240)

mainly of small cells are characterized by less mature lymphocytes with greater irregularities of the nuclear contour (Fig. 11.8). The cells show a greater variation of their size and shape than that noted in WDL, and display small, multiple nucleoli (Fig. 11.9).

BURKITT'S LYMPHOMA

Undifferentiated lymphomas are usually subclassified into Burkitt's and non-Burkitt's varieties. Burkitt's lym-

phoma may present either as small-size or medium-size cells. As noted previously, it is not always possible to classify a lymphoma by cytologic means alone, but Burkitt's lymphoma is an exception to this rule. This tumor is characterized by medium-sized cells with tendency toward necrosis and karyorrhexis and an abundant cytoplasm with frequent lipid vacuoles which may also involve the nuclei. Burkitt's lymphoma may also present exclusively as small cells in the pediatric age group. The cells in this neoplasm have a small amount of cytoplasm which may contain lipid in the form of very small vacuoles (Fig. 11.10). The nuclei are non-

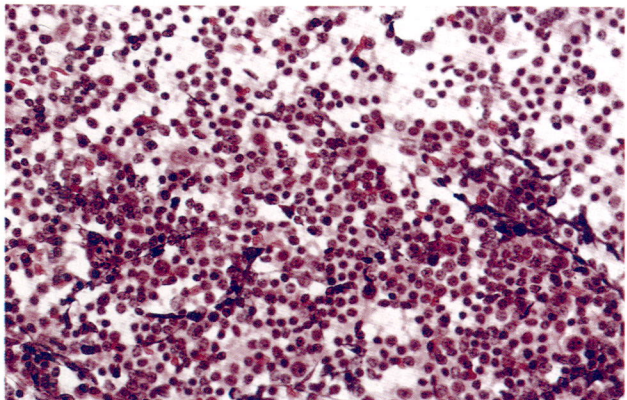

FIGURE 11.8 Poorly differentiated lymphocytic lymphoma composed mainly of small cells. A few large lymphocytes are also present, creating a less monotonous cell population than that noted in WDL. (Pap× 90)

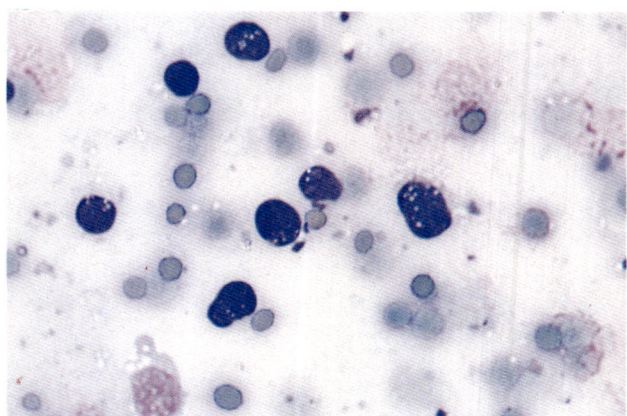

FIGURE 11.10 Peritoneal fluid showing undifferentiated lymphoma, Burkitt's type. Small to medium-sized cells display vacuolization, well demonstrated by Wright's stain. (Wright× 240)

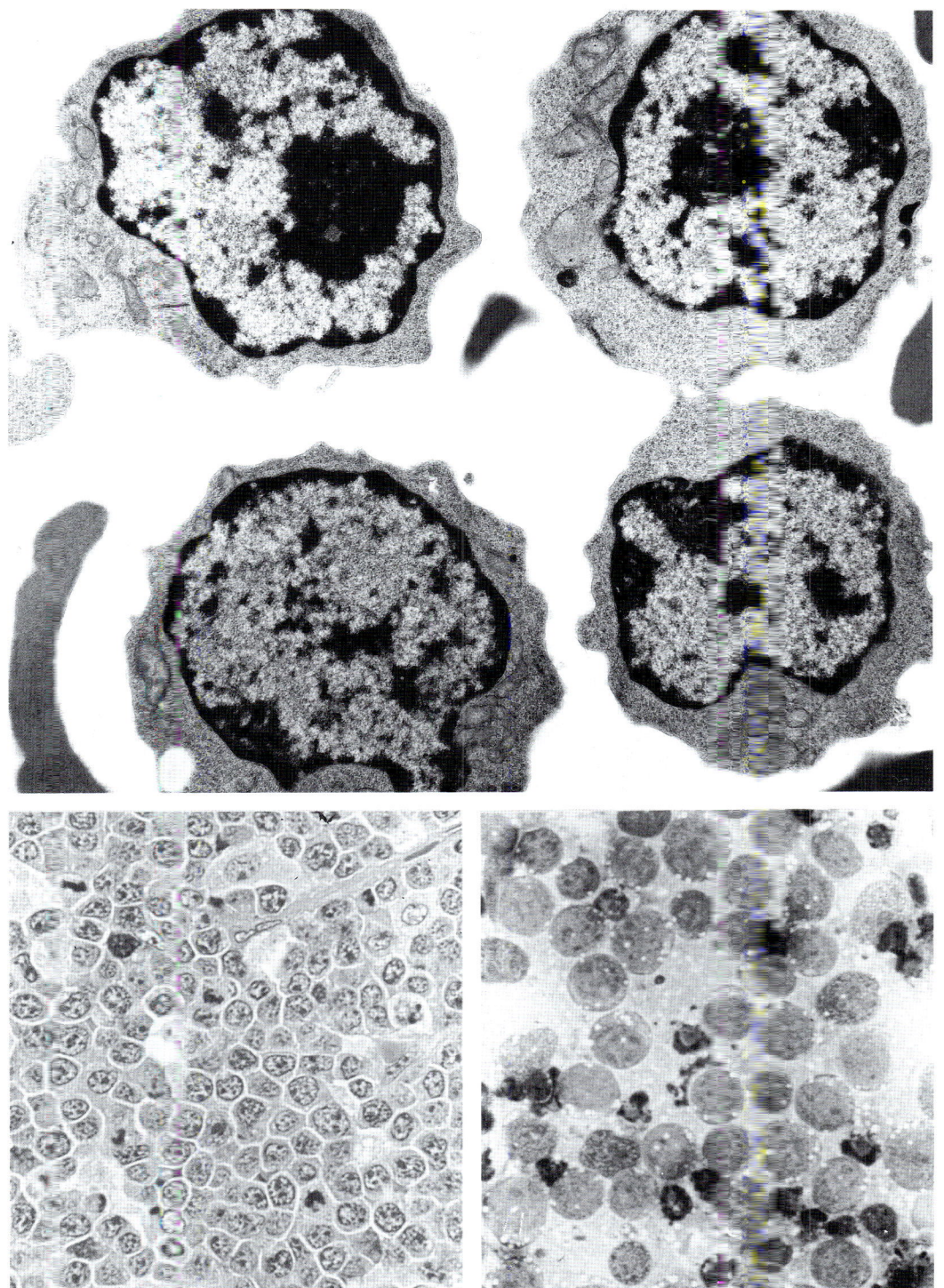

FIGURE 11.11 **Burkitt's lymphoma: Top, left:** Histologic section shows small undifferentiated lymphocytes. (H&E × 200). **Bottom, left:** Cytologic preparation showing vacuolization in cytoplasm and in the nucleus (Diff Quik × 300). **Right:** EM shows cells without intercellular junctions and occasional small lipid vacuoles (EM × 8,000) (Courtesy M. Akhtar, MD).

cleaved and the cytoplasm stains pale blue with the Diff-Quik stain. With this stain nuclei may also demonstrate vacuoles but they are not well appreciated with the pap stain.

In undifferentiated non-Burkitt's lymphoma the picture is cytologically similar but the process affects adults and should be differentiated from the large cell lymphoma because of their size variability. Non-Burkitt's undifferentiated lymphoma yields lymphocytes that appear malignant by cytologic nuclear criteria, but its exact classification is not possible beyond placement in the small cell lymphoma category. By marker studies these lymphocytes are immature B cells, usually TdT negative and positive for CD9, CD10, CD19, CD20, CD22, and CD24. Ultrastructural studies have little to contribute except for the demonstration of lipid vacuoles in the cytoplasm of tumor cells (Fig. 11.11).

LYMPHOMAS OF MEDIUM SIZED CELLS

These lymphomas are arbitrarily separated from small cell lymphomas mostly by the appearance rather than the size of lymphocytes. They are more easily distinguished from large cell lymphomas, characterized by considerably larger cells. Beyond that, they are difficult to recognize cytologically without a previous histologic diagnosis which often subclassifies them either as peripheral T-cell lymphomas or as lymphoblastic lymphomas.

PERIPHERAL T-CELL LYMPHOMAS

Peripheral T-cell lymphomas are only infrequently accompanied by effusion. The proliferating lymphocytes are discohesive T cells with rather convoluted nuclei and a negligible amount of cytoplasm (Fig. 11.12). Nuclei range from small to medium-sized, but are invariably markedly irregular or they may appear elongated (Fig. 11.13). These cells are rather fragile, leading to easy fragmentation of the cytoplasm which may appear as rather sparse "lympho-glandular" bodies in smears prepared from the sediment of effusions (Fig. 11.14). Those tumors presenting with a cutaneous component—*Mycosis fungoides*—display the greatest degree of nuclear irregularity. These T cells are unique by their punctate pattern of acid phosphatase reactivity and positivity for UCHL-1, T26, and other T-cell markers, in cell blocks. If the process is of long duration reactive

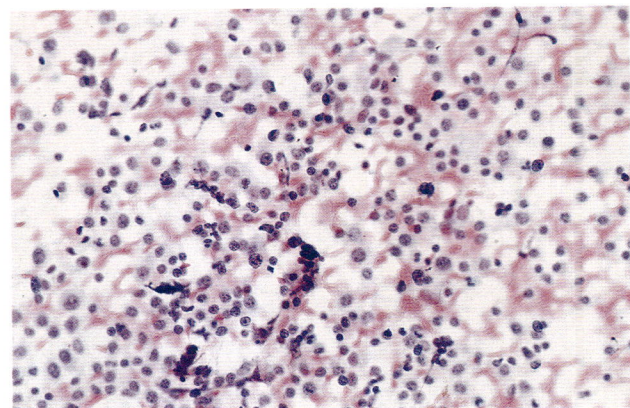

FIGURE 11.12   Peripheral T-cell lymphoma, in a pleural effusion. Note the small to medium-sized discohesive cells in a background containing RBCs. (Pap × 40)

lymphocytes, polys and eosinophils may become part of the cytologic picture and hamper interpretation. Special caution should be exercised not to confuse the process with Hodgkin's lymphoma (Fig 11.15).

LYMPHOBLASTIC LYMPHOMAS

The lymphoblastic lymphomas occur in children and are characterized by effusions containing medium-sized lymphocytes with a moderate degree of pleomorphism (Fig. 11.16). Nuclei are less convoluted and elongated than in peripheral T-cell lymphoma and the chromatin

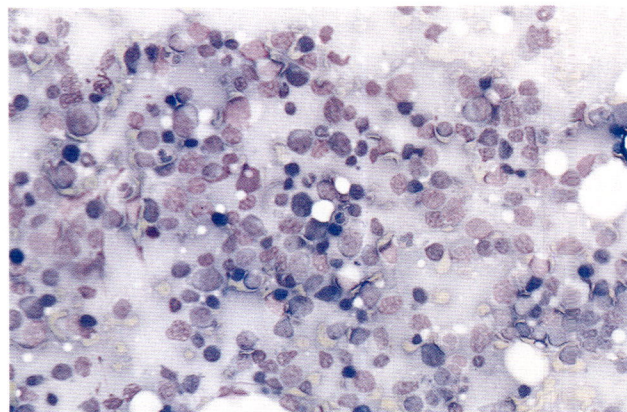

FIGURE 11.13   Same case as in Figure 11.12, stained by MGG. The neoplastic cells are pale with elongated or round nuclei. Reactive lymphocytes are also noted. (MGG × 90)

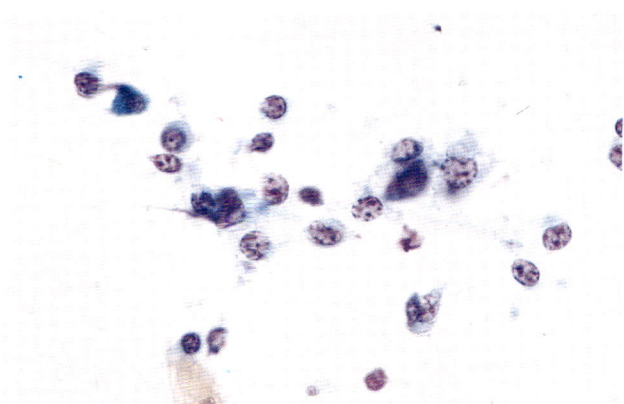

FIGURE 11.14 Typical peripheral T cells showing slight elongation of the nuclei. The cytoplasm ranges from dense to wispy and shows evidence of fragmentation. (Pap × 120)

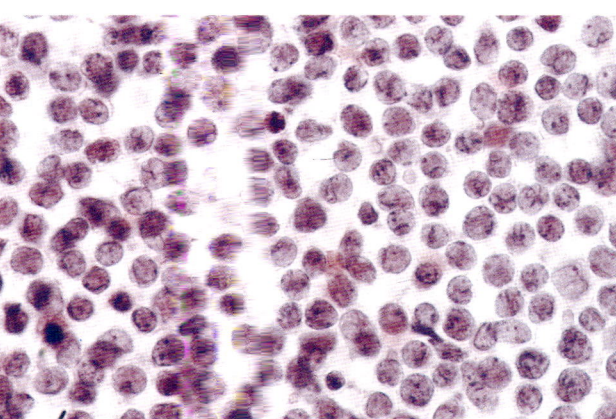

FIGURE 11.16 Lymphoma of medium-sized cells, lymphoblastic type. Note the stripped nuclei with small, multiple nucleoli. (Pap × 120)

pattern tends to be clear with multiple, small nucleoli (Fig. 11.17). The lymphocytes mark as T cells, are TdT positive and express CD2, CD7, and CD71. Expression of CD1, 3, 4, 5, 8, 10, and 38 depends on the stage of development of the malignant cells. Most express CD1 and CD5. Positivity for these markers and focal positivity for acid phosphatase allow distinction of lymphoblastic lymphoma from Burkitt's lymphoma. In doubtful cases, formation of E-rosettes with sheep RBCs confirms the T-cell nature of the lymphoblasts.

LARGE CELL LYMPHOMAS

Both nodular and diffuse large cell lymphomas may uncommonly be complicated by effusion, but it is not possible to distinguish these entities on a cytologic basis alone. The cells of large cell lymphoma are twice the size of histiocytes with a more homogeneous distribution of the chromatin clumps. In contrast with tuberculosis, where the lymphoid cells occur in the absence of mesothelial cells, large cell lymphomas maybe

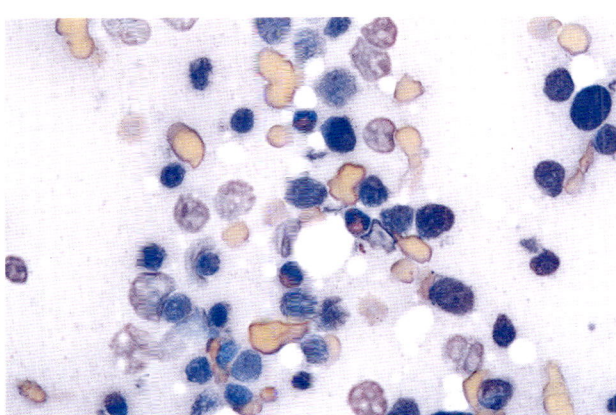

FIGURE 11.15 Peripheral T-cell lymphoma accompanied by reactive leukocytosis. Note the bilobed eosinophils near the center. (Wright × 120)

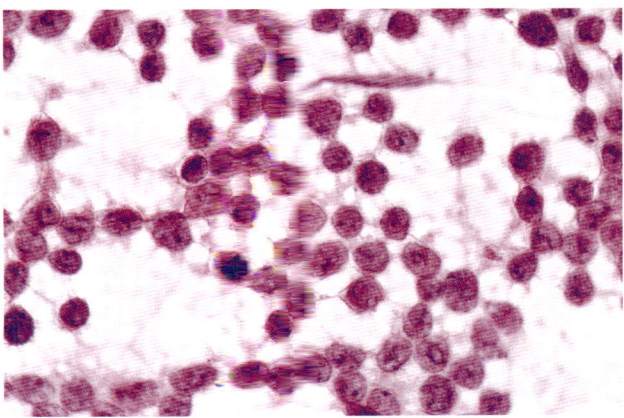

FIGURE 11.17 Same cases in Figure 11.16 showing a monotonous population of small to medium-sized cells. The chromatin pattern is clear and the multiple nucleoli are rather small. (Pap × 120)

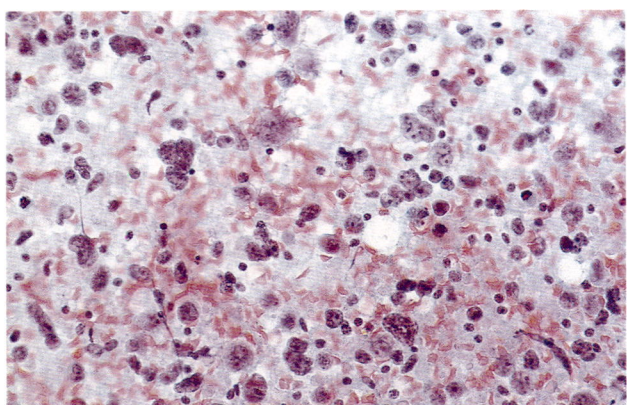

FIGURE 11.18 Large cell lymphoma, follicular center cell type. The malignant cells are large and pleomorphic. The nuclei are irregular, but there are no prominent nucleoli. (Pap× 40)

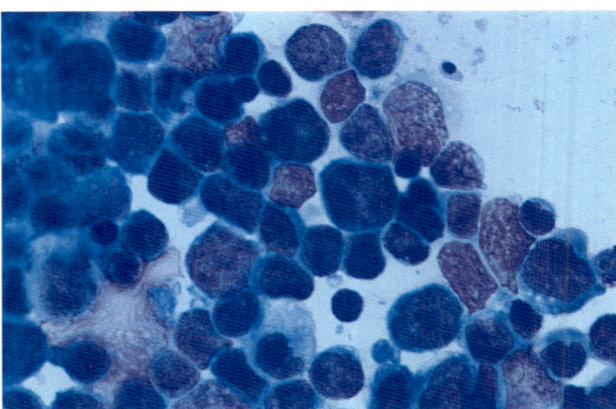

FIGURE 11.20 With Wright's stain, the chromatinic structure of this large cell lymphoma is not well appreciated. However, large, discohesive cells are noted, dwarfing small lymphocytes in the background. (Wright× 240)

accompanied by reactive mesothelial cells. Large cell lymphomas are believed to derive from follicular center cells (FCC), which tend to be pleomorphic when examined cytologically (Fig. 11.18). The danger is to confuse these cells with histiocytes or other large cells (Fig. 11.19). Large lymphocytes display unusually irregular nuclei with frequent clefts, blebs, and protrusions of the nuclear envelope, a phenomenon that appears enhanced in effusions. These large cells are usually noted against a background of smaller reactive lymphocytes (Fig. 11.20). The proportion of large lymphocytes is greatest in high grade, diffuse large cell lymphomas, but it is not prudent to judge the grade of the lymphoma by cytologic examination of effusions (Fig. 11.21). Marker studies in high grade lymphoma show an almost pure population of either B cells or T cells. B cells are usually positive for IGG, with either kappa or lambda expression but not both.

Large cell lymphomas may show progressive differentiation toward an immunoglobulin-producing cell population. When the majority of cells are recognizable as immunoblasts, an immunoblastic lymphoma is diag-

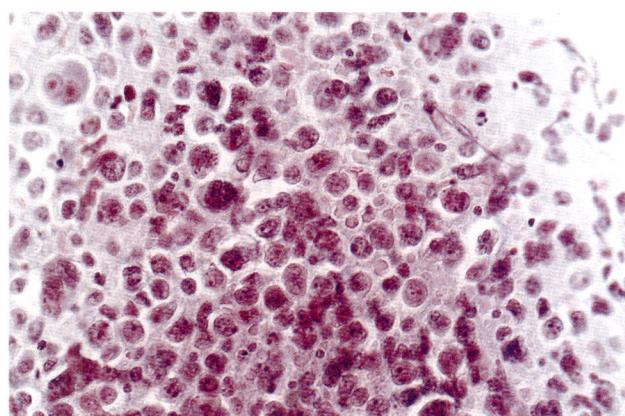

FIGURE 11.19 Same case shown in Figure 11.18. Note the nuclei with contour irregularity, nuclear pockets, and multiple small nucleoli. Binucleate cells at the upper left have features reminiscent of the Reed-Sternberg cells. (Pap× 100)

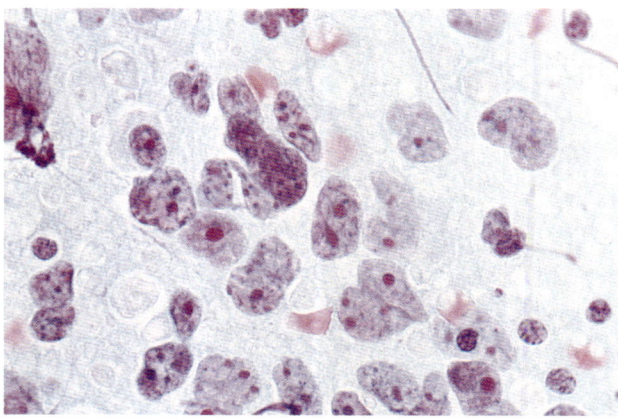

FIGURE 11.21 Large cell lymphoma, high grade. Note the extreme irregularity of the nuclei and the multiple large, brightly eosinophilic nucleoli. (Pap× 400)

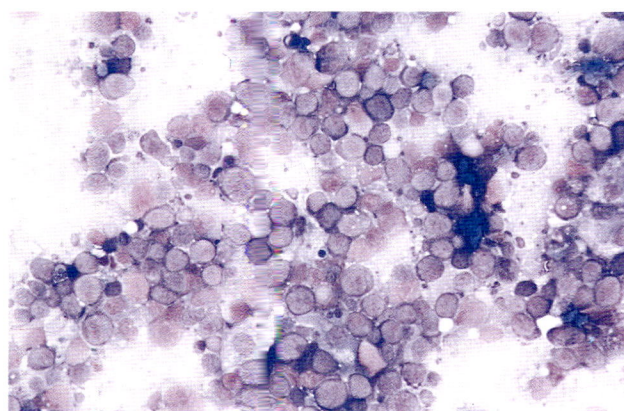

FIGURE 11.22   Immunoblastic lymphoma stained by Wright's method. Note the irregular size and shape of the large cells crowding one another, and the moderate amount of cytoplasm. (Wright × 100)

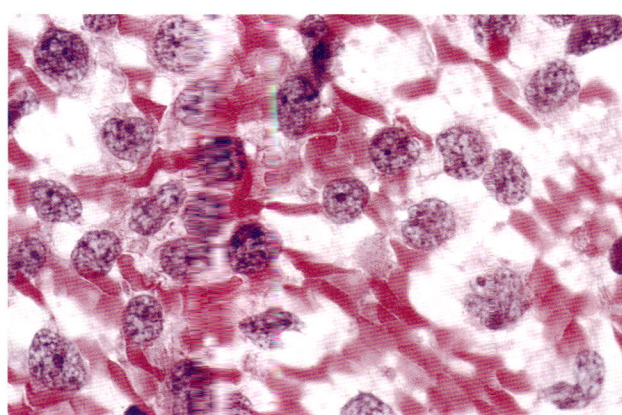

FIGURE 11.24   Same case as that shown in Figure 11.23. The H&E stain is helpful in demonstrating the chromatinic structure the prominent nucleoli, and the fragile nature of the cytoplasm. (H&E × 240)

nosable by cytologic criteria (Fig. 11.22). Immunoblasts are characterized by regular, eccentrically located nuclei and a pale area of the cytoplasm marking the location of the Golgi apparatus. The methyl green pironin (MGP) stain is useful to document immunoglobulin synthesis that may be only suspected with the MGG stain (Fig. 11.23). In cell blocks the cytoplasm of immunoblasts tend to fragment and be lost (Fig. 11.24). Nucleoli are very prominent and the cytoplasm may occasionally contain closely packed immunoglobulin crystals, seldom demonstrable with the Papanicolaou

stain. A rare case has been described with unequivocal Mott cells present in the malignant pleural effusion.

Large cell lymphomas may also present as an intermediate-grade malignancy, lacking pleomorphism or differentiation towards immunoglobulin production. These tumors display a mixture of cleaved and noncleaved large cells, easily confusible with histiocytes (Fig. 11.25). Nucleoli are not as prominent as in pleomorphic large cell lymphoma and the cytoplasm is not as abundant as in the immunoblastic variety of large cell lymphoma (Fig. 11.26). Cell blocks are useful for

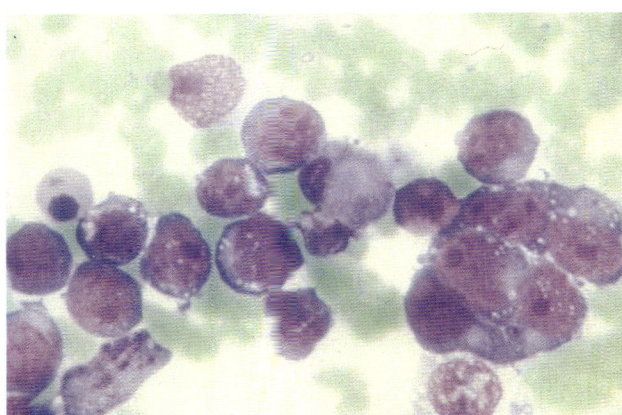

FIGURE 11.23   Immunoblastic lymphoma stained by MGG. The abundant vacuolated cytoplasm is compatible with immunoglobulin synthesis by the neoplasm. (MGG × 100)

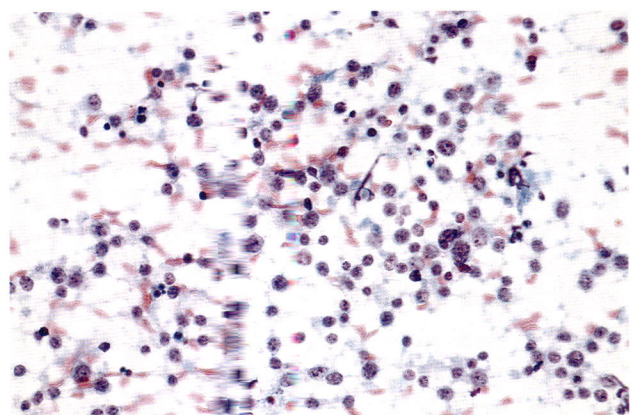

FIGURE 11.25   Large cell lymphoma, intermediate grade, with a mixture of cleaved and noncleaved cells. Note the nuclei shaped like those of histiocytes, hence the old term "histiocytic" applied to this neoplasm. (Pap × 90)

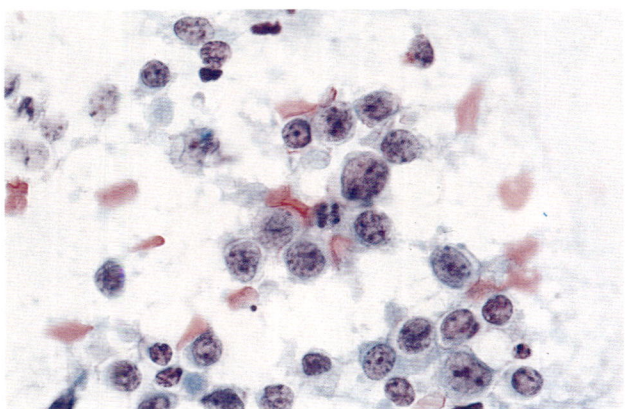

FIGURE 11.26   Same case as in Figure 11.25. Non-cleaved cells are large, with clearing and clumping of the chromatin and multiple small nucleoli. Also noted are small cleaved cells with grooves and indentations of their nuclei. Note one cell in mitosis. (Pap× 120)

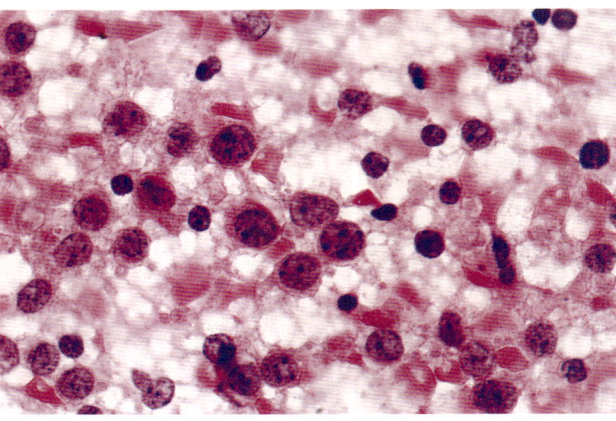

FIGURE 11.28   Same case as Fig 11.27. Note the combination of cleaved and noncleaved cells and RBCs in the background. (Pap× 120)

obtaining preparations easily comparable to preexisting surgical specimens and allowing the use of immunocytochemical markers. At times, epithelial and lymphoid markers have to be used to rule out carcinomas masquerading as large cell lymphoma (Fig. 11.27 and 11.28). Another process resembling large cell lymphoma is "hairy-cell leukemia." Only rarely this process leads to serous fluid accumulation. The effusion is bloody and the neoplasic cells are rich in cytoplasmic projections but they are not readily noticeable in smears (Fig. 11.29). The danger in cases of hairy-cell leukemia

occurs when only a small number of malignant cells is present in cell blocks. Because of their cytoplasmic projections, these cells resemble mesothelial cells (Fig. 11.30). A helpful maneuver in cases such as these is to compare the atypical cells with mesothelial cells from other areas of the cytologic preparations (Fig. 11.31). Hairy-cell leukemia gives consistently positive reactions for CD19, CD20, CD22, and CD37.

It is clear now that most lymphomas with cells resembling tissue histiocytes are in reality of B-cell derivation. However, there remains a small proportion of true histiocytic lymphomas that cause generalized lymphoadenopathy which may occasionally result in malig-

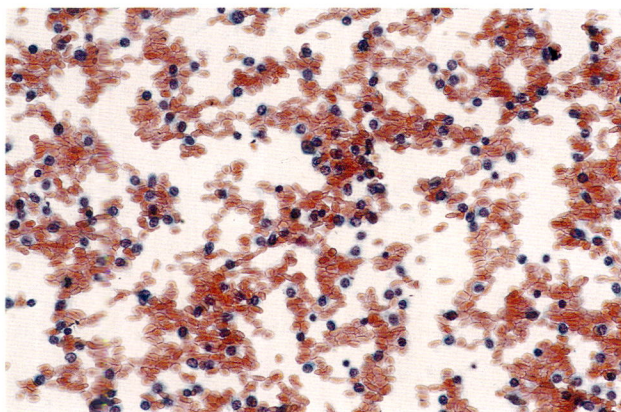

FIGURE 11.27   Intermediate lymphoma in ascitic fluid. Small lymphoid elements in a rather noncohesive distribution are noted against a background of numerous RBCs. (Pap× 40)

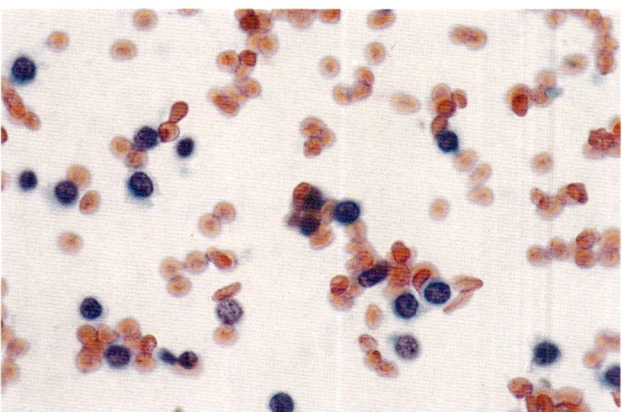

FIGURE 11.29   Ascitic fluid in patient with hairy cell leukemia. Note the occasional elongated elements and many RBCs in the background. (Pap× 90)

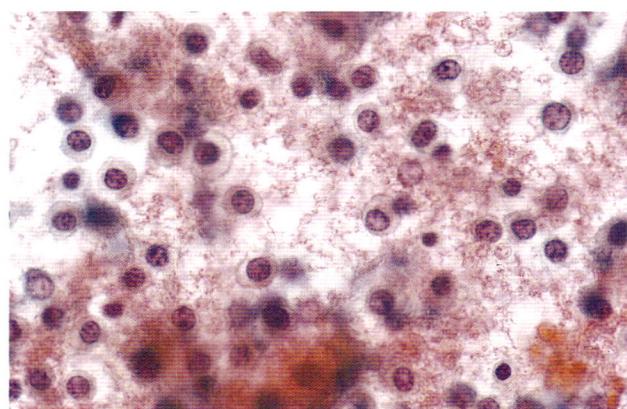

FIGURE 11.30 H&E preparation from the specimen shown in Figure 11.29. The artificial lacunae are a consequence of the long cytoplasmic extensions of the hairy cells. (H&E × 90)

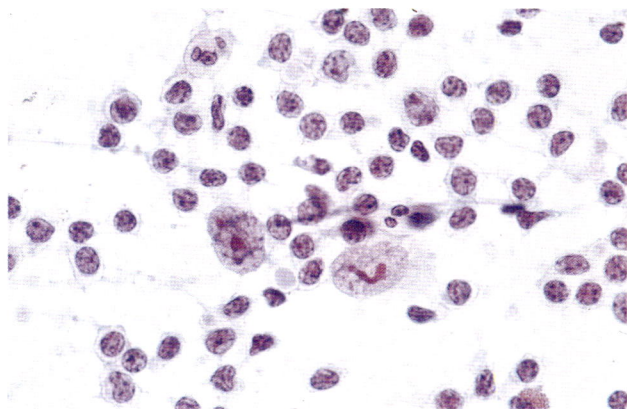

FIGURE 11.32 Hodgkin's disease. Note the lymphocytes with variable degrees of maturation and large, single, atypical cells. These have prominent nucleoli and are colloquially referred to as "mononuclear" Reed-Sternberg cells. (Pap × 180)

nant effusions. Marker studies for leucocyte common antigen (LCA), B-cell and T-cell markers are negative, but the cells are positive for α_1-AT, α_1-ACT, and lysozyme. True histiocytic lymphoma are positive for CD11, CD15, CD25, and CD68. In malignant histiocytosis the culprit cell is the macrophage, which dominates the cytologic picture. A large number of mononuclear cells correspond to the cells of monocytic origin that failed to differentiate fully into histiocytic elements. The latter are characterized by phagocytosis of RBCs, neutrophils, and lymphoid elements while a small proportion of cells

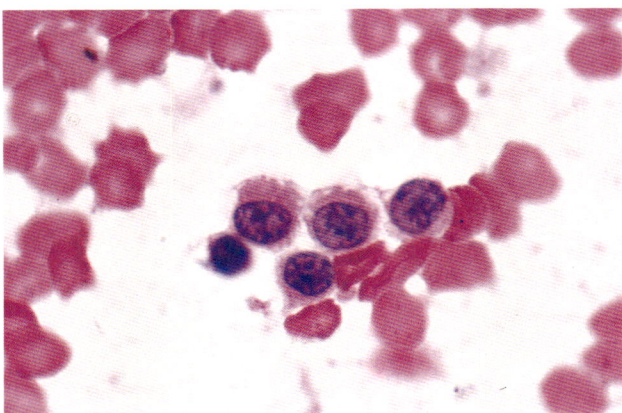

FIGURE 11.31 Hairy cells with dense eosinophilic cytoplasm and ruffled borders. Even though these cells are small, they must be distinguished from mesothelial cells. (H&E × 90)

appear bizarre and immature, hence the old term "reticulum cell sarcoma" applied to these neoplasms.

HODGKIN'S DISEASE

Untreated Hodgkin's disease may lead to pleural effusion, but modern forms of therapy have rendered this complication a rather uncommon event. The cytologic picture is pleomorphic with a mixed population of mature and immature lymphocytes and various proportions of eosinophils, plasma cells, neutrophils and large mononuclear cells (Fig. 11.32). The mesothelial cells are reactive and there is also an increase in the number of macrophages so that the initial impression is invariably one of an inflammatory process. Knowledge of a previous diagnosis of Hodgkin's disease and the presence of unequivocal Reed–Sternberg cells greatly facilitate the clinching of the diagnosis.

Two presentations of Reed–Sternberg cells can be recognized cytologically. The classic Reed–Sternberg cell is binucleated with very large eosinophilic nucleoli that are mirror images of each other. In the polyploid variety, multinucleated Reed–Sternberg cells show multilobed nuclei with prominent nucleoli. Reed–Sternberg cells are negative for LN1, LN2 and UCHL-1 but are positive for Leu M-1, and the Ki-1 antigen. The presence of Reed–Sternberg cells alone, in an effusion, is not sufficient for the diagnosis of Hodgkin's disease. Other lymphomas, particularly immunoblastic lym-

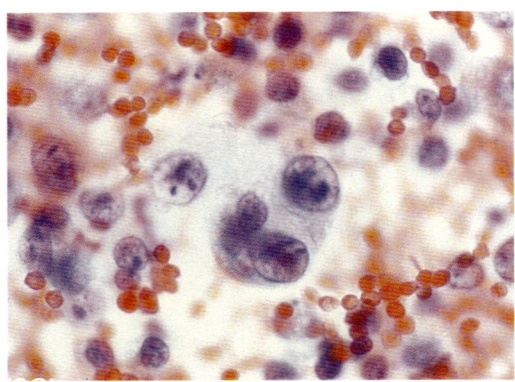

FIGURE 11.33 Hodgkins disease in pleural fluid. Note the mononuclear cells and a binucleate cell fulfilling the criteria for Reed-Sternberg cells. (Pap × 240)

phoma, may present with Reed–Sternberg–like cells as may other processes, including nonlymphomatous conditions.

Reed-Sternberg cells vary tremendously in the nuclear size and amount of the surrounding cytoplasm, which is faintly basophilic with MGG stain and lacy green or blue with Papanicolaou's method (Fig. 11.33). Nuclei have regular, arcuate contours without angulations or protrusions. Nucleoli are rather large, particularly in nuclei that are mirror images of each other (Fig. 11.34). By MGG stain, nuclei of Reed-Sternberg have the texture of those seen in blast cells, whereas with the Papanicolaou stain they are characterized by

finely dispersed chromatin clumps. Polyploid Reed–Sternberg cells should not be confused with multinucleated mesothelial cells, histiocytic giant cells, or megakaryocytes, from which they can be distinguished by morphologic criteria (Fig. 11.35). Doubtful cases may be helped by immunocytochemistry with antibodies against keratin, EMA, A1AT, A1ACT and Factor VIII. However, immunocytochemical markers do not replace expert recognition of cytologic criteria which remains the golden standard in the diagnosis of Hodgkin's disease.

PLASMA CELL DYSCRASIAS

Of all plasma cell dyscrasias, multiple myeloma is the one most commonly accompanied by an effusion. Effusion is more frequent in extraskeletal multiple myeloma, but involvement of the vertebrae may extend to pleural or pericardial effusions. Plasma cell myelomas may be composed entirely of cellular elements resembling mature plasma cells (Fig. 11.36). Myelomas may also be rather anaplastic with large multinucleated elements and single box-shaped cells with eccentric nuclei and granular cytoplasm. These cells are positive for immunoglobulins and also stain strongly positive with methyl green pironin (MGP). In poorly differentiated plasma cell myelomas the cells must be differentiated from anaplastic tumors such as high grade lymphomas or large cell carcinomas (Fig. 11.37). This task may be difficult since the myeloma may be a poor producer of immunoglobulin. Immunocytochemically malignant plasma cells show monoclonality for kappa or lambda, and CD38, PC1, and PCA-1. The characteristic nuclear features of the plasma cells in anaplastic tumors are lost because of the poorly differentiated nature of the neoplasm. However, the cytoplasm retains its amphophilia and the paranuclear hole noted in a few cells serves as a clue to the plasmacytic nature of the process. Plasma cell tumors may also be so undifferentiated that they enter the differential diagnosis of small blue round cell tumors, discussed in the next chapter.

MEGAKARYOCYTIC PROCESSES

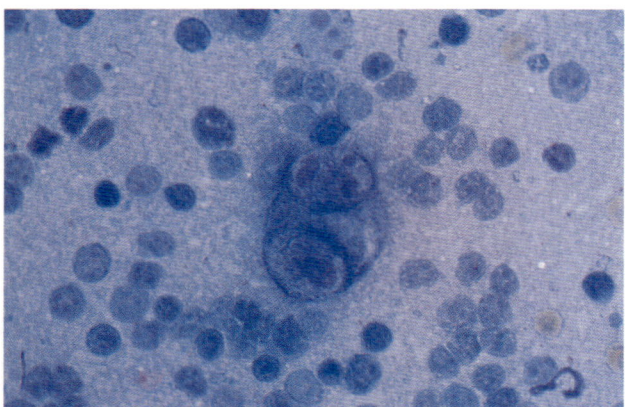

FIGURE 11.34 Same specimen as in Fig. 11.33 with typical Reed-Sternberg cell. disease. Each nucleus is a mirror image of the other, and both contain large nucleoli. (MGG × 240) (Courtesy of S. Rollins, MD)

Megakaryocytes have been noted in a number of cytologic specimens, particularly needle aspirates from an unintentionally punctured vertebra or rib. The most frequent cytologic presentation, however, is the finding of

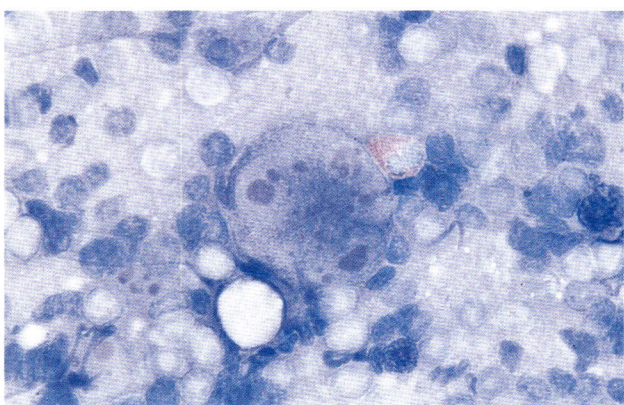

FIGURE 11.35 Another Reed-Sternberg cell stained by MGG. There are multiple nuclei displaying enormous nucleoli (MGG × 240) (Courtesy of S. Rollins, MD)

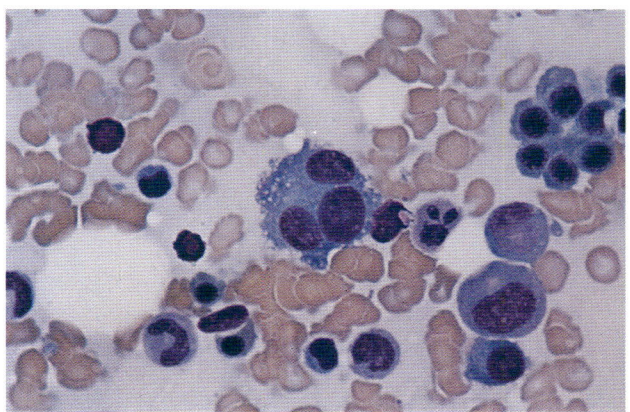

FIGURE 11.37 Multiple myeloma with Diff-Quik stain. Notice malignant, multinucleated plasma cells with little resemblance to plasma cells. (Diff-Quik × 180)

megakaryocytes in serous effusions due to lymphoproliferative disorders. The ascitic fluid is a common site for megakaryocytes to occur in association with agnogenic myeloid metaplasia and extramedullary hematopoiesis that affects the mesentery. With the Papanicolaou stain, megakaryocytes display multilobed nuclei and may attain a bizarre cytologic appearance. To avoid confusion with metastatic carcinomas, reactive mesothelial cells, or multinucleated histiocytes Romanowsky-stained smears can be prepared in which the appearance of megakaryocytes may be more familiar to the pathologist. Positivity for factor VIII-related antigen is confirmatory of the megakaryocytic nature of these cells.

ANCILLARY METHODS

It is our practice to "triage" specimens with wet films stained by toluidine blue, as recommended by Naylor. Whenever possible, effusion material is also stained by H&E to facilitate comparison with histologic sections of lymphoma. Effusions are also ideally suitable for marker studies capable of defining and characterizing lymphomas. DNA ploidy studies distinguish lymphoma from benign lymphocytosis monoclonality also defines a lymphoma and can be determined by immunocytochemical stainings of cytospin preparations. There are currently reliable markers that work well in alcohol- or formalin-fixed cell blocks and allow the subclassification of lymphomas (Table 11.2).

We prefer to apply the markers to B5/formalin-fixed cell blocks and there is usually a good correlation between marker studies in the cell blocks and cell suspensions of unfixed material. In contrast, electron microscopy has little to offer in the diagnosis and classification of lymphomas. The characteristic cytologic feature of large cell lymphoma is irregularity of the nuclear membrane. Certain tumors are recognized as cleaved or noncleaved, but it is extremely difficult to determine a B-cell or a T-cell origin by cytology alone. If the nuclei are elongated and convoluted, a peripheral T-cell origin can be surmised. Most small lymphocytic lymphomas are of B-cell origin. True histiocytes contain bean-shaped nuclei and stain positive for one or more of those enzymes: α_1-AT, α_1-ACT, or lysozyme. Very little can be accomplished by cytology alone to determine the degree of differentiation of a lymphoma.

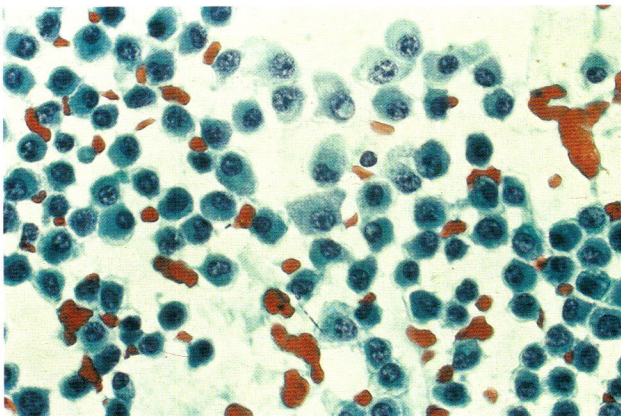

FIGURE 11.36 Pleural fluid in advanced multiple myeloma. The majority of the cells bear resemblance to mature plasma cells. (Pap × 240)

TABLE 11.2 Selective Lymphohistiocytic Markers Applicable to Cytologic Material

Antigen/Antibody	Cells Recognized	Diagnostic Applications
LCA (T29/33; PD7/26)	Lymphocytes, granulocytes, macrophages, monocytes	Lymphoid versus nonlymphoid neoplasms
LN-1	FCC lymphocytes, erythroid cells	FCC, lymphomas
LN-2[a]	Pan-B (except plasma cells), monocyte series	B cell lymphomas, monocytic leukemias
L-26	Pan-B (includes mantles zone)	B cell lymphomas
UCHL-1	Pan-T, macrophages, neutrophils, thymocytes	Peripheral T cell lymphoma versus carcinoma
Anti-Ig (G,M,D,E)	Lymphoid and plasmacytoid cells (intracytoplasmic immunoglobulin)	Multiple myeloma, plasmacytoid lymphoma
λ, κ, and heavy chains	Lymphoid and plasmacytoid cells (clonality)	Multiple myeloma, plasmacytoid lymphoma
Lysozyme	Granulocytes, monocytes, macrophages	Granulocytic and monocytic leukemias
α_1-Antitrypsin, α_1-Antichymotrypsin	Monocytes, macrophages, granulocytes	Malignant histiocytosis, true histiocytic lymphoma
S100	Neutral tissue, Langerhans cells, melanocytes	Histiocytosis X, melanoma
Leu M_1	Myelocytes	Reed-Sternberg cells, adenocarcinoma
Leu 7 (HNK_1)	Natural killer cells, neuroendocrine cells	FCC lymphomas, melanoma, oat cell carcinoma
Antihemoglobin A	Erythroid cells	Erythroleukemias

[a]LN-2 may react with epithelial cells, melanocytes, and other nonlymphoid cells.
From Bedrossian CWM: Immunocytochemistry. In Astarita RW, ed. Practical Cytopathology. New York, Churchill & Livingston, 1990. Chap 14 pp 403–457, with permission.

There are antibodies that define clusters of differentiation (CD antigens) but require fresh cell suspensions or frozen sections of excised lymph nodes for reliable results. It is our practice to submit a part of each effusion for CD antigen analysis in all cases suspicious for lymphoma and leukemia or previously diagnosed as such.

BIBLIOGRAPHY

Normal Lymphocytes

Cardozo PL, Harting MC. On the function of lymphocytes in malignant effusions. *Acta Cytol.* 1972;4:307–313.

Domagala W, Emeson EE, Koss LG. T and B lymphocyte enumeration in the diagnosis of lymphocyte rich pleural fluids. *Acta Cytol.* 1981;25:108.

Ghosh AK, Spriggs AI and Mason DY. Immunocytochemical staining of T and B lymphocytes in serous effusions. *J Clin Pathol.* 1985;38:608.

Peterson T. Acid alpha-naphthyl acetate esterase staining of lymphocytes in pleural effusions. *Acta Cytol.* 1982;26:109–114.

Kay NE, Ackerman SK, Douglas SD. Anatomy of the immune system. *Semin Hematol.* 1979;16:252–382.

O'Hara MF, Cousar JB, Glick AD, et al. Multiparameter approach to the diagnosis of hematopoietic lymphoid neoplasms in body fluids. *Diagn Cytopathol.* 1985;1:33.

Robey SS, Cafferty LL, Beschorner WE, et al. Value of lymphocyte marker studies in diagnostic cytopathology. *Acta Cytol.* 1987;31:453–459.

Taylor CR, Burns I. The demonstration of plasma cells and other immunoglobulin containing cells in formalin fixed, paraffin embedded tissues using peroxidase labelled antibody. *J Clin Pathol.* 1974;27:14–19.

Yam L. Diagnostic significance of lymphocytes in pleural effusions. *Ann Intern Med.* 1967;66(5):972–982.

Lymphoid Hyperplasia

Bollum FJ. Terminal deoxynucleotidyl transferase as a hematopoietic cell marker. *Blood.* 1979;54:1203–1215.

Catovsky K, Pittman S, O'Brien M, et al. Multiparameter studies in lymphoid leukemias. *Am J Clin Pathol.* 1979;72:736–745.

Domagala W, Emerson EE, Koss LG. T and B lymphocyte enumeration in the diagnosis of lymphocyte-rich pleural fluids. *Acta Cytol.* 1981;25:108–110.

Glick AD, Paniker K, Flexner J, et al. Acute leukemia of adults: Ultrastructural cytochemical and histologic observations in 100 cases. *Am J Clin Pathol.* 1980;73:459–470.

Glick AD, Vestal BK, Flexner JM, et al. Ultrastructural study of acute lymphocytic leukemia: Comparison with immunologic studies. *Blood.* 1978;52:311–322.

Groman GS, Castele RJ, Altose MD, et al. Lymphocyte subpopulations in sarcoid pleural effusion. *Ann Intern Med.* 1984;100:75–77.

Johnson EJ, Scott CS, Parapia LA, et al. Diagnostic differentiation between reactive and malignant lymphoid cells in serous effusions. *Eur J Cancer Clin Oncol.* 1987;23:245–250.

Kim YK, Mohsenifar Z, Koerner SK. Lymphocytic pleural effusion in postpericardiotomy syndrome. *Am Heart J.* 1988;115:1077–1079.

McKenna RW, Parkin J, Brunning RD. Morphologic ultrastructural characteristics of T-cell acute lymphoblastic leukemia. *Cancer.* 1979;44:1290–1297.

O'Hara MF, Bedrossian CWM, Johnson TS, et al. Flow cytometry in cancer diagnosis. In: *Progress in Clinical Pathology.* New York: Grune & Stratton; 1983;9(6):135–153.

Non-Hodgkin's Lymphoma

Boccato P, Saran B, Pasine L, et al. Immunology of lymphocytes in pleurisy and in effusions due to pleural infiltration by chronic lymphocytic leukemia cells. *Acta Cytol.* 1978;22:284–285.

Cartun R, Coles FB, Pastuszak W. Utilization of monoclonal antibody L26 in the identification and confirmation of B-cell lymphomas. *Am J Pathol.* 1987;129(3):415–421.

Das DK, Gupta SK, Ayyagari S, et al. Pleural effusions in non-Hodgkin's lymphoma: A cytomorphologic, cytochemical and immunologic study. *Acta Cytol.* 1987;31:119–124.

Janckila AJ, Yam LT, Li CY. Immunocytochemical diagnosis of acute leukemia with pleural involvement. *Acta Cytol.* 1985;29:67–72.

Katz RL, Raval P, Manning JT, et al. A morphologic, immunologic and cytometric approach to the classification of non-Hodgkin's lymphoma in effusions. *Diagn Cytopathol.* 1987;3:91.

Krajewski AS, Dewar AE, Ramage EF. T and B lymphocyte markers in effusions of patients with non-Hodgkin's lymphoma. *J Clin Pathol.* 1982;35:1216–1219.

Krause JR, Dekker A. Hairy cell leukemia (leukemic reticuloendotheliosis) in serous effusions. *Acta Cytol.* 1978;22:80–82.

Melamed MR. The cytological presentation of malignant lymphomas and related diseases in effusions. *Cancer.* 1963;16:413.

Melo JV, Robinson DSF, de Oliveira MP, et al. Morphology and immunology of circulating cells in leukaemic phase of follicular lymphoma. *J Clin Pathol.* 1988;41:951.

Menarguez-Palanca FJ, Lacruz-Pelea C, Echeverria V, et al. Cytomorphologic differentiation of common acute lymphoblastic leukemia from other immunologic subtypes. *Acta Cytol.* 1985;29:842–845.

Miliauskas JR, Berard CW, Young RC, et al. Undifferentiated non-Hodgkin's lymphomas (Burkitt's and non-Burkitt's type): The relevance of making this histologic distinction. *Cancer.* 1982;50:2115–2121.

Nathwani BN, Kim H, Rappaport H. Malignant lymphoma, lymphoblastic. *Cancer.* 1976;38:964–983.

Qizilbash AH, Elavathil LJ, Chen V, et al. Aspiration biopsy cytology of lymph nodes in malignant lymphoma. *Diagn Cytopathol.* 1985;1:18–22.

Seidel T, Garbes A. Cellules Grumelees: Old terminology revisited regarding the cytologic diagnosis of chronic lymphocytic leukemia and well differentiated lymphocytic lymphoma in pleural effusions. *Acta Cytol.* 1985;29(5):775–780.

Spriggs AI, Vanhegan RI. Cytological diagnosis of lymphoma in serous effusions. *J Clin Pathol.* 1981;34:1311–1325.

Spriggs AI, Vanhegan RI. Cytological diagnosis of lymphoma in pleural effusions. *J Clin Pathol.* 1982;35:1311–1325.

Strobel SL, Brandt JT. The value of the Wright-Giemsa stain for diagnosing hairy cell leukemia in body cavity fluids. *J Surg Oncol.* 1986;33:182–185.

Ueshima Y, Fukuhara S, Nagai K, Takatsuki K and Uchino H. Cytogenetic studies and clinical aspects of patients with plasma cell leukemia and leukemic macroglobulinemia. *Cancer Res* 1983;43:905–912.

Wilkerson JA. Intraoperative cytology of lymph nodes and lymphoid lesions. *Diagn Cytopathol.* 1985;1:46–52.

Yam LT, Lin DG, Janckila AJ, et al. Immunocytochemical diagnosis of lymphoma in serous effusions. *Acta Cytol.* 1985;29:833–841.

Yutani C, Maeda H, Takajima T, et al. Primary ovarian lymphoma associated with Meig's syndrome. *Acta Cytol.* 1982;26:44–48.

Hodgkin's Disease

Billingham ME, Rawlinson DG, Berry PF, et al. The cytodiagnosis of malignant lymphomas and Hodgkin's disease in cerebrospinal, pleural and ascitic fluids. *Acta Cytol.* 1975;19:547–556.

Byrne GE: Histopathologic diagnosis of Hodgkin's disease. *Semin Oncol.* 1980;7:103–113.

Das DK, Gupta SK, Ayyagari S, et al. Pleural effusions in

non-Hodgkin's lymphoma. A cytomorphologic, cytochemical and immunologic study. Acta Cytol. 1987;31:119–124.

Tindle B. Malignant lymphomas. Am J pathol. 1984; 116:119–174.

Volpe R, Carbone A. Reed-Sternberg cells in pericardial fluid. Acta Cytol. 1982;26:61–64.

Weick JK, Kiely JM, Harrison EG Jr., et al. Pleural effusion in lymphoma. Cancer. 1973;31:848–853.

Histiocytic and Granulocytic Processes

Volkman A. Disparity in origin of mononuclear phagocyte populations. J Reticuloendothel Soc. 1976;19:249.

Yam LT. Granulocytic sarcoma with pleural involvement. Acta Cytol. 1985;29:63–66.

Plasma Cell Dyscrasias

Kapadia SB. Cytologic diagnosis of malignant pleural effusions in myeloma. Arch Pathol Lab Med. 1977;101:534–535.

Safa AM, Van Orstrand HS. Pleural effusion due to myeloma. Chest. 1973;64:246–248.

Young J, Crocker J. Pleural fluid cytology in lymphoplasmacytoid lymphoma with numerous intracytoplasmic immunoglobulin inclusions. Acta Cytol. 1984;28:419–424.

Megakaryocytic Processes

Bartiziota EV, Naylor B. Megakaryocytes in a hemorrhagic pleural effusion caused by anticoagulation overdose. Acta Cytol. 1986;30:163–165.

Billingham ME, Rawlinson DG, Berry PF, et al. The cytodiagnosis of malignant lymphomas and Hodgkin's disease in CSF, pleural and ascitic fluids. Acta Cytol. 1975;19:547–556.

Calle S. Megakaryocytes in an abdominal fluid. Acta Cytol. 1968;12:78–80.

Chen KTK. Megakariocytes in a fine needle aspirate of the lung. Acta Cytol. 1987;31:81–82.

Higby DJ, Ohnuma T. Plasmacytoma cell ascites. N Y State J Med. 1975;75;1074–1076.

Kumar ND, Naylor B. Megakaryocytes in pleural and peritoneal fluids and prevalence, significance, morphology and cytohistological correlations. J Clin Pathol. 1980;33:1153–1159.

Pedio G, Krause M, Jansova I. Megakaryocytes in ascitic fluid in a case of agnogenic myeloid metaplasia. Acta Cytol. 1986;30:163–165.

Silverman J. Extramedullary hema ascitic fluid cytology in myelofibrosis. Am J Clin Pathol. 1985;84:125–128.

Sprigg AI, Boddington MM. Absence of mesothelial cells from tuberculous pleural effusions. Thorax. 1960;15:169–176.

Vilaseca J, Arnau JM, Tallada N, et al. Megakariocytes in serous effusions (Letter). J Clin Pathol. 1981;34:939–

Yazdi H. Cytopathology of extramedullary hemopoiesis in effusions and peritoneal washings. Diagn Cytopathol. 1986; 2:326–329.

Ancillary Methods

Katz RL, Raval P, Manning JT, et al. A morphologic, immunologic and cytometric approach to the classification of non-Hodgkin's lymphoma in effusions. Diagn Cytopathol. 1987; 3:91–101.

Linder J, Ye Y, Armitage J, et al. Monoclonal antibodies marking B-cell non-Hodgkin's lymphoma in paraffin-embedded tissue. Mod Pathol. 1988;29(1):29–34.

CHAPTER TWELVE

Small Blue Round Cell Tumors

This category of neoplasms known as small blue round cell tumors (SBRCT) is a challenging problem in effusions. The differential diagnosis encompasses benign lymphocytosis versus a lymphoma versus a number of tumors presenting with noncohesive blue cells in the range of 15 to 25 microns in diameter. These tumors can roughly be subdivided into neuroendocrine and nonneuroendocrine SBRCTs (Table 12.1). Neuroendocrine tumors may present predominantly epithelial or predominantly neural features but their appearance is decidedly neuroepithelial and one is hard pressed to further classify them without ancillary methods. Cytomorphology alone also falls short in the subclassification of nonneuroendocrine SBRCTs, including both the mesenchymal and the lymphohistiocytic category. The nuclear membrane irregularities (noselike protrusions) exhibited by lymphocytes are not sufficient to justify a diagnosis of malignancy because they may occur in atypical lymphoid hyperplasia. A combination of flow cytometry for DNA ploidy studies and cell surface markers establishes a definitive diagnosis of lymphoma. Leucocyte common antigen and a number of antibodies are helpful in the staining of lymphomas in paraffin-embedded cell blocks, particularly, if the material is fixed in B-5 formalin and postfixed in alcohol. Markers of the LN lineage will recognize B cell–derived lymphomas whereas UCHL-1 functions as a pan-T marker. Lymphoid markers are invariably negative in neuroendocrine carcinomas even though LN2 may be positive in some other carcinomas. Monoclonal antibodies applied to fresh cell suspensions or frozen sections from acetone-treated cell blocks allow a more precise classification of lymphomas. This same goal is attained by flow cytometry as noted in the previous chapter.

Recognition of non-lymphomatous SBRCTs' pre-supposes that the neoplasm is non-reactive for leucocyte common antigen. A large proportion of these neoplasms are neuroendocrine tumors. Neuron-specific enolase (NSE) recognizes this broad category of neuroendocrine neoplasms. However, polyclonal NSE antibodies are rather nonspecific and will react positively with nonneuroendocrine tumors, including Ewing's sarcoma and lymphomas. Electron microscopy reveals typical electron-dense granules in tumors of neuroendocrine lineage. Oat cell carcinomas lack neurofilament whereas neuroblastoma expresses this intermediate filament in the cytoplasm. The mesenchymal SBRCTS are common in the pediatric age groups. They affect the soft tissues and certain parenchymal organs such as the kidney. All of them may be the cause of malignant effusions. Ewing's sarcoma is rich in glycogen and should not display neuroendocrine activity with a monoclonal NSE antibody. Cells from Wilm's tumor lack the rosettes exhibited by neuroblastoma and do not show abundant glycogen in the cytoplasm. Vimentin is negative in neuroblastoma but is of no help in distinguishing between Wilm's tumor and Ewing's sarcoma, both of which are vimentin positive. Most SBRCTs of adults fall into the epithelial-like neuroendocrine category including carcinoid and small cell carcinomas of the lung. Oat cell carcinoma sheds cells with a slight tendency toward cohesiveness; consequently, small tridimensional groups or short stacks of cells are recognized in effusions. This is not the case in Ewing's sarcoma, which sheds mostly single cells. Neuroblastoma, on the other hand, may reveal pseudorosettes or rosettelike cell groups in effusions (Table 12.2). Neuroblastoma may occur both in the pediatric and in the adult age group. In contrast, pheochromocytoma and paraganglioma rarely occur in children. As it will

177

TABLE 12.1 Differential Diagnosis of Small Blue Round Cell Tumors

Tumor Category		NE	Ker	NF	Hormone	LCA	LN1 or 2	ACT	VIM
Neuroendocrine									
Epithelial:	Carcinoid	+	+	+	+	−	−	−	−
	Intermediate	+	+	+	+	−	−	−	−
	NE carcinoma	+	+	+	−	−	−	−	−
Neural:	Neuroblastoma	+	+	+	−	−	−	−	−
	Pheochromocytoma	+	+	+	−	−	−	−	−
	Paraganglioma	+	+	+	−	−	−	−	−
Nonneuroendocrine									
Lymphohistiocytic:	Lymphoma	−	−	−	−	+	+	±	±
	Plasmacytoma	−	−	−	−	−	+	−	±
	Histiocytic	−	−	−	−	+	±	+	+
Mesenchymal:	Wilm's tumor	−	−	−	−	+	±	+	+
	Ewing's sarcoma	±	±	−	−	−	−	−	+
	Rhabdomyosarcoma	−	−	−	−	−	−	−	+

NE = neuroendocrine marker; Ker = keratin; NF = neurofilament; LCA = leukocyte common antigen; ACT = antichymotrypsin; VIM = vimentin.
From: Bedrossian CWM. Immunocytochemistry. Astarita RW, ed. *Practical Cytopathology.* New York: Churchill Livingstone; 1990: chap 14, 403–457. With permission.

be emphasized throughout this chapter, clinical history is essential to classify SBRCTs, an exercise facilitated by the use ancillary methods.

THYMOMA

Thymomas are relatively uncommon SBRCTs of the anterior mediastinum which may present in a nonmalignant (encapsulated) or malignant (invasive) form. Tumors that manifest invasiveness have a tendency to extend to lymph nodes, pleura, and pericardium, therefore precluding surgical extirpation. The aggressiveness of the tumor may be evidenced by its recurrence, even following apparently successful radiation therapy. Not infrequently, the first sign of recurrence is a malignant effusion into either the pericardial sac or the pleural cavities. This tumor differs from the other SBRCTs in which it commonly presents with a two-cell population. In fact, the salient cytologic feature of thymoma is a mixture of small dark lymphocyte-like cells with larger pale, epithelial-like cells (Fig. 12.1). Thymomas shed individual cells but have also a great tendency to appear in the form of small tissue fragments. These can be grossly observed as specks within a bloody effusion and are very often strikingly observed in the cell block but not in the filters or smears (Fig. 12.2). The groups of

cells are rather compact, composed of mature lymphocytes intermixed with paler, larger epithelial cells. The cytologic appearance of thymoma is an exact recapitulation of the pattern noted in tissue biopsies of the neoplasm. In mediastinoscopical biopsies thymomas show frequent necrosis so that cytomorphology is best appreciated in imprints.

The lymphocyte-like cells of thymoma typically display dark hyperchromatic nuclei and resemble mature lymphocytes. Occasional transformed elements are also identified. Nuclei of epithelial-like cells are large, round to oval or irregular, with finely dispersed chromatin and several small nucleoli. Occasionally the epithelial cells are degenerated, in which case they may appear hypervacuolated. No secretory material can be demonstrated in these cells, however. In very rare examples, the epithelial cells may have squamoid features manifested by greater pleomorphism and elongation of their nuclei. Not infrequently, the epithelial element is immature and requires immunocytochemistry for its demonstration (Fig. 12.3). Most difficult to recognize are thymomas in which the epithelial cells either regress or fail to invade the serosal cavity. In these cases, a lymphocytosis or a lymphoma is suspected and the tumors require ancillary methods for their recognition. No other neoplasm accompanied by mediastinal involvement presents with biphasic pattern of malignant cells in effusion specimens. Consequently, in classic cases the diag-

TABLE 12.2 Differential Diagnosis of Small Cell Tumors

Tumor Type	Cytopathology	Electron Microscopy	Immunocytochemistry
Thymoma	Mixture of dark lymphocyte-like cells and large, epithelial-like elements	Intercellular junctions and intermediate filaments in epithelial cells	Keratin, EMA, LCA, T cell markers, T6, Leu 11
Wilms' tumor	Biphasic cell pattern, large, pale cells, small spindle cells, primitive tubules	Tubular lumina, basal lamina, frequent cell junctions, projecting microvilli	Vimentin Keratin/EMA
Neuroblastoma	Loose, small clusters, pseudorosettes, fibrillary background	True neuritic processes, microtubules, neurofilaments, small NE granules, common cell junction	NSE S-100 GFAP NF
Ewing's tumor	Small cell groups, uniform single cells, clear spaces in cytoplasm, PAS + PASD −	Abundant glycogen, occasional cell junctions, heterochromatinic nuclei	Vimentin PAS, NSE Keratin/Leu7
Rhabdomyosarcoma	Pleomorphic small cells, punctate glycogen, multinucleated cells,	Thick & thin filaments, single-file ribosomes, Z-band material, myofilaments, rare cell junctions, Z-protein	Vimentin HHF-35 Desmin Myoglobin Creatine kinase
Lymphoma/Leukemia	Discohesive cells, lymphoglandular bodies, irregular nuclei, no cell junctions, lipid droplets	Peripheral chromatin, nuclear protrusions, paucity of organelles markers	LCA (T200) vimentin B-cell, T-cell markers
Neuroendocrine carcinoma	Small cell groups with nuclear molding	Small number of neuroendocrine (NE) granules, mainly in cytoplasmic extensions	NSE, synaptophysin
Carcinoid tumor	Greater amount of cytoplasm than NE carcinoma	Widely distributed numerous NE granules in cytoplasm	NSE, chromogranin
Merkel cell neoplasm	Small cells with eccentrically-placed nuclei	Tufts of intermediate filaments push the nucleus aside	NSE, Keratin, N-F

Modified from: Bedrossian CWM. Small blue round cell tumors. In: Proceedings of WHO Training Course on the Application of Electron Microscopy in Biomedical Research and Diagnosis of Human Diseases, Beijing, 1990. WHO. With permission.

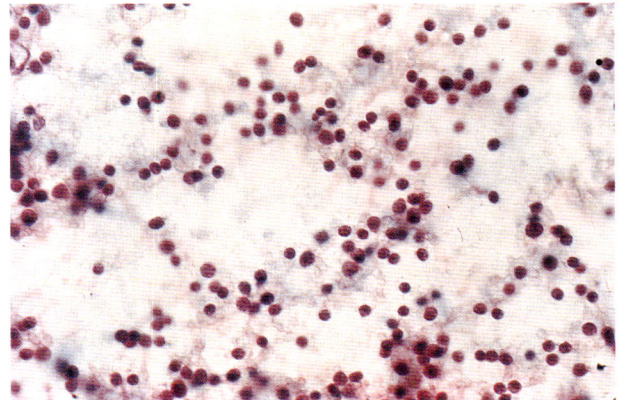

FIGURE 12.1 Thymoma in pericardial fluid. Note the small dark blue cells intermixed with occasional paler, epithelial-like elements. (Pap × 40)

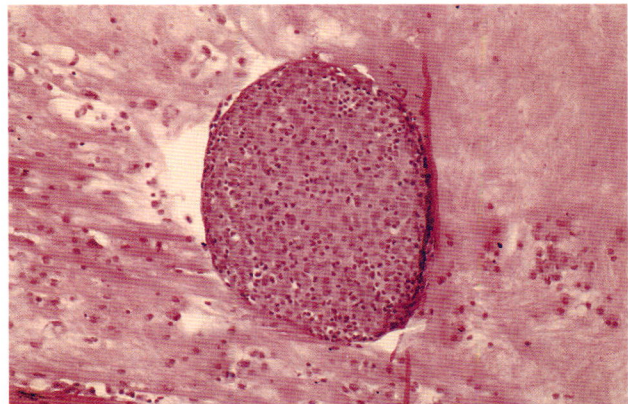

FIGURE 12.2 Cell block from a thymoma. A rounded tissue fragment clearly shows the mixture of lymphocyte-like and epithelial-like cells. (H&E × 120)

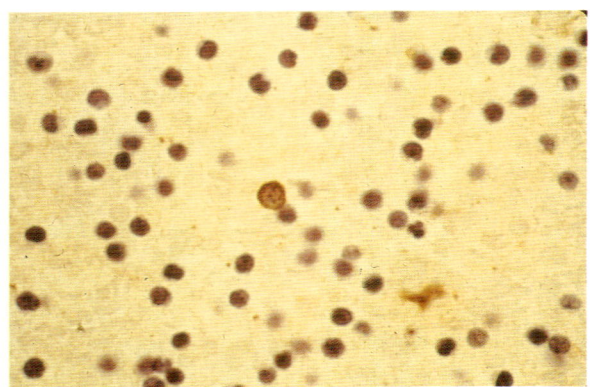

FIGURE 12.3   Keratin stain of thymoma. The large, pale cells are positive for this marker of epithelial differentiation. Note the negative lymphocytes and RBCs in the background. (P.A.P. × 90)

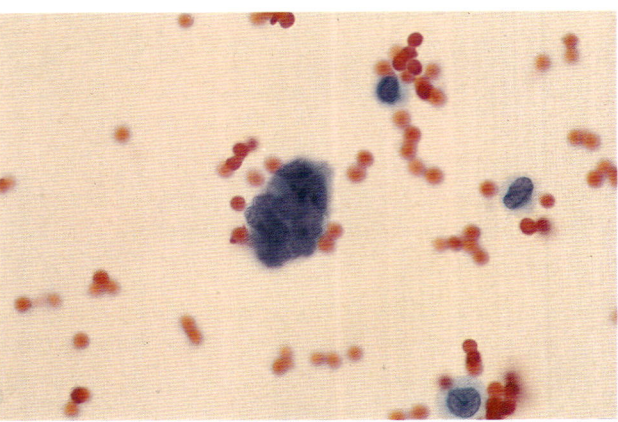

FIGURE 12.4   Wilms' tumor in peritoneal fluid. The groups of small blue, round cells contrasts with the mesothelial cells and RBCs in the background. (Pap × 120)

nosis of thymoma is readily accomplished. In doubtful cases, leukocyte common antigens, L26 or UCHL1 are sufficient to demonstrate the lymphocytic component whereas cytokeratins of broad specificity are useful in the recognition of the epithelial component. Specific markers for thymocytes such as T6 and LU11 can be used to demonstrate the lymphocytic component, but they work best in fresh cells. Ultrastructurally, one needs to demonstrate evidence of epithelial differentiation including intercellular junctions, in order to accept the diagnosis of thymoma.

WILMS' TUMOR

Wilms' tumor is a common pediatric neoplasm affecting the kidneys and the retroperitoneal space. Also known as nephroblastoma, this is a tumor with developmental overtones. Immature spindle cell elements intermixed with organoid structures characterize the primary site. Any of these components can become invasive, most often penetrating the retroperitoneal space. In disseminated metastasis malignant effusions may occur in any of the body cavities, but most frequently they appear in ascitic fluid or pleural effusions. The immature undifferentiated round and blue cells are difficult to distinguish from those of the other SBRCTs. However, Wilms' tumor lacks the prominent glycogenation typical of Ewing's sarcoma and embryonorhabdomyosarcoma. Groups of round blue cells, smaller than mesothelial

cells are typical of Wilms' tumor (Fig. 12.4). Nuclei are round to oval, with dark, evenly distributed chromatin granules. Nucleoli are inconspicuous. The tumor may form small spaces surrounding a small lumen, often empty of secretion. Occasionally, the cell population is represented by larger, pale-staining cells attempting to form tubules. The immature cells are smaller, more elongated; they are considerably more hyperchromatic, and fail to form any organoid configuration. By electron microscopy Wilms' tumors reveal frequent cell junctions in contrast to neuroblastoma and Ewing's sarcoma. Ultrastructural study of FNAs have demonstrated cells surrounded by basal lamina and showing tubular differentiation (Fig. 12.5) not noticeable by light microscopy. Immunocytochemically, however, Wilms' tumor lacks the distinctiveness of neuroblastoma, which is NSE positive, and rhabdomyosarcoma, which is commonly positive for desmin and myoglobin. Wilms' tumors are only positive for vimentin but may even fail to express this marker, an indication of their primitive nature.

NEUROBLASTOMA

Neuroblastoma is a frequent neoplasm occurring in the suprarenal portion of the kidney of infants. The tumor may also occur in dispersed neuroendocrine cells both in the retroperitoneum and in distant sites. The neoplasm may appear in adults in rare instances, but no example accompanied by malignant effusion has been

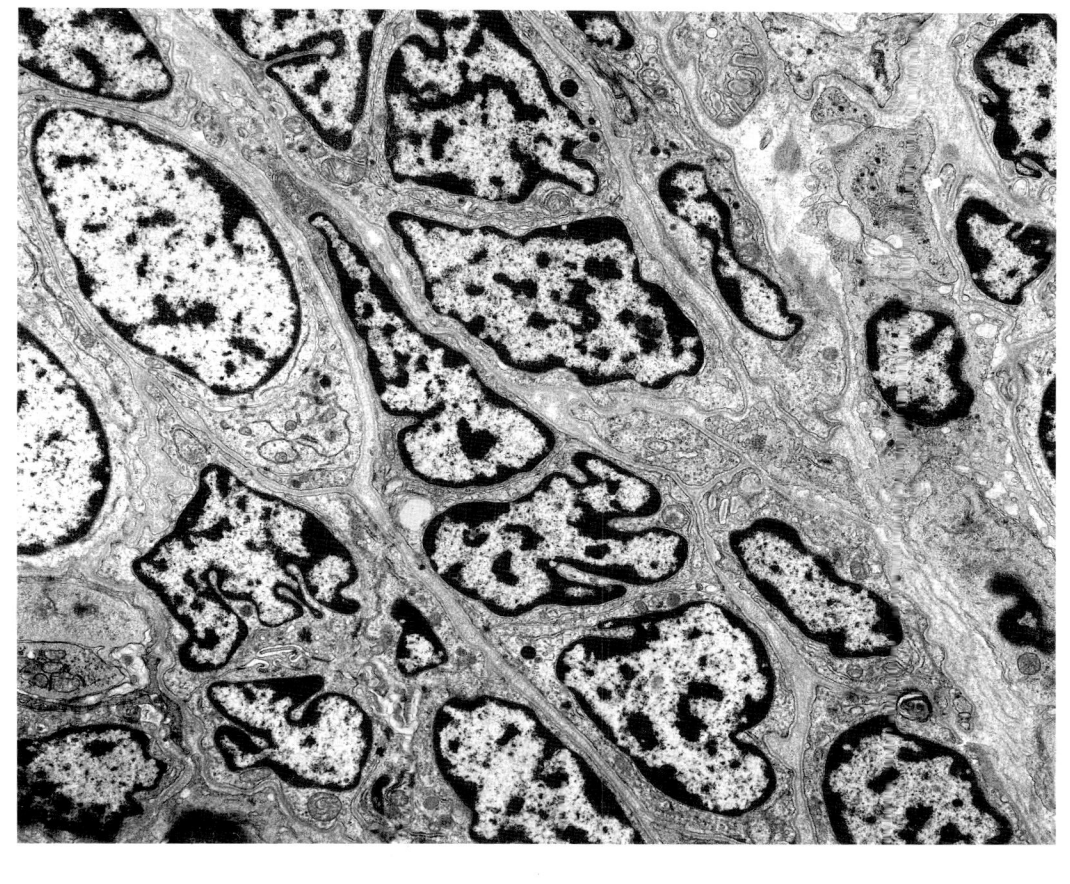

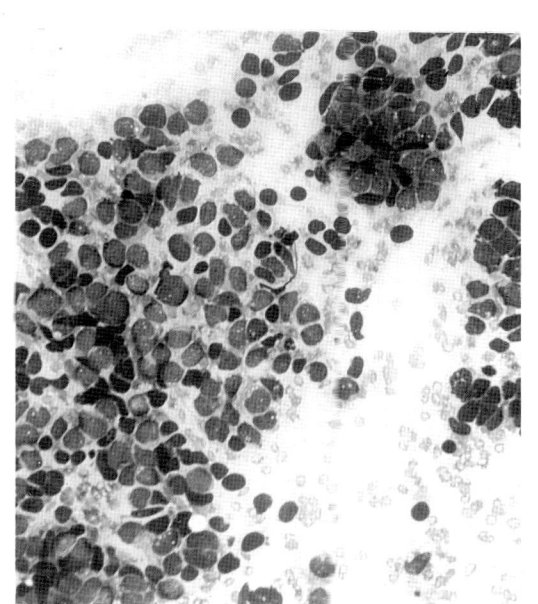

FIGURE 12.5 Wilms' tumor. **Top, left:** Neoplasm composed of tightly packed small blue cells. (H&E × 150) **Bottom, left:** Cytologically, cells of SBRCS appear mostly isolated. (D-Q × 200) **Right:** By EM the tumor shows packed cells surrounded by basal lamina. (EM × 5,000) (Courtesy of M. Akhtar, MD)

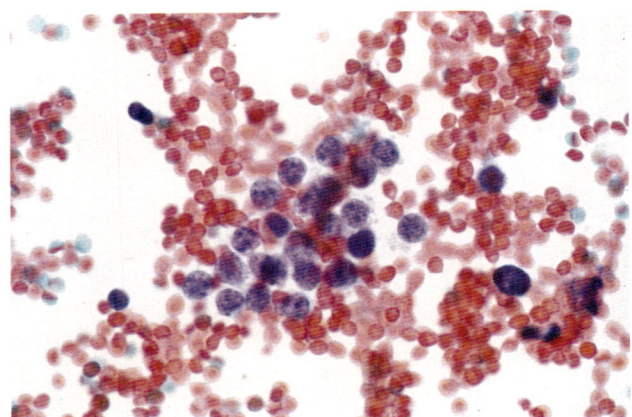

FIGURE 12.6 Well-preserved preparation of neuro-blastoma demonstrating clearly the nuclear features. Dark, evenly distributed chromatin in the absence of nucleoli is a hallmark of neuroendocrine neoplasms. (Pap × 120)

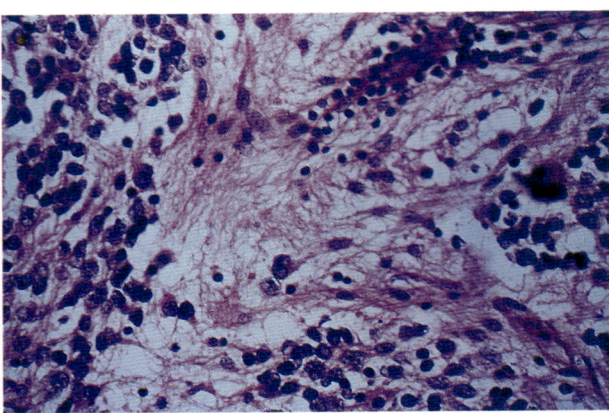

FIGURE 12.8 Resected specimen. In histologic sections, the nature of the neuropile is well demonstrated, in the form of pinkish fibrillary material separating the tumor into nests of small blue cells. (H&E × 120)

described to date. Aspirated specimens have shown rudimentary rosettes, but in effusions the cells most often are either totally dispersed or aggregated in small groups of cells (Fig. 12.6). As with other neuroendocrine tumors, the nuclear:cytoplasmic ratio is extremely elevated and the chromatin distribution is even, creating a very dark, hyperchromatic appearance. Nucleoli are inconspicuous. In cell blocks the tumor cells tend to appear only as undifferentiated small aggregates, with greater resemblance to tissue specimens (Fig. 12.7). In histologic sections, the fibrillary background is typical of

neuroblastoma (Fig. 12.8). When well preserved material is obtained by fine needle aspiration the cells appear crisper than in effusions of long duration and a greater amount of cytoplasm may be appreciated (Fig. 12.9). These fresh specimens are ideally suited for electron microscopy. At the ultrastructural level, neuroblastoma lacks desmosomes and other junctional complexes. The tumor is characterized by elongated cell processes within which microtubules and the neurofilament can be identified (Fig. 12.10). The neuroendocrine granules are small and inconspicuous, never reaching the num-

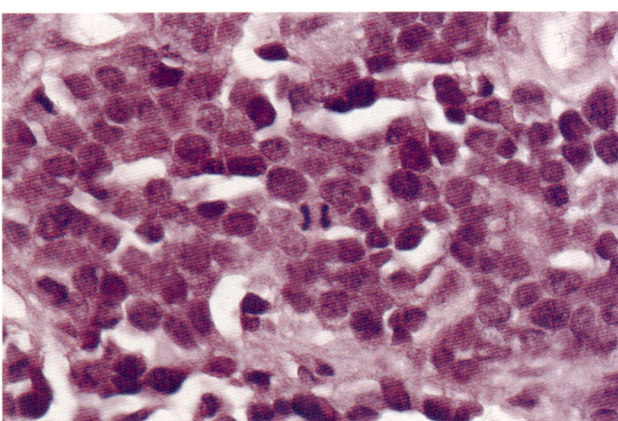

FIGURE 12.7 Cell block of neuroblastoma demonstrating a mitotic figure. Despite their apparent cohesiveness, the tumor cells fall short of forming tubules, or pseudorosettes. (H&E × 240)

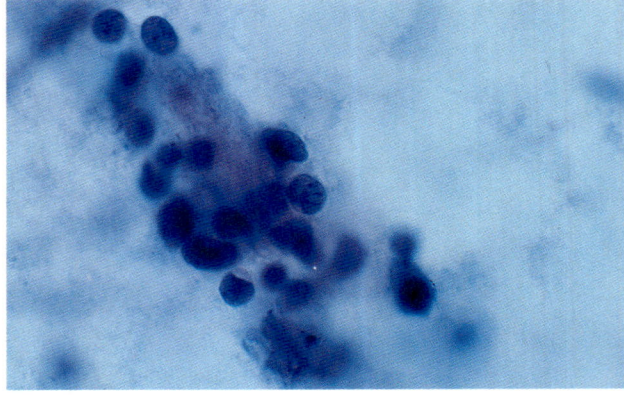

FIGURE 12.9 Neuroblastoma in a fine needle aspirate of a retroperitoneal mass. In this type of preparation the cells show more abundant cytoplasm and appear more cohesive, held together by tangles of neuropiles. (Pap × 180)

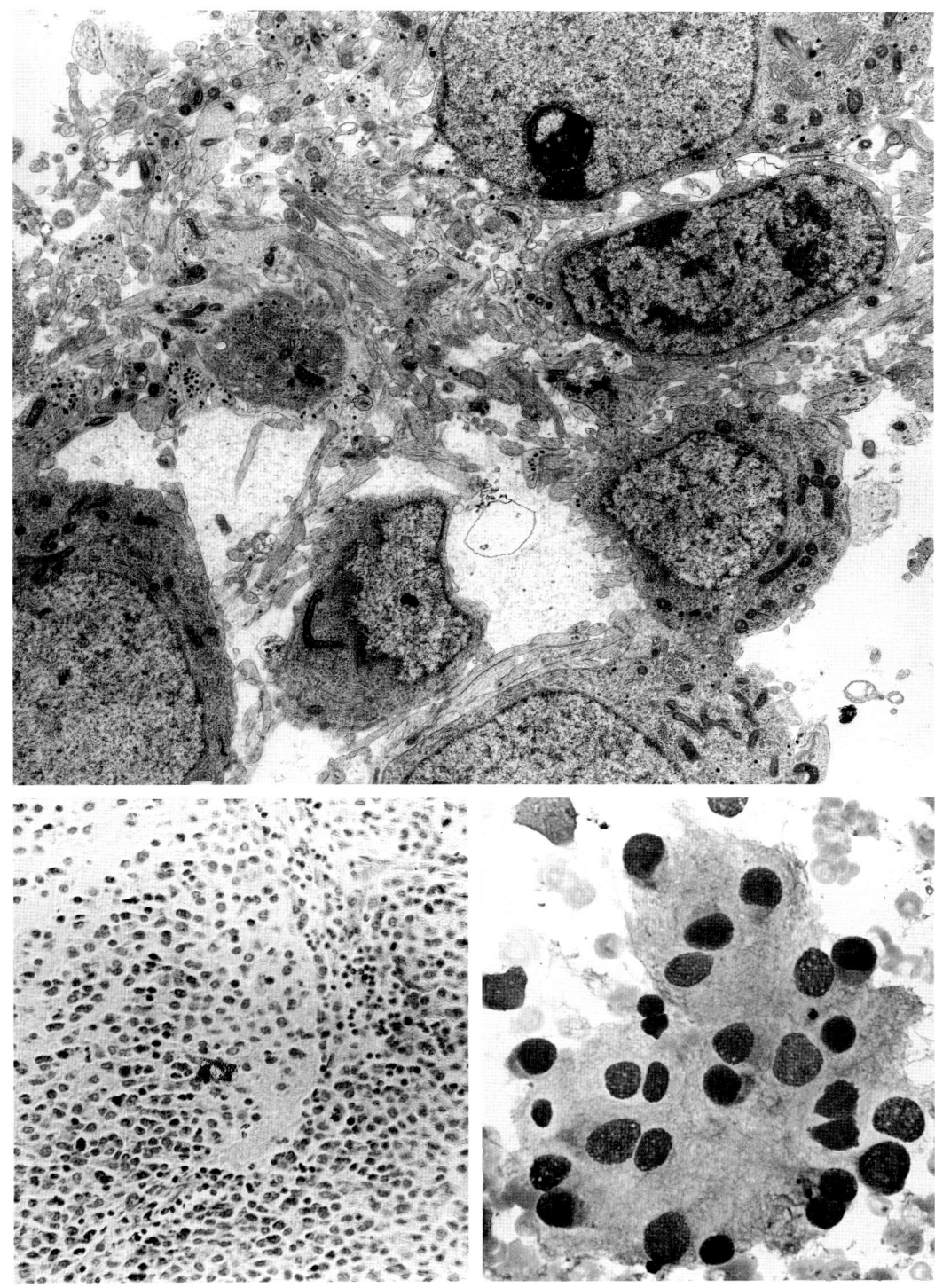

FIGURE 12.10 Neuroblastoma. **Top, left:** Neoplasm showing small cells against a fibrillary background. (H&E × 150) **Bottom, left:** Cytologic preparation stained by Diff-Quick. Notice fibrillary cytoplasm and interspersed small nuclei. (D-Q × 300) **Right:** Corresponding ultrastructure shows cytoplasmic cell processes with scattered neuroendocrine granules. (Courtesy of M. Akhtar, MD)

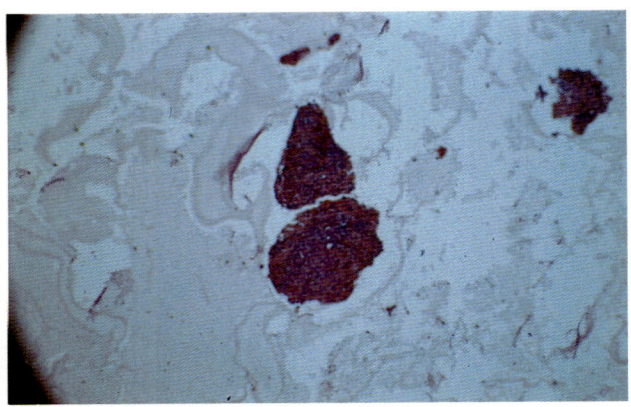

FIGURE 12.11 Neuroblastoma stained immunocytochemically for NSE. The strong positivity of the tissue fragment attests to the suitability of cell blocks for this type of examination. (P.A.P. × 90)

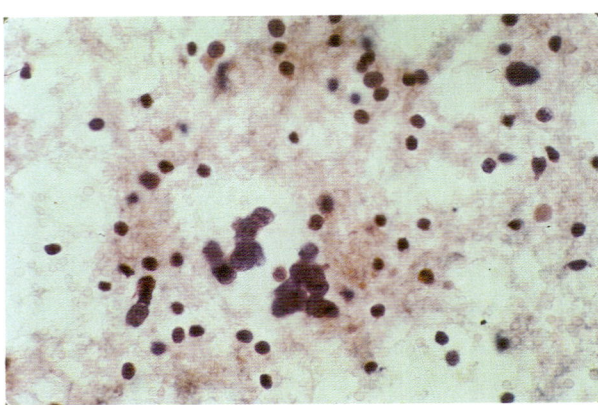

FIGURE 12.12 Ewing's sarcoma. Small, blue, round cells loosely arranged and demonstrating a high nuclear: cytoplasmic ratio. Note the small, punctate vacuoles in the cytoplasm. (Pap × 90)

bers seen in carcinoid tumors. The neoplasm is positive for NSE but negative for chromogranin and for the neuropeptide hormones (Fig. 12.11). The tumor cells may be faintly positive for neurofilament, but this marker is not easily demonstrable in cytologic material.

EWING'S SARCOMA

This primary malignant tumor of bone of unknown histogenesis is gaining notoriety since its description in the adult age group and presentation in soft tissues. The tumor is composed of uniformly round tumor cells without any evidence of differentiation. The neoplasm may invade locally and may appear in malignant effusions (Fig. 12.12). Abundant glycogen in the cytoplasm is a characteristic feature, although not totally specific for Ewing's sarcoma. It does, however, allow the identification of this tumor and its differentiation from Wilm's tumor, thymoma, and lymphoma. Controversy exists regarding the amount of glycogen in neuroblastoma, whereas rhabdomyosarcoma may present with a moderate amount of glycogen in the cytoplasm. Cytologically Ewing's sarcoma sheds cells with perfectly round or oval nuclei, as well as tumor cells with indented nuclei, a feature that can be noted even with the Pap stain. The cytoplasm is wispy, but the tumor fails to form rosettes or rudimentary tubular structures. At the ultrastructural level cytoplasmic extensions may be

identified, but they are never as elongated as a neuroblastoma, and they also lack microtubules and neurofilaments (Fig. 12.13). The tumor is positive for vimentin but negative for NSE, desmin, and myoglobin.

RHABDOMYOSARCOMA

Embryonal rhabdomyosarcoma, a SBRCT of the pediatric age group may develop in the retroperitoneum and mediastinum from where it may spread to the peritoneal and peritoneal cavities. The neoplastic cells are small, slightly elongated or may show the abundant cytoplasm without the features typical of full rhabdomyoblastic differentiation (Fig. 12.14). However, following chemotherapy the cells may develop eosinophilic cytoplasm or even cross-striations. In the embryonal variety, the cells tend to be pleomorphic, noncohesive, without pseudorosettes or any other cellular groupings (Fig. 12.15). With the MGG stain, the cytoplasm appears wispy or vacuolated, due to the presence of glycogen (Fig. 12.16). The cells are positive for vimentin and may also be positive for desmin or another myogenic marker in cytologic specimens (Fig. 12.17). Ultrastructurally, the true nature of the cytoplasm is revealed by myogenous-like bundles of thick and thin filaments. Z bands, however, are noted only in the better differentiated neoplasms (Fig. 12.18).

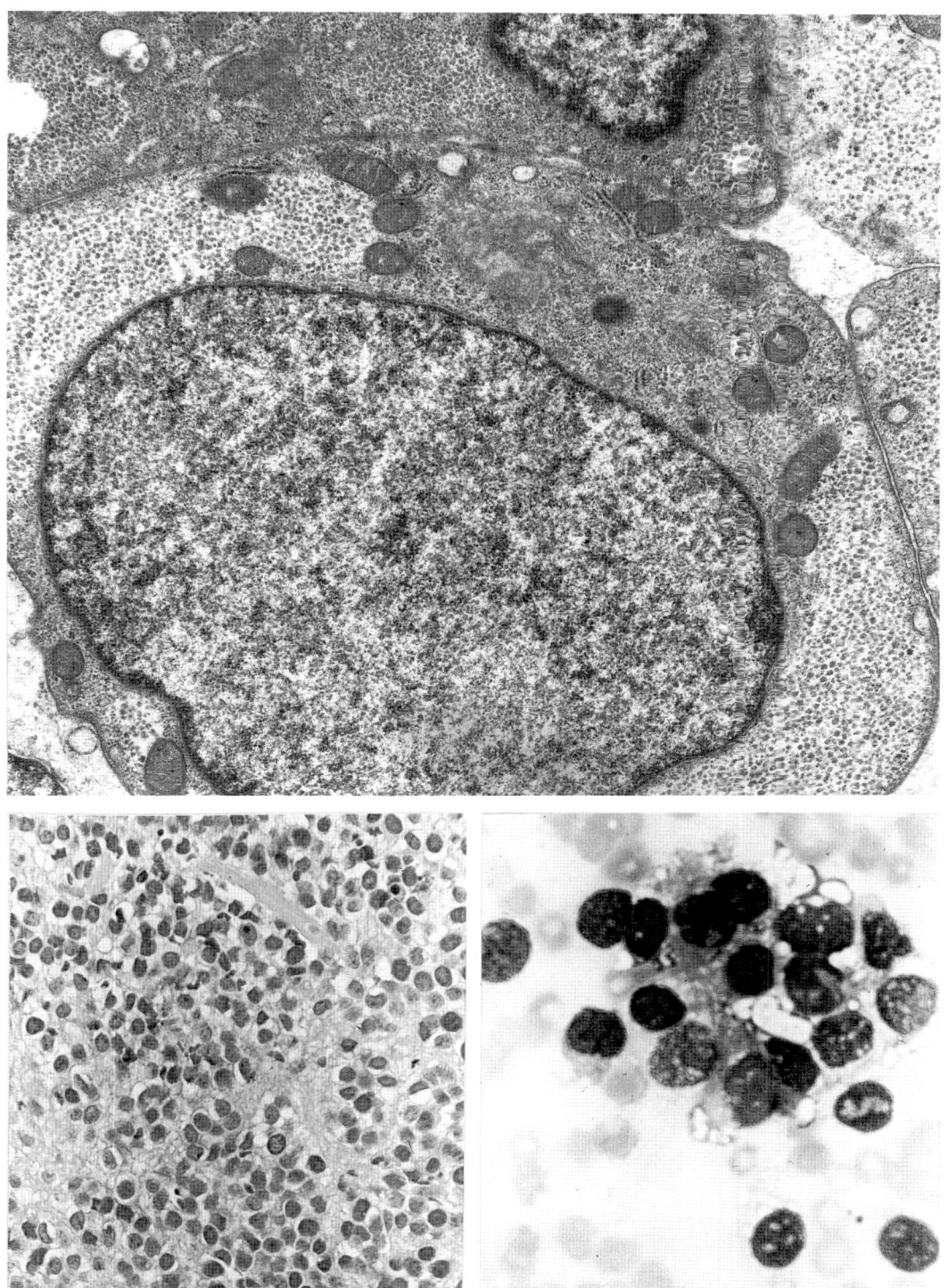

FIGURE 12.13 Ewing's sarcoma. **Top, left:** Neoplasm with delicate septa surrounding compartments filled with SBRCT cells. (H&E × 150) **Bottom, left:** Cytologically the cells display glycogen-like vacuolization of the nucleus and cytoplasm. (D-Q × 350) **Right:** By EM, notice rare mitochondria and abundant glycogen and intermediate filaments in the cytoplasm. (EM × 12,000) (Courtesy of M. Akhtar, MD)

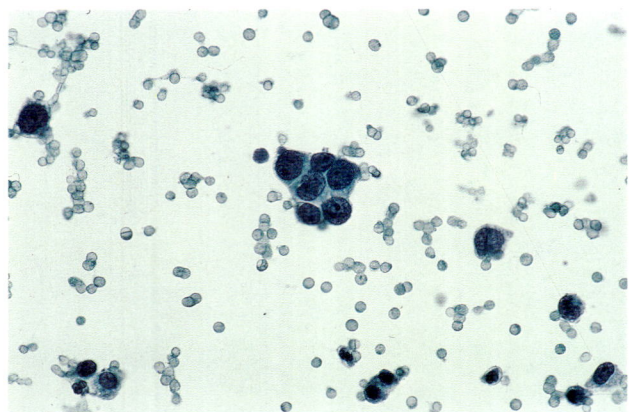

FIGURE 12.14 Papanicolaou-stained preparation of embryonal rhabdomyosarcoma. The group of tumor cells shows greater variation in the size and shape of the nuclei. Note the RBCs in the background. (Pap × 90)

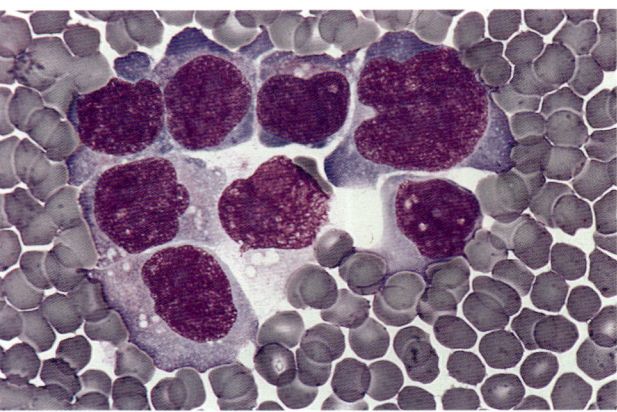

FIGURE 12.16 Vacuolization in Ewing's sarcoma. Vacuoles in the nuclei correspond to glycogen containing invaginations of the cytoplasm. (MGG × 800)

NEUROENDOCRINE CARCINOMA

Oat cell carcinoma is the prototype of this group of tumors capable of expressing neural and endocrine differentiation in the same cell. Neural capability is represented by the elaboration of neuron-specific enolase and neurofilament. Hormone production ranges from the elaboration of neuropeptides such as bombesin and synaptophysin to complete hormones such as calcitonin and antidiuretic hormone. Carcinoid tumors are considered the better differentiated members of this group of tumors, whereas oat cell carcinoma is the least differentiated. Intermediate types occur in the lung, but current evidence suggests that neuroendocrine carcinomas are more prevalent than previously believed. Examples in extrapulmonary sites have been described, including the breast, salivary gland, and prostate. A characteristic feature is that neuroendocrine carcinomas have an aggressive biologic behavior that may lead to effusions. The cytologic appearance of neuroendocrine carcinoma is characteristic, with a predominance of SBRCs. Neurendocrine differentiation in tumors composed of large cells cannot be detected cytologically.

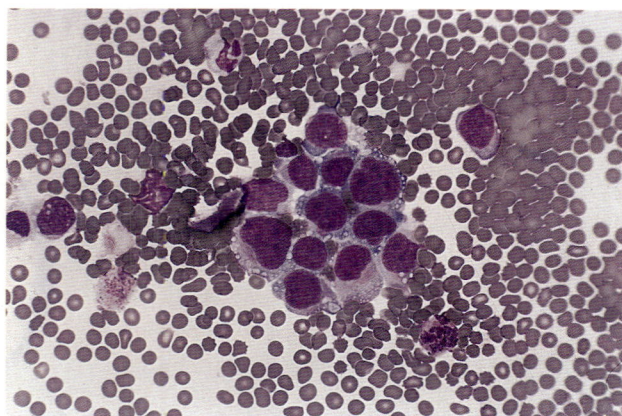

FIGURE 12.15 Ewing's sarcoma. Stained by Diff-Quik. Notice SBRCT cells arranged as a mosaic. Note absence of rosette formation and lack of nuclear detail. (Diff-Quik × 180)

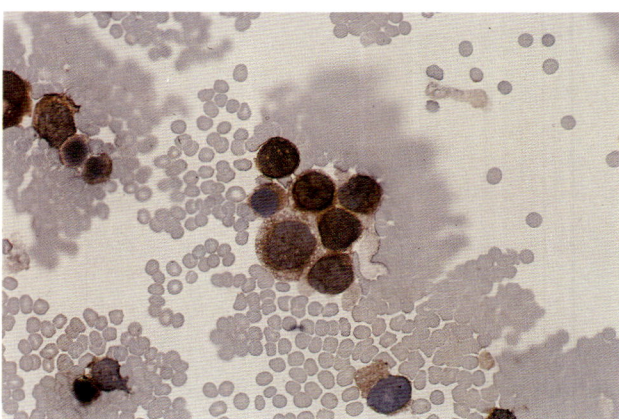

FIGURE 12.17 Desmin reactivity in embryonal rhabdomyosarcoma. Positivity is stronger in intact, more viable cells than in those with raggedy cytoplasm. (P.A.P. × 120) (Figs. 12.14 through 12.17, courtesy of L. Ellwood, MD)

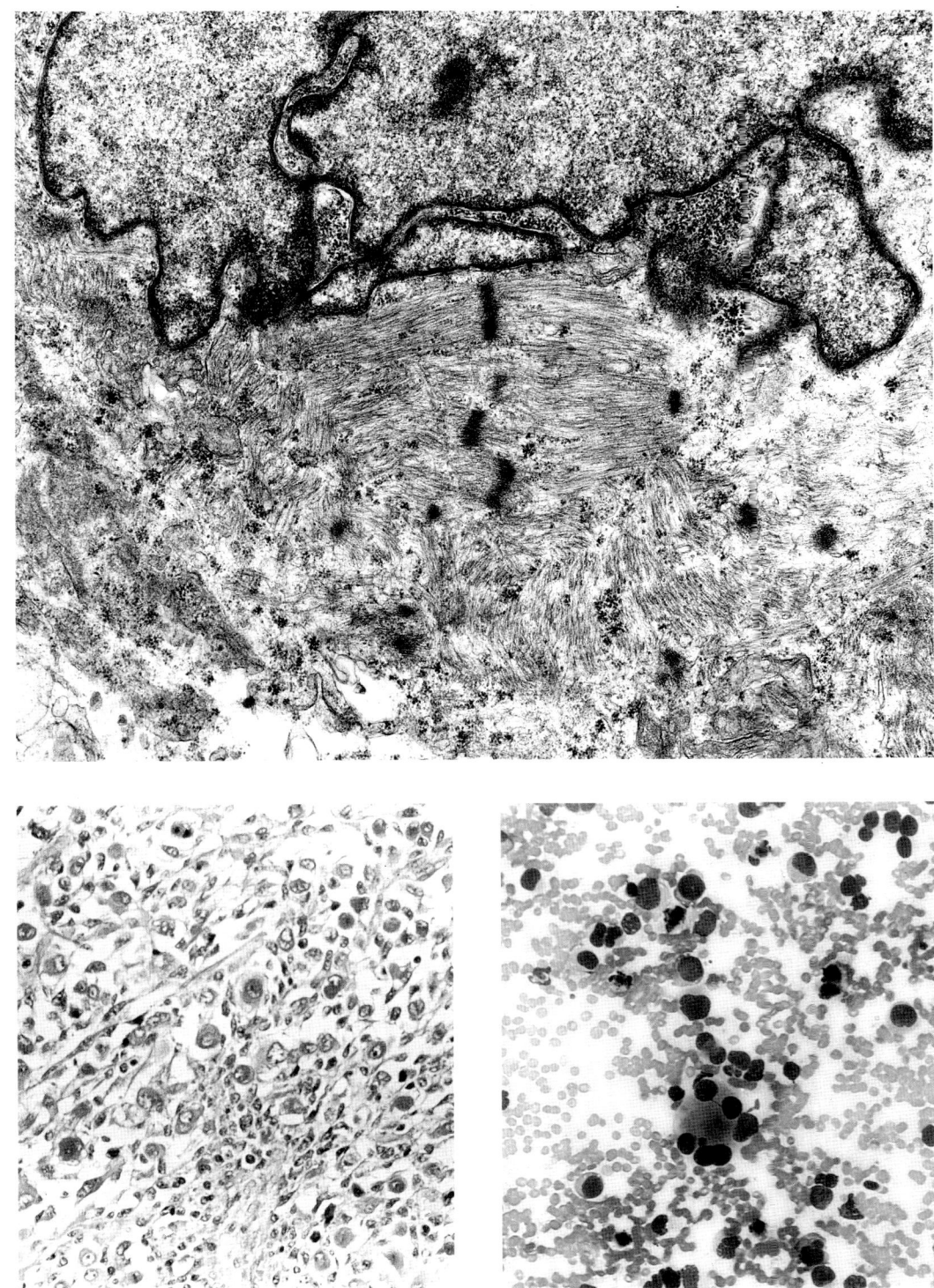

FIGURE 12.18 Embryonal rhabdomyosarcoma. **Top, left:** The neoplasm show a mixture of SBRCT cells, and larger cells with more abundant cytoplasm. (H&E × 150) **Bottom, left:** Diff-Quick stained cells show small, round to oval nuclei. (D-Q × 150) **Right:** By EM the cytoplasm shows a mixture of thick and thin filaments. Also note Z bands near the center. (EM × 12,000) (Courtesy of M. Akhtar, MD)

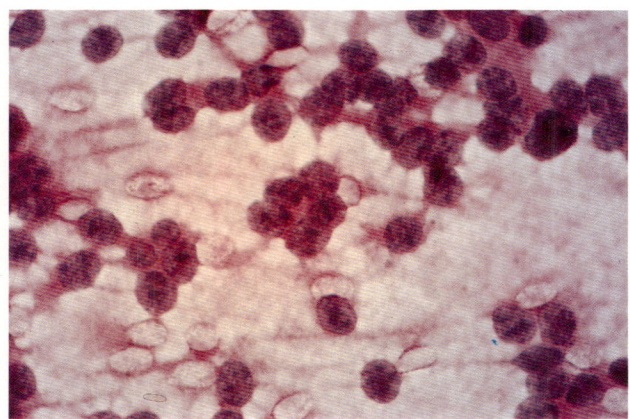

FIGURE 12.19 Carcinoid tumor metastatic to the liver and the peritoneal cavity. The cells are small, with eccentric nuclei pushed aside by pinkish, homogeneous cytoplasm. (H&E × 240)

Despite their common name, "small cell" carcinomas actually shed cells that are larger than lymphocytes. The nuclear diameter is approximately one-and-a-half times that of a small lymphocyte, but the negligible amount of cytoplasm makes the entire cell about the same size of a large lymphocyte. The nucleus of neuroendocrine carcinoma cells is characteristically dark and hyperchromatic, with evenly distributed chromatin granules and no nucleoli in the majority of the cells. In B5-fixed preparations the cells display a tendency toward molding, with small groups forming irregular clusters having no microacinar or papillary formations. Cells of small cell carcinoma shed differently in effusions when compared with lung specimens. In the liquid medium of serous effusions they appear as small onion-like groups of cells showing molding of their nuclei. Occasionally, chance arrangements may mimic the rouleaux phenomenon but at times the cells appear as discrete elements resembling the distribution of cells in lymphoma.

The cells of intermediate size neuroendocrine carcinoma are slightly larger, with appreciable cytoplasm and similar nuclear characteristics, except that a few more cells display nucleoli. They can be distinguished from lymphoma because of their slightly more elongated shape and the absence of the prominent nucleoli present in lymphoma. Neuroendocrine carcinomas can be identified by markers that demonstrate various aspects of the differentiation process: (1) enzymes important in the neuroendocrine secretory chain, such as alpha and gamma neuron-specific enolase; (2) proteins which constitute the supporting matrix of the secretory granules, such as chromogranin; and (3) the secretory product itself, such as synaptophysin, bombesin, or any of the polypeptide hormones. NSE is the most ubiquitously expressed, being very common in oat cell carcinoma, intermediate neuroendocrine carcinoma, and carcinoid tumors. Chromogranin is almost always negative in oat cell carcinoma but is commonly positive in carcinoid tumors. The secretion products and the hormones are variably positive in a wide range of neuroendocrine tumors.

CARCINOID TUMOR

The carcinoid tumors have a distinctive histologic appearance in the form of vascularized compartmentalization and no tendency toward necrosis or crushing artifact as demonstrated by oat cell carcinoma. However, carcinoid cells share the neuroendocrine property of oat cells and also their cytoplasmic fragility and nuclear characteristics. Even though the cytoplasm is abundant in well-fixed material, it is commonly lost during smear preparation (Fig. 12.19). Stripped nuclei resemble those of the intermediate type of neuroendocrine carcinoma, both in size and in the tendency to display nucleoli. Because the carcinoids that cause effusion are aggressive in their behavior, the cells may appear elongated and are slightly more pleomorphic than typical carcinoids. Nucleoli may be more prominent, but the "neuroendocrine" character of the chromatin is still noted in carcinoid tumors. These tumors are strongly positive for NSE and may also be positive for chromogranin, serotonin and other hormonelike substances. By electron microscopy the granules are larger and more pleomorphic than in oat cell carcinoma. They are also extremely more abundant and more evenly distributed throughout the cytoplasm than in oat cell carcinoma.

MERKEL CELL NEOPLASM

This uncommon neuroendocrine tumor of the skin may disseminate widely and present as a malignant effusion. However, without clinical knowledge of the primary site, it is often impossible to arrive at a specific diagnosis. The tumor cells resemble those of other neuroendocrine carcinomas. Occasionally, the cytoplasm may display a dot-like dense inclusion next to the nucleus, composed of intermediate filaments at the ultrastructural level. However, without immunocytochemistry it is not possible to ascertain the exact nature of the substance making up the inclusion.

BIBLIOGRAPHY

Thymoma

Venegas RJ, Sun NCJ. Cardiac tamponade as a presentation of malignant thymoma. *Acta Cytol.* 1988 32:257–262.

Zirkin HJ. Pleural fluid cytology in invasive thymoma. *Acta Cytol.* 1985;29:1011–1014.

Wilms' Tumor

Hajdu SI. Exfoliative cytology of primary and metastatic Wilms' tumor. *Acta Cytol.* 1971;15:339–342.

Drut R. Neuron-specific enolase positive rosettes in nephroblastoma. *Diagn Cytopathol.* 1987;3:74–76.

Neuroblastoma

Jobst S, Ljung B, Gilkey F, et al. Cytologic diagnosis of olfactory neuroblastoma. *Acta Cytol.* 1983;27:299–305.

Akhtar M, Ali MA, Sackey K, et al. Aspiration cytology of neuroblastoma: Light and electron microscopy with TEM and SEM correlations. *Diagn Cytopathol.* 1988;4:323–327.

Ewing's Sarcoma

Akhtar M, Ali MA, Sabbah R. Aspiration cytology of Ewing's sarcoma light and electron microscopy correlations. *Cancer* 1985;56:2051–2060.

Geisinger KR, Hajdu SI, Helson L. Exfoliative cytology of non-lympho-reticular neoplasms in children. *Acta Cytol.* 1984;28:16–28.

Akhtar M, Bedrossian CWM, Ali MA, et al. FNA-biopsy of pediatric neoplasms: correlation between EM and ICC in diagnosis and classification. *Diagn Cytopathol* 1992;258–265.

Rhabdomyosarcoma

Hajdu SI, Koss LG. Cytologic diagnosis of metastatic myosarcomas. *Acta Cytol.* 1969;13:545–551.

Seidal T, Walaas L, Kindblom LG, et al. Cytology of em-

bryonal rhabdomyosarcoma. *Diagn Cytopathol.* 1988;4:292–299.

Oat Cell Carcinoma

Banner BF, Warren WF, Gould VE. Cytomorphology and marker expressions of malignant neuroendocrine cells in pleural effusions. *Acta Cytol.* 1986;30:99–104.

Salhadin A, Nasiell M, Nasiell K, et al. The unique cytologic picture of oat cell carcinoma in effusion. *Acta Cytol.* 1976;20:298–302.

Spriggs A, Boddington MM. Oat-cell bronchial carcinoma: Identification of cells in pleural fluid. *Acta Cytol.* 1976;20:525–529.

Yam LT, Winkler CP. Immunocytochemical diagnosis of oat cell carcinoma in pleural effusion. *Acta Cytol.* 1984; 28:425–429.

Carcinoid Tumor

Khorsand J, Katz FL, Savaraj N. Malignant carcinoid of the pancreas: A cytologic, ultrastructural and immunocytochemical study of a case diagnosed by FNA of supraclavicular node metastasis. *Diagn Cytopathol.* 1987;3:222–227.

Gephardt GN, Belovich DM. Cytology of pulmonary carcinoid tumors. *Acta Cytol.* 1982;26:433–438.

Pheochromocytoma

Traub YM, Rosenfeld JB. Malignant pheochromocytoma with pleural metastasis of unusually long duration. *Chest.* 1970;58:546–550.

Koss LG, Zajicek J. Aspiration biopsy requiring image-guidance. In: Koss LG (ed) Diagnostic cytology and its histopathologic basis, 4th ed. Philadelphia: JB Lippincott; 1992:1336–1402.

Other Neuroendocrine Tumors

Watson C, Freidman K Cytology of metastatic neuroendocrine (Merkel-cell) carcinoma in pleural fluid. *Acta Cytol.* 1985;29:397–402.

Domagala W, Lubinski J, Lasota J, et al. Neuroendocrine (Merkel-cell) skin carcinoma: Cytology, intermediate filament typing, and ultrastructure of tumor cells in FNA. *Acta Cytol.* 1987;31:267–275

Hagood P, Johnson F, Bedrossian CWM. Small cell carcinoma of the prostate: a case report with evaluation of tumor markers. *Cancer* 1991;69:1046–1050.

CHAPTER THIRTEEN

In Search of the Primary Site

When considering the primary site of a metastatic malignancy, three factors are crucial: (1) the type of cell present in the effusion, (2) the location of the effusion in relation to the age and sex of the patient, and (3) the presence and nature of a tumor in a possible primary site. If these three pieces of information are available, diagnosis of the primary site often falls into place without the need of sophisticated techniques. If any of these three crucial pieces of information are missing, the puzzle may be resolved by astute interpretation of cytologic detail and use of ancillary methods, especially immunocytochemistry and electron microscopy (EM).

The two major cell types most frequently found in effusions are (1) secretory or glandular cells, which indicate adenocarcinomas, and (2) nonsecretory cells, which, depending on their size and shape, may indicate a variety of neoplasms. The former far outnumber the latter. However, adenocarcinoma cells are difficult to distinguish from reactive mesothelial cells, which creates a more basic dilemma: is there a malignant effusion at all? In addition, simply arriving at a diagnosis of adenocarcinoma has little meaning in the absence of a known primary site. Even though statistics considerably narrow the diagnostic possibilities, the source of the neoplasm is often hard to discern by routine cytology alone. For nonsecretory cells, the possibilities are even more numerous; it is difficult to determine if the primary tumor is a sarcoma or a carcinoma—for instance, when the neoplastic elements are "small round blue cells" or fall into the anaplastic category. We follow a systematic approach in evaluating a malignant effusion of cryptic origin, underpinned by establishing categories of malignant cells, based on their cytologic appearance.

PINPOINTING THE ORIGIN OF MALIGNANT CELLS

As is clear from previous chapters, tumors originating in various primary sites may bear a striking resemblance to each other. The challenge, when a clinical history is available, is to ascertain whether the cytologic appearance of the effusion corresponds with the known primary source of the neoplasm. This task is relatively simple if one is familiar with the nuances of the cytologic appearances exhibited by the various primary neoplasms; the spectrum of these appearances has been described for each body site. Much more difficult, however, is to interpret cytologic data when the clinical history provides no clue to the primary origin of the neoplasm. This task is problematic because it is often fraught with subjectivity, but a sensible approach may make it considerably more reasonable. Our approach is to consider the differential diagnosis based on the predominant cytologic feature displayed by the malignant cells. The first important decision is to place the tumor cells in one of the several major categories based on size and shape of the cells, and, secondarily, on texture and contents of the cytoplasm (Table 13.1). These features are quite characteristic, and, when matched to the age and sex of the patient, they may direct attention to certain possible primary sites that can then be investigated more thoroughly. Table 13.1 is not a histogenetic classification related to the cell of origin of various types of malignant tumors; rather, it is a system used to group cells that share certain common features, or "look alike," in the terminology popularized by Bibbo.

ISOLATED CELLS

Noncohesive malignant cells may be difficult to distinguish from mesothelial cells, particularly when they present as a single cell population in the absence of the latter. This phenomenon often occurs in carcinomas of the breast, stomach, kidney, and prostate (Fig. 13.1). However, the same pattern may be present in less common tumors from other primary sites (Table 13.2). It is

TABLE 13.1   Categorization of Neoplasms According to Their Predominant Cytologic Features

Predominantly noncohesive cells
    Large single cells
    Small single cells
    Signet ring cells
    Pigmented cells
    Pleomorphic large cells
    Multinucleated giant cells
Predominantly cohesive cells
    Cell balls
    Nonvacuolated cell clusters
    Vacuolated cell clusters
    Papillary formations
    Tall columnar fronds
    Indian file arrangement
    Free-floating acini

TABLE 13.2   Differential Diagnosis of Effusions Composed of Large, Noncohesive Tumor Cells

Breast carcinoma
Gastric carcinoma
Renal-cell carcinoma
Prostatic carcinoma
Hepatocellular carcinoma
Malignant melanoma
Ovarian carcinoma
Large-cell carcinoma of lung
Squamous-cell carcinoma of lung
Round-cell sarcoma
Multiple myeloma
Malignant mesothelioma
Reactive mesothelial cells
Extraneous hepatocytes

important to recognize features in these cells that are not displayed by mesothelial cells in order to recognize them as an alien, malignant population. Age, sex, and symptoms are very helpful when considering a malignant origin for these cells. The distinction between alien and native cell populations is aided by ancillary procedures, including special stains and immunocytochemistry (Fig. 13.2). Rare mesothelial cells staining positively for keratin may serve as a striking contrast to keratin-negative tumor cells (Fig. 13.3). Strong positivity for neutral mucins favors a gastrointestinal origin. Strong positivity for CEA rules out a mesothelial origin for the

malignant cell (Fig. 13.4). Breast and prostate tumors can be detected using immunocytochemical markers: lactalbumin and estrogen receptors, and prostate-specific antigens and prostatic acid phosphatase, respectively. Noncohesive cells may also be present as isolated single elements that stand out from mesothelial cells in the background (Fig. 13.5). At times a few dominant malignant cells stand out from a field of numerous malignant cells but it should not become the object of undue attention (Fig. 13.6). Hepatocellular and renal-cell carcinomas display isolated malignant cells, which tend to be larger than mesothelial cells. Malignant cells in both types of tumor lack mucin-type vacuoles; they

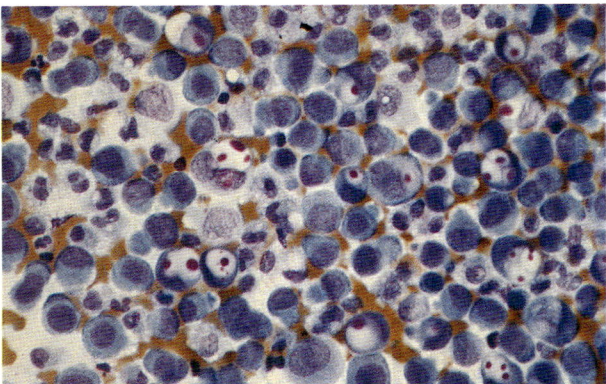

FIGURE 13.1   Isolated malignant cells from a breast adenocarcinoma. Note the intracytoplasmic lumen formation and the inspissated secretion pushing the nuclei aside. (DQ × 90)

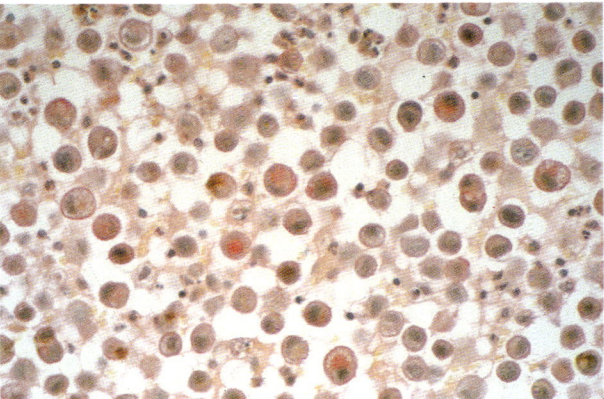

FIGURE 13.2   Same cell population as in Figure 13.1 stained with mucicarmine. Many of the cells are positive for mucin, which is in keeping with the adenocarcinomatous origin of the neoplasm. (Mucicarmine × 90)

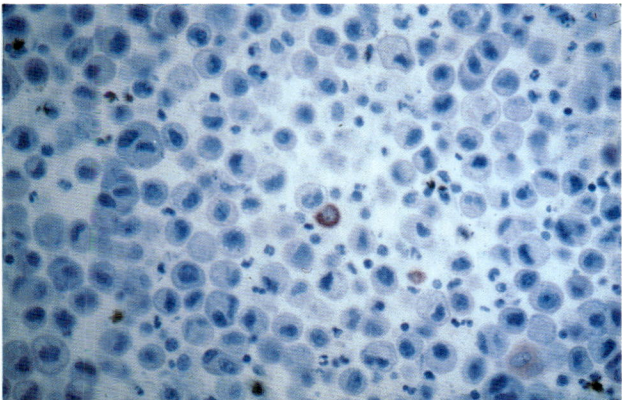

FIGURE 13.3 Single cell population of malignant cells staining negatively for keratin. Only a solitary mesothelial cell in the center is positive for this marker. (P.A.P. × 90)

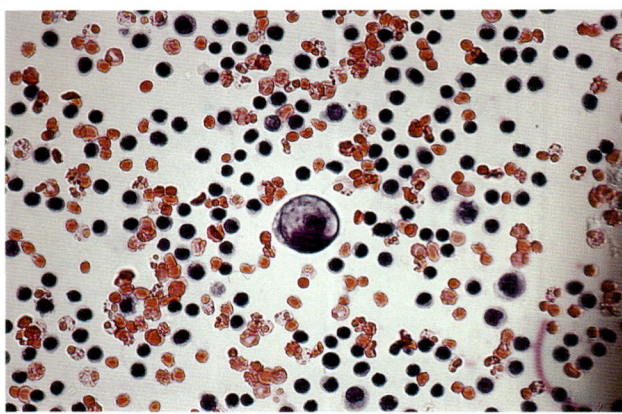

FIGURE 13.5 Single malignant cell many times larger than the benign mesothelial and inflammatory cells in the background. The primary neoplasm was a carcinoma of the lung. (Pap × 100)

present with either a flocculent or a granular-textured cytoplasm (Fig. 13.7). These cytoplasmic features are so dissimilar to mesothelial cells that they allow their identification as malignant cells. Squamous cell carcinoma also sheds single cells in malignant effusions with cytoplasmic features nowhere resembling mesothelial cells (Fig 13.8). Small, noncohesive cells are characteristic of a number of neoplasms that are predominantly of nonepithelial origin. They fall in the general category of small blue round-cell tumors (Table 13.3). These neoplasms are reviewed in Chapter 12.

PIGMENTED CELLS

Pigmented cells represent a unique presentation of noncohesive cells in effusions. Malignant melanoma is the obvious condition to be considered when entertaining the differential diagnoses of malignant pigmented cells. Not uncommonly, melanoma present with multinucleated cells displaying faint pigmentation (Fig. 13.9). The cells, however, may be predominantly nonpigmented; a diligent search is therefore needed to disclose the mel-

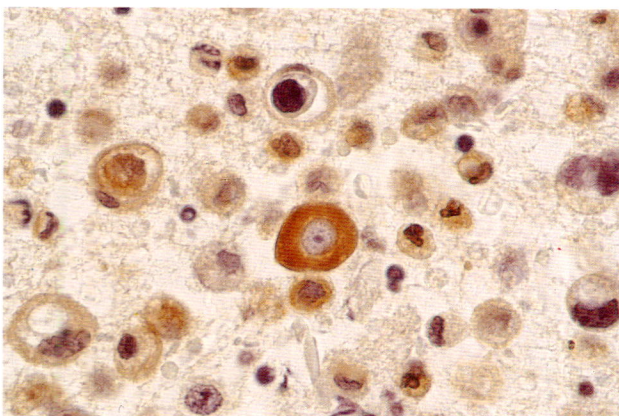

FIGURE 13.4 Adenocarcinoma stained for CEA. Not all cells are positive for this marker, including some with the signet ring appearance. (Pap × 100)

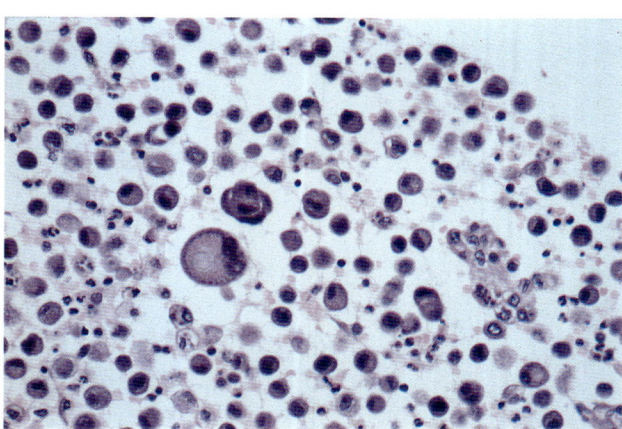

FIGURE 13.6 Single cell population where all elements are malignant cells derived from breast carcinoma. The cell block shows two dominant single cells several times larger than their neighbors. (H&E × 100)

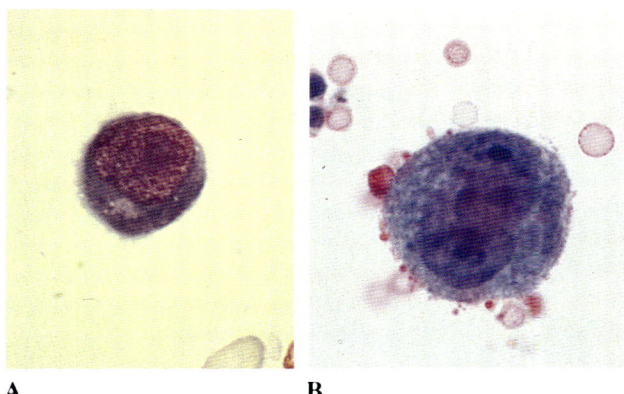

A   **B**

FIGURE 13.7   Peritoneal fluid in an hepatocellular carcinoma. (A) Note the large, centrally placed nucleolus and absence of secretion in the cytoplasm of the single cell. (MGG × 120) (B) Binucleated, isolated malignant cell. Despite the foaminess of the cytoplasm, no large vacuole is identified. (Pap × 120)

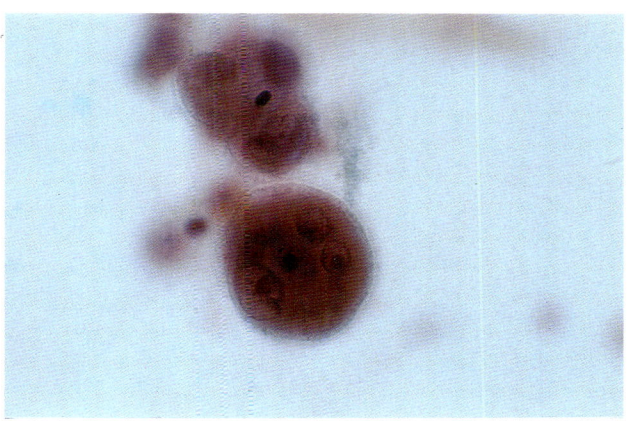

FIGURE 13.9   Pigmented cell from malignant melanoma. Notice dusky pigmentation and prominent nucleoli. (Pap × 240)

anomatous nature of the process. Clues to this diagnosis include a dusky, finely textured cytoplasm that sometimes displays discrete vacuoles. Special care should be exercised not to interpret hemosiderin-laden macrophages as originating from melanoma (Fig. 13-10). Melanoma cells are often binucleate, with mirror-image nuclei and prominent nucleoli, a feature reminiscent of Hodgkin's disease. However, Hodgkin's disease can be easily ruled out by the lack of other distinguishing features, such as the polymorphous lymphocytic popula-

TABLE 13.3   Differential Diagnosis of Effusions Composed of Small, Noncohesive Cells
Lymphoma
Leukemia
Plasmacytoma
Ewing's sarcoma
Rhabdomyosarcoma
Neuroblastoma
Melanoma
Small-cell osteosarcoma

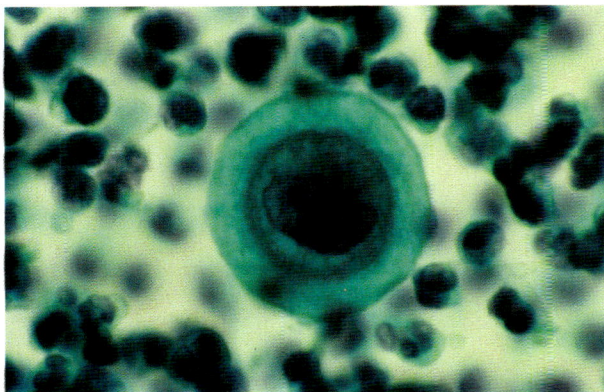

FIGURE 13.8   Not all large, non-cohesive malignant cells represent adenocarcinomas. This single cell derived from a squamous-cell carcinoma of the lung displays a rather dense cytoplasm, which indicates keratinization. (Pap × 240)

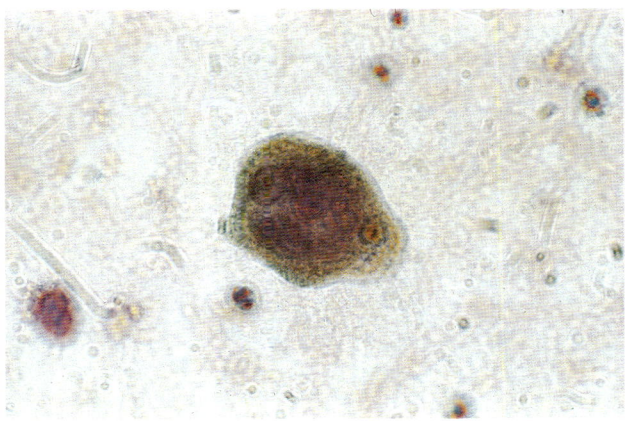

FIGURE 13.10   Hemosiderin-laden macrophage from long-standing bloody effusion. The faint brown pigment should not be confused with melanin. (Pap × 240)

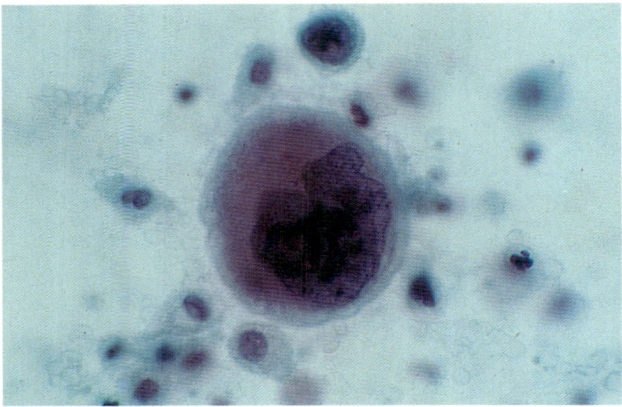

FIGURE 13.11 Undifferentiated large-cell carcinoma of the lung. The bizarre tumor cell has a nucleus with intense hyperchromatism and a markedly irregular contour. (Pap× 240)

TABLE 13.4 Differential Diagnosis of Effusions Containing Pigmented Cells

Malignant melanoma
Pigmented macrophages
Hepatocellular carcinoma
Extraneous vegetable cells

tion and eosinophils in the background. Caution should be exercised in making the diagnosis of melanoma based only on the presence of pigmented cells. As indicated in Table 13.4, other conditions in addition to melanoma lead to accumulation of pigment in cells; these conditions should not be misinterpreted to indicate melanoma.

PLEOMORPHIC LARGE CELLS

Pleomorphic large cells can also originate from anaplastic neoplasms prone to shed noncohesive cells. Anaplastic large-cell neoplasms run the gamut between epithelial and nonepithelial neoplasm, as well as melanoma and large-cell lymphomas. The list of diagnostic possibilites based on the presence of these cells is quite extensive (Table 13.5). Large cell anaplastic carcinoma of the lung sheds enormous cells with bizarre shaped nuclei (Fig. 13.11). The cells of the so-called "anaplastic" type of giant cell carcinoma of the pancreas may

TABLE 13.5 Differential Diagnosis of Effusions Containing Pleomorphic Large Cells

Giant-cell carcinoma of lung
Renal cell carcinoma
Pancreatic carcinoma
Hodgkin's disease
Trophoblastic neoplasms
Pleomorphic sarcomas
Anaplastic myeloma
Malignant melanoma
Malignant mesothelioma
Multinucleated histiocytes
Megakaryocytes
Multinucleated mesothelial cells

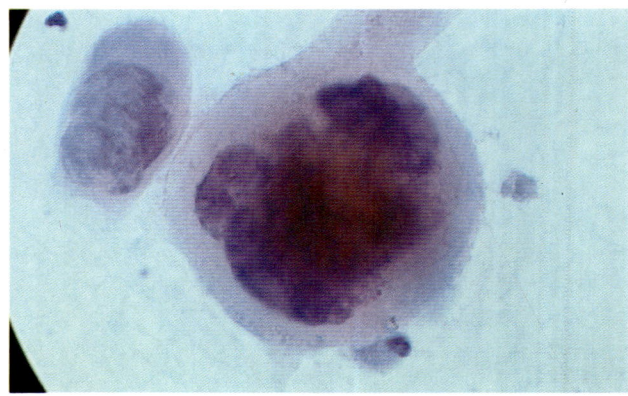

FIGURE 13.12 Bizarre malignant cell from anaplastic carcinoma, primary in the pancreas. Multiple-lobed nuclei show irregular chromatin distribution. (Pap× 240)

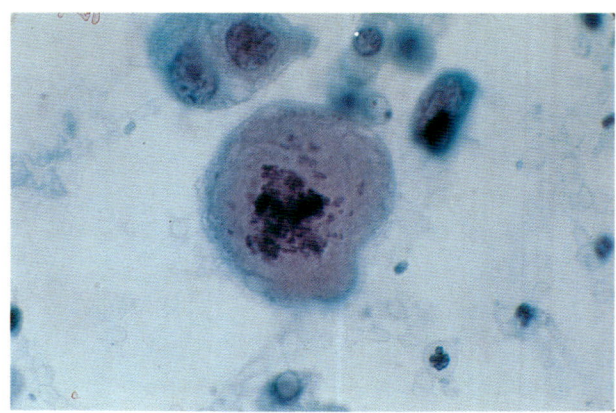

FIGURE 13.13 Single malignant cell from a mesothelioma. Note the multipolar mitotic figure and other tumor cells dwarfed in the background. (Pap× 240)

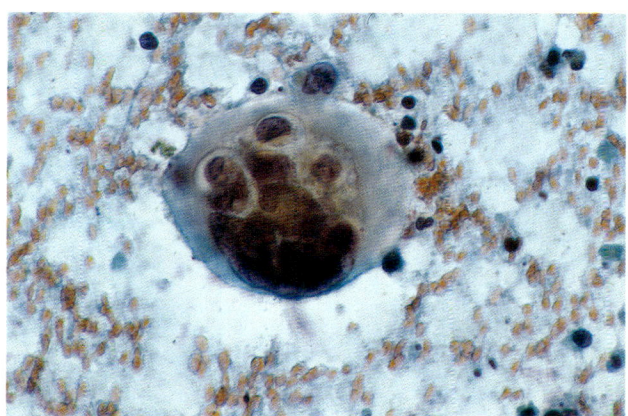

FIGURE 13.14 Multinucleated malignant cell resembling an osteoclast. The primary tumor was in the pancreato-biliary area and extended to the retroperitoneum. (Pap × 240)

FIGURE 13.15 Renal-cell carcinoma with a bizarre giant cell. The nuclei are arranged peripherally, and the cytoplasm displays a tendency toward fragility. (Pap × 240)

attain even a greater size (Fig. 13.12). Not uncommonly, rapidly proliferating large cells may display abnormal mitoses (Fig. 13.13). Neither the frequency of mitosis nor any other cytologic feature of pleomorphic cells allow recognition of the primary site. Unless there is a prior history of the primary tumor or previous cytologic or histologic material for comparison with the effusion, the source of the malignant cells cannot be pinpointed.

MULTINUCLEATED GIANT CELLS

Multinucleated epithelial elements should be distinguished from giant cells of histiocytic origin, megakaryocytes, and multinucleated mesothelial cells (Table 13.6). Cytomorphology may be helpful in recognizing cell products in the cytoplasm of cells, such as melanin in

melanomas, bile in hepatocellular carcinomas, or mucin in large-cell adenocarcinomas. Of all carcinomas, lung tumors present most commonly with giant cells, even though pancreatic tumors may have osteoclast-like elements (Fig. 13.14). Less commonly, undifferentiated thyroid neoplasm may show spindle and giant cells but we have not seen this tumor in an effusion specimen. Renal cell carcinomas are known as the great imitators and as such they often present with giant cells indistinguishable from those of other carcinomas (Fig. 13.15). Tumors with multinucleated giant cells may be recognized by their secretory products. As previously noted, melanomas shed large mononuclear or pleomorphic

---

TABLE 13.6 Differential Diagnosis of Effusions Containing Multinucleated Giant Cells

Giant-cell carcinoma
Pleomorphic sarcoma
Malignant fibrous histiocytoma
Hepatocellular carcinoma
Multiple myeloma
Malignant melanoma
Renal-cell carcinoma
Trophoblastic neoplasms

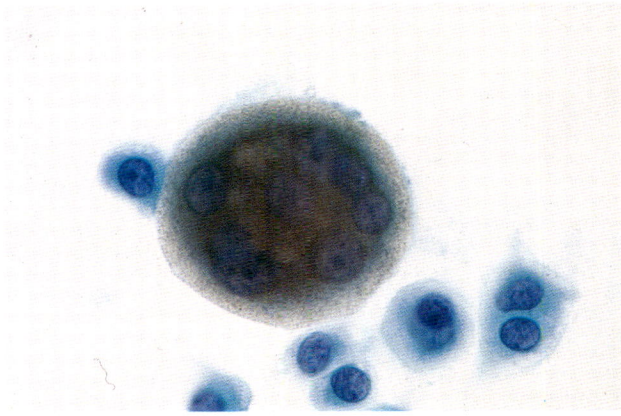

FIGURE 13.16 Multinucleated cell from malignant melanoma. Notice the partially pigmented cytoplasm and nuclei with prominent nucleoli. (Pap × 240)

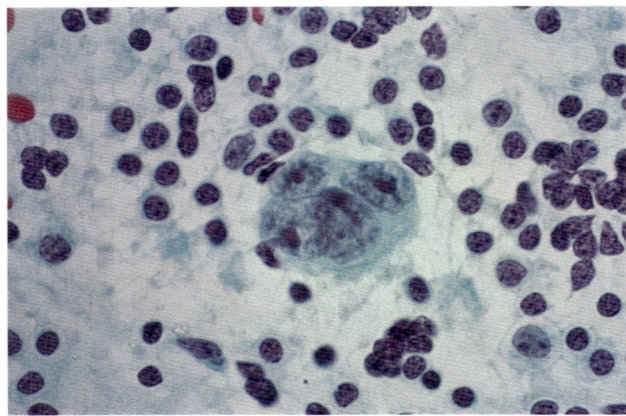

FIGURE 13.17 Reed-Sternberg cell from patient with Hodgkin's disease and a malignant effusion. Notice atypical lymphocytes in the background. (Pap × 240)

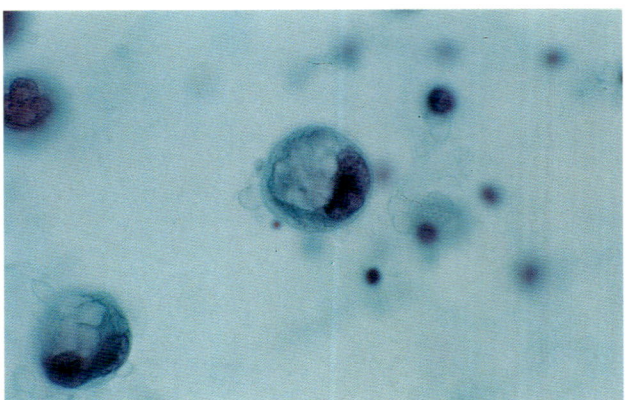

FIGURE 13.19 Malignant cells from gastric adenocarcinoma. The signet-ring appearance is a result of secretory products accumulated in the cytoplasm. (Pap × 240)

cells in effusions but may also be accompanied by multinucleated giant cells (Fig. 13.16). Even when these cells are nonpigmented, they are positive by Fontana-Masson stain and for S-100 and HMB-45 by immunoperoxidase. Germ-cell tumors with syncitio-cytotrophoblasts are positive for BHCG, whereas embryonal carcinomas are positive for alpha-fetoprotein (AFP) and yolk-sac tumors show positivity for A1AT. Aggressive high grade lymphomas may be exceptionally present with multinucleated giant cells. Large-cell lymphomas are mostly of B-cell lineage, but a small proportion are of true histiocytic origin. These tumors are positive for A1AT, A1CT, and lysozyme.

Hodgkin's disease is the only neoplastic condition to be present with classical Reed-Sternberg cells (Fig. 13.17). Other hematopoietic malignancies, however, may display multinucleated elements, including plasma cell myeloma. As noted in chapter 10, sarcomas are often present with multinucleated giant cells. In general, multinucleated cells are noncohesive and tend to attain a rounded configuration in effusion. This tends to occur regardless of the epithelial or nonepithelial nature of the parent neoplasm (Fig. 13.18). For this reason, the differential diagnosis of malignant effusions containing multinucleated giant cells often requires the use of ancillary methods.

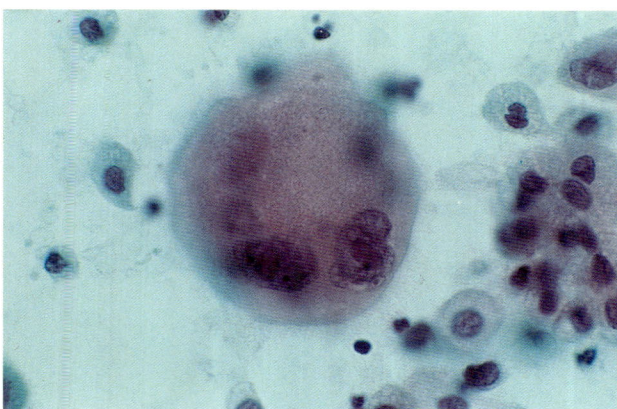

FIGURE 13.18 Multinucleated giant cell in effusion from autopsy subject. The patient had a diagnosis of malignant fibrous histiocytoma. (Pap × 240)

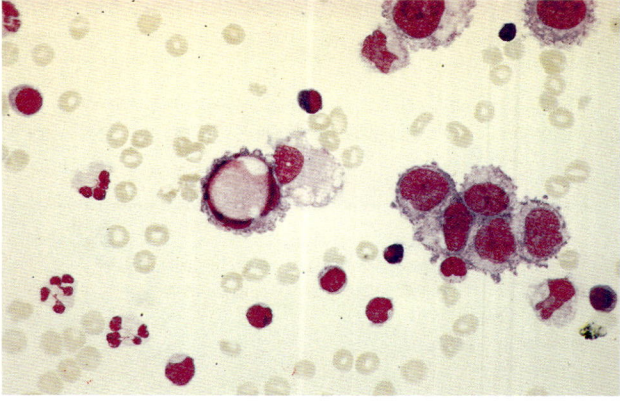

FIGURE 13.20 Signet-ring adenocarcinoma of the stomach in pleural fluid. The secretory product in the tumor cell creates a contrast with neighboring reactive mesothelial cells. (DQ × 90) (Courtesy S. Zaleski, CT)

TABLE 13.7   Differential Diagnosis of Effusions
Containing Signet Ring Cells

Gastric adenocarcinoma
Colonic adenocarcinoma
Pancreatic adenocarcinoma
Ovarian adenocarcinoma
Mammary adenocarcinoma
Degenerated mesothelial cells

SIGNET RINGS

Signet-ring cells are a special form of isolated cells that denote a mucin-secreting adenocarcinoma. Stomach, colon, pancreas, and gallbladder tumors should be included in the differential diagnosis whenever these cells dominate the cytologic features of the effusion (Table 13.7). Signet-ring cells typically display a nucleus pushed toward the periphery by secretory product accumulated in the cytoplasm (Fig. 13.19 and 13.20. The nature of the secretory product may vary but most often it represents a mucosubstance. Lipid and immunoglobulin may also accumulate and cause a cell to assume a signet-ring appearance. When mesothelial cells assume this configuration it is usually as a result of degeneration. The signet-ring appearance of the tumor cells may be elucidated by mucicarmine or another special stain, including immunostains (Fig. 13.21). We have used alcian blue in association with carcinoembryonic

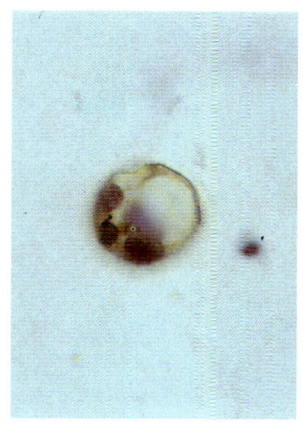
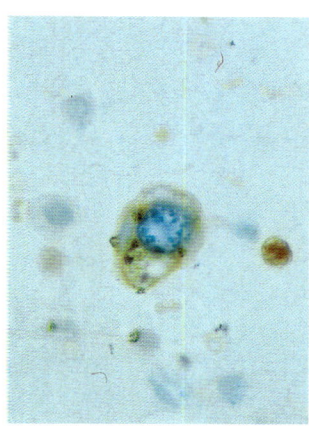

FIGURE 13.22   Same case as shown in Figure 13.21. Left: The CEA stain is positive but fails to react with the secretory product. Right: CEA/Alcian Blue reaction showing positivity of the secretory product with Alcian Blue. (P.A.P. × 180)

antigen (CEA) to demonstrate signet ring cells in effusions and needle aspirates (Fig. 13.22). Signet-ring cells should be distinguished from degenerated mesothelial and lipid-filled cells, particularly in cell blocks. Neither of these two cell types will stain for mucin or CEA, but they will be positive for vimentin. Although lipid-filled cells may be positive for S-100, they are easily identifiable by fat stains if renal cell carcinoma is suspected and air-dried slides are prepared.

PSEUDOMYXOMA PERITONEI

Another special form of mucin-secreting neoplasms constitutes one of the most enigmatic presentations of malignant effusions: pseudomyxoma peritonei. In this condition, the effusion has a high content of mucin within which free-floating malignant cells appear, either singly or in clusters (Fig. 13.23). The ovary and the appendix are the most common sites, but in many patients the primary source of the neoplasm cannot be discerned. With the Diff-Quik stain mucin appears as a light blue amorphous material surrounding the cells (Fig. 13.24). In Pap-stained preparations, free-floating mucin is not readily appreciated, but it can be highlighted by special stains (Fig. 13.25); or a combination of immunocytochemical and histochemical stains (Fig. 13.26). Not all pseudomyxoma peritonei result from a malignant process. A ruptured viscus may also result in this same cytologic appearance (Fig. 13.27).

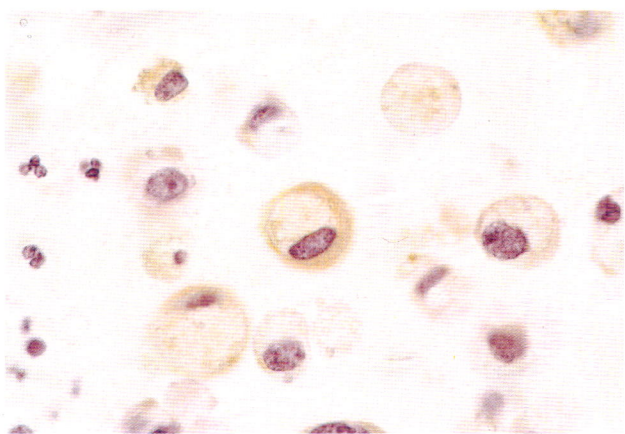

FIGURE 13.21   Gastric carcinoma stained for EMA. There is only a faint positivity of the distended cytoplasm of signet rings (P.A.P. × 90)

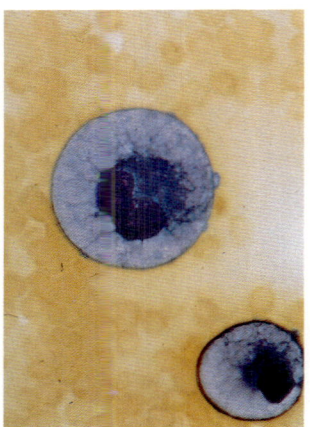
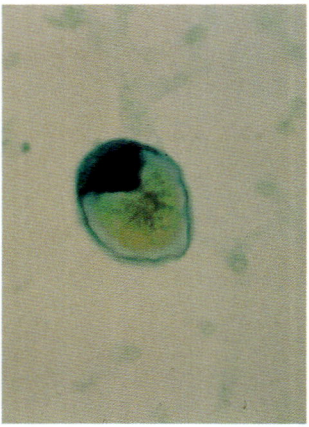

FIGURE 13.23   Contrast in the cytologic appearance of mucus-filled cells. Left: With the Diff-Quik. The flocculent nature of the secretion is readily appreciated (DQ × 240). Right: With the Pap stain the secretory material appears inspissated (Pap × 240)

SOLID CELL BALLS

The solid cell ball configuration is a rather typical presentation of breast, ovary, and lung carcinomas, in decreasing order of frequency (Table 13.8). This cytologic appearance is, therefore, commonly seen in effusions of elderly women. The number of cells in the cell ball ranges from a few to several hundred, but it never attains the incredibly large number seen in mesotheliomas. The cells are compact and fit tightly around one another. The individual tumor cells in the ball formation

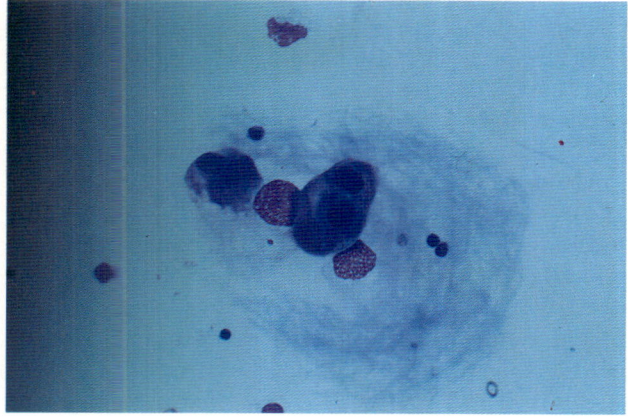

FIGURE 13.24   Pseudomyxoma peritonei. Note malignant cells enmeshed in a background of faint secretory material. (DQ × 180)

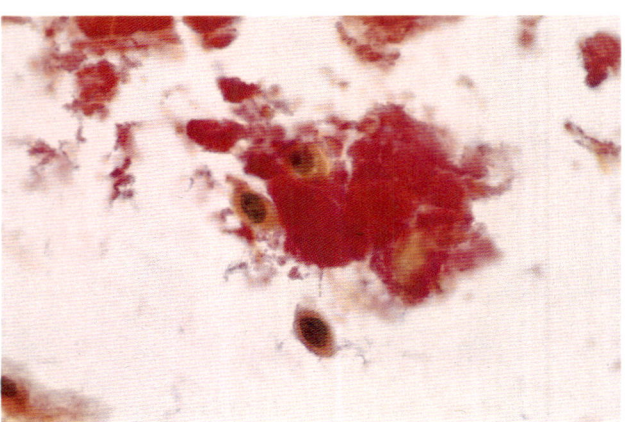

FIGURE 13.25   Blob of secretory material positive for mucicarmine. Notice scarcity of tumor cells. (Mucicarmine × 180)

are considerably larger than the neighboring groups of mesothelial cells (Fig. 13.28). The cell balls immediately stand out even under low-power examination not only because of their size, but also because of their distinct configuration. The perception that the cells are alien to the effusion is the most important decision necessary to clinch a malignant diagnosis (Fig. 13.27). Observation of the nuclei in the cell ball to distinguish between the ball and the mesothelial cells in the background also contributes to precise diagnosis of malignancy.

In paraffin- and plastic-embedded cell blocks, it is possible to appreciate that some of the cell balls are actually hollow spheres. The apical pole of the tumor cells faces the outside and not the lumen in the center of the sphere, as is the case in free-floating acini. Most often, cell balls are not composed of vacuolated elements but contain rather non-descript cells that are small and compactly arranged (Fig. 13.29). In general, nuclear detail is best appreciated with the Papanicolaou stain than with the Diff-Quik method. Diff-Quik, however, offers a better appreciation of the cytoplasm (Fig.

TABLE 13.8   Differential Diagnosis of Effusions Composed Predominantly of Cell Balls

Breast carcinoma
Ovarian carcinoma
Adenocarcinoma of lung
Adenocarcinoma of stomach
Prostatic carcinoma
Malignant mesothelioma
Reactive mesothelial cells

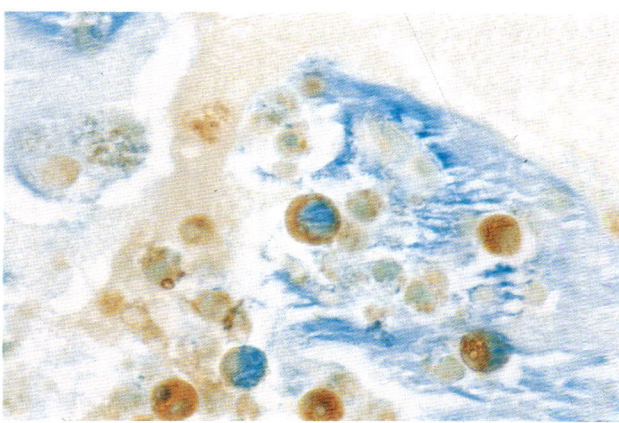

FIGURE 13.26 Special stains in pseudomyxoma peritonei. The cells are positive for CEA; the scretory material is
positive for Alcian Blue (Alcian Blue-CEA × 180).

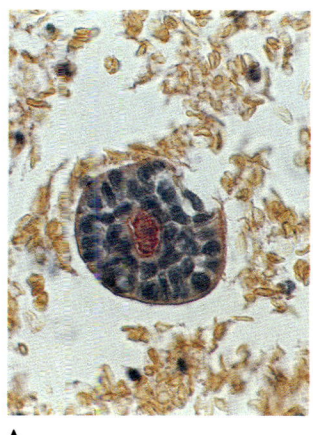

A

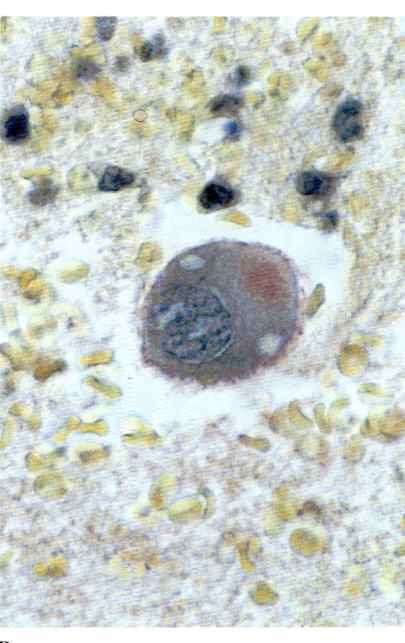

B

FIGURE 13.27 Pseudomyxoma peritonei secondary to
a ruptured appendix. (A) An intact tissue fragment is noted
against a bloody background (Mucicarmine × 180). (B) Single malignant cell shows a blush of positivity in the cytoplasm (Mucicarmine × 180).

13.30). Before accepting that the cell balls indicate carcinoma, the possibility that they represent either mesothelial hyperplasia or mesothelioma should be ruled
out. If this is not possible on the basis that the cells
appear alien to the effusion, the process may be facilitated by special stains and immunocytochemical methods. With immunocytochemistry, it is often possible to
delineate the internal architecture of the cell ball. Mesothelial cells may also be differentiated from adenocarcinomatous cells on the basis of their ultrastructural
features. The use of electron microscopy and immunocytochemistry is discussed in more detail in chapters 14
and 15, respectively.

PAPILLARY FORMATIONS

Papillary formations differ from solid cell balls because
of their fibrovascular core. Whereas solid cell balls may
exfoliate from a tumor that is not papillary on histologi-
cal examination, papillary formations originate from
predominantly papillary neoplasms. The exact mechanism of solid cell ball formation is not clear, and no
clues are offered by the predominantly solid pattern of
certain carcinomas. Very possibly the cell balls represent nests of tumor cells that detach from the main tumor and illustrate the growing and invasive edge of
the neoplasm. In contrast, it is commonly accepted that
papillary formations in cytologic specimens represent
broken tips of papillae in predominantly papillary neoplasms. At times, a large papillary frond is found intact

in effusion specimens, but it is not possible to appreciate
its vascular core (Fig. 13.31). The presence of endothelial cells or RBCs and positivity for Factor VIII are helpful in demonstrating a vascular core. Not infrequently,
it is possible to visualize or surmise the presence of a
core, on a purely cytologic basis (Fig. 13.32). The nuclei
in a papillary formation are polarized; their parallel ar-

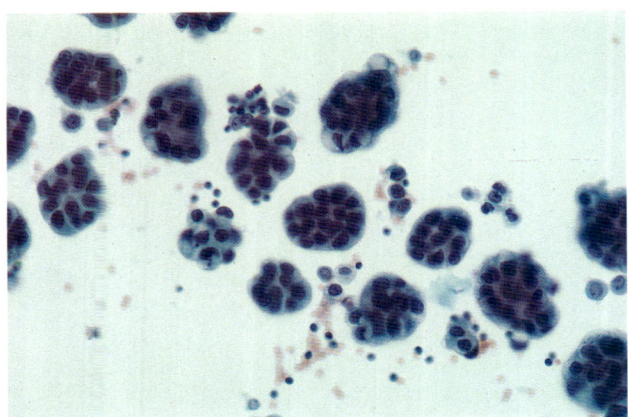

FIGURE 13.28 Numerous cell balls in a pleural effusion secondary to a breast carcinoma. Note the variable size of the groupings; (proportional to the number of individual cells in the cell balls). (Pap × 80)

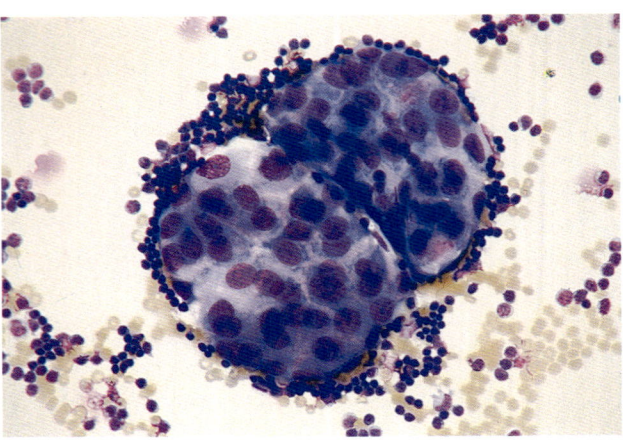

FIGURE 13.30 Breast carcinoma in pleural effusions. A. With the Diff-Quik stain the cytoplasmic texture of a tight group of cells is clearly identified (Diff-Quik, × 180)

rangement converges toward the center, as opposed to the irregular or nonpreferential distribution of nuclei in cell balls. Papillary formations are common in neoplasms arising in ovary, thyroid, and lung, among others (Table 13.9).

In papillary formations arising from the thyroid, no vacuolated or mucus-filled cells are identified, whereas lung and ovary neoplasms usually show a mixture of vacuolated and nonvacuolated cells. It is important to scrutinize very carefully a preparation containing papil-

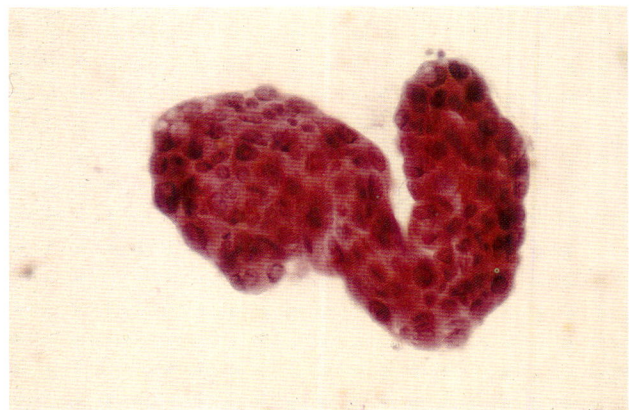

FIGURE 13.31 Large papillary cluster from serous cystadenocarcinoma of the ovary. Notice nonvacuolated cells tightly arranged around a barely perceptible core. (Pap × 180)

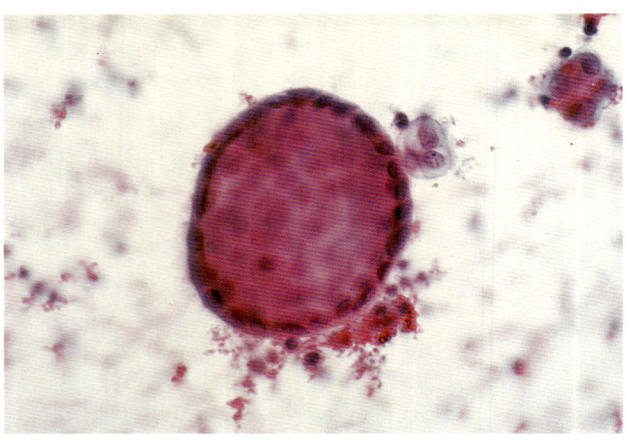

FIGURE 13.29 Tight cell ball from a breast carcinoma. These cell groupings may be solid or hollow, but this cannot always be verified using cytologic preparations alone. (Pap × 120)

TABLE 13.9 Differential Diagnosis of Effusions Containing Papillary Formations

Ovarian carcinoma
Papillary carcinoma of thyroid
Bronchioloalveolar carcinoma
Transitional-cell carcinoma
Malignant mesothelioma
Reactive mesothelial cells

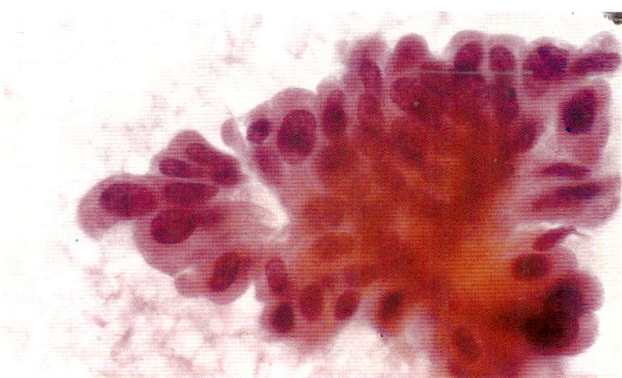

FIGURE 13.32   Same case as shown in Figure 13.31. The malignant cells show long axis radiating towards the center of the core. (Pap × 240)

lary formations for the presence of psammoma bodies (Fig. 13.33). Without the help of ancilary studies it is not possible to pinpoint the site of origin. Bronchioloalveolar carcinomas present with a large number of papillary groups and neoplastic cell balls. The cell groups may coalesce further and form large, multilobed conglomerates of spherical and oval cell balls that are clearly distinguishable from the mesothelial cells in the background. Isolated tumor cells accompanying the cell groups are bland but still show malignant characteristics and are also clearly different from individual mesothelial cells. In mesothelioma and mesothelial hyperplasias, the papillary formations are composed of cells that bear a striking resemblance to the isolated mesothelial cells in the background. The greatest challenge is to distinguish between hyperplasia and neoplasia of mesothelial cells, as discussed in Chapter 7.

PSAMMOMA BODIES

Psammoma bodies are curious structures that represent degeneration and calcification of cells commonly arranged in papillary clusters. Although most frequently associated with a neoplastic process, psammoma bodies may form in the peritoneal space following intra-abdominal surgery. A malignant diagnosis should not be made unless well-preserved neoplastic cells are clearly identified. Ovarian, thyroidal, pulmonary, and, less frequently, other types of adenocarcinomas are accompanied by psammoma bodies (Table 13.10). However, it should be remembered that other neoplasms, including oat cell carcinoma of the lung may exceptionally be

TABLE 13.10   Differential Diagnosis of Effusions Containing Psammoma Bodies
Ovarian carcinoma
Papillary carcinoma of thyroid
Breast carcinoma
Gastric carcinoma
Bronchioloalveolar carcinoma
Benign mesothelial hyperplasia

accompanied by psammoma bodies. The calcific concretions are usually larger and more irregular than calcospherites and commonly fragment along straight fracture lines (Fig. 13.34). A psammomatous form of serous carcinoma has been described in which the ovary contains thousands of these concretions. Benign and malignant mesothelial proliferations may be accompanied by calcific concretions that fulfill the criteria of psammoma bodies; therefore, they cannot be interpreted as unequivocal evidence of malignancy. Caution is particularly indicated when interpreting peritoneal washes obtained during second-look operations for ovarian carcinomas. Adhesions, old scars, and areas of hyperplasia may all shed light papillary clusters of mesothelial cells alongside psammoma bodies.

NONVACUOLATED CELL CLUSTERS

Malignant effusions may be composed of small, partially cohesive tumor cells that do not have overt differentiat-

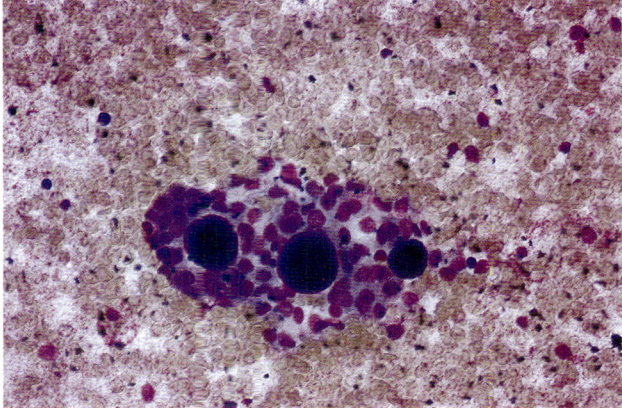

FIGURE 13.33   Metastatic papillary carcinoma. Notice multiple psammoma bodies in the supportive stroma of the neoplastic cells. (MGG × 180)

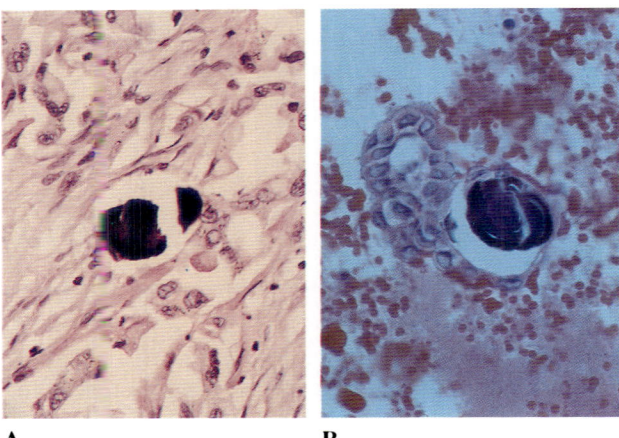

A   **B**

FIGURE 13.34 Psammoma bodies in a papillary ovarian adenocarcinoma. (*A*) In the tissue specimen, the psammoma body occupies a hollow space within the neoplasm. (H&E × 120) (*B*) The cell block demonstrates a fracture line that splits the concretion. (Pap × 120)

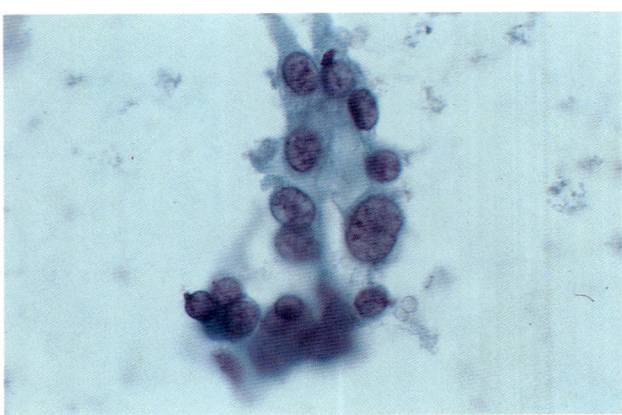

FIGURE 13.35 Adenocarcinoma of the lower esophagus. The poorly cohesive group of cells show only faint vacuolization of the cytoplasm. (Pap × 240)

ing features noted in the cytoplasm. There is only a small amount of nonvacuolated cytoplasm exhibited by these cells and they lack a tight-ball, acinar, or papillary configuration (Fig. 13.35). The cell cluster may break up into smaller groups that have no consistent pattern of size and shape. Some refer to this configuration as small-sized "mini-biopsies" and stress that some molding occurs between the tumor cells, in contrast to the clumps of lymphocytes and histiocytes artificially thrown together. Neoplasms most likely to exhibit nonvacuolated cell clusters include breast carcinoma, oat-cell carcinoma of the lung, carcinoid tumor, prostatic carcinoma, and a few nonepithelial tumors (Table 13.11). As noted in chapter 12, SBRCTs often present with similar groups of small partially cohesive tumor cells. In carcinoid, the molding among nuclei is reminiscent of the onion-skin effect present in oat-cell carci-

noma, but the cytologic atypia is not as pronounced (Fig. 13.36). Breast carcinoma can be distinguished from oat-cell carcinoma if the nonvacuolated cell clusters display nucleoli, in sharp contrast with the absent nucleoli in the latter. Prostatic carcinomas may show a cribriform pattern, which resembles the configuration noted in histopathologic preparations. In cholangiocarcinoma, the predominant cell type in the cluster is nonvacuolated but occasionally cells show vacuolization (Fig. 13.37). This same phenomenon occurs in ovarian carcinoma so that it is not always possible to distinguish mucinous from serous carcinomas (Fig. 13.38). Not all non-vacuolated cell clusters derive from adenocarci-

TABLE 13.11 Differential Diagnosis of Neoplasms Composed of Small Partially Cohesive Tumor Cells

Breast carcinoma
Oat-cell carcinoma of lung
Carcinoid
Prostatic carcinoma
Wilms' tumor
Thymoma

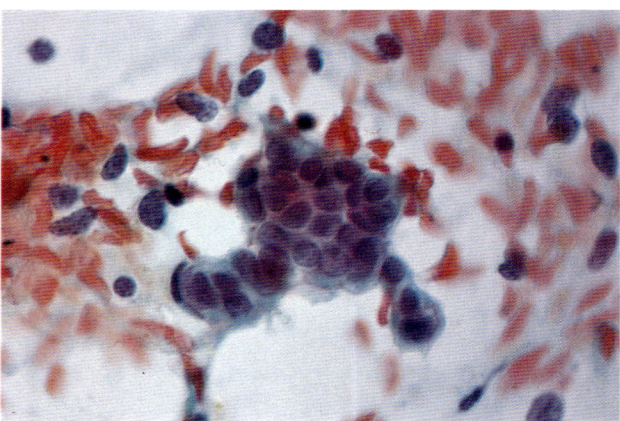

FIGURE 13.36 Metastatic carcinoid tumor. Small tissue fragment showing a tendency towards molding of the neoplastic cells. (Pap × 200)

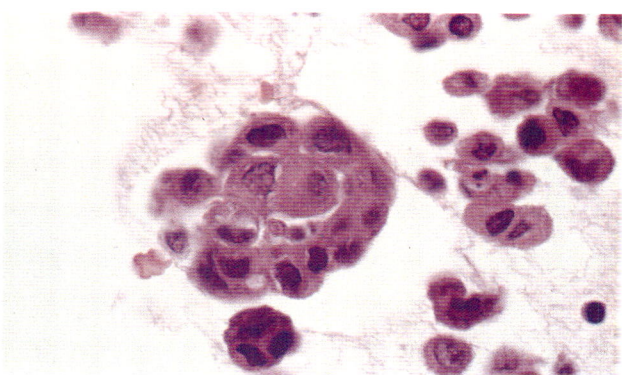

FIGURE 13.37 Cholangiocarcinoma in cell block from ascites. The cell group is composed predominantly of nonvacuolated tumor cells. (H&E × 120)

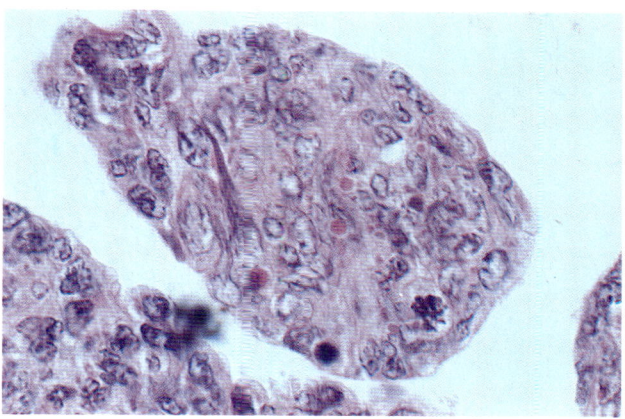

FIGURE 13.39 Cell block from Oat-cell carcinoma treated by chemotherapy. The more abundant cytoplasm reflects attempted differentiation. (H&E × 180)

noma. Oat-cell carcinoma of the lung sheds cell groups with layered nuclei, a configuration resembling onion skin. The layering of the cells and acquisition of cytoplasm are accentuated in effusions of patients who responded partially to chemotherapy (Fig. 13.39). Not infrequently, partially differentiated clusters of oat-cell carcinoma contain mitotic figures. The exact explanation for this cytologic appearance is not known but may be related to continued multiplication of tumor cells in the liquid milieu represented by the effusion. Squamous cell carcinoma tends to shed individual cells in effusions. In the rare instances when cell clusters are present, they resemble waterlogged keratin pearls.

VACUOLATED CELL CLUSTERS

This most common form of presentation of malignant cells in effusions seldom causes diagnostic difficulties. Vacuolated cell clusters are indicative of adenocarcinomatous differentiation, reflected by a moderate to abundant amount of cytoplasm that shows evidence of secretory activity. The presence of vacuolated cytoplasm renders the clusters considerably larger than groups of mesothelial cells and nonvacuolated cell clusters. Vacuolated cell clusters are the most frequent presentation of adenocarcinomas, and are present either as the predominant component or as part of a cytologic picture dominated by other elements. Table 13.12 is a partial list of the tumors that show this pattern in malignant effusions. Vacuolated cell clusters favor a gastrointesti-

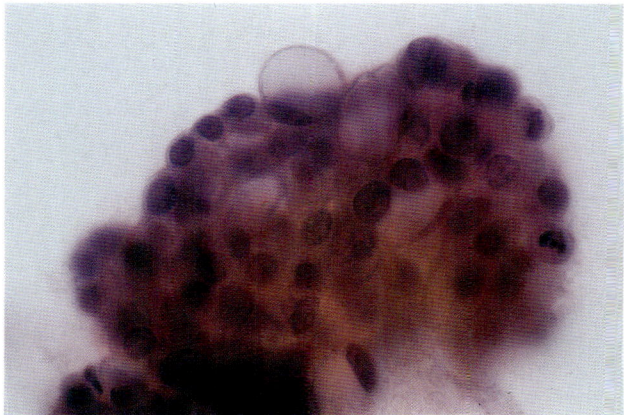

FIGURE 13.38 Mixture of vacuolated and nonvacuolated tumor cells in ovarian carcinoma. The important task is to distinguish the group from degenerating mesothelial cells. (Pap × 180)

TABLE 13.12 Differential Diagnosis of Effusions Containing Vacuolated Cell Clusters

Adenocarcinoma of lung
Adenocarcinoma of ovary
Adenocarcinoma of breast
Adenocarcinoma of gastrointestinal tract
Adenocarcinoma of pancreas
Renal-cell carcinoma
Malignant mesothelioma
Degenerated mesothelial cells
Degenerated histiocytes
Irradiated mesothelial cells
Chemotherapy effect

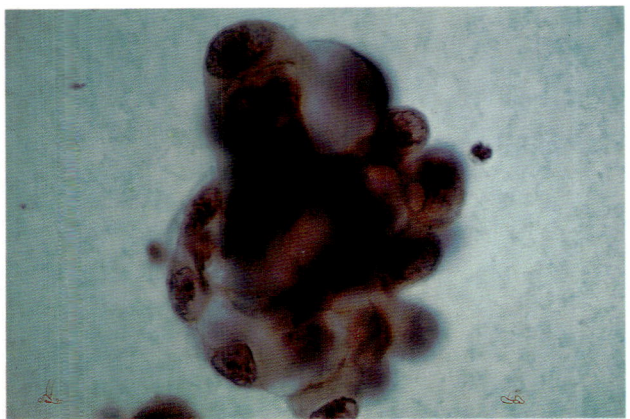

FIGURE 13.40   Vacuolated cell cluster from a pancreatic adenocarcinoma. Note the tridimensional effect created by overlapping nuclei and the scalloped contour of the cell grouping. (Pap × 180)

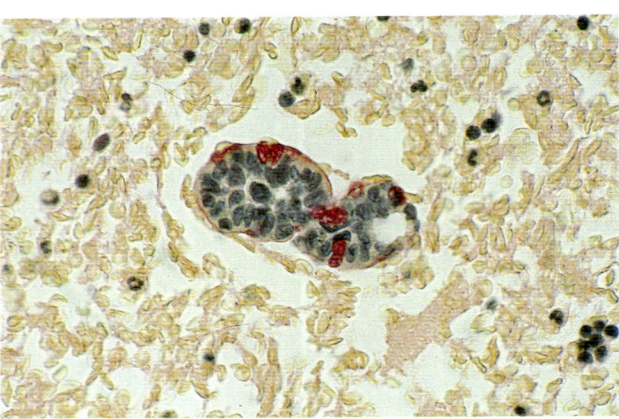

FIGURE 13.42   Free-floating acini in an ovarian adenocarcinoma. Luminal spaces may be difficult to distinguish from edematous cores of papillary groups. (Mucicarmine × 180)

nal, pulmonary, or ovarian origin for the malignant effusion; however, depending on its degree of mucinous differentiation, the same pattern may be mimicked by adenocarcinomas of multiple primary sites. In the typical case, the cells fit closely together, nuclear molding is identified, and the abundant cytoplasm displays vacuoles of various sizes (Fig. 13.40). Even when the nuclei are pushed aside by a large vacuole, appeciation of mucin production is not always possible with the Pap stain. With the Diff-Quik stain, however, a fluffy texture is rather characteristic of mucosubstances (Fig. 13.41). Confirmation of mucin production is achieved by the use of special stains. The maneuver is more successful in cell blocks where various special stains can be utilized in multiple sections at different levels (Fig. 13.42). Positivity is greatest in carcinomas of the lung, the gastrointestinal tract, the ovary, and the pancreas and weakest in carcinomas of the breast and the gallbladder. Mucin production may be of such degree that the mucosubstance accumulates extracellularly. In these cases, the mucosubstance may adhere to the outer surface of the cells or the cell cluster may appear enmeshed in a glob of mucosubstance (Fig. 13.43). Using EM, pleomorphic, electron-dense secretory granules are noted to engorge the cytoplasm and to extrude from the cell. Abundant but short microvilli cover the free surface of the

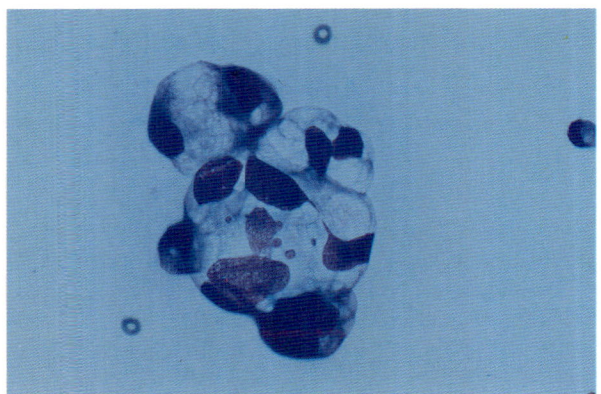

FIGURE 13.41   Same case as shown in Figure 13.40, stained with Diff-Quik. Even though nuclear detail is lost, large vacuoles are clearly demonstrated in the cytoplasm. (DQ × 250)

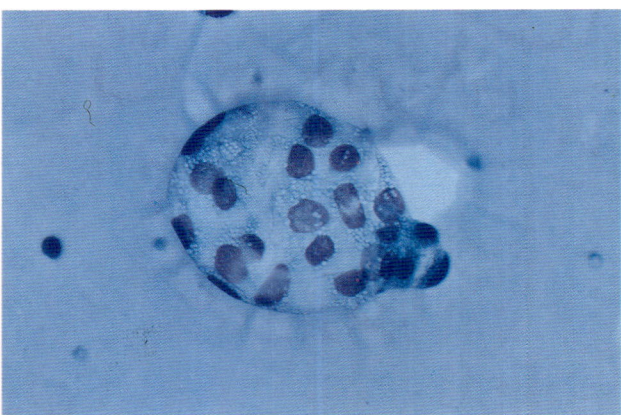

FIGURE 13.43   Mucus-producing adenocarcinoma. The tumor cells are contained in a matrix of mucosubstance. Note mucosubstance material with flocculent texture in the cytoplasm of neoplastic cells. (MGG × 200)

cells, connected to each other by complex interdigitating and scattered intercellular junctions.

Vacuolated cell clusters may be associated with individual cells, small pseudoacinar groups, or large papillary fronds. Frequently, however, they are associated with tridimensional clusters of tumor cells. Although certain tumors have a propensity for one combination more than another, it is difficult to ascertain the cell of origin by cytomorphology alone. We rely on electron microscopy and antibody panels for such distinction, as elaborated in Chapters 14 and 15. Special stains, however, should not be eschewed in favor of immunocytochemistry in every case. Demonstration of glycogen (PAS), mucin (PAS-D, mucicarmine, alcian blue), lipid (Oil red-0), and bile (Hall's) help to identify the cell of origin of certain adenocarcinomas. Kreyberg's stain recognizes a combined adenosquamous differentiation, whereas Grimelius identifies an associated neuroendocrine component.

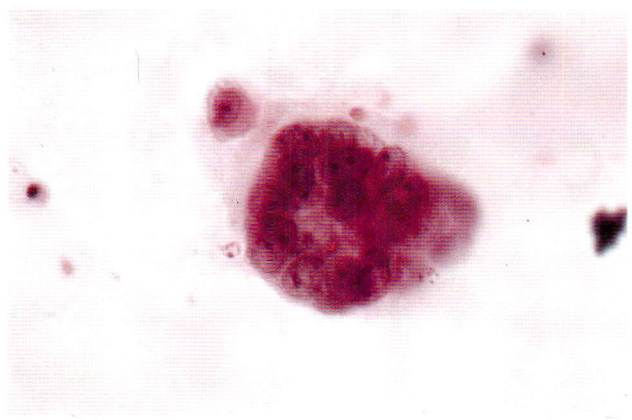

FIGURE 13.45   Gastric adenocarcinoma with a cohesive and irregular grouping of cells. This specimen originated from a poorly differentiated neoplasm. (Pap × 120)

FREE-FLOATING ACINI

Occasionally, free-floating acini are present in adenocarcinomas with or without secretion in the lumina. Similar hollow structures may also derive as a result of epithelial cells sloughing off their stalk (Fig. 13.44). This feature is present most frequently in carcinomas of the colon, lung, and ovary, where the acini are not always perfectly formed. In cell blocks, oval or irregularly shaped acini show eccentric lumina or may connect

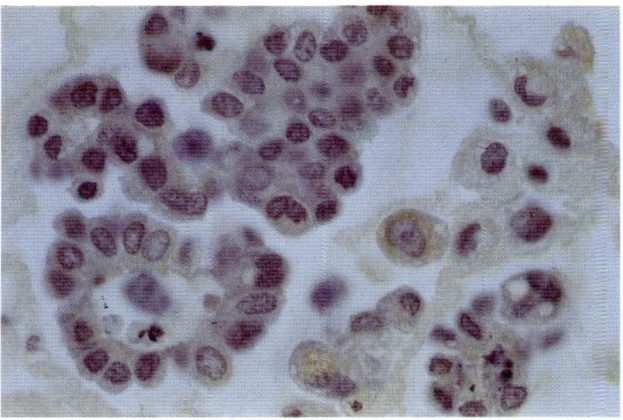

FIGURE 13.44   Irregular grouping in an adenocarcinoma of the gallbladder. Not all cholangiocarcinomas look the same. This grouping shows a combination of papillary and acini-like formations. (H&E × 180)

themselves with cell balls or the tangential cuts of neighboring acini. Cells at the edge of the acini are molded or may display a signet ring appearance or be filled with mucin-like contents. This appearance is common in tumors of gastrointestinal and pancreatic origin. It may not be possible to detect the contents of acinar structures particularly if they are deformed during the process of exfoliation (Fig. 13.45). Similar rudimentary acini is also noted in tumors of prostatic and mammary origin. In general, the shape of the cells is not completely distinctive of a certain origin, even though tall cells are noted in colonic and endocervical carcinomas. Whereas, cuboidal cells are more common in carcinomas of the breast and prostate.

TALL COLUMNAR FRONDS

Groups of elongated tumor cells perpendicular to a central core are typical of carcinomas of the colon. Depending on their preservation, either strips of columnar cells or nearly intact fronds are observed (Fig. 13.46). At the base of these tall columnar fronds, vacuolated cells sometimes are present, helping to distinguish them from transitional-cell carcinomas. The large fronds are accompanied by smaller vacuolated cell clusters or by cell clusters of elongated cells in which the individual cells frequently curve around their neighbors. The spatial arrangement of vacuolated and non-vacuolated tumor cells in the frond may be highlighted by special stains (Fig. 13.47).

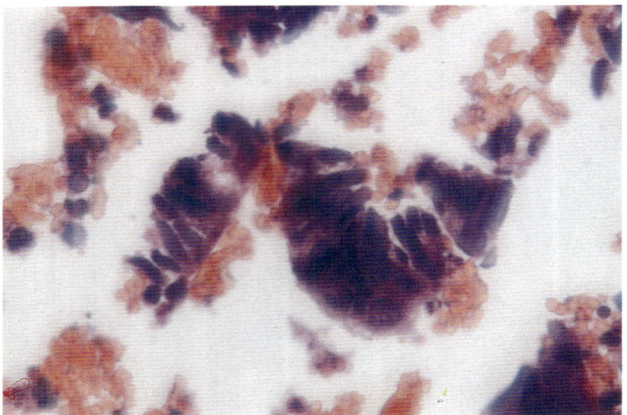

FIGURE 13.46   Tall columnar frond from a colonic adenocarcinoma. Despite the tendency of the effusion specimens to ball up, cells of a colonic carcinoma often display their elongated appearance. (H&E × 180)

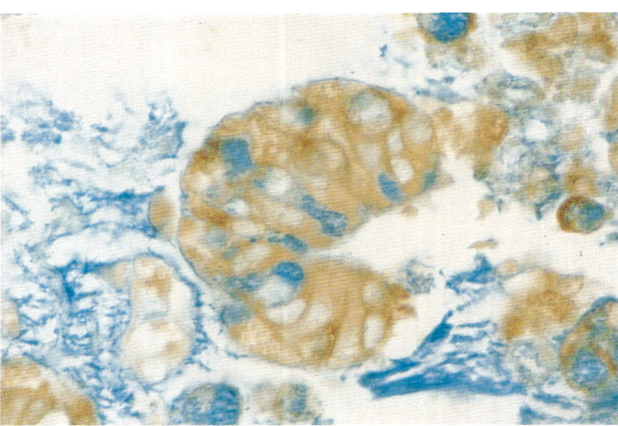

Figure 13.47   Same fluid as figure 13.46. The Alcian Blue shows mucosubstances in the tall columnar cells. (Alcian Blue-CEA × 180)

INDIAN FILE

Tandem formations of tumor cells are known as "Indian files," a phenomenon that occurs commonly in breast and oat-cell carcinomas of the lung (Table 13.13). In histologic sections, the arrangement in rows is understandable, the tumor cells appear to fall in line because of the surrounding stroma of the neoplasm. Even though this external pressure is missing in exfoliated cells, intact tandems of malignant cells may still be identified in effusions (Fig. 13.48). That the rows of cells do not come together randomly, can be verified by EM, which clearly shows the intercellular connections between the various members of the rows. However, this same phenomenon can occur by chance arrangement of neoplastic and mesothelial cells, particularly in degenerated specimens.

SPINDLE CELLS

Spindle cells are found primarily in association with sarcomas (Table 13.14), which are discussed in more detail in Chapter 10. Sarcomatous spindle cells in effusions have a tendency to plump up and attain an oval or rounded configuration (Fig. 13.49). However, similar spindle cells may derive from the submesothelial layer and from benign, localized mesotheliomas. It is rare to find this pattern in naturally accumulated effusions, but procedures such as pelvic washes and cell collection during pleuroscopy may yield plumpish spindle cells of traumatic mesothelial origin. Spindle cells should not be immediately assumed to originate from a sarcoma.

TABLE 13.13   Differential Diagnosis of Effusions Containing Cells in Indian File Arrangement

Breast adenocarcinoma
Lung adenocarcinoma
Small-cell carcinoma of lung
Neuroendocrine carcinoma of extrapulmonary origin

TABLE 13.14   Differential Diagnosis of Effusions Composed of Spindle-Shaped Cells

Leiomyosarcoma
Fibrosarcoma
Malignant fibrous histiocytoma
Neurofibrosarcoma
Rhabdomyosarcoma
Synovial sarcoma
Localized benign mesothelioma

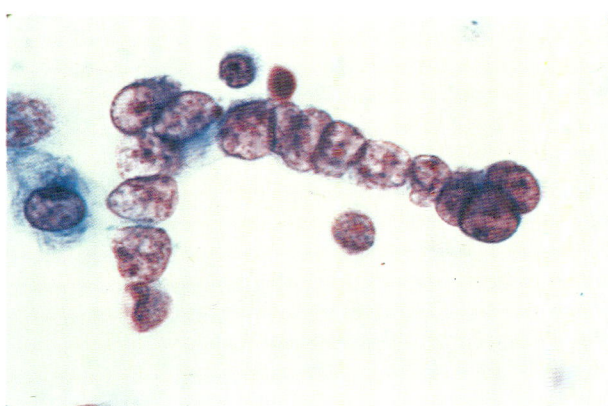

FIGURE 13.48   Indian file in a pleural effusion. Even though best seen in tissue and in needle aspirates, effusion sometimes exhibit this phenomenon, which is typical breast carcinomas but not exclusive of other types. (Pap × 120) (Courtesy Y. Erozan, MD)

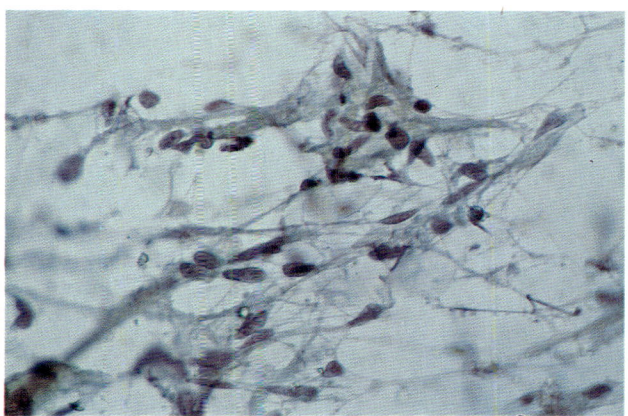

FIGURE 13.49   Spindle cells in cul-de-sac aspirate. The cells originated in a uterine sarcoma that extended into the pelvic soft tissues. (Pap × 180)

EFFUSIONS OF CRYPTIC ORIGIN

Some patients have effusions that tend to reaccumulate and resist every attempt at further clarification. In some instances, extensive clinical and radiographic investigations fail to identify a possible source of the effusion. Conversely, despite all clues that indicate a primary site, it is not always possible to verify the diagnosis using light microscopy alone. Furthermore, pinpointing the origin of the neoplasm may not provide any guidance for further treatment or reliable predictions of therapeutic outcome. As a result of these uncertainties, two techniques have emerged as adjuncts to diagnosis and classification of malignant effusions: EM and immunocytochemistry. The latter method is also emerging as a means to anticipate the success of treatment, thanks to numerous recently developed prognostic markers.

BIBLIOGRAPHY

Pinpointing the Primary Site

Foot NC. Identification of types and primary sites of metastatic tumors from exfoliated cells in serous fluids. *Am J Pathol.* 1954;30:661–677.

Grunze H. The comparative diagnostic accuracy, efficiency and specificity of cytologic technics used in the diagnosis of malignant neoplasm in serous effusions of the pleural and pericardial cavities. *Acta Cytol.* 1964;8:150–163.

Murphy W, Ng A BF. Determination of primary site by examination of cancer cells in body fluids. *Am J Clin Pathol.* 1972; 58:479–488.

Spieler P, Gloor F. Identification of types and primary sites of malignant tumors by examination of exfoliated tumor cells in serous fluids. *Acta Cytol.* 1985;29:753–774.

Menard S, Rilke F, Della Torre, et al. Sensitivity enhancement of the cytologic detection of cancer cells in effusions by monoclonal antibodies. *Am J Clin Pathol.* 1985;83:571–576.

Hanna W, Kahn HJ. The ultrastructure of metastatic adenocarcinoma in serous fluids: An aid in identification of the primary site of the neoplasm. *Acta Cytol.* 1985;29:202–210.

Large Single Cells

Graham JB, Graham RM, Schueller EF. Preclinical detection of ovarian cancer. *Cancer* 1964;17:1414.

Woyke S, Domagala W, Olszewski W. Ultrastructure of hepatoma cells detected in peritoneal fluid. *Acta Cytol.* 1974; 18:130.

Spriggs AI, Jerrome DW. Intracellular mucous inclusions: A feature of malignant cells in effusions in the serous cavities, particularly due to carcinoma of the breast. *J Clin Pathol.* 1975;28:929–936.

Danner DE, Gmelich JT. A comparative study of tumor cells from metastatic carcinoma of the breast in effusions. *Acta Cytol.* 1975;19:509–518.

O'Brien MJ, Kirkham SE, Burke B, et al. CEA, ZGM and EMA localization in cells of pleural and peritoneal effusion: A preliminary study. *Invest Cell Pathol.* 1980;3:251.

Gupta PK, Albritton N, Erozan YS, et al. Occurrence of cilia in exfoliated ovarian adenocarcinoma cells. *Diagn Cytopathol.* 1985;1:228.

Nguyen G-K, Schnitka TK, Jewell LD, et al. Exfoliative cytology of clear-cell sarcoma metastases in pleural fluid. *Diagn Cytopathol.* 1986;2:144.

Small Single Cells

Melamed MR. The cytological presentation of malignant lymphomas and related diseases in effusions. *Cancer* 1963; 16:413–431.

Naylor B. The exfoliative cytology of diffuse malignant mesotheliomia. *J Pathol Bacteriol.* 1963;86:293–298.

Weick JF, Kiely JM, Harrison EG, et al. Pleural effusion in lymphoma. *Cancer* 1973;31:848–853.

Hajdu SI, Nolan MA. Exfoliative cytology of malignant germ cell tumors. *Acta Cytol.* 1975;19:255–260.

Kapadia SB. Cytological diagnosis of malignant pleural effusion in myeloma. *Arch Pathol. Lab Med* 1977;101:534–535.

Spriggs AI, Vanhegan RI. Cytological diagnosis of lymphoma in serous effusions. *J Clin Pathol.* 1981;34:1311–1325.

Geisinger KR, Hajdu SI, Helson L. Exfoliative cytology of nonlymphoreticular neoplasms in children. *Acta Cytol.* 1984;28:16–28.

Spieler P, Kradolfer D, Schmidt U. Immunocytochemical characterization of lymphocytes in benign and malignant lymphocyte-rich serous effusions. *Virchows Arch [A].* 1986; 409:211–221.

Katz RL, Raval P, Manning JT, et al. A morphologic immunologic and cytometric approach to the classification of non-Hodgkin's lymphoma in effusions. *Diagn Cytopathol.* 1987;3:91.

Sasser RL, Yam LT, Li CY. Myeloma with involvement of the serous cavities. Cytologic and immunochemical diagnosis and literature review. *Acta Cytol.* 1990;34:479–485.

Pigmented Cells

Yamada T, Itou U, Watanabe Y, et al. Cytologic diagnosis of malignant melanoma. *Acta Cytol.* 1972;16:70–76.

Hajdu SI, Savino A: Cytologic diagnosis of malignant melanoma. *Acta Cytol.* 1973;17:320–327.

Weaver KM, Novak PM, Naylor B. Vegetable cell contaminants in cytologic specimens. Their resemblance to cells associated with various normal and pathologic states. *Acta Cytol.* 1981;25:210–214.

Johnston WW, Borowitz MJ, Stuhlmiller GM, et al. Expression of a melanoma tumor-associated antigen as demonstrated by a monoclonal antibody (D.6.1) in cytopathologic preparations of human tumor cells from effusions and needle aspirates. *Anal Quant Cytol Histol.* 1985;7:72.

Walts AE: Malignant melanoma in effusions: A source of false-negative cytodiagnoses. *Diagn Cytopathol* 1986;2:150.

Angeli S, Koelma IA, Fleuren GJ, et al. Malignant melanoma in fine needle aspirates and effusions. An immunocytochemi-

cal study using monoclonal antibodies. *Acta Cytol.* 1988; 32:707–712.

Gibson LE, Goellner JR. Amelanotic melanoma: Cases studied by Fontana stain, S-100 immunostain, and ultrastructural examination. *Mayo Clin Proc.* 1988;63:777–782.

Martinez F, Merenda G, Bedrossian CWM. Fine needle aspiration of a lipid rich metastatic balloon cell melanoma. *Diagn Cytopathol.* 1990;6:427–433.

Pleomorphic Large Cells

Gorshein D, Brauer MJ. Ascites in myeloid metaplasia due to ectopic peritoneal implantation. *Cancer.* 1969;23:1408.

Krause JR, Dekker A. Hairy cell leukemia (leukemia reticuloendotheliosis) in serous effusions. *Acta Cytol.* 1978;22:80.

Vernon SE, Rosenthal DL. Sezary cells in ascitic fluid. *Acta Cytol.* 1979;23:408–411.

Geisinger KR, Naylor B, Beals TF, et al. Cytopathology, including transmission and scanning electron microscopy, of pleomorphic liposarcomas in pleural fluids. *Acta Cytol.* 1980;24:435.

Aozasa K, Kurokawa K, Kabori Y, et al. Malignant histiocytosis showing ascites and recurrent meningeal infiltration. *Acta Cytol.* 1980;24:228–231.

Yam LT. Granulocytic sarcoma with pleural involvement: Identification of neoplastic cells with cytochemistry. *Acta Cytol.* 1985;29:63–66.

Miller RT, Baker KI, Moga D. Multilobated B-cell lymphoma. Report of a case with immunocytologic diagnosis in pleural fluid. *Acta Cytol.* 1987;31:785–790.

Wilson MS, Theil KS, Goodwin RA, et al. Comparison of Papanicolaou's and Wright-Giemsa stains in the examination of body fluids for Hodgkin's disease. *Arch Pathol Lab Med.* 1988;112:612–615.

Multinucleated Giant Cells

Kumar NB, Naylor B. Megakaryocytes in pleural and peritoneal fluids: Prevalence, significance, morphology and cytohistological correlation. *J Clin Pathol.* 1980;33:1153.

Geisinger HR, Naylor B, Beals TF, et al. Cytopathology, including transmission and electron microscopy, of pleomorphic liposarcoma in pleural fluids. *Acta Cytol.* 1980;24:435–441.

Yang H-Y, Weaver LL, Fonti PR. Primary malignant fibrous histiocytoma of the pleura. A case report. *Acta Cytol.* 1983;27:663–687.

Yazdi HM. Cytopathology of extramedullary hemopoiesis in effusions and peritoneal washings. *Diagn Cytopathol.* 1986;2:326.

Bartziota EV, Naylor B. Megakaryocytes in a hemorrhagic pleural effusion caused by anticoagulant overdose. *Acta Cytol.* 1986;30:163.

Silverman JF, Gardner J, Larkin EW, et al. Ascitic fluid cytology in a case of metastatic mixed mesodermal tumor of the ovary. *Acta Cytol.* 1986;30:173.

Satake T, Matsuyama M. Cytologic features of ascites in malignant fibrous histiocytoma of the colon. *Acta Pathol Jpn.* 1988;38:921–928.

Signet Rings

Spriggs AI, Jerome DW. Intracellular mucous inclusions. A feature of malignant cells in effusions in the serous cavities, particularly due to carcinoma of the breast. *J Clin Pathol.* 1975:28:929–936.

Kim H, Dofman RF, Rappaport H. Signet ring lymphoma: A rare morphologic and functional expression of nodular (follicular) lymphoma. *Am J Surg Pathol.* 1978;2:119–132.

Young JA, Crocker J. Pleural fluid cytology in lymphoplasmacytoid lymphoma with numerous intracytoplasmic immunoglobulin inclusions. A case report with immunocytochemistry. *Acta Cytol.* 1984;28:419–424.

Pseudomyxoma Peritonei

Green N, Gancedo H, Smith R, et al. Pseudomyxoma peritonei—nonoperative management and biomedical findings: A case report. *Cancer.* 1975;36:1834–1837.

Rammou-Kinia R, Sirmakechian-Karra T. Pseudomyxoma peritonei and malignant mucocele of the appendix. *Acta Cytol.* 1986;30:169–172.

Solid Cell Balls

Ramsey SJ, Tweeddale DN, Bryant LR, et al. Cytologic features of pericardial mesothelium. *Acta Cytol.* 1970;14:283.

Whitaker D. Cell aggregates in malignant mesothelioma. *Acta Cytol.* 1977;21:236–239.

Carlon G, della Giustina D. Atypical mesothelial cells in peritoneal dialysis fluid. *Acta Cytol.* 1983;27:706.

Spriggs AI. The architecture of tumor cell clusters in serous effusions. In Koss LG, Coleman DV, eds. *Advances in Clinical Cytology,* vol 2. New York: Masson. 1984;267–290.

Carlson GJ, Samuelson JJ, Dehner LP. Cytologic diagnosis of florid peritoneal endosalpingiosis. *Acta Cytol.* 1986;30:494.

Papillary Formations

Julian CG, Woodruff D. The biologic behavior of low-grade papillary serous carcinoma of the ovary. *Obstet Gynecol.* 1972;40:860–867.

Becker SN, Papin DW, Rosenthal DL. Mesothelial papilloma. A case of mistaken identity in a pericardial effusion. *Acta Cytol.* 1976;20:266.

Malkasian GD Jr, Melton LJ, O'Brien PC, et al. Prognostic significance of histologic classification and grading of epithelial malignancies of the ovary. *Am J Obstet Gynecol.* 1984; 149:274–282.

Coffin CM, Adcock LL, Dehner LP. The second-look operation of ovarian neoplasms: A study of 85 cases emphasizing cytologic and histologic problems. *Int J Gynecol Pathol.* 1985;4:97–109.

Rubin SC, Dulaney ED, Markman M, et al. Peritoneal cytology as an indicator of disease in patients with residual ovarian carcinoma. *Obstet Gynecol.* 1988;71:850–853.

Mills SE, Andersen WA, Fechner RE, et al. Serous surface papillary carcinoma. A clinicopathologic study of 10 cases and comparison with stage III–IV ovarian serous carcinoma. *Am J Surg Pathol.* 1988;12:827–834.

Psammoma Bodies

Burmeister RE, Fechner RE, Franklin RR. Endosalpingiosis of the peritoneum. *Obstet Gynecol.* 1969;34:310–318.

Kern WH. Benign papillary structures with psammoma bodies in culdocentesis fluid. *Acta Cytol.* 1969;13:178–180.

Bennington JL, Smith JV, Lagunoff D. Calcification in psammoma bodies of the human meningioma. *Lab Invest.* 1970;22:241–244.

Gupta PK, Verma K. Calcified (psammoma) bodies in alveolar cell carcinoma of lung. *Acta Cytol.* 1972;16:59–62.

Beyer-Boon ME. Psammoma bodies in cervicovaginal smears: An indicator of the presence of ovarian carcinoma. *Acta Cytol.* 1974;18:41–44.

Bauer T, Erozan Y. Psammoma bodies in small cell carcinoma of the lung. *Acta Cytol.* 1982;26:327–330.

Bell DA, Weinstock MA, Scully RE. Peritoneal implants of ovarian serous borderline tumors: Histologic features and prognosis. *Cancer.* 1988;62:2212–2222.

Young OH, Bellingson JL, Papillo JL, et al. Psammoma bodies in peritoneal washings. *Acta Cytol.* 1982;26:233–236.

Covell JL, Carry JB, Feldman PS. Peritoneal washings in ovarian tumors: Potential sources of error in cytologic diagnosis. *Acta Cytol.* 1985;29:310–316.

Nonvacuolated Cell Clusters

Labay GR, Feiner E. Malignant pleural endometriosis. *Am J Obstet Gynecol.* 1971;110:478–480.

Hajdu SI. Exfoliative cytology of primary and metastatic Wilms' tumors. *Acta Cytol.* 1971;15:339.

Farr GH, Hajdu S. Exfoliative cytology of metastatic neuroblastoma. *Acta Cytol.* 1971;16:203–206.

Wilson LM, Kinnier J, Draper GJ. Neuroblastoma, its natural history and prognosis: A study of 487 cases. *Br Med J.* 1974;3:301–307.

Salhadin A, Nasiell M, Nasiell K, et al. The unique cytologic picture of oat cell carcinoma in effusions. *Acta Cytol.* 1976;20:298.

Lozowski W, Hajdu SI, Melamed MR. Cytomorphology of carcinoid tumors. *Acta Cytol.* 1979;23:360–365.

Jobst SB, Ljung B-M, Gilkey FN, et al. Cytologic diagnosis of olfactory neuroblastoma. Report of a case with multiple diagnostic parameters. *Acta Cytol.* 1983;27:299–305.

Yam LT, Winkler CF. Immunocytochemical diagnosis of oat-cell carcinoma in pleural effusion. *Acta Cytol.* 1984;28:425.

Zirkin HJ. Pleural fluid cytology of invasive thymoma. *Acta Cytol.* 1985;29:1011–1014.

Sears D, Hajdu SI. The cytologic diagnosis of malignant neoplasms in pleural and peritoneal effusions. *Acta Cytol.* 1987;31:85–97.

Spriggs AI, Boddington MM. Oat-cell bronchial carcinoma. Identification of cells in pleural fluids. *Acta Cytol.* 1976; 20:525–529.

Akhtar M, Bedrossian CWM, Ali MA, et al. Fine-needle aspiration biopsy of pediatric neoplasms: Correlation between electron microscopy and immunocytochemistry in diagnosis and classification. *Diagn Cytopathol.* 1992;8:258–265.

Vacuolated Cell Clusters

Woyke S, Domagala W, Olszewski W. Alveolar cell carcinoma of the lung: An ultrastructural study of the cancer cells detected in the pleural fluid. *Acta Cytol.* 1972;16:63–69.

Tsukamoto N, Matsukuma K, Diamauru Y, et al. Cytologic presentation of ovarian adenosquamous carcinoma in ascitic fluid. A case report. *Acta Cytol.* 1984;28:703–705.

Kobayashi TK, Teraoka S, Tsujioka T, et al. Ciliated ovarian adenocarcinoma cells in ascitic fluid cytology: Report of a case with immunocytochemical features. *Diagn Cytopathol.* 1988;4:234–238.

Roncalli M, Gribaudi G, Simoncelli D, et al. Cytology of yolk-sac tumor of the ovary in ascitic fluid. Report of a case. *Acta Cytol.* 1988;32:113–116.

Free-floating Acini

Spriggs AI. The architecture of tumor cell clusters in serous effusions. In Koss LG, Coleman DV. eds. *Advances in Clinical Cytology,* vol 2. New York: Masson. 1984:267–290.

Sneige N, Fernandez T, Copeland LJ, et al. Mullerian inclusions in peritoneal washings. Potential source of error in cytologic diagnosis. *Acta Cytol.* 1986;30:271.

Tall Columnar Fronds

Whitaker D, Shilkin KB. Diagnosis of pleural malignant mesothelioma in life—a practical approach. *J Pathol.* 1984; 143:147.

Cobb CJ, Wynn J, Cobb SR, et al. Cytologic findings in an effusion caused by rupture of a benign cystic teratoma of the mediastinum into a serous cavity. *Acta Cytol.* 1985;29: 1015–1020.

Indian File

Naylor B. The elimination of ribbing effect in cytologic smears. *Am J Clin Pathol.* 1958;30:143–144.

Ashton PR, Hollingsworth AS Jr, Johnston WW. The cytopathology of metastatic breast cancer. *Acta Cytol.* 1975;19:1–6.

Yazdi HM, Hajdu SI, Melamed MR. Cytopathology of pericardial effusion. *Acta Cytol.* 1980;24:401–406.

Spriggs AI. The architecture of tumor cell clusters in serous effusions. In Koss LG, Coleman DV, eds. *Advances in Clinical Cytology,* vol 2. New York: Masson. 1984:267–290.

Spindle Cells

Hong S: The exfoliative cytology of endometrial stromal sarcoma in peritoneal fluid. *Acta Cytol.* 1981;25:277.

Nguyen G-K, Jeannot A: Cytology of synovial sarcoma metastases in pleural fluid. *Acta Cytol.* 1982;62:517.

Gaba AR, Fine G, Raju UB. Malignant angioendothelioma. Cytologic, histologic and ultrastructural findings. *Acta Cytol.* 1983;27:76–80.

Effusions of Cryptic Origin

Light RW, Erozan YS, Ball WC. Cells in pleural fluid. Their value in differential diagnosis. *Arch Intern Med* 1973; 132:854–860.

Bakalos D, Constantakis N, Tsicricas T. Recognition of malignant cells in pleural and peritoneal effusions. *Acta Cytol.* 1974;18:118–121.

Dines DE, Pierre RV, Franzen SI. The value of cells in the pleural fluid in the differential diagnosis. *Mayo Clin Proc.* 1975;50:571–572.

Wuerker RB, Guglietti LC, Nations ED. Comparison of light and transmission electron microscopy for the evaluation of body cavity effusions. *Acta Cytol.* 1983;27:614–624.

Yam LT, Lin DG, Janckila AJ, et al. Immunocytochemical diagnosis of lymphoma in serous effusions. *Acta Cytol.* 1985;29:833–841.

Bedrossian CWM. Immunocytochemistry. In Astarita R, ed. *Practical Cytopathology,* New York: Churchill-Livingstone. 1990:403–457.

CHAPTER FOURTEEN

Electron Microscopy

The greatest limitation of electron microscopy (EM) is the small size of the sample. If the sample is not representative, it virtually negates any advantage gained by the high magnification afforded by EM. However, sampling error can be minimized by light microscopic evaluation of the plastic-embedded cell blocks. Great morphologic detail can be appreciated in the thick sections prepared from these cell blocks, in particular: the configuration of cell surfaces, the size and shape of secretory granules, the distribution of accumulated substances in the cytoplasm, and the presence of intracytoplasmic lumina. Careful correlation between light microscopy and transmission electron microscopy (TEM) has proved most useful in (1) the distinction between mesothelioma and adenocarcinoma; (2) the distinction between lymphoid and epithelial malignancies; (3) the differential diagnosis of small, round, blue cell tumors; (4) the identification of certain types of adenocarcinomas; and (5) the separation of nonepithelial tumors into various categories of sarcoma. Scanning electron microscopy (SEM) has a somewhat more limited applicability but has been used to study solid and hemopoietic tumors. SEM is most useful to (1) distinguish between epithelial cells, mesothelial cells, and macrophages; (2) recognize certain types of lymphoid neoplasms; and (3) distinguish between certain types of adenocarcinomas. Less frequently, EM has been used in the study of benign, inflammatory, and infectious conditions accompanied by effusions in the serous cavities. Neither TEM nor SEM are very useful in establishment of a malignant diagnosis, even though there are some reliable ultrastructural hallmarks of malignant transformation. The impediment for using ultrastructural features to diagnose malignancy derives from the fact that the sample may not contain the crucial cellular elements. Once the malignant diagnosis is established by classic cytology, however, EM has an important role in the classification of neoplasms.

Malignant effusions are ideally suited for ultrastructural examination. Not only do they contain a large number of cells, but also they are often composed of a single cell population. The cells are protected from degeneration by the nutrients in the effusion, which also allow for cellular multiplication and renewal. In addition, tumor cells are easily contrasted against the background of mesothelial cells, which are rather unique and easy to discern with ultrastructural examination. When used in combination with immunocytochemistry, EM becomes a powerful tool for identification of the primary site of metastatic neoplasms. Tumor cells may display distinctive ultrastructural features, including intercellular junctions, surface specializations, cytoplasmic and secretory peculiarities of the cytoplasm, as well as nuclear alterations (Table 14.1). Some of these ultrastructural features are more helpful than others. Accordingly, EM has emerged as a crucial diagnostic tool in certain types of tumors, such as neuroendocrine neoplasms, malignant mesothelioma, and sarcomas of various degrees of differentiation. The differential diagnosis between spindle-cell carcinomas and sarcomas is also helped by EM, whereas the method is not as critical in separating the various types of carcinomas. However, even in patients in whom cytomorphology and immunocytochemistry have already identified the primary site, EM can elucidate the nature of the cytologic features observed by light microscopy.

BENIGN CONDITIONS

As with other areas of cytopathology, the tendency exists to overlook benign conditions when examining serous effusions by cytologic means. The euphemistic designation ''reactive'' is nearly worthless when applied to the interpretation of effusions. Because exfoliation of

TABLE 14.1 Assessment of Malignant Cells
by Ultrastructural Analysis

Intercellular relationships
    Basal and external lamina
    Desmosomes and desmosome-like structures
    Tight junctions and terminal bars
    Subplasmalemmal linear densities
Surface specializations
    Straight and interdigitated boundaries
    Microvilli and their core rootlets
    Glycocalyceal bodies
    Brush border
    Cytoplasmic processes
Nuclear features
    Nuclear size and shape
    Nuclear contour, grooves and pockets
    Intranuclear inclusion bodies
    Heterochromatin and euchromatin
    Chromatin margination
    Nucleolar number, size, and shape
Cytoplasmic characteristics
    Glycogen and lipid deposits
    Rough endoplasmic reticulum
    Mitochondria size and appearance
    Prominence of the golgi complex
    Lysosomes and secretory granules
    Intracytoplasmic lumina
    Distribution of cytoskeletal filaments

mesothelial cells will not occur in the absence of fluid accumulation, these cells are always reactive if not malignant when encountered in effusions. Unfortunately, EM contributes little to recognition of the benign nature of mesothelial cells, even though quiescent are less rich in microvilli than their malignant counterparts (Fig. 14.1). Ultrastructural studies are useful in the demonstration of cytoplasmic contents in mesothelial cells. The amount of glycogen, lipid and hyaluronic acid is not a good criterion to distinguish benign from malignant mesothelial cells. Benign mesothelial cells differ from their malignant counterparts mainly by their nuclear features and the sparsity of microvilli on their surface (Table 14.2). Quiescent mesothelial cells display bland, round nuclei with a smooth contour and may totally lack microvilli. The cytoplasm is rich in intermediate filaments, particularly surrounding the immediate perinuclear area (Fig. 14.2). Reactive mesothelial cells begin to sprout microvilli and often display glycogen vacuoles beneath the cell membrane. These cells also show blebs amidst their microvilli which contribute to the empty appearance of windows between mesothelial cells (Fig.

14.3). As mesothelial cells become more reactive, the microvilli cover a greater portion of their surface area and the windows between them is more pronounced. (Fig. 14.4). The more reactive the cells, the longer and more complex the microvilli are on their surface. As mesothelial hyperplasia progresses, so does their tendency to clasp one another and form scalloped cell groups (Fig. 14.5). This inability to intimately mold, is the hall-mark of mesothelial cells, observable even in doublets of reactive cells (Fig. 14.6).

The SEM electron micrographs in this chapter (provided by Dr. Gonzalez-Devesa) illustrate the application of this method in the study of serous effusions. Both TEM and SEM have been utilized to demonstrate microorganisms, such as viruses, fungi, and protozoa, in cytologic specimens, but very seldom in effusion samples. We have observed cytomegalovirus in the pericardial fluid of a renal transplant patient; Katz observed *Varicella* in pleural fluid; the diagnosis was confirmed by immunocytochemistry. *Pneumocystis carinii* has now been observed in pleural, peritoneal, and pericardial fluid. Correlation of TEM and SEM findings assists in elucidating the characteristics of these yeast-like fungi, which have long been misinterpreted as protozoa. Hidvegi illustrated histiocytes engulfing lymphocytes and the beginnings of the lupus erythematosus phenomenon in the pleural fluid of a patient with systemic lupus erythematosus. As illustrated in chapter 5, Geisinger documented the origin of spindle and giant cells in rheumatoid arthritis by correlating TEM and SEM findings with the cytologic appearance of the same cells in pleural fluid.

MALIGNANT TUMORS

A peculiar phenomenon noted in tumor cells is alterations of the cell surface that accompany neoplastic transformation. Tumor cells also alter their intercellular relationships, often with loss of junctions or penetration of the surrounding base or lamina. The cytoskeleton of malignant cells is also quite different from their benign counterpart. Profound changes of the intermediate filaments take place in tumors undergoing different types of differentiation. Classifying carcinomas depends on the variable nature of their accumulated secretory products, which lend themselves well to ultrastructural identification. A number of nuclear criteria of malignancy are well demonstrated by EM, including enlarged nuclear size, increased nuclear to cytoplasm (N/C) ratio, nuclear pleomorphism, irregular distribution of hetero-

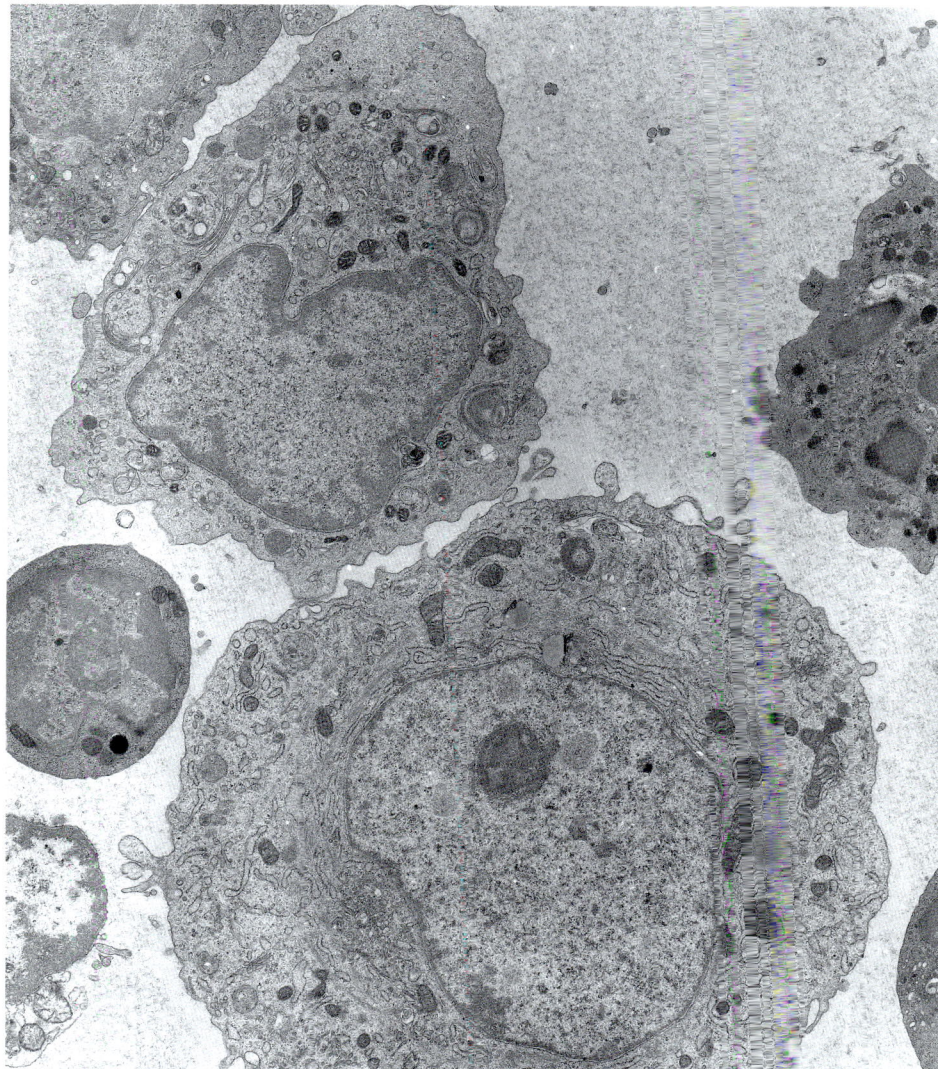

FIGURE 14.1   Quiescent mesothelial cells. Notice absence of microvilli on the cell surface. The cytoplasm contains sparse organelles including lipid droplets and mitochondria. (EM× 10,000)

chromatin, prominent nucleolization, peripheral chromatin clumping, and increased mitotic rate. In addition, certain subsets of neoplasms may exhibit special nuclear features of malignancy, such as persistent nucleoli that fail to disappear during mitosis; intranuclear annulate lamellae; and a variety of nuclear bodies, including ring-shaped nucleoli, "zebra" bodies, and intranuclear rodlets. Nucleolar abnormalities demonstrated by EM correlate well with high counts of silver impregnation of nuclear organizing regions (AgNOR) of malignant cells. In malignant lymphomas, the nuclear membrane is rather irregular (i.e., blebbing, protrusions, and

pockets), but these changes are also noted in atypical lymphocytes. In general, nuclear criteria of malignancy are unreliable at the ultrastructural level. This is particularly noticeable in mesotheliomas where nuclei can be extremely bland (Fig. 14.7)

INTERCELLULAR RELATIONSHIPS

When cells exfoliate in an effusion, they lose their involucrum of basal and external lamina, even though bits

TABLE 14.2   Ultrastructural Distinction Between Benign and Malignant Mesothelial Cells

	Benign Mesothelial Cells	Malignant Mesothelial Cells
Cell surface	Sparse, blunt cytoplasmic projections	Florid, slender, elongated microvilli
Cytoplasm	Paranuclear intermediate filaments; clusters of glycogen granules; no mucus, minimal lipid	Intermediate filaments; glycogen granules and vacuoles; absent mucus; variable amount of lipid
Nuclei	Oral or round shape; regular contour	Irregular shape; deep cerebriform indentations

of basement membrane—like material may occasionally be seen ultrastructurally on the surface of tumor cells suspended in malignant effusions. A mesh represented by myoepithelial cells is wrapped around epithelial cell groups and is frequently noted in benign fine-needle aspirates, but we have not observed it in cell groups present in effusions. Malignant cells have low concentrations of fibronectin, a surface glycoprotein that promotes cellular adhesion among nontransformed cells. This finding may explain distant metastasis and migration of malignant cells. A helpful aid in identifying and classifying tumor cells is observation of various types of cell-to-cell junctions on the surface of malignant cells. The type of junction connecting neighboring cells represents the basis of subclassifying epithelial neoplasms

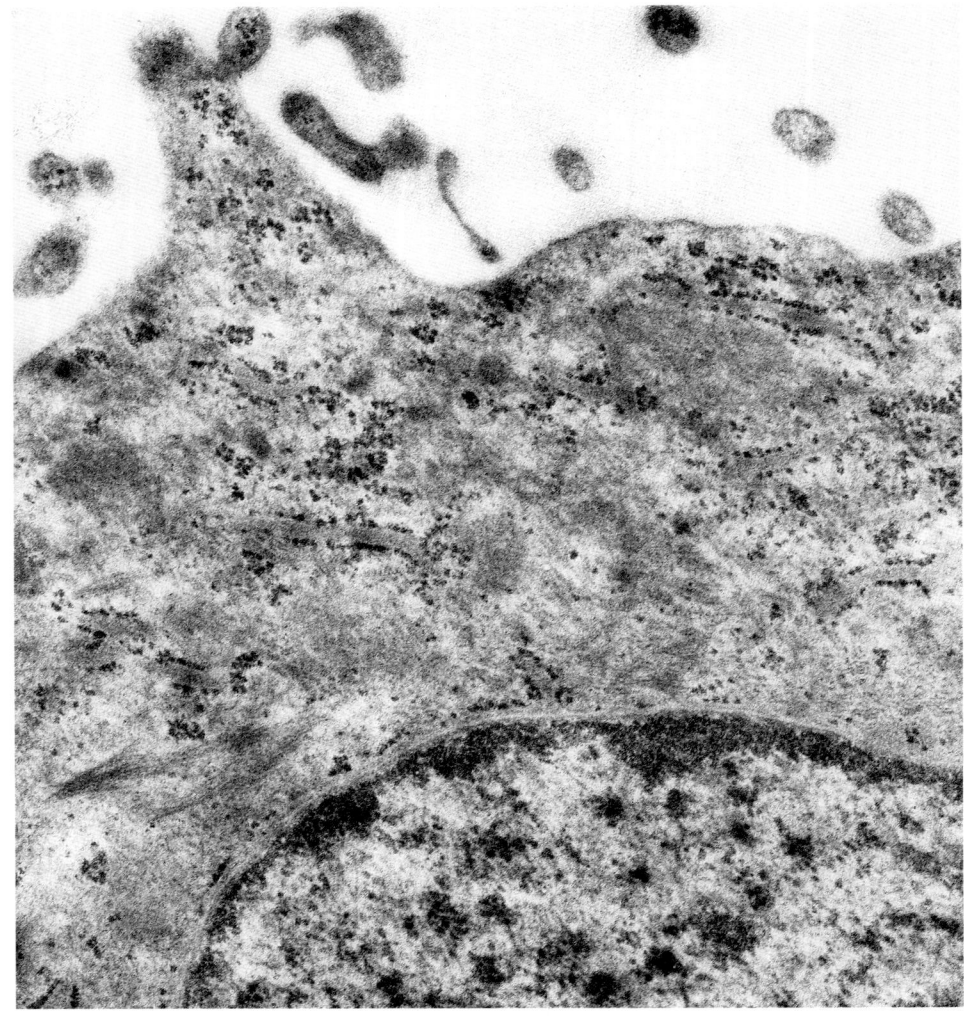

FIGURE 14.2   Detail of cytoplasm of quiescent mesothelial cell. Notice abundant intermediate filaments, glycogen particles and dilated endoplasmic reticulum. (EM × 36,000)

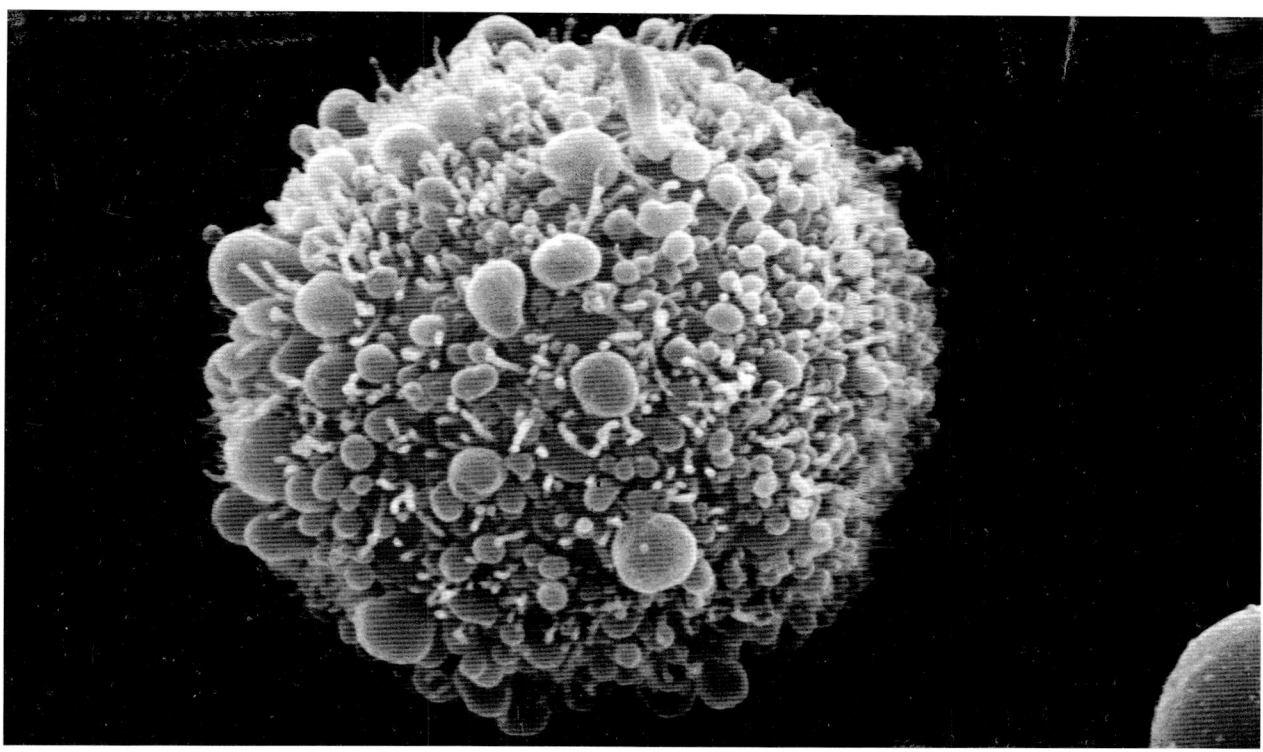

FIGURE 14.3 Reactive mesothelial cell. The surface of the cell is covered by numerous blebs and sparse microvilli (SEM× 2,500)

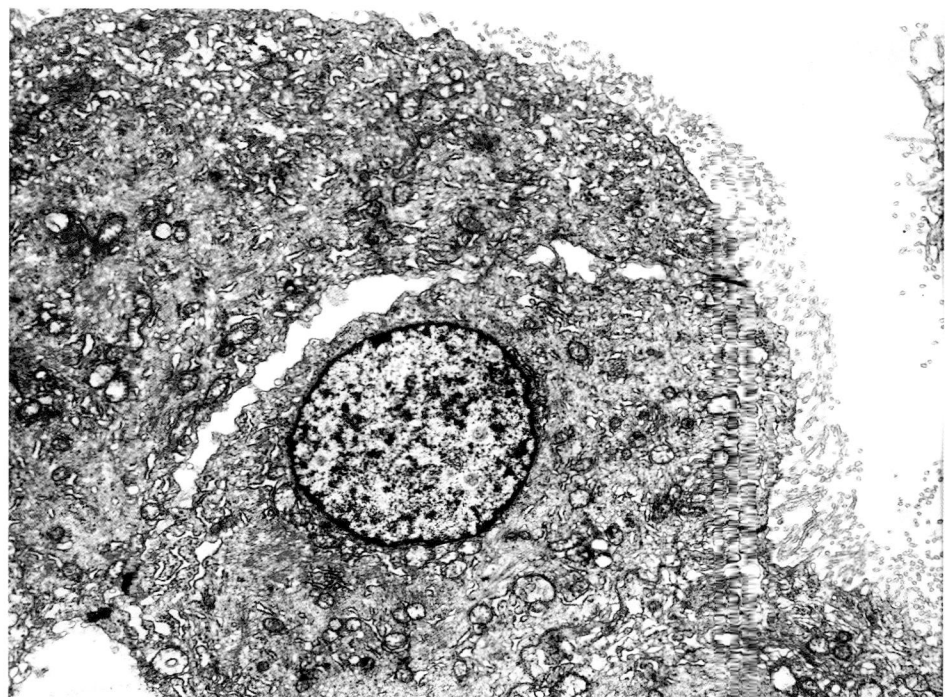

FIGURE 14.4 Doublet of reactive mesothelial cells. One cell attempts to clasp another but leaves a narrow slit between the two cells, (EM× 12,000) (Courtesy Dr. J. Reilova)

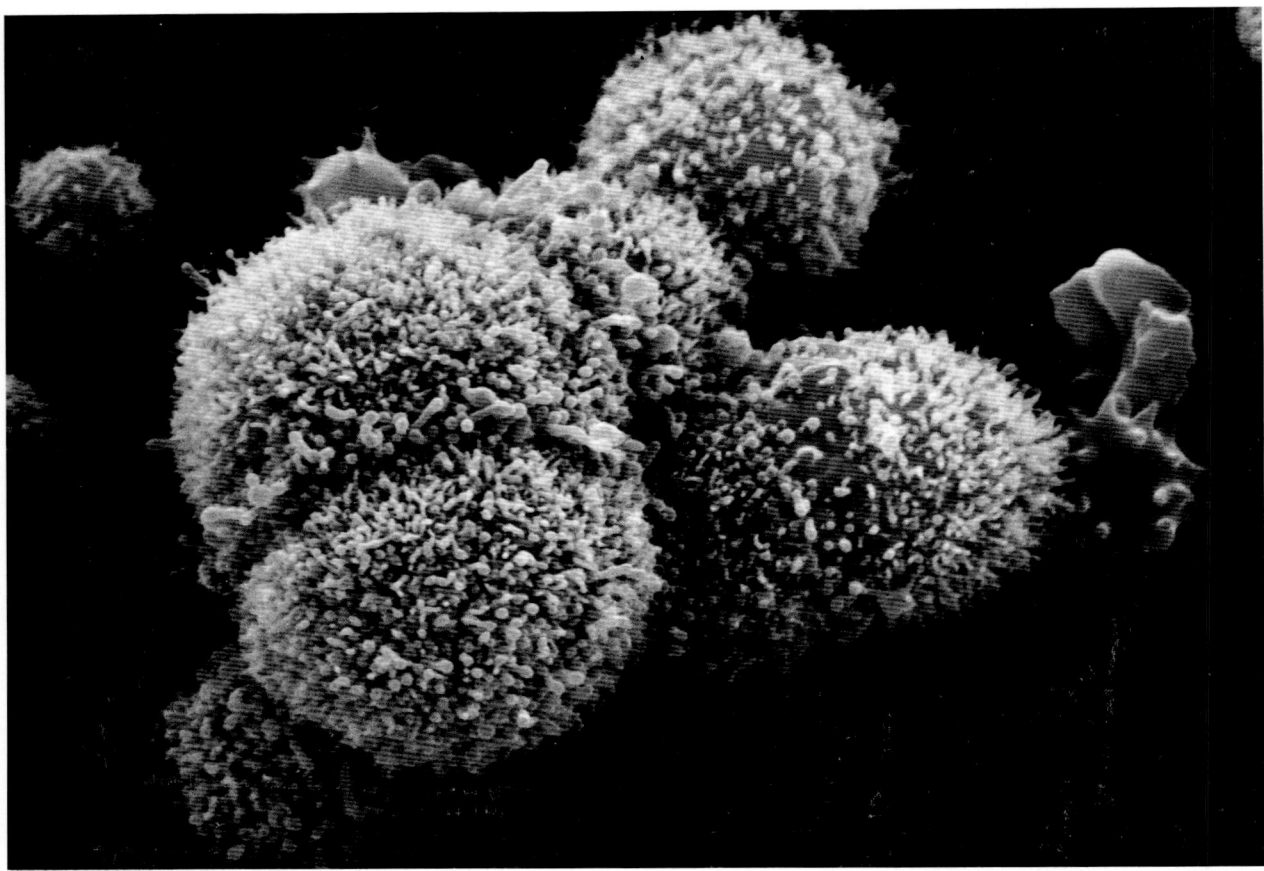

FIGURE 14.5 Group of reactive mesothelial cells with attempted clasping. Notice the gaps created between adjacent cells (SEM × 1,250)

into squamous, adenocarcinomatous, and undifferentiated categories.

Clusters and sheets of cells in effusions are helpful in the study of cell-to-cell junctions. These structures have been extensively studied in neoplasms, and clearly defined ultrastructural criteria exist for the various types of interconnecting devices. Malignant epithelial cells exfoliated in effusions are rich in intercellular junctions. These structures are responsible for the strong cell-to-cell cohesion noted in cellular groupings of metastatic carcinomas. Spriggs has studied this phenomenon and illustrated the architectural relationship of neoplastic epithelial in contrast to mesothelial cells. Carcinomas shed cohesive groups of cells arranged as cell balls, microacini, tandems or mosaic-like sheets. Cell balls range from very tight structures to looser groups that still maintain molding between individual cells. Not infrequently, a combination of groupings is noted in the same sample such as cell balls and tandems in adenocarcinoma. The mosaic-like pattern is possible because the cell-to-cell contact in epithelial cells is often through straight cell membranes connected by tight junctions. This intimate contact between the cells leads to flat areas shared by several neighbours (Fig. 14.8). Adenocarcinomatous cells may also demonstrate interdigitating cell membranes connected by desmosomes. Near their apical pole, adenocarcinomatous cells are connected to one another by terminal bars. Desmosomes or desmosome-like junctions are characteristic of epithelial neoplasms found in squamous-cell carcinomas, adenocarcinomas of various sites, urothelial carcinomas, and epithelial thymomas. Desmosomes are also found in Ewing's sarcomas, pheochromocytomas, chordomas, meningiomas, synovial sarcomas, and neuroendocrine neoplasms.

Mesotheliomas show a combination of structures in

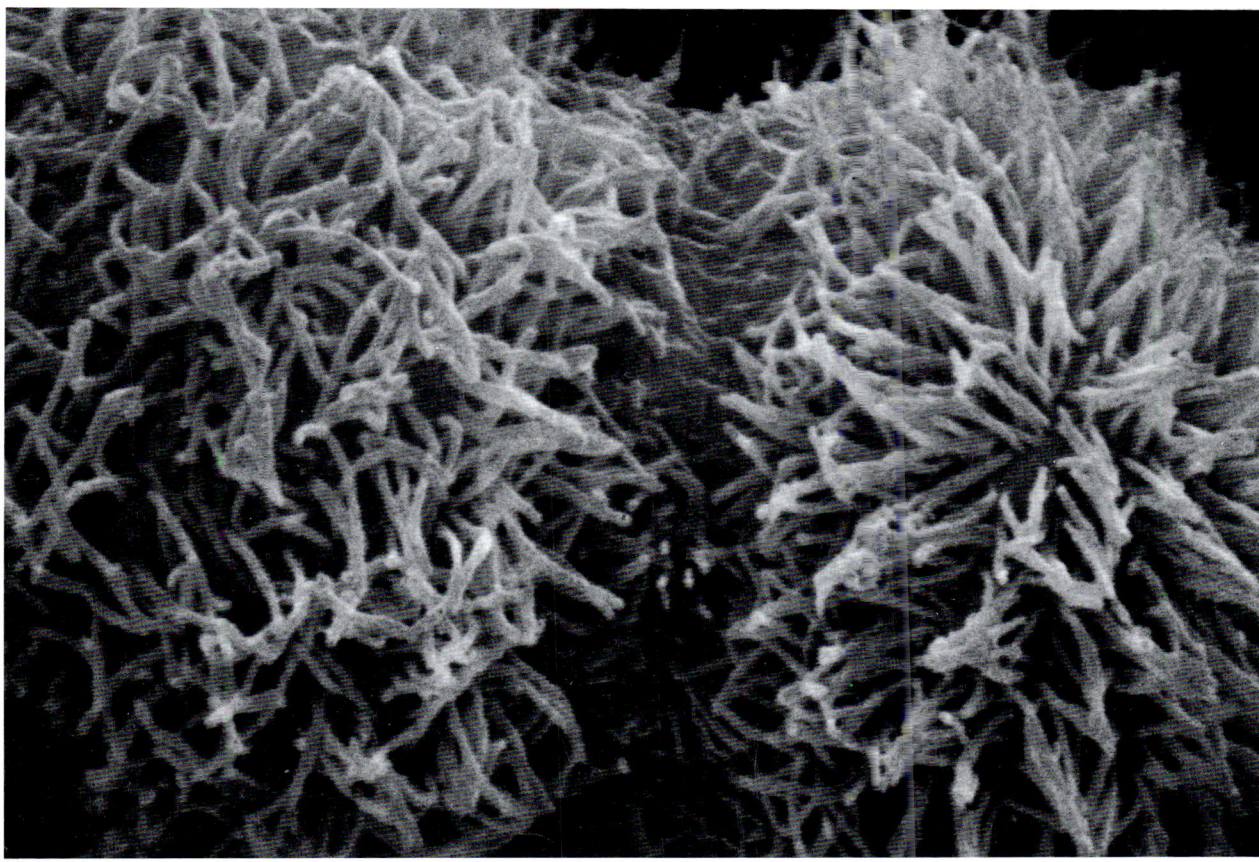

FIGURE 14.6   Doublet of cells from mesothelioma. The ridge between the cells is traversed by microvilli and corresponds the windows seen by light microscopy. Notice microvilli stuck to one another near their tips. (SEM × 2800)

their junctional complexes, including desmosomes, tight junctions, and interspersed gap junctions. However, the microvilli on the surface of mesotheliomatous cells do not allow their close juxtaposition (Figs. 14.9 and 14.10). Even when large cells appear to create a relatively flat area on the boundary a cluster, other smaller cells project above its surface (Fig. 14.11). The desmosomes of mesothelioma are indistinguishable from those of adenocarcinoma. However, some authors have observed a high frequency of desmosomes that are longer than usual in mesothelioma. Tight junctions are typical of adenocarcinomas; they are often associated with rudimentary desmosomes near the apex of the tumor cells and well-formed terminal bars. Tumors with prominent abluminal terminal bars and a profuse microvilli are almost invariably adenocarcinomas. In the absence of microvilli, however, tight junctions have been seen in a variety of other tumors, such as vasoformative neo-

plasms (i.e., lymphangiomas, angiosarcomas, and hemangioperacytomas), as well as synovial sarcomas, transitional cell tumors, and meningiomas.

The absence of cell junctions is a very significant ultrastructural feature in effusions. In small, round, blue cell tumors, this picture is highly suggestive of lymphoma or leukemia. Theoretically, however, a very poorly differentiated carcinoma may have no readily evident cell junctions. Sarcomas may also have cell-to-cell junctions, such as Ewing's sarcomas, epithelioid sarcomas, synovial sarcomas, and chordomas, which can be differentiated from carcinomas by immunocytochemistry. Both lymphomas and sarcomas may present with condensation of the plasma membrane, known as subplasmalemmal linear densities, which should not be confused with tight junctions or desmosomes. Similar condensations have been described in Ewing's sarcomas, alveolar soft-part sarcomas, leiomyomas, leio-

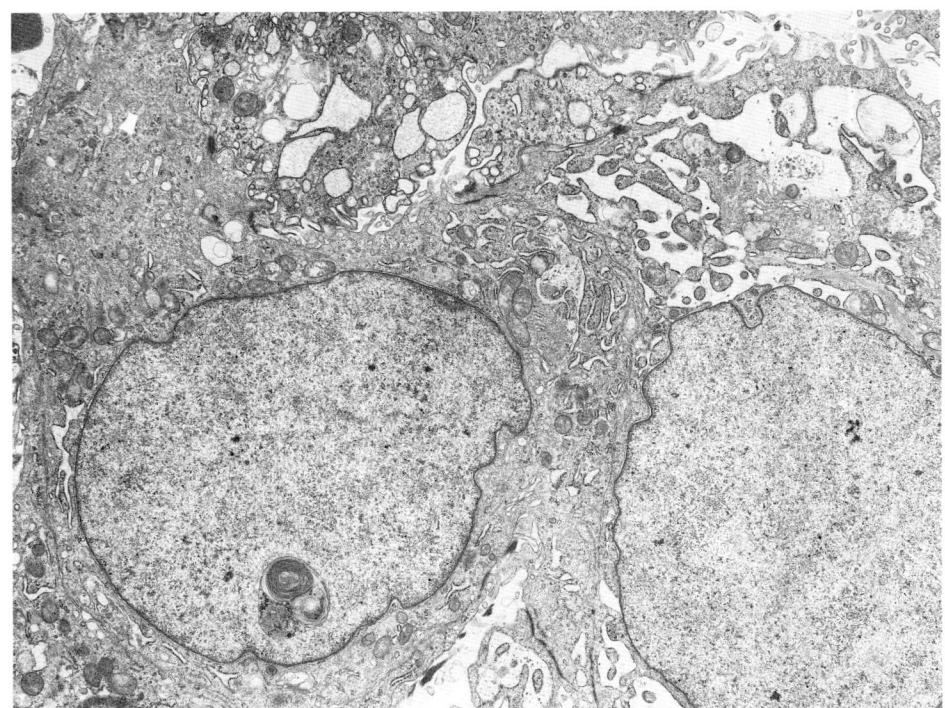

FIGURE 14.7 Adjacent cells from mesothelioma. Notice bland appearing nuclei with smooth nuclear envelope and evenly dispersed chromatinic material. A cytoplasmic pseudoinclusion containing lipid protrudes through one of the nuclei. (EM × 48,000)

myoblastomas, rhabdomyosarcomas, Schwannomas, malignant fibrocystis cytomas, and neuroblastomas.

SURFACE SPECIALIZATIONS

Mesothelial cells are unique because they are covered with copious amounts of microvilli along the entire perimeter of the cell surface. The microvilli are characterized by complex intertwining and considerable overlap reflected at the light microscopic level by dense staining with either histochemical or immunocytochemical methods. With the May-Grunwald-Giemsa stain, mesothelial cells demonstrate a rim of pink apron-like spikes. The microvilli are not as noticeable with the Pap stain, but occasionally one may appreciate a fuzzy rim blending with the peripheral vacuoles typical of mesothelial cells (Fig. 14.12). At the ultrastructural level, the fuzzy border correspond to the bushy microvilli, each of which is extremely elongated and has a very narrow

cross-sectional diameter (Fig. 14.13). Intermixed with the microvilli one may see the bleb-like protrusions containing glycogen with similar ultrastructural appearance as the peripheral vacuoles (Fig. 14.14). These microvilli measure up to 50 nm long, but are no more than 4 nm wide even though they may end in bulbous tips (Fig. 14.15). By TEM microfilaments run the length of the microvilli but they lack a glycocalyx (Fig. 14.16). The most dramatic expression of the microvillous profusion of mesothelial cells is the so-called thick membrane pattern of immunostaining for epithelial membrane antigen (EMA) by mesotheliomas. This strong apical membrane positivity is sufficient to separate mesotheliomas from adenocarcinomas, which also give a linear pattern of positive staining in addition to a more diffuse positive EMA stage of the cytoplasm.

SEM is ideally suited to illustrate the surface characteristics of adenocarcinomatous cells often found in clusters (Fig. 14.17). Depending on the number of cells, rather large or small groups are formed but the gaps beween cells are considerably narrower than between

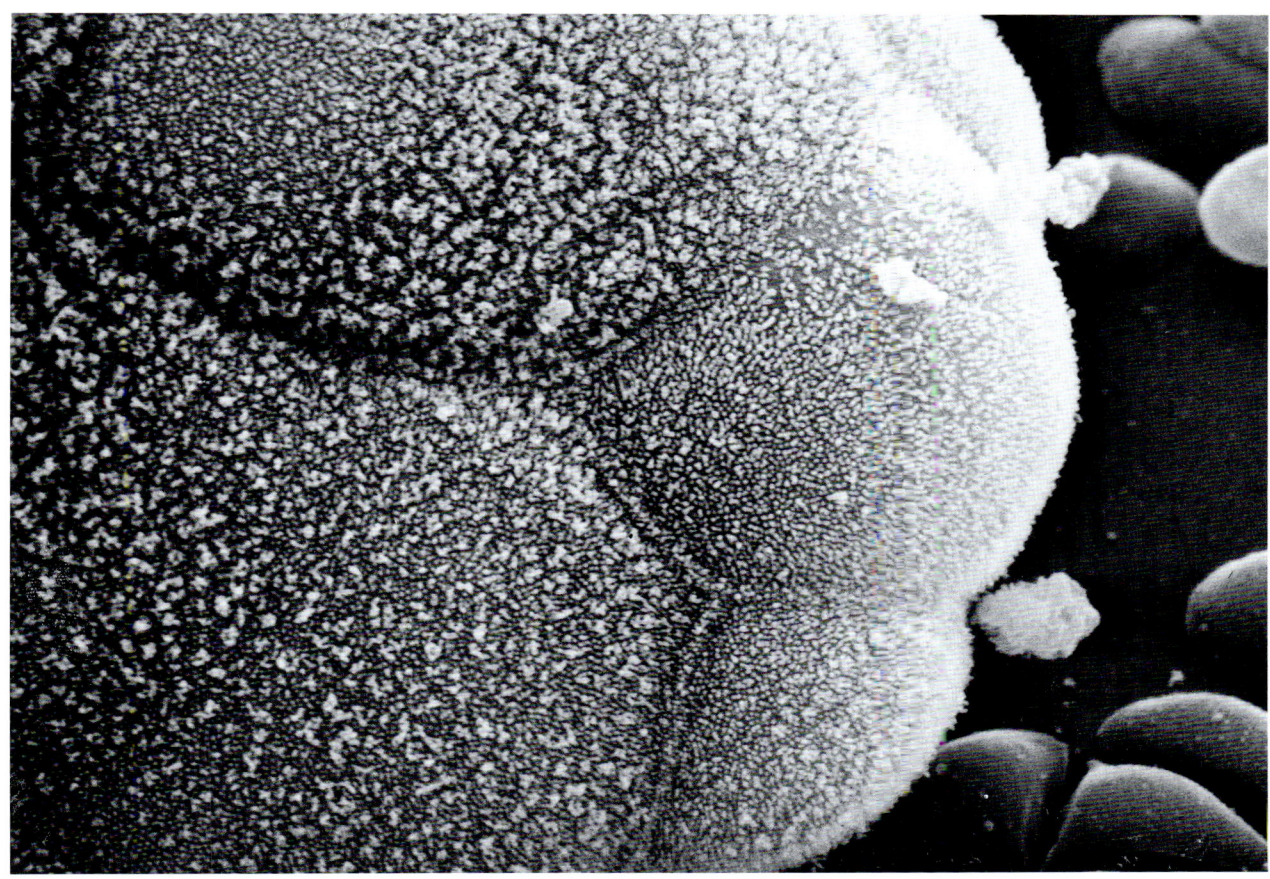

FIGURE 14.8 Flat community border shared by cells from breast carcinoma. The microvilli are short and there is virtually no space between adjacent cells (SEM × 2,500)

mesothelial cells (Fig. 14.18). In contrast to mesothelial cells, adenocarcinomatous cells may connect either with straight membranes or interdigitating cytoplasmic processes. These cells lack the wide intercellular spaces or windows noted between mesothelial cells. The surface of adenocarcinomatous cells varies from neoplasm to neoplasm. Most are covered by short to medium-length microvilli, but these may be attenuated in cytologic samples (Fig. 14.19). By SEM, the microvilli extend over the entire surface of the cells but do not interfere with their close contact (Fig. 14.20). Both TEM and SEM are helpful in distinguishing the various neoplasms, based on the length and the density of their microvillous projections. Table 14.3 lists various neoplasms according to the characteristics of their microvilli, which are roughly classifiable into (1) microvilli with filamentous cores and glycocalyceal bodies, typical of intestinal type adenocarcinomas and moderate in length; (2) microvilli without core rootlets and without glycocalyceal bodies that are short and are represented by adenocarcinomas arising in sites other than the aerodigestive tract; and (3) microvilli with glycocalyceal bodies without filamentous cores, variable in length, and typical of certain carcinomas and nonepithelial neoplasms.

Tumors of the gastrointestinal trace have very long rootlets, and show glycocalyceal bodies along the microvilli and near the cell surface (Fig. 14.21). Other tumors showing this so-called intestinal type of microvilli include the ovary, the pancreas, the gallbladder, the lung, and the bladder. Nonintestinal type microvilli are associated with adenocarcinomas originating in the breast, the thyroid, the prostate, the kidney, and the liver. Lymphocytes have microvilli on their surfaces that may become rather prominent during malignant trans-

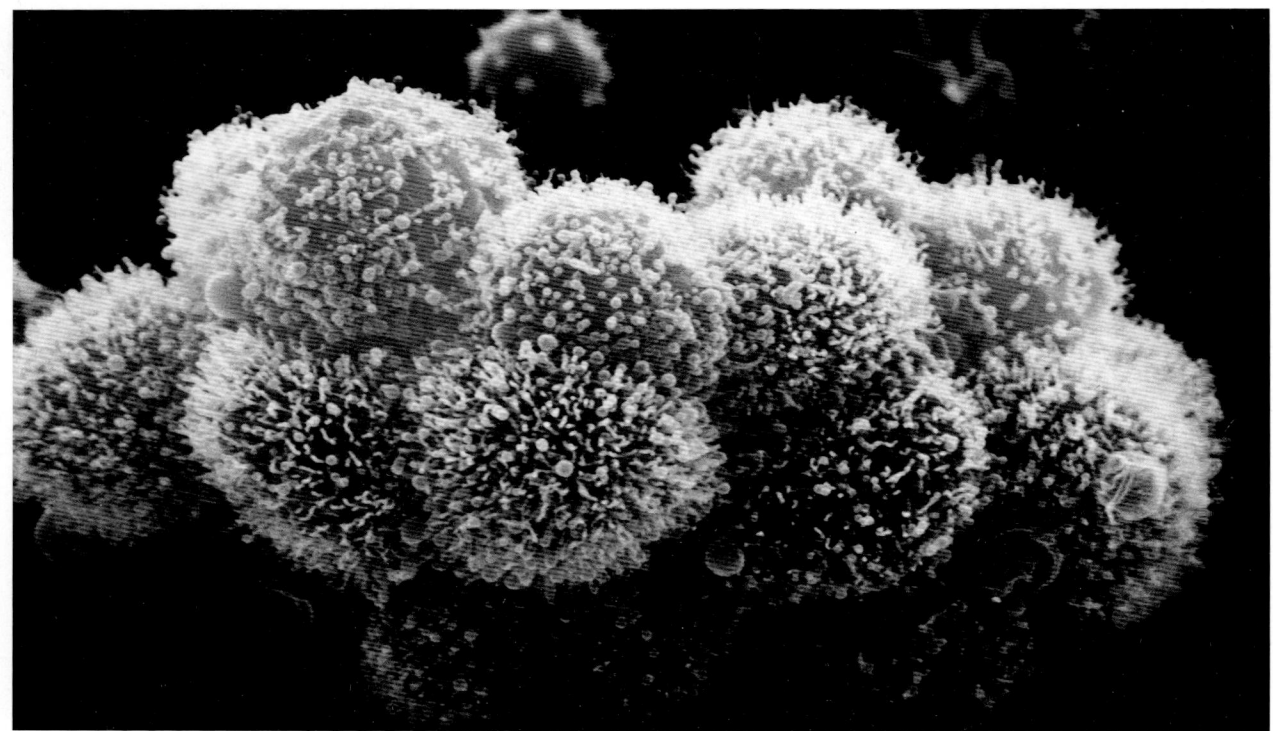

FIGURE 14.9   Reactive group of mesothelial cells. The scalloped contour is characteristic of mesotheliomatous groupings. (SEM× 1,200)

formation, as is noted in hairy-cell leukemias. In general, malignant cells lack cilia, but ciliated malignant cells have been observed in ovarian and pulmonary carcinomas. Neurogenic tumors present with cytoplasmic processes that can be very long and interdigitating, as in neuroblastoma.

ULTRASTRUCTURAL CORRELATES OF EPITHELIAL DIFFERENTIATION

Malignant transformation leads to the appearance of new cellular products, including oncofetal antigens, differentiation antigens, tumor-associated antigens, and virus-associated antigens, all of which can be detected by immunocytochemistry. The effect of oncogenes may result in accumulation of abnormal gene products, which can also be detected by immunocytochemistry. These abnormal antigens are rarely visible by EM. A

much more rewarding application of EM is the search for abnormal substances secreted or accumulated in tumor cells as a result of malignant transformation. These products form the basis of a cytologist's ability to classify or gauge the degree of differentiation of neoplastic cells from the observation of the cytoplasmic contents.

Glycogen

Virtually all neoplasms contain glycogen, but a large amount of glycogen is characteristic of seminomas; adenocarcinomas of the kidney, the cervix, and the lung; and rhabdomyosarcomas. Minimal or absent glycogen is characteristic of carcinomas of the breast, the pancreas, and the gastrointestinal tract. In contrast, mesothelial cells contain moderate to large amounts of glycogen demonstrable with the PAS stain followed by diastase digestion. The peripheral vacuolization of mesotheliomatous cells is not seen in any other glycogen-

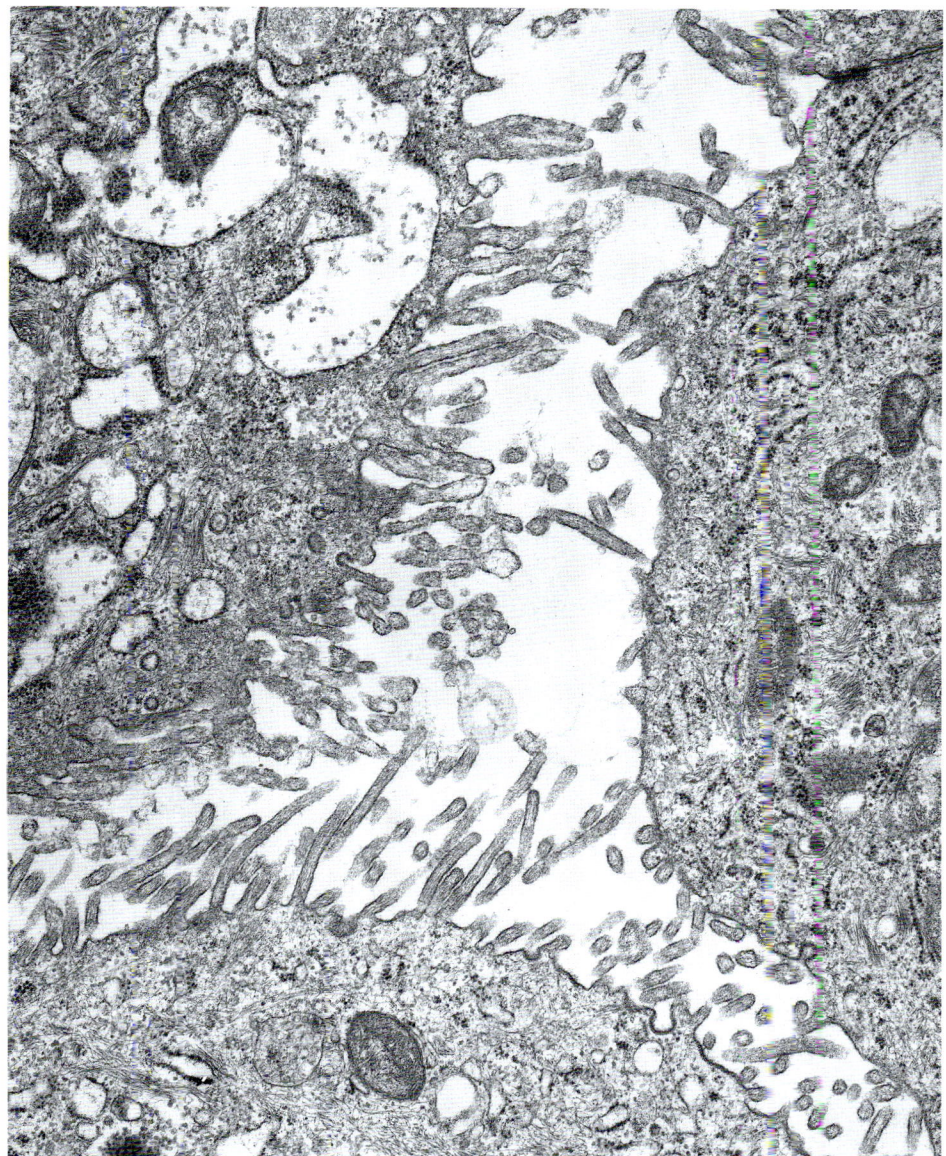

FIGURE 14.10 Semi-triangular intercellular space between mesotheliomatous cells. The space is traversed by microvilli cut tangentially and longitudinally. Notice a clear bleb at right center. (EM × 52,000)

containing neoplasm. Ultrastructurally, the clear spaces correspond to glycogen and dilated vesicles of E.R. Most of the glycogen is in its free form; it has a tendency to leak out into the fixative solution so that glycogen-rich tumors often have a clear-cell appearance on light microscopy. The glycogen content of tumor cells may be so great that the cells may raise above their neigh-bors, resulting in the typical peg-like configuration of clear-cell neoplasms.

Secretory Granules

Secretory granules may run the entire gamut of electron density, ranging from virtually electron-lucent to ex-

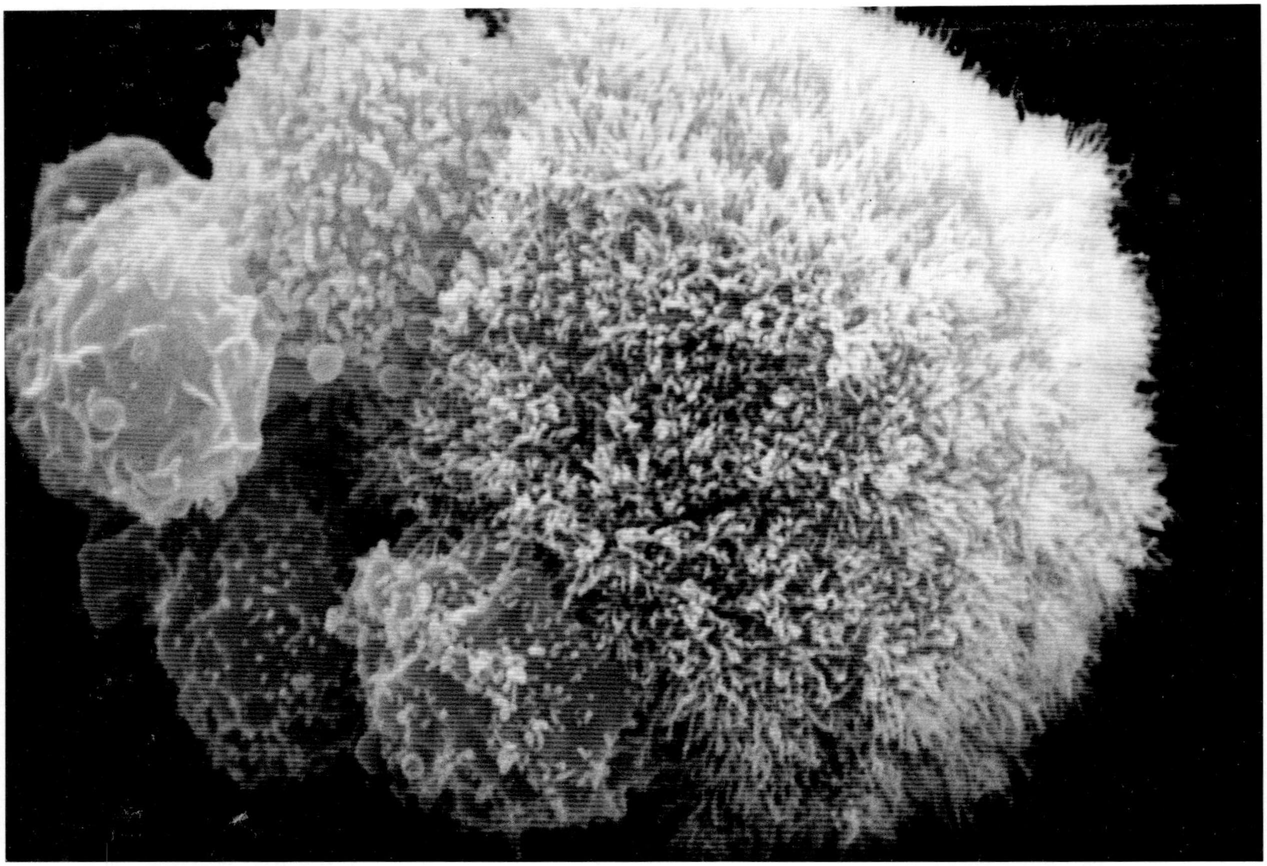

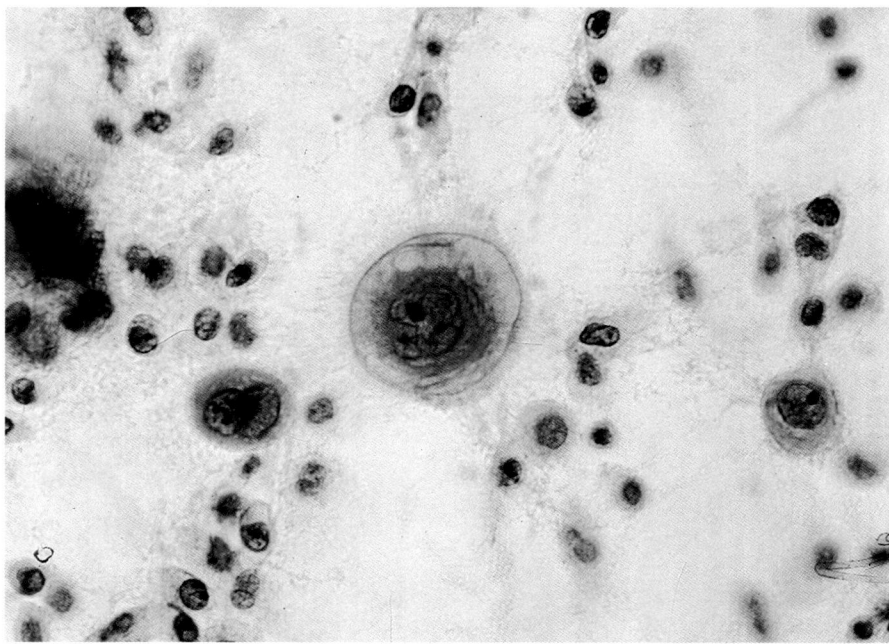

FIGURE 14.11 Large group of cells from mesothelioma. Their surface is covered by microvilli while the cytoplasm projects into large protrusions and small blebs. (SEM× 2,400)

FIGURE 14.12 Malignant mesothelioma cells in pleural effusion. Light microscopy shows peripherally situated vacuoles. Notice also a crown of microvilli on the surface of the cell. (Pap× 800)

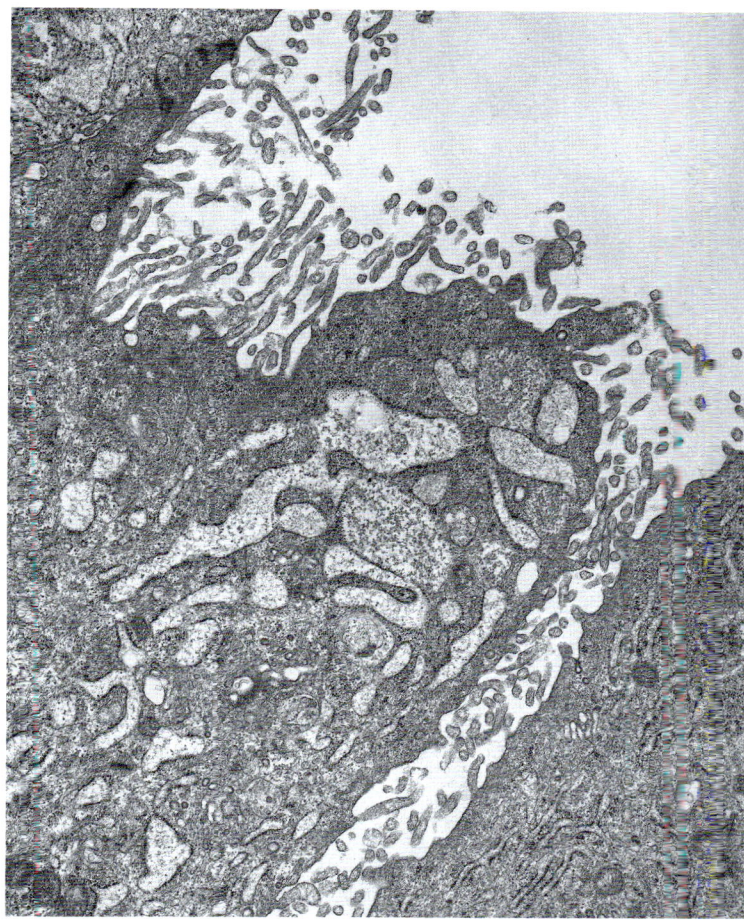

FIGURE 14.13   Same case as 14.12. The edge of the cytoplasm has a combination of glycogen accumulation and dilated vesicles of ER. The sum of these is responsible for the clear cell appearance at the periphery of mesothelial cells. (EM × 48,000)

tremely electron-dense structures, such as those represented by neuroendocrine granules. They also cover a wide range of size and distribution within the cell cytoplasm and are largely responsible for its texture by light microscopy. Finely vacuolated cells display small secretory granules with a fluffy matrix (Fig. 14.22); whereas larger, coalesced granules correspond to more coarsely vacuolated tumor cells (Fig. 14.23). Despite the distinctiveness of secretory granules, it is very seldom possible to utilize them for the purpose of tumor classification. One exception is the specific granules that allow distinction between subtypes of bronchioalveolar carcinomas. Mucinous, Clara cell, and type 2 granules (lamellar bod-

ies) have a distinct ultrastructural appearance which serve as the basis for their subclassification (Fig. 14.24). A few other ultrastructural appearances may be suggestive of certain types of neoplasms: (1) medium to small granules distributed preferentially beneath the apical plasma membrane (ovarian carcinoma) (Fig. 14.25); (2) large pleomorphic neuroendocrine granules (rectal carcinoids); (3) sparse, small neuroendocrine granules within cytoplasmic processes (oat-cell carcinoma); (4) large, fluffy secretory granules corresponding to mucin secretion (lung and gastrointestinal tract carcinomas); and (5) lysosome-like granules in the luminal pole of tumor cells containing short microvilli (thyroid carci-

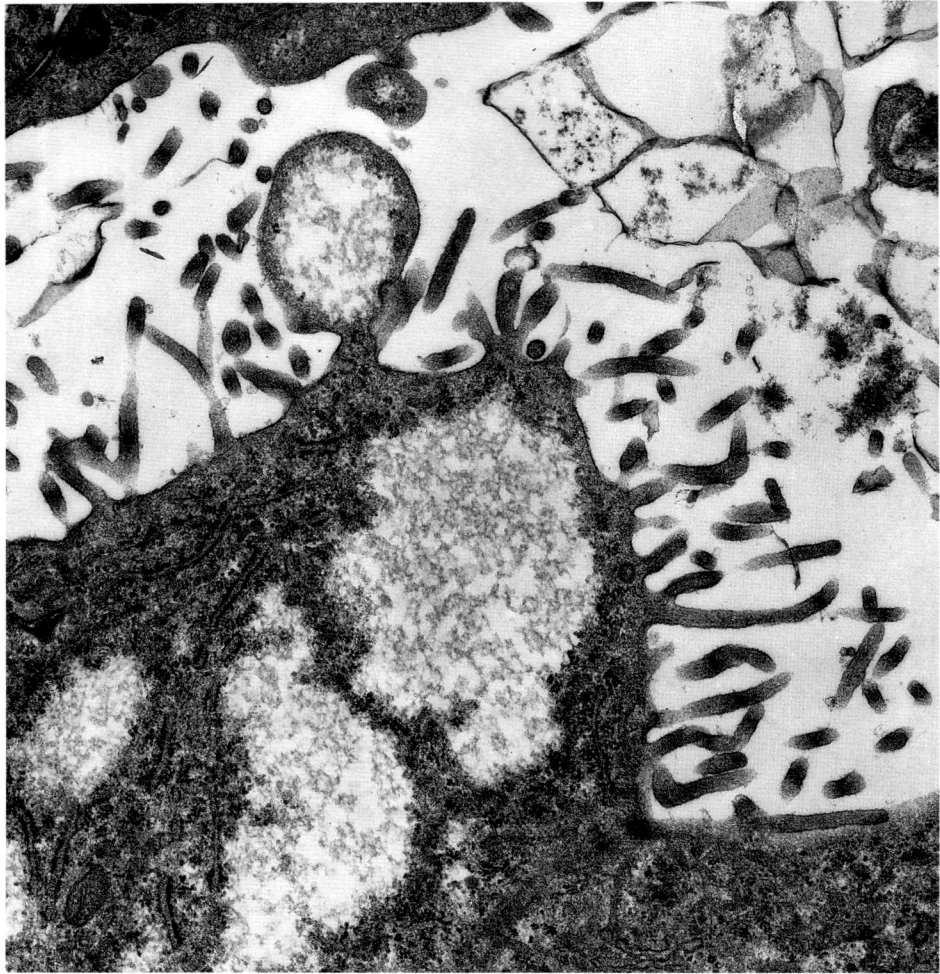

FIGURE 14.14   Detail of reactive mesothelial cells. Microvilli are noted on the surface, beneath which there are dilated clear spaces. In top center notice blebs with empty contents. (EM× 22,000)

noma). None of these features, however, are completely specific and require correlation with light microscopic and clinical information to be useful in classifying neoplasms.

Intracytoplasmic Lumina

Intracytoplasmic lumina should not be confused with large vacuoles or accumulation of secretion. Lumina are actually a specialization of the cellular excretory apparatus and protect both the cytoplasm of the tumor cells and the extracellular space from the cell's own secretory products. Typical examples include the intracytoplasmic lumina of gastric chief cells, which keep hydrochloric acid away from cells in the immediate vicinity, thus delivering the product directly into the lumen of the stomach. Carcinomas of the breast are frequently associated with intracytoplasmic lumina, but this feature is by no means exclusive to breast carcinoma (Fig. 14.26). Other tumors that show intracytoplasmic lumina in cytologic preparations include mesotheliomas and carcinomas of the lung, the kidney, and the liver. The contents of intracytoplasmic lumina may offer some clues regarding the primary site of the carcinoma. Lactalbumin is pathogenic of breast carcinoma, and alpha-fetoprotein is characteristic of liver-cell carcinomas. However, other

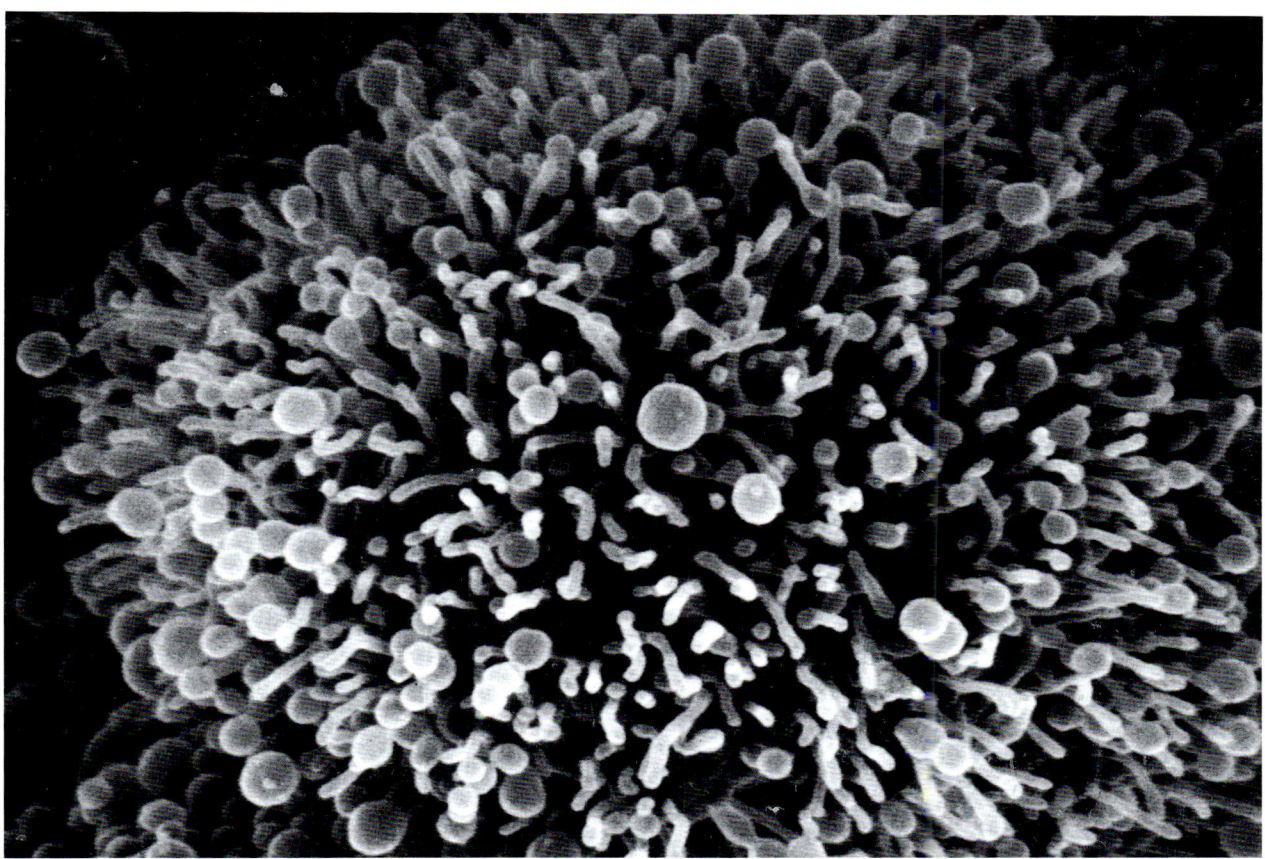

FIGURE 14.15 Surface projections from reactive mesothelial cells. In this example, the microvilli out-number the cytoplasmic blebs (SEM × 5,000)

products may be accumulated in these structures (e.g., alpha-1 antitrypsin and albumin in hepatocellular carcinomas). It cannot be assumed that intracytoplasmic lumina are exclusively found in carcinomas, because they are also present in meningiomas. The list of neoplasms showing intracytoplasmic lumina on EM grows every year; therefore, this finding cannot be considered a specific phenotypic hallmark for any type of malignancy (Table 14.4).

Endoplasmic Reticulum

A rough endoplasmic reticulum (RER) is usually more prominent in tumor cells than in their benign counter-

part. A large amount of RER occurs in sarcomas secreting extracellular material and in plasma-cell neoplasms engaged in the secretion of immunoglobulins (Fig. 14.27). Prominent mitochondria are typical of granular cell tumors originating in the thyroid, the salivary glands, the kidney, and other less frequently noted locations. The golgi complex is dilated and pale in plasma cells and immunoblasts. An enlarged golgi complex is typical of lymphomas with punctate PAS positivity and acid phosphatase activity. Large pleomorphic lysosomes are typical of tumors with Schwann-cell differentiation. They are also present in the so-called granular cell myoblastomas and other tumors with a granular appearance. Small lipid droplets are ubiquitous in many sarcomas and a few carcinomas, whereas large coalescent vacuoles are the rule in liposarcomas. Adipocytes

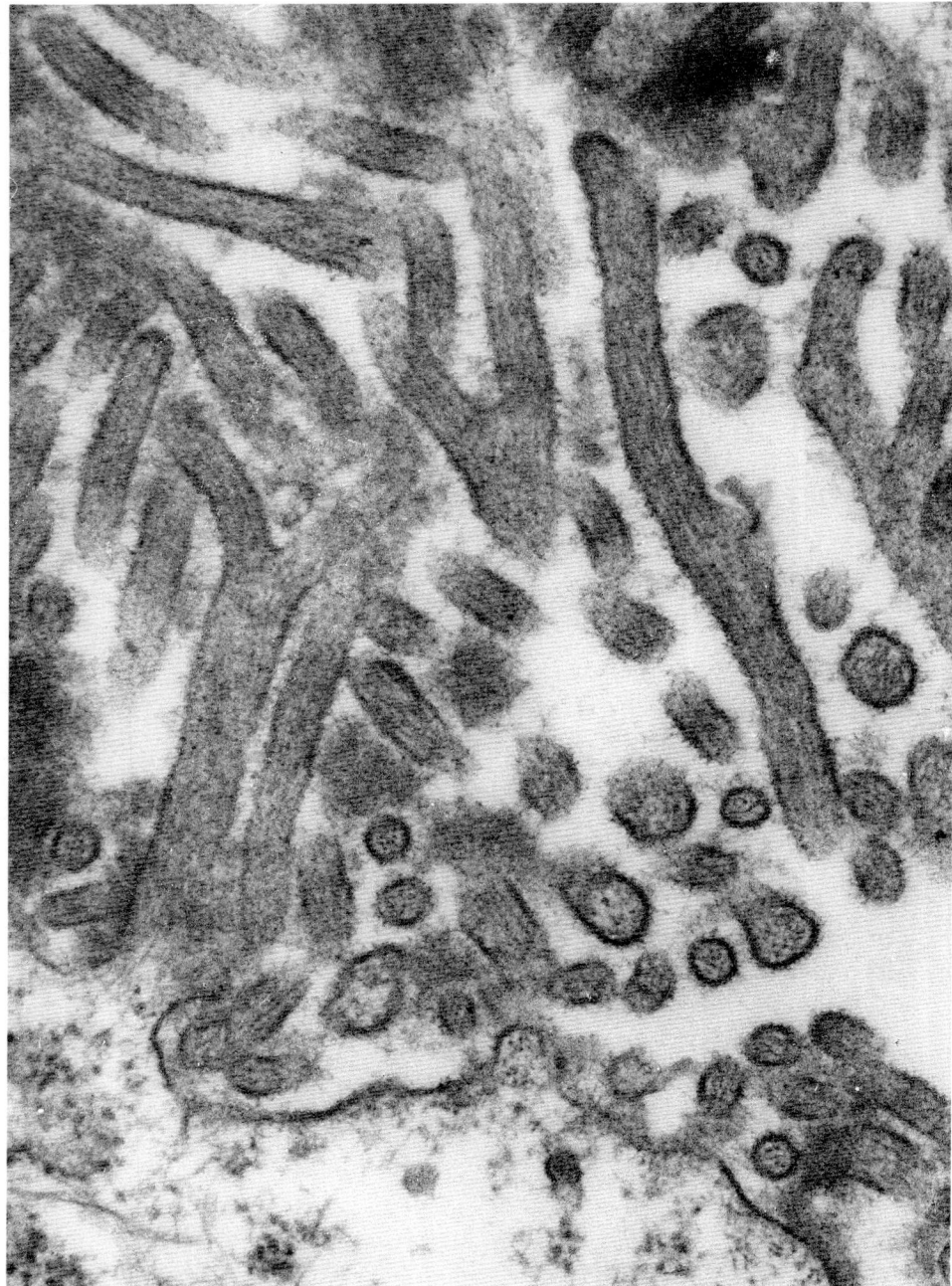

FIGURE 14.16 High power view of cell surface in mesothelioma. Notice branching elongated microvilli with thin filaments running along its length. (EM× 77,000) (Courtesy of S. Bonsib, MD)

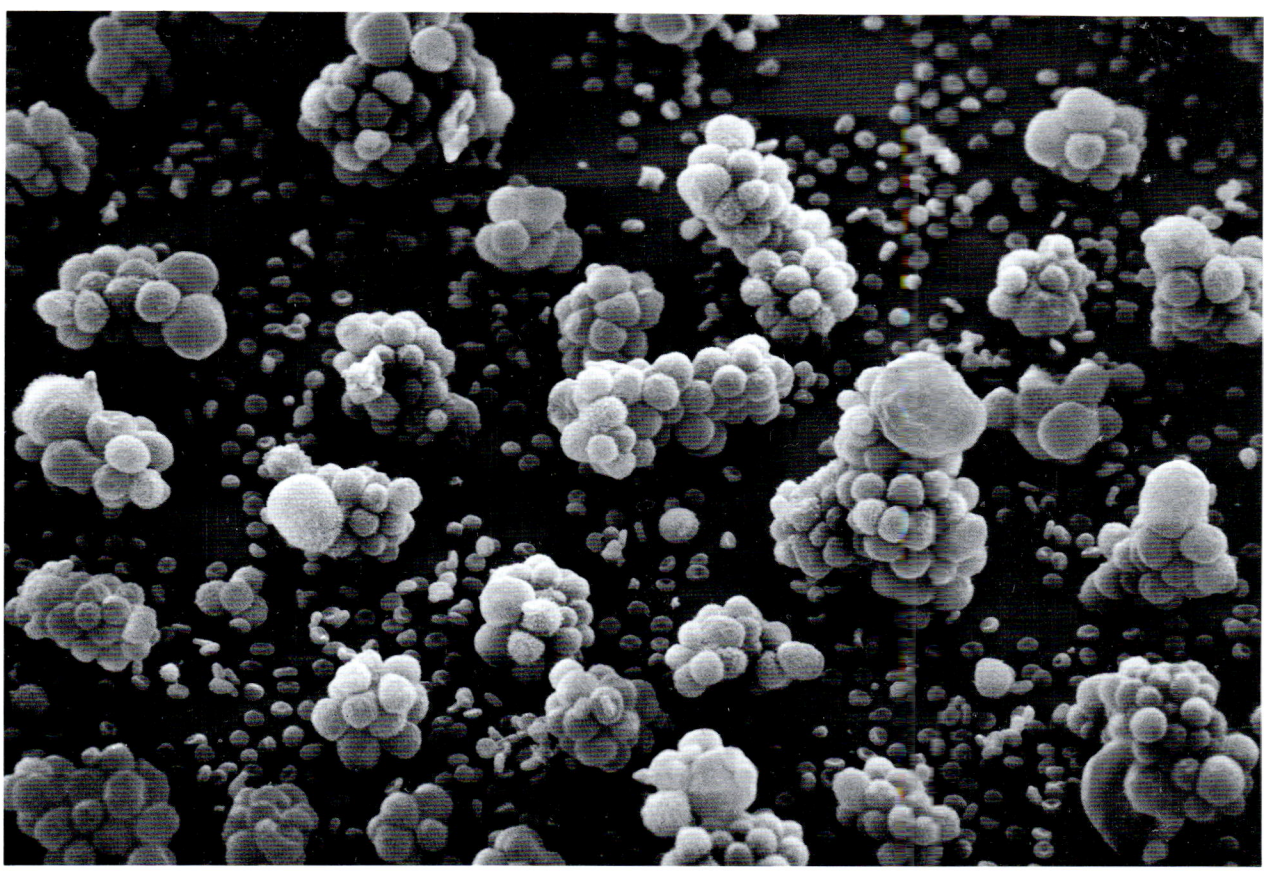

FIGURE 14.17   Pleural fluid is disseminated adenocarcinoma of the fluid. The numerous groups of malignant cells dwarf the RBC's in the background (SEM× 480)

with abundant lipid are known as lipoblasts, and they characteristically have indentations of the nuclei secondary to lipid accumulation.

Cytoskeleton

Cytoskeletal differences exist between mesothelial and neoplastic cells. Mesothelial cells have a distinct paranuclear distribution of intermediate filaments (IFs) responsible for the typical sharp demarcation between the ectoplasm and the endoplasm. Tufts of IFs are noted in a paranuclear localization in certain types of neuroendocrine carcinomas, such as Merkel-cell tumors of the skin and neuroendocrine carcinomas of the lung. How-

ever, mesothelial cells may also occasionally form such tufts. Abundant keratin-type IFs may oppose each other laterally in the form of tonofilaments. These filaments converge on desmosomes and are typical of epithelial neoplasms, including mesotheliomas. In certain types of carcinomas, the filament converging to the desmosome may be vimentin.

A concentric distribution of IFs is typical of all mesothelial cells and is displayed by mesotheliomas. This peculiar ultrastructural feature allows the distinction of mesotheliomas from tumors shedding simple malignant cells, such as breast carcinomas and melanomas. In both these tumors, IFs are sparse and not arranged concentrically around the nucleus. These subtle differences cannot always be appreciated by routine stains such as Papanicolaou and MGG; however, they are highlighted

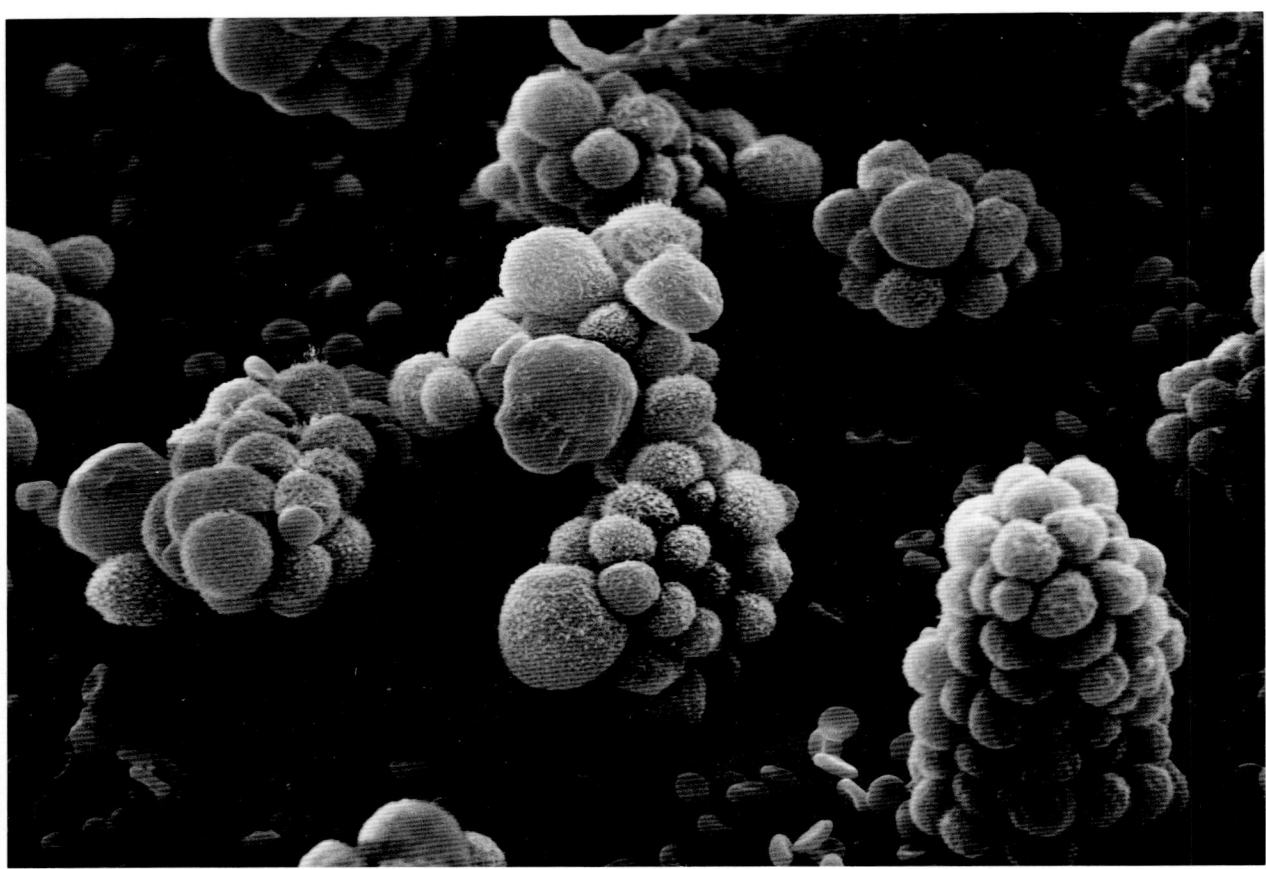

FIGURE 14.18   Same fluid as Figure 14.17. The groups vary in size and shape but show tight molding among tumor cells. (SEM × 800)

by immunostains. Keratin, for example, gives a targetoid or onion-ring pattern in mesotheliomas, and a very intense perinuclear halo makes the positive cells stand out from their neighbors. In contrast, the keratin pattern of positivity in carcinomas is diffuse, or arborizing, and rather faint, if positive at all in melanomas. The ER of the cell, which harbors its secretory apparatus, is homogeneously distributed throughout the entire cytoers. Cytologic appearances of mesotheliomas that vary from the classic cases have been described but appear rather uncommonly. In one variant, large clear cells with features of macrophages have been encountered and interpreted either as the progeny of conventional mesothelial cells or a granulomatous reaction to the presence of tumor cells. Another variant accumulates a large amount of crystalloids in the RER, similar to the

phenomenon of immunoglobulin accumulation (Russell bodies) displayed by plasma cells.

Mitochondria

Malignant cells have an increased respiratory metabolism secondary to uncoupling of oxidative phosphorylation. Ultrastructurally, this increase may be reflected by excessive accumulation of mitochondria in the cytoplasm of tumor cells, which occurs frequently in certain cell types, such as oncocytoma and Hürthle-cell tumors. The exact significance of this change, however, is not altogether clear since tumors other than these two types may also present with abundant mitochondria (Fig. 14.28). Crowded mitochondria may show crystalline inclusion bodies and structural abnormalities, such as ab-

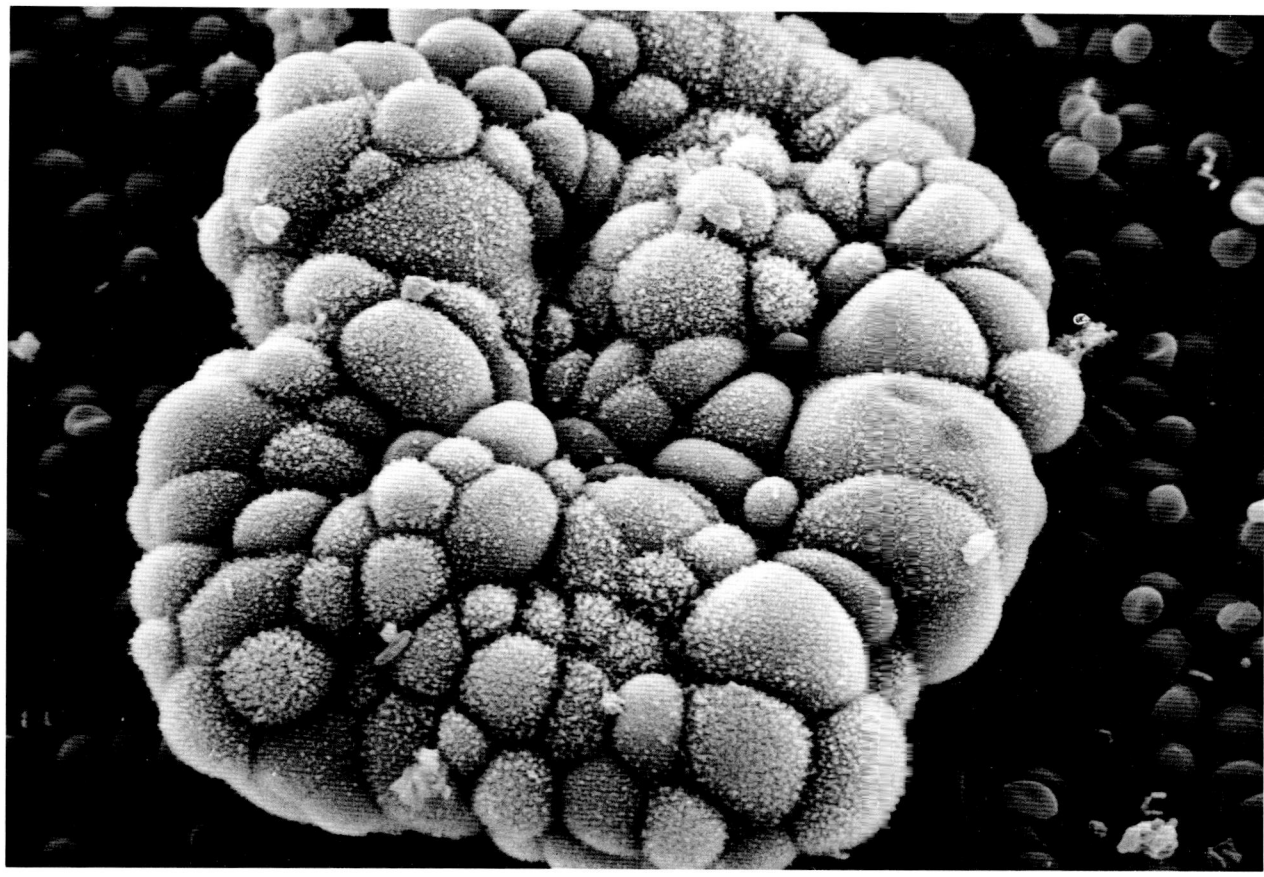

FIGURE 14.19   Malignant group of cells from adenocarcinoma. Not only the group is enormous in size but several cells share a community border. Some cells protrude above the surface, but the gaps among cells is very narrow. (SEM × 640)

TABLE 14.3   Microvillous Ultrastructure of Metastatic Tumors in Malignant Effusions

Filamentous core rootlets *plus* glycocalyceal bodies	No filamentous core rootlets; *no* glycocalyceal bodies
Ovary	Breast
Gastrointestinal tract	Thyroid
Pancreas	Liver
Gall bladder	Kidney
Lung	Adrenal
Bladder	Prostate
Filamentous core rootlets; *no* glycocalyceal bodies	
Nasal adenocarcinoma	
Carcinoid tumor	
Yolk sac tumor	
Synovial sarcoma	
Schwannoma	

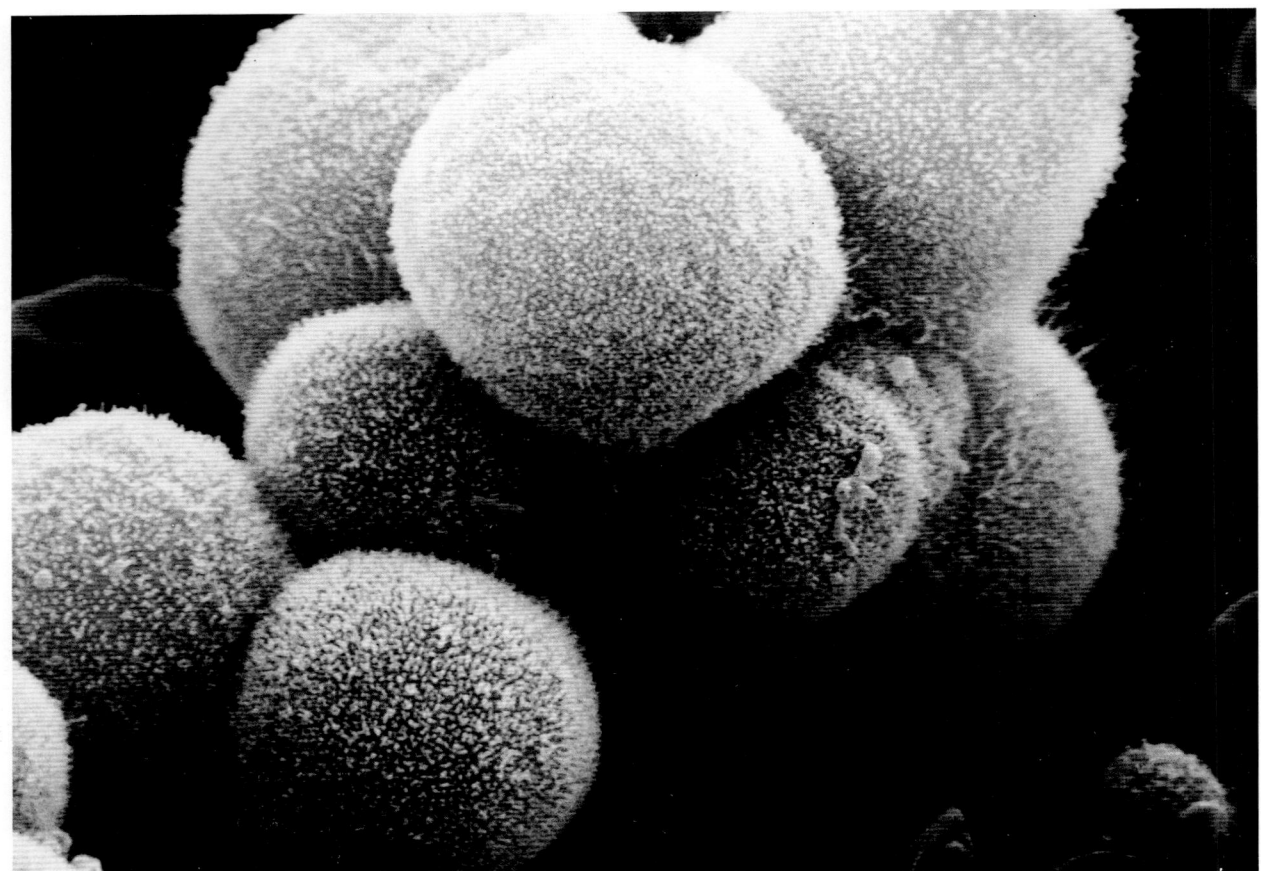

FIGURE 14.20 Group of cells from ovarian adenocarcinoma. The microvilli are closely cropped but elongated microvili are sparsely identified (SEM × 2,000)

normal orientation, matrial swelling, decreased or absent cristae, intercristal fusion, and intramitochondrial dense bodies. Unfortunately, none of these changes are sufficiently specific to allow subclassification of tumors based on the ultrastructural appearance of their mitochondria.

Lysosomes

Certain neoplasms may accumulate lysosomes that may be abnormally large. An increased number of lamellated lysosomes is typical of bronchioloalveolar cell carcinomas, whereas giant autophagosomes occur in granular cell tumors. Carcinomas of the bladder and the renal pelvis occasionally present with accumulation

of lysosomes in the cytoplasm of urothelial cells. Muramidase and alpha-one antitrypsin (A1AT) are detected in the lysosomes of neoplastic histiocytes in malignant histiocytosis. No specific ultrastructural appearance has been linked to loss of common histiocytic markers or acquisition of unusual immunopositivity by malignant cells.

ULTRASTRUCTURAL CORRELATES OF NONEPITHELIAL DIFFERENTIATION

The vast majority of malignant effusions are secondary to epithelial neoplasms; however, mesenchymal tumors

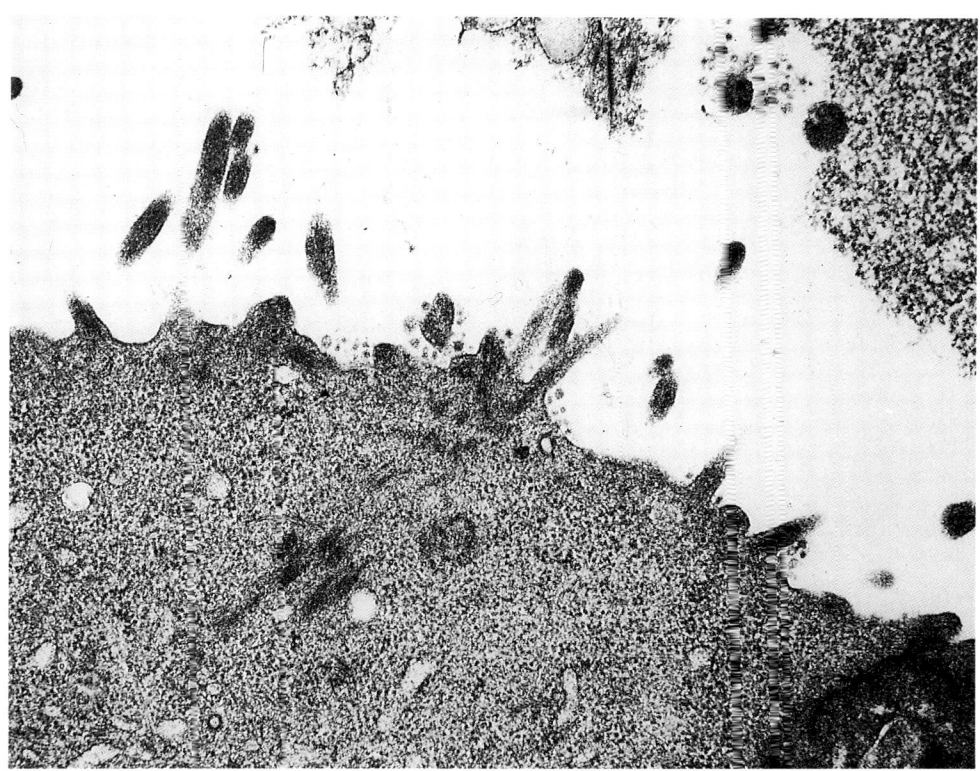

FIGURE 14.21 Adenocarcinoma of colon. Notice deep seated core rootless and relatively short microvilli on the surface. (EM × 60,000) (Courtesy Dr. Bruce MacKay)

may sometimes be accompanied by effusions, as discussed in Chapters 10 and 13. We use a morphologic categorization of these tumors into (small cell, large cell, pleomorphic cell, and spindle cell) groups that facilitate their differential diagnosis. Whenever possible, ultrastructural features are interpreted in correlation with cytomorphologic observations in routinely stained cytologic preparations (Table 14.5). EM is also interpreted in light of immunocytochemical results if available, as depicted in Chapter 10 (Table 10.5). Only a small number of sarcomas, however, have been studied by EM examination of cytologic specimens. Fig. 14.29 illustrates myogenous differentiation in a leiomyosarcoma diagnosed by cul-de-sac aspirate.

SCANNING ELECTRON MICROSCOPY

Effusions are a favorite target of studies using SEM. Effusions of serous fluid are not only a ready source of

malignant cells, but also they tend to be quite different from the built-in internal control represented by mesothelial cells, lymphocytes and RBCs. Mesothelial cells are unique under SEM because of their florid microvillous surfaces. In practice, SEM very elegantly demonstrates the differences between the surface topography of mesothelial cells versus cells of lymphohistiocytic origin, as well as between mesothelial cells and malignant cells of epithelial and nonepithelial origin. Table 14.6 summarizes the salient surface characteristics of various neoplasms studied by SEM. The method has been applied to cell suspensions obtained directly from the effusion or indirectly from slides containing cells obtained after centrifugation. The latter method has the advantage of selecting only cells of interest for study, whereas direct preparations are ideal for visualization of the contrast between various cell types.

The surface configuration of mesothelial cells has been extensively studied in effusions by Domagala and Gonzalez-Devesa. As can be expected from TEM and light microscopy, the surface of mesothelial cells is

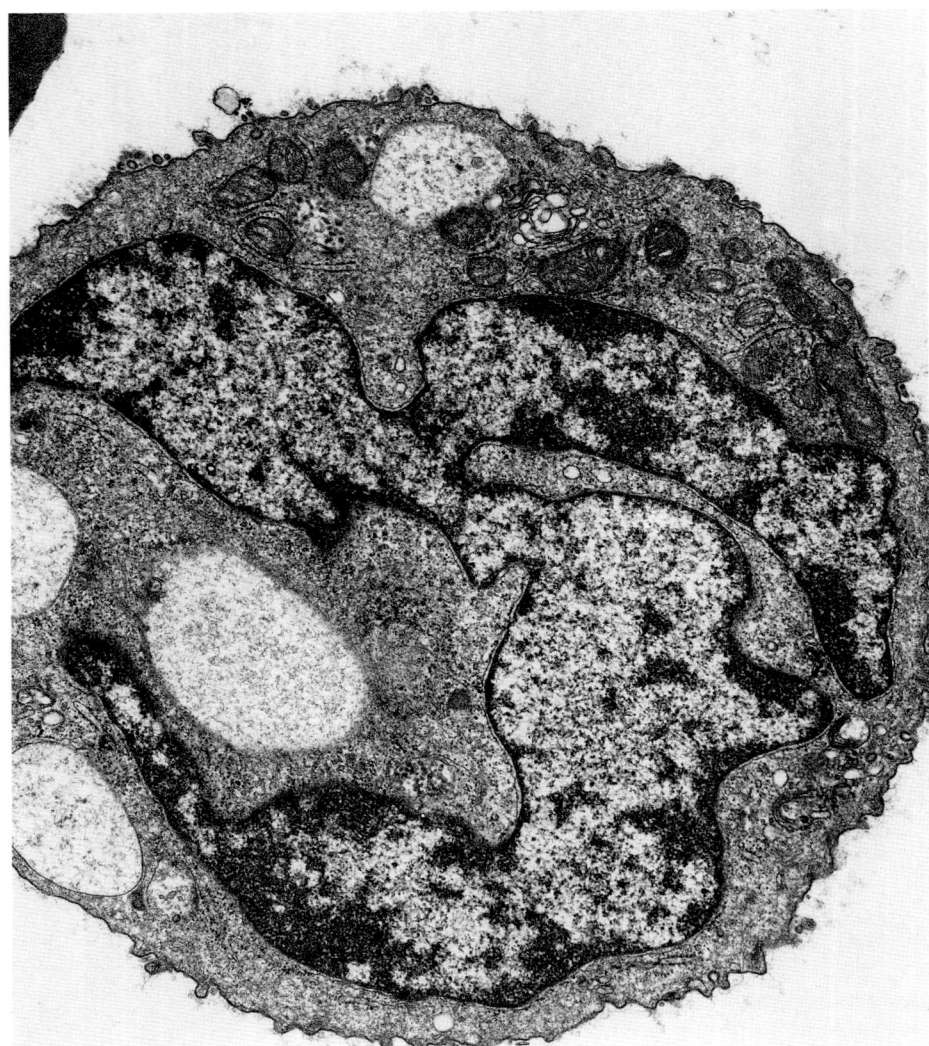

FIGURE 14.22   Mucin-producing breast carcinoma. Notice smooth cellular surface with only blunt, stubby cytoplasmic extensions. The cytoplasm shows secretory granules. (EM × 48,000)

prickly and demonstrates the complex branching pattern of the microvilli. Unlike macrophages, however, they lack ruffles and ridges, and unlike epithelial cells they lack bald spots. With *freeze fracture* EM, mesothelial cells exhibit some differences in relation to carcinomatous cells (Fig. 14.30). In carcinoma, a rich network of tight junctions is the rule, while in mesothelioma, gap junctions are included within the tight junction network (Fig. 14.31). By transmission EM terminal bars similar to those seen in adenocarcinoma are present in mesothelioma (Fig. 14.32). Desmosomes, however, are considerably longer in mesothelioma than in adenocarcinoma (Fig. 14.33). Fibrous mesotheliomas are difficult to distinguish from spindle-cell sarcomas of the pleura, such as fibrosarcomas and leiomyosarcomas. At the ultrastructural level, the mesothelioma exhibits considerable epithelial differentiation despite its sarcomatoid appearance. These tumors are rich in IFs on immunocytochemistry and have been shown to coexpress keratin and vimentin. In tissue fragments, their microvillous surfaces come into direct contact with collagen, which is helpful in recognizing their mesotheliomatous nature.

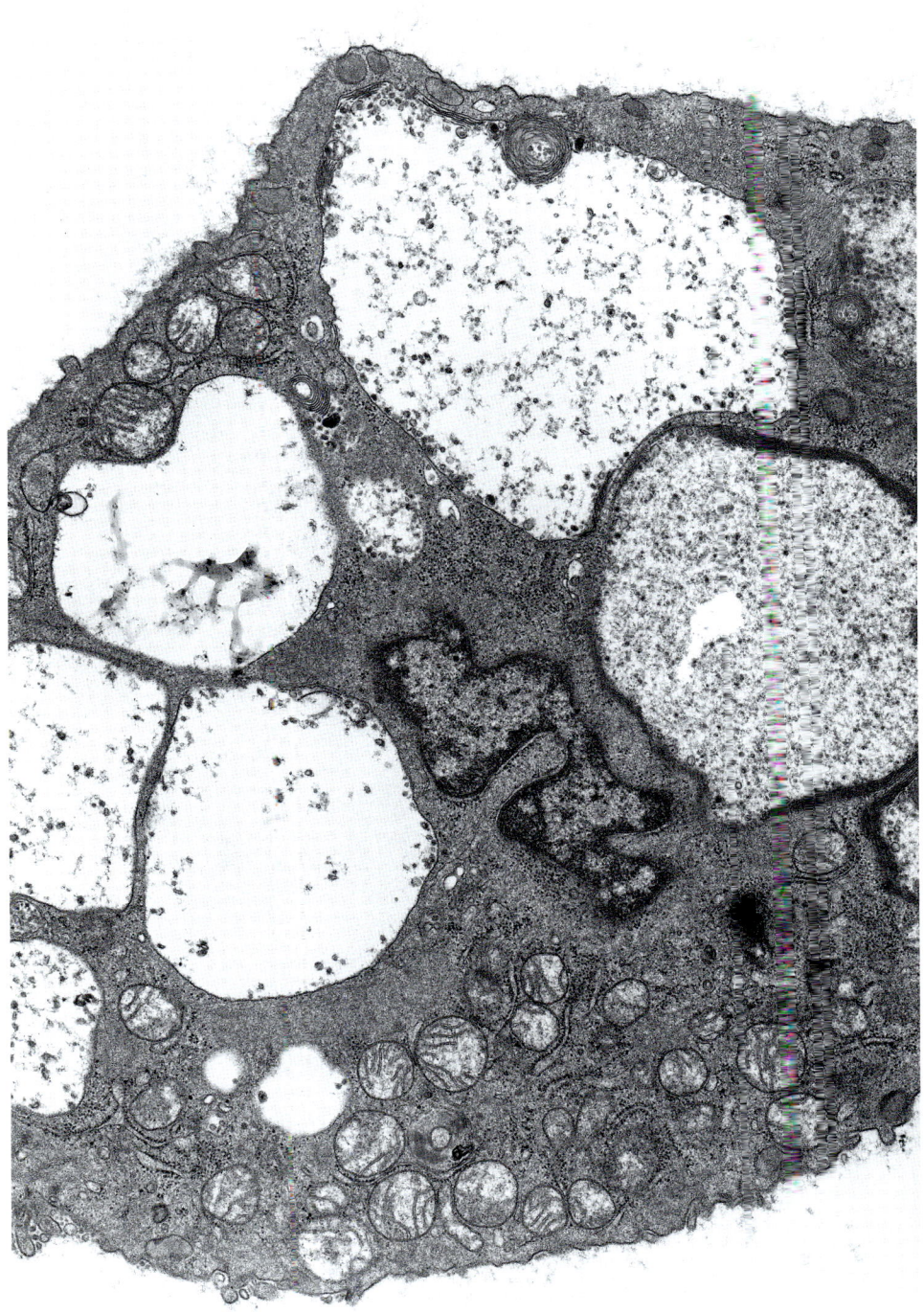

FIGURE 14.23 Mucin-secreting adenosarcoma of the stomach. Several secretory vacuoles are identified. Notice variable electrodensity ranging from totally clear vacuoles to those containing fluffy mucosubstances. (EM × 48,000).

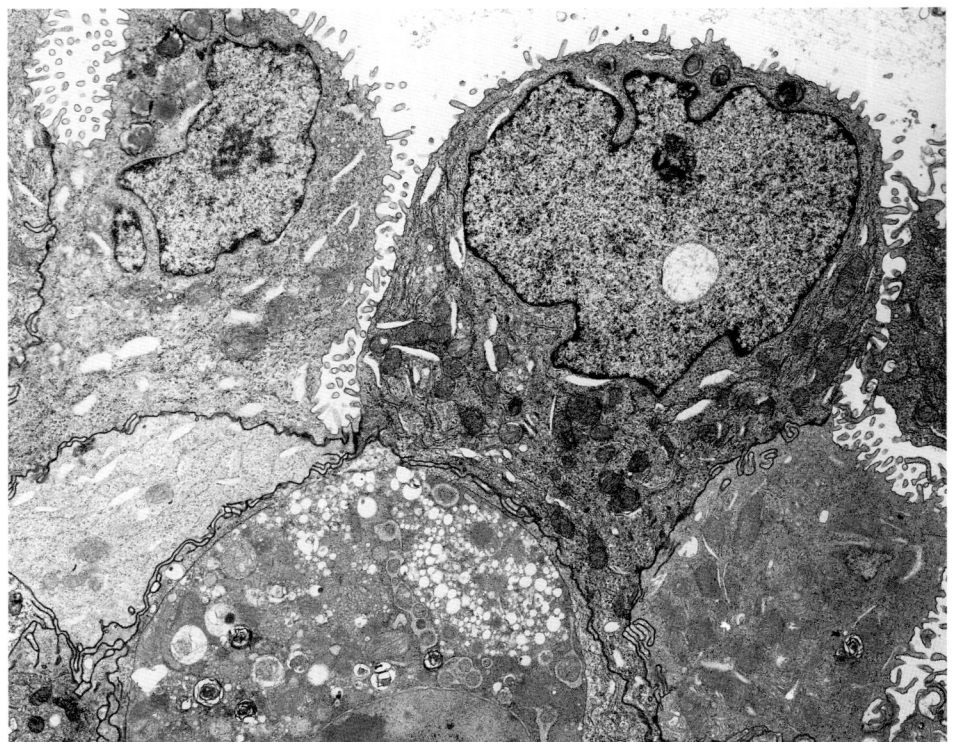

FIGURE 14.24 Cluster of cells from adenocarcinoma of the lung. Notice microvilli restricted to one pole of the cells that connect to one another by complex interdigitations. (EM × 9,000)

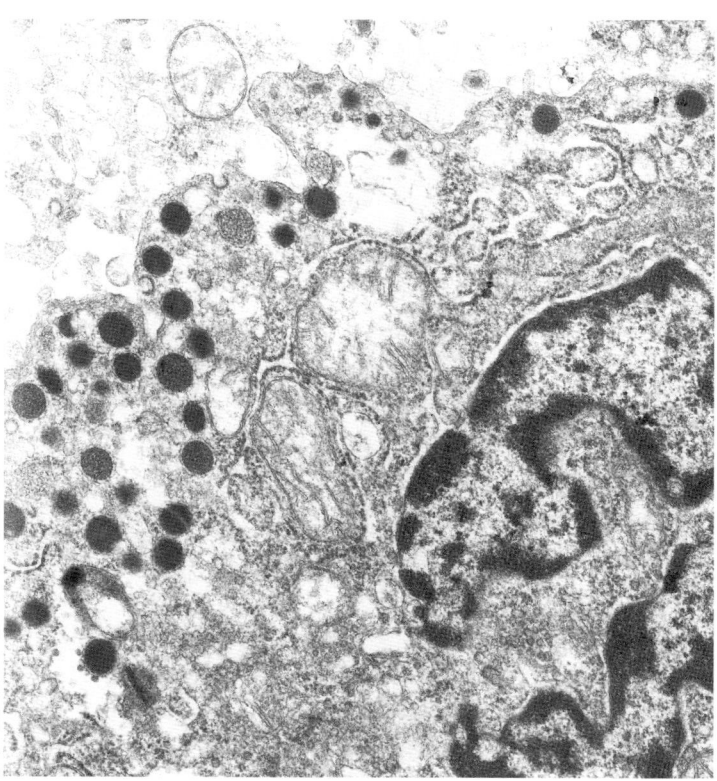

FIGURE 14.25 Malignant cell from ovarian carcinoma. The microvilli are short or absent and secretory products are abundant just beneath the plasma membrane (TEM × 6,600)

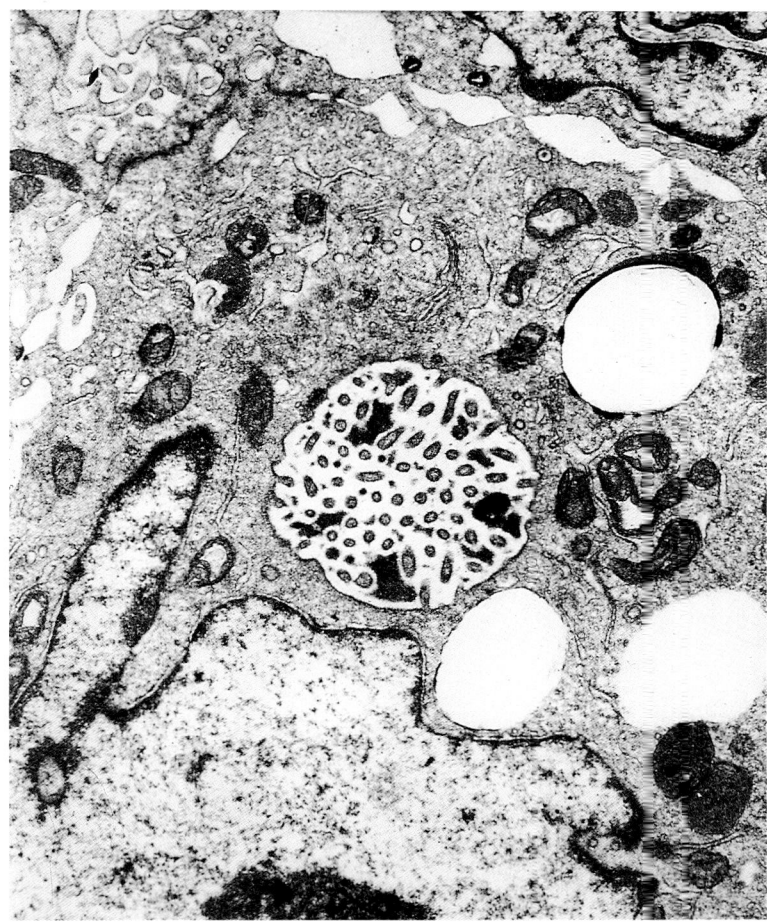

FIGURE 14.26 Junction between several cells from breast carcinoma. They are connected by terminal bars and the cytoplasm is dominated by an intracellular lumen. (TEM × 4,800)

TABLE 14.4 Neoplasm and Other Conditions Displaying Intracytoplasmic Lumina at the Ultrastructural Level

Normal and Reactive Cells	Pancreatic carcinoma
Hepatocytes	Renal-cell carcinoma
Pancreatic acinar cells	Ovarian (serous and mucinous) carcinoma
Corpus luteum cells	Skin adnexal carcinomas (several types)
Breast epithelium	Prostatic carcinoma
Follicular cells of the thyroid	Gastric carcinoma
Urothelium	Lung carcinoma
Nasal mucosa	Salivary gland carcinomas (several types)
Carcinomas	Hepatocellular carcinoma
Breast carcinoma	Other Neoplasms
Clear-cell carcinoma of endocervix	Mesothelioma
Thyroid (follicular and papillary) carcinoma	Pheochromocytoma
Hurthle cell tumor of thyroid	Paraganglioma

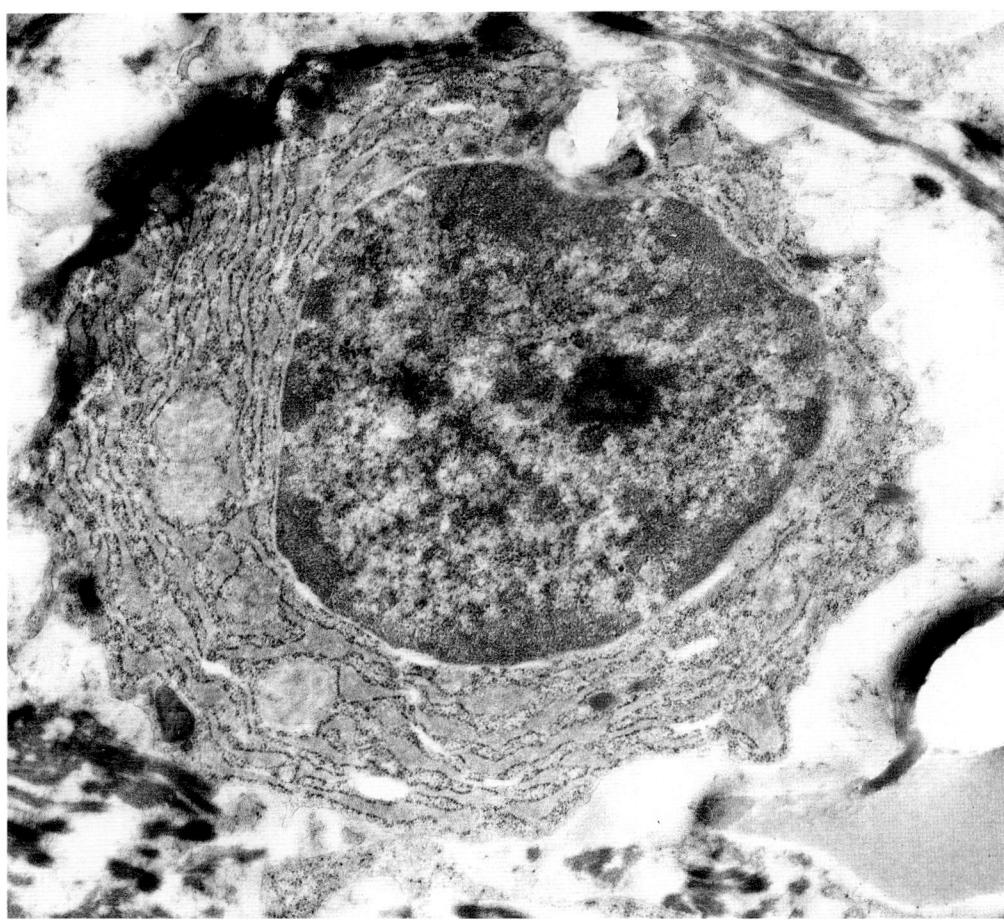

FIGURE 14.27 Effusion with lymphohistiocytic predominance. Notice plasma cells with numerous parallel stacks of rough endoplasmic reticulum throughout the cytoplasm. (EM × 24,000)

Little is known about the surface characteristics of sarcomatous mesotheliomas on SEM.

Lymphocytes appear relatively smooth at the light microscopic level; however, both TEM and SEM accurately reveal the complex surface morphology of lymphocytes. They lack the ridges of macrophages but may display a considerable amount of microvillous projections, particularly in B-cell lymphomas. This finding explains the fact that lymphomatous cells in long-standing effusions may degenerate in the form of small cellular aggregates. The contact among lymphocytes and between lymphocytes and macrophages may be very close and may give rise to subplasmalemmal linear densities that are mirror-images of one another and may mimic desmosomes. They lack an association

with IFs, however, which assists in their correct identification.

DIAGNOSTIC APPLICATIONS

EM is seldom the primary method used to establish a malignant diagnosis in the study of effusions. Slightly more than 700 cases of serous fluids studied by TEM have been reported to date (Table 14.7). Because the cost of instrumentation has remained high and the method requires special training, EM is rapidly being supplanted by immunocytochemistry and other ancillary techniques. The major applications of EM concern

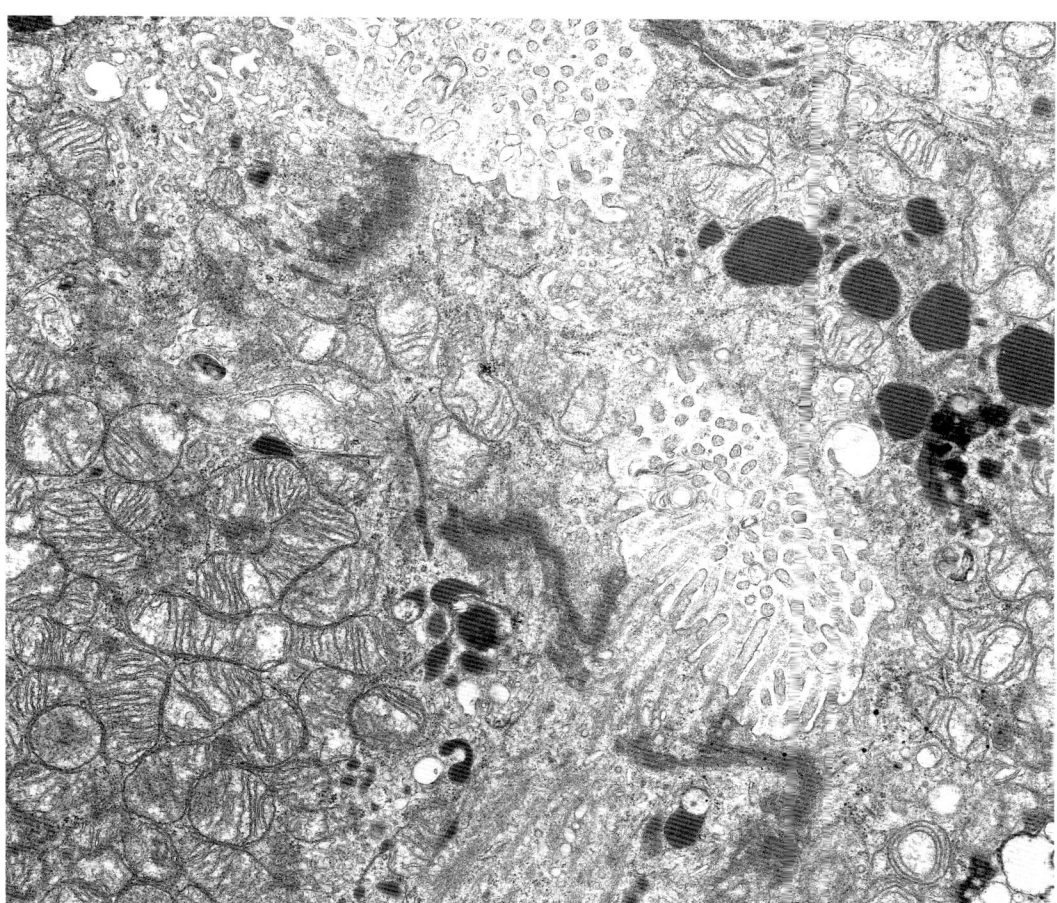

FIGURE 14.28 Renal cell carcinoma in body fluid. Mitochondria and lipid in the cytoplasm rendered a granular appearance to the cytoplasm. Notice microvilli on the surface of the cells. (EM × 18,000)

finding specific cytoplasmic markers indicative of peculiar forms of phenotypic differentiation. These markers range in specificity from very low to very high, so EM should be chosen judiciously, either as the only special study to clarify diagnostic dilemmas or in conjunction with other methods (Table 14.8). In general, if these ultrastructural hallmarks are exhibited by the primary tumor, they will also be present in malignant effusions resulting from the same neoplasm. If they are not detected during the first trial of EM but are suspected from the light microscopic appearance of the tumor cells, repeat taps should be obtained for more careful handling of the sample for EM.

The specificity of immunocytochemistry can be coupled with the precision of EM to identify the location and nature of subcellular alterations. The resulting technique, known as immuno-EM, has found its way into the study of cytologic specimens. Using immuno-EM, it has been possible to verify the exact localization of CEA (within the RER) and EMA (predominantly along the microvilli). Likewise, antikeratin antibodies are distributed according to the concentration of IFs in the various cell types, thus explaining the different patterns of immunopositivity noted by light microscopy. Immuno-EM has also shown that the amount of CEA in mesothelial cells is insufficient for a reliable interpretation of immunopositivity by immunocytochemistry.

TABLE 14.5 Cytomorphologic and Ultrastructural Features of Nonepithelial Tumors

Sub-Type	Cytomorphology	Ultrastructure
Small cells		
Neuroblastoma	Single cells; rosette-like formations; filamentous and granular material in the group	Tangles of elongated processes; neurosecretory granules; microtubules and IF; primitive intercellular junctions
Ewing's sarcoma	Single cells loosely cohesive; punctate vacuoles in cytoplasm PAS+ (glycogen)	Primitive cytoplasm; glycogen lakes; sparse lipid droplets; well-dispersed euchromatin in nuclei
Wilms' tumor	Biphasic pattern; large mole cells and dark spindle cells; primitive tubules	Tubular lumina with microvilli; basal lumina; frequent cell junctions; tufts of IF
Rhabdomyosarcoma	Single cells; showing anisocytosis; eccentric, eosinophilic cytoplasm PAS+ (glycogen)	Z-bands; thick and thin filaments; irregular nuclear profile; prominent RER
Large cells		
Melanoma	Single cells; dusky vacuolated or pigmented cytoplasm; binucleation; prominent nucleoli	Premelonosomes; lipid droplets; coated intracysternal tubules
Histiocytic neoplasm	Single cells; plump shape, moderate amount of cytoplasm	Loosely cohesive cells; variable lysosomal content; cell surface projections; Birbeck granules (histiocytosis X)
Paraganglioma	Loosely cohesive cells; polygonal, granular cytoplasm; lattice-like strands	Angulated cell shape; profuse IF; focal basal lamina and sparse cell junctions
Alveolar soft part sarcoma	Single cells; abundant clear/granular cytoplasm; crystalloids in some cells	Mesenchymal cells; rhomboid crystals in cysternae of RER
Pleomorphic cells		
Liposarcoma	Clustered and single cells; vacuolated cytoplasm; association with capillaries	Indented nuclei; coalesced lipid droplets; fuzzy cellular surfaces
MFH	Large bizarre cells; spindle cells; plump cells; foamy cells	Mixed cells population; spindle, undifferentiated, giant lipid droplets; proteoglycans in stroma
Cell tumor	Abundant, granular cytoplasm; stripped nuclei; extracellular granular materials	Aggregates of lysosomes; angulate residual bodies microtubules; redundant membranes
Spindle cells		
Fibrosarcoma	Isolated cells; needle-shaped nuclei; collagenous background	Separated cells; prominent RER; no myofilaments; intercellular proteoglycans
Leiomyosarcoma	Simple or clustered spindle cells; cigar-shaped nuclei	Closely associated cells; basal lamina; linear dense bodies; thin filaments (6–8 nm)
Schwannoma	Intimately associated cells; palisading nuclei	Intertwining cell processes; reduplicated basal lamina; elongated crystaes
Synovial Sarcoma	Cohesive spindle and plump cells; round to ovoid nuclei; scarce intercellular material	Rudimentary acinar lumina; focal basal lamina; intercellular junctions

MFH = malignant fibrous histiocytome; IF = intermediate filament; RER = rough endoplasmic reticulum.

TABLE 14.6 SEM Characteristics of Cell Types Found in Malignant Effusions

Cell Type	Ultrastructural Features	Cell Type	Ultrastructural Features
Mesothelial cells	Spiked surface; florid microvilli; majority long and narrow. Some blebes and short microvilli noted; no ridges or craters	Lymphocytes	T cells: smooth surface; moderate number of short, stub-like projections (digitations)
Carcinoma cells	Adenocarcinoma; short, stubby microvilli; some variability ranging from fuzzy border (liver) to elongated microvilli (ovary) Squamous cell carcinoma: flat cells with sparse projections		B cells: ruffled surface; large number of long projections resembling epithelial cells
		Macrophages	Ridged surfaces; variable number of pseudopods, depending on cell activation. Blebes; crater-like indentations

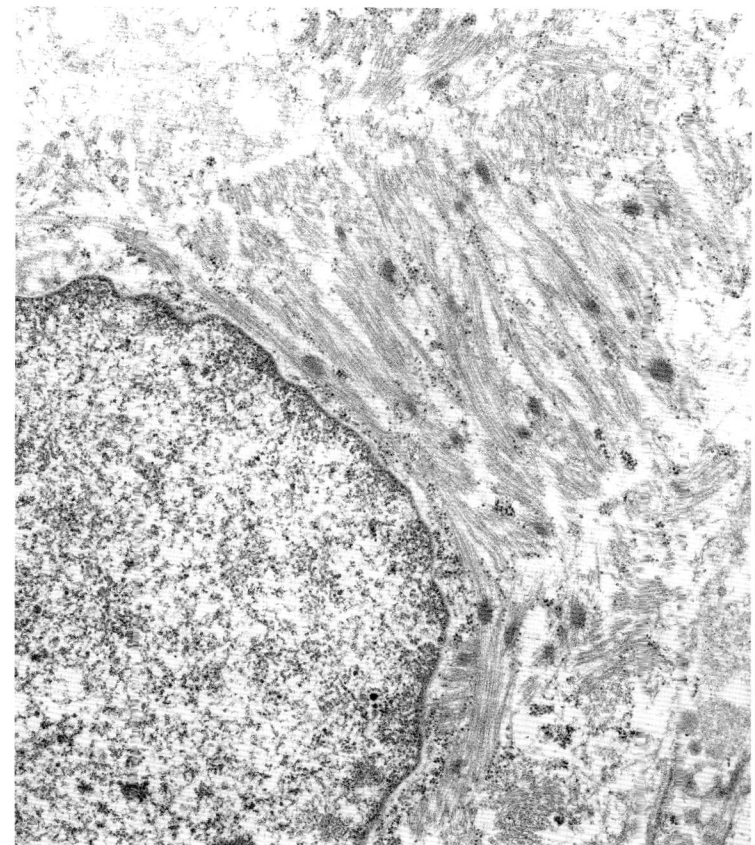

FIGURE 14.29 Cytoplasm of lyomyosarcoma cell. Notice thick and thin filaments and glycogen granules and darker dense bodies. (EM × 30,000)

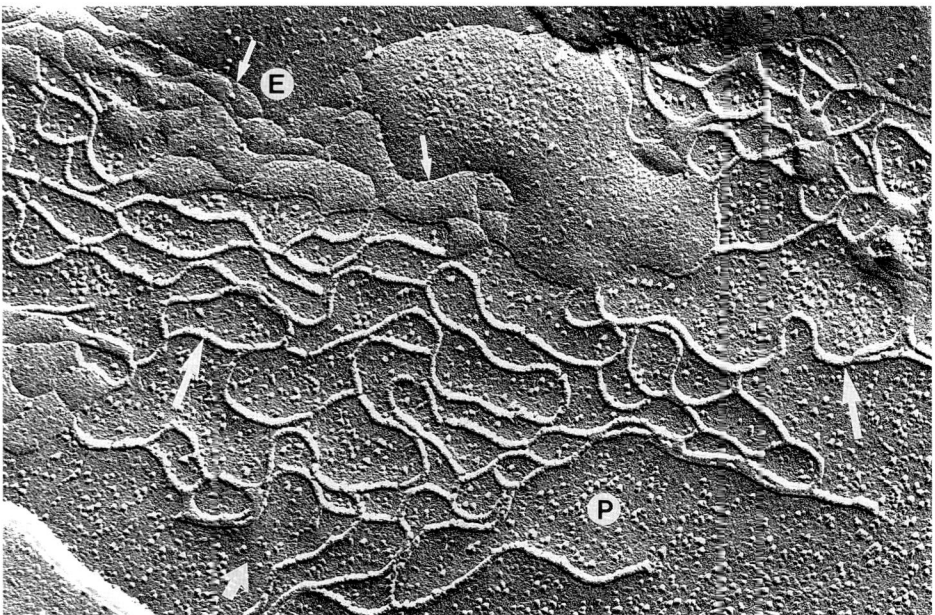

FIGURE 14.30 Freeze fracture EM from adenocarcinoma. Notice rich meshwork of tight junctions appearing either as ridges (large arrows) or furrows (short arrow). (FF × 60,000) (Courtesy Dr. T. Mukherjee)
E: E-face; P: P-face

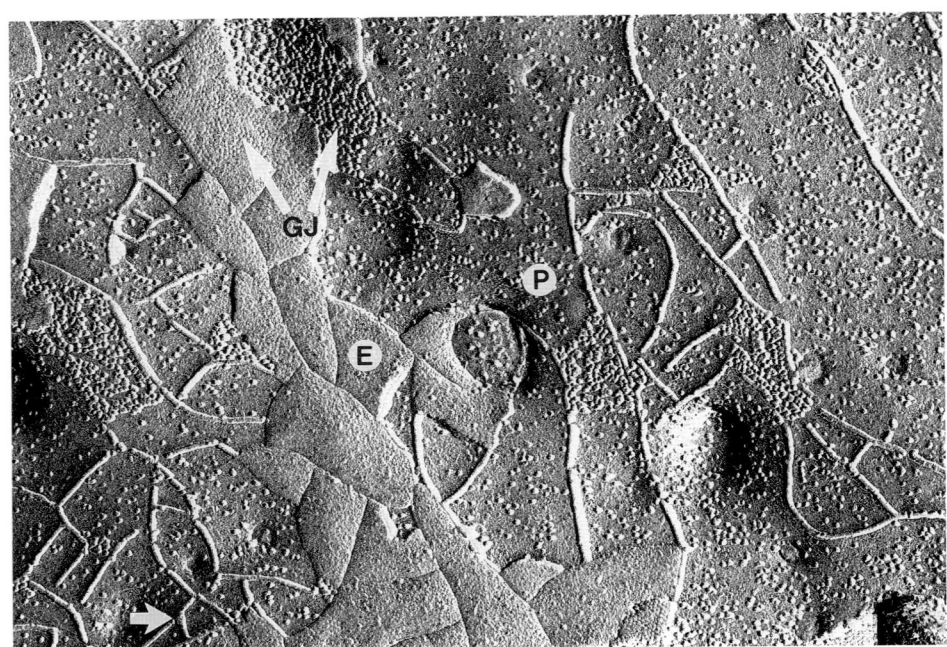

FIGURE 14.31 Mesothelioma examined by freeze fracture EM. Amidst a network of tight junctions notice scattered gap junctions (arrows). (FF × 60,000) (Courtesy Dr. T. Mukherjee)
E: E-face; P: P-face

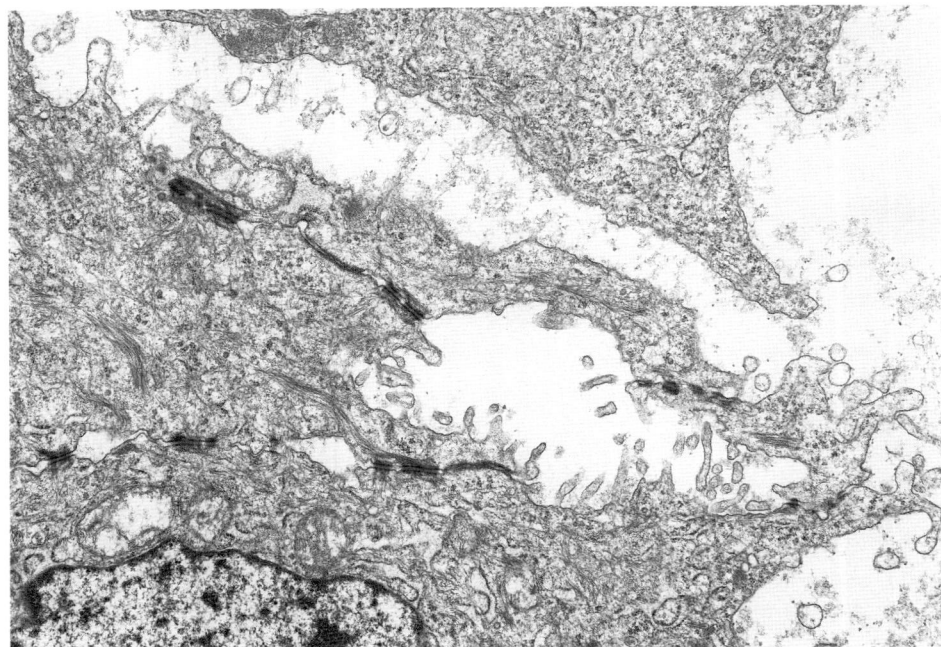

FIGURE 14.32 Junctional complexes in mesothelioma. Confluence of several mesothelial cells show numerous desmosomes in a row near their apex. Notice extracellular lumen with protruding microvilli and cytoplasm with abundant intermediate filaments. (EM × 12,000)

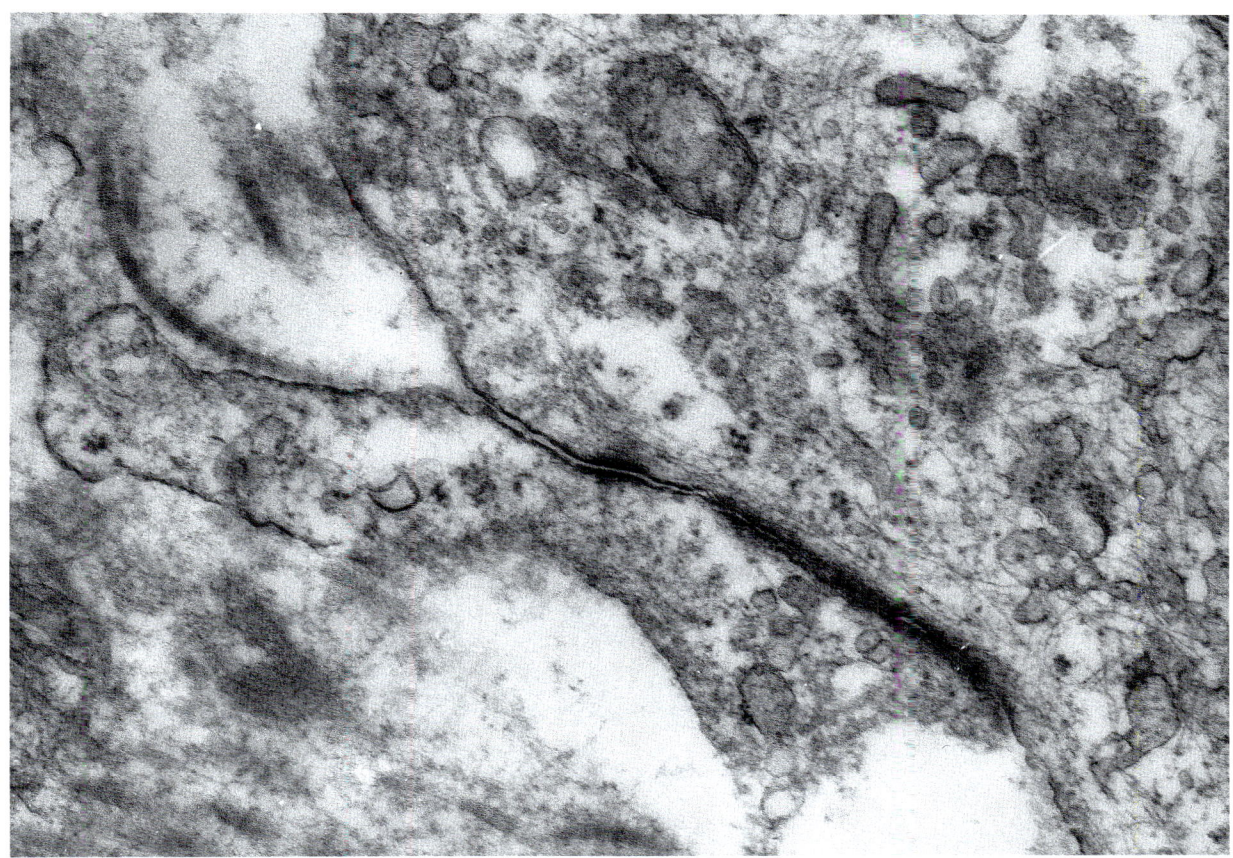

FIGURE 14.33   Very large desmosome connecting cells from mesothelioma. Notice elongated lamina densa with attendant intermediate filaments. (EM × 16,000).

TABLE 14.7   Ultrastructural Study of Serous Effusions

Author, Year	Total Patients Cases (Malignant)	Source of Fluid	Diagnosis				
			Mes	Lymph	Mel	Ca	Other
Murad, 1973	42 (28)	Pl Pt	. . .	7	3	17	1
Legrand, 1974	32 (32)	Pl	32	. . .	. . .	. . .	. . .
Domagala, 1975	82 (52)	Pl	. . .	3	. . .	44	. . .
Gondos, 1978	42 (23)	Pl Pc Pt	. . .	1	2	17	3
Wuerker, 1983	282 (79)	Pl Pt	12	8	2	57	2
Herrera, 1985	104 (69)	Pl Pc Pt	4	3	4	58	0
Bewtra, 1985	28 (12)	Pl Pc Pt	2	. . .	. . .	10	0
Kobzik, 1985	17 (16)	Pl Pt	. . .	. . .	. . .	9	1
Hanna, 1985	16 (16)	Pl Pt Pc	. . .	. . .	. . .	16	. . .

Mes = mesothelioma; Lymph = lymphoma; Mel = melanoma; Ca = Carcinoma; Pl = pleural; Pt = peritoneal; Pc = pericardial.

TABLE 14.8 Ultrastructural Hallmarks with High Phenotypic Specificity

Epithelial Tumors	Nonepithelial tumors
Acinar-cell carcinoma: zymogen granules	Malignant melanoma: premelanosomes
Alveolar cell carcinoma: lamellated bodies	Histiocytosis-X: Birbeck granules
Bronchiolar cell carcinoma: Clara cell granule	Rhabdomyosarcoma: Z bands
Leydig/Hilus cell tumors: Reinke crystals	Dermatofibrosarcoma protuberans: "satellite nuclei"
Islet-cell tumor (insulinoma): clear-haloed NE granule	Leiomyosarcoma: dense bodies/contractile nuclei
Juxtaglomerular carcinoma: rhomboid protogranules	Malignant fibrous histiocytoma: branching cysternae of RER
Merkel cell tumor: paranuclear tuft of IF	Hairy-cell leukemia: ribosome-lamella complex
Malignant mesothelioma: long and tortuous microvilli	Liposarcoma (lipoblasts): lipid-related nuclear indentations
Oncocytoma: mitochondria with lamelliform cristae	Lymphoblastic lymphoma: convoluted nuclear contour
Benign "sugar" tumor (lung): membrane-bound glycogen	Mycosis fungoides/Sezary syndrome: cribriform nuclei
Arhenoblastoma: Charcot-Bottcher crystalloids	Osteosarcoma: hydroxyapatite crystals
Neuroendocrine tumors: neuroendocrine granules	Schwannoma: pseudomesaxon-like structures
Colonic adenocarcinoma: deep-seated rootlets	Vascular neoplasms: Weibel-Palade body
Breast carcinoma: intracytoplasmic lumen	Alveolar soft-part sarcoma: rhomboid crystals
	Granular cell tumor: residual bodies (lysosomes)

NE = neuroendocrine; IF = intermediate filament; RER = rough endoplasmic reticulum.

BIBLIOGRAPHY

Electron Microscopy Use in Effusions

Murad TM. Electron microscopic studies of cells in pleural and peritoneal effusions. *Acta Cytol.* 1973;17:401–409.

Domagala W, Woyke S. Transmission and scanning electron microscopic studies of cells in effusions. *Acta Cytol.* 1975;19:214–224.

Legrand M, Pariente R. Electron microscopy in the cytological examination of metastatic pleural effusions. *Thorax.* 1976;31:443–449.

Kaneshima S, Kiyasu Y, Kudo H, et al. Application of SEM to cytodiagnosis of pleural and peritoneal fluids. *Acta Cytol.* 22:490–499.

Mukherjee TM. The role of electron microscopy in the diagnosis of neoplastic cells in effusion fluids. *J Submicrosc Cytol.* 1982;14:717–743.

Wuerker RB, Guglietti LC, Nations ED. Comparison on light and transmission electron microscopy in the definitive diagnosis of effusions. *Acta Cytol.* 1983;22:297–304.

Benign Conditions

Halter SA, Hunt LS, Roche B, Riedal RD. Backscatter electron imaging of cells from effusions. *Scan Electron Microsc.* 1984;4:1883–1892.

Geisinger K, Vance R, Prater T, et al. Rheumatoid pleural effusion: a transmission and scanning electron microscopic evaluation. *Acta Cytol.* 1985;29:239–247.

Hidvegi DF, Gurley AM. Electron microscopy. In Bibbo M, ed. *Comprehensive Cytopathology.* Philadelphia: Sanders. 1990:917–945.

Bedrossian CWM. Ultrastructure of pneumocystis carinii: a review of internal and surface characteristics. *Semin Diagn Pathol.* 1989;6:245–261.

Malignant Tumors

Martinez-Palomo A. Ultrastructural modifications of intercellular junctions in some epithelial tumors. *Lab Invest.* 1970;22:605–614.

Hanna W, Kahn H. The ultrastructure of metastatic adenocarcinoma in serous fluids. *Acta Cytol.* 1985;29:202–210.

Bewtra C, Greer K. Ultrastructural studies of cells in body cavity effusions. *Acta Cytol.* 1985;29:226–238.

Herrera GA, Wilkerson JA. Ultrastructural studies of malignant cells in fluids. *Diagn Cytopathol.* 1985;1:272–285.

Mesothelioma

Wang N-S. Electron microscopy in the diagnosis of pleural mesotheliomas. *Cancer.* 1973;27:1455–1464.

Butler EB, Johnson JF. The use of electron microscopy in the diagnosis of diffuse mesotheliomas using human pleural effusions. *In* Wagner JC, ed. *Biological Effects of Mineral Fibers,* vol 30. Lyon: IARC. 1980;409–418.

Warhol MJ, Hickey WF, Corson JM. Malignant mesothelioma: ultrastructural distinction from adenocarcinoma. *Am J Surg Pathol.* 1982;6:307–314.

Kobzik L, Antman K, Warhol M. The distinction of mesothelioma from adenocarcinoma in malignant effusions by electron microscopy. *Acta Cytol.* 1985;29:219–225.

Walts AE, Said JW, Shintaku IP. Epithelial membrane antigen in the cytodiagnosis of effusions and aspirates: immunocytochemical ultrastructural localization in benign and malignant cells. *Diagn Cytopathol.* 1987;3:41–49.

Adenocarcinoma

Woyke S, Domagala W, Olszewski W. Alveolar cell carcinoma of the lung: an ultrastructural study of the cancer cells detected in the pleural fluid. *Acta Cytol.* 1972;16:63–69.

Woyke S, Domagala W, Olszewski W. Ultrastructure of hepatoma cells detected in peritoneal fluid. *Acta Cytol.* 1974; 18:130–136.

Hickey WF, Seiler M. Ultrastructural markers of colonic adenocarcinoma. *Cancer.* 1981;47:140–145.

Posalaky Z, McGinley D, Posalaky IP. Electron microscopic identification of the colorectal origins of tumor cells in pleural fluid. *Acta Cytol.* 1983;27:45–48.

Hanna W, Kahn H. The ultrastructure of metastatic adenocarcinoma in serous fluids. *Acta Cytol.* 1985;29:202–210.

Duane G, Kanter M. Light and electron microscopic characteristics of signet-ring adenocarcinoma cells in serous effusions and their distinction from mesothelial cells. *Acta Cytol.* 1985;29:211–218.

Bedrossian CWM, Weilbaecher DG, Bentnick DC, Greenberg SD. Ultrastructure of human bronchiolo-alveolar carcinoma. *Cancer* 1975;36:1399–1413.

Other Tumors

Melamed MR, Wolinska WH. On the significance of intracytoplasmic inclusions in the urinary sediment. *Am J Pathol.* 1961;38:711.

Woyke S, Domagala W, Olszewski W. Ultrastructure of hepatoma cells detected in peritoneal fluid. *Acta Cytol.* 1974; 18:130–136.

Domagala W. The hairy cell. *Hum Pathol.* 1975;6:760–761.

Rosai J, Sumner HW, Kostianovski M, Perez-Mesa C. Angiosarcoma of the skin: a clinicopathologic and fine structural study. *Hum Pathol.* 1976;7:83–109.

Scanning Electron Microscopy

Polliack A, Lampen N, Clarkson B, et al. Identification of human B and T lymphocytes by scanning electron microscopy. *J Exp Med.* 1973;138:607–624.

Bahr GF, Bibbo M, Mikel U, et al. Correlation of light and scanning electron microscopy: a new method for exfoliative cytology. *Acta Cytol.* 1976;20:239–242.

Berliner JA, Jansser M, McLatchie C. The use of scanning electron microscopy in the diagnosis of malignancy in human serous effusions. *Scan Electron Microsc.* 1978;2:797–802.

Domagala W, Koss LG. Surface configuration of mesothelial cells in effusions. *Virchows Arch [B].* 1979;30:231–243.

Gondos B, Lai C, King EB. Distinction between atypical mesothelial cells and malignant cells by scanning electron microscopy. *Acta Cytol.* 1979;23:321–326.

Domagala W, Koss LG. Configuration of surfaces of cells in effusions by scanning electron microscopy. In Koss LG, Coleman DV, eds. *Advances in Clinical Cytology.* London: Butterworths. 1981, pp 270–313.

Beals T. Scanning electron microscopy of body fluids. *Diagn Cytopathol.* 1992;8:266–271.

Diagnostic Applications

Peven DR, Gruhn JD. The development of electron microscopy. *Arch Pathol Lab Med.* 1985;109:683–691.

Koss L. Electron microscopy in cytology. *Acta Cytol.* 1986; 30:195–196.

Duffy A, Stevens M, McLennan G. The immunogold staining technique for the measurement of lymphocyte subpopulations in bronchoalveolar lavage fluid. *Acta Cytol.* 1986;30: 152–156.

Bedrossian CWM. Electron microscopy: the neglected tool of cytopathology. *Diagn Cytopathol.* 1992;8:vi–viii.

Immuno-EM

Kahn HJ, Hanna W, Baumal R. Immunohistochemical localization of prekeratin filaments in benign and malignant cells in effusions: comparison with intermediate filament distribution by electron microscopy. *Am J Pathol.* 1982;109: 206–214.

Walts AE, Said JW, Shintaku IP. Epithelial membrane antigen in the cytodiagnosis of effusions and aspirates: immunocytochemical and ultrastructural localization in benign and malignant cells. *Diagn Cytopathol.* 1987;3:41–49.

CHAPTER FIFTEEN

Immunocytochemistry

Malignant effusions often constitute evidence of widespread metastasis that may preclude surgical therapy or even radiotherapy. A malignant effusion commonly mandates chemotherapy with profound therapeutic and prognostic implications. As such, it is a diagnosis that cannot be made lightly. Morphologic analysis of the cells recovered from an effusion may not be sufficient for arriving at a malignant diagnosis. Not uncommonly, the distinction between hyperplastic mesothelial cells and metastatic carcinomas is impossible because of the notorious reactivity of mesothelial cells. Some carcinomas shed single cells that are difficult to distinguish from macrophages and mesothelial cells. In sarcomas, there may not be enough cells in the effusion; even when present, they may not be familiar to the examiner, due to the relative infrequency of these neoplasms.

Ancillary methods have been employed in an attempt to improve the diagnostic accuracy of recognizing and classifying malignancy in effusions. As discussed in detail in Chapter 16, many of the ancillary techniques provide quantitative data but add little to the appreciation of cytomorphology. In contrast, immunocytochemistry relies on visual appreciation of cellular detail by ordinary light microscopy, a task familiar to every cytologist. Consequently, it has enjoyed enormous popularity, backed by various studies beginning in the early 1980s. Currently, the greatest difficulty with this technique concerns choosing the best antibodies applicable to effusions from the burgeoning repertoire currently on the market. Markers are currently available that specifically enhance every structural and functional component of the cell.

When coupled with a counterstain that renders the usual morphology of the cell appreciable, immunocytochemistry becomes one of the most powerful tools for cytologic examination of clinical specimens. This combination is called immunocytopathology because both immunophenotyping and cytologic scrutiny can be accomplished in the same preparation. A crucial element of this approach is the opportunity to survey nuclear features indicative of malignancy. Immunocytopathology is different from the immunophenotyping of cell suspensions and frozen sections with immunofluorescence or immunoperoxidase techniques. With these techniques, morphologic detail is lost and cytologic appreciation of the distribution of the immunostain is not possible. Immunocytopathology is also superior to cytomorphology alone because it allows more precise classification of cell types by identifying specific membrane, cytoskeletal, cytoplasmic, and nuclear products. A crucial step is to utilize the peroxidase-antiperoxidase (P.A.P.) method alongside a good cytologic counterstain such as Lillie-Mayer's hematoxylin. Immunocytochemistry is very effective when combined with EM because it allows elucidation of precise subcellular localization, in addition to recognizing a specific marker. Because of their appreciation of subtle morphologic features and their understanding of cellular mechanisms, cytopathologists are uniquely equipped to take advantage of this method for both diagnostic and investigative purposes. Immunocytopathology can also be utilized beyond its diagnostic applications as a result of a number of recently described prognostic markers.

DIAGNOSTIC APPLICATIONS

There have been a number of studies of effusion specimens performed using immunocytochemistry that used at least 50 different markers. Some of these markers are not commercially available or have been used in relatively few specimens; reproducibility and reliability is therefore difficult to ascertain. Many, however, have emerged as particularly useful in the study of effusions and have been categorized according to their ability to demonstrate various structural elements of the cell (Table 15.1).

TABLE 15.1 Immunocytochemical Characterization
of Cells in Cytologic Preparations

Epithelial Cells
  Epithelial membrane antigens
  Oncofetal markers
  Secretory markers
  Neuroendocrine markers
  Squamous markers
  Germ-cell markers
  Organ-related markers
Nonepithelial Cells
  Collagen fibrils
  Myogenous markers
  Neurogenic markers
  Vascular markers
  Lipocytic markers
  Osteochondrocytic markers
  Melanocytic markers
Lymphohistiocytic Markers
  Leucocyte-common antigens
  Cell-lineage markers
  Cell-surface markers
  Immunoglobulins
  Histiocytic markers
  Megakaryocytic markers
  Erythroleukemic markers

Cytoskeletal markers are most useful in the distinction between mesotheliomas and carcinomas. Cytokeratins expressed by mesothelial cells differ significantly from those expressed by carcinoma cells; however, little difference exists in the cytokeratins expressed by benign and malignant mesothelial cells. Some differences exist also between the expression of keratin by various types of carcinomas in effusions, and this phenomenon has undergone limited investigation regarding elucidation of primary sites of neoplasms responsible for malignant effusions. A much greater number of studies have relied on the differential expression of epithelial membrane antigens (EMAs), secretory products, and oncofetal markers for detection and classification of carcinomas in effusions. Lymphohistiocytic markers have also been extensively and successfully applied to effusion specimens on the basis of their success in the study of biopsy material from lymph nodes. Mesenchymal markers have not been as thoroughly studied in effusions as in biopsy and fine-needle aspiration biopsy specimens. The same is true of antibodies that identify infective agents, as discussed in Chapter 6. In this chapter, lymphomas and leukemias are discussed to the extent

that they may enter the differential diagnosis of solid neoplasms. The following comments, however, apply to more common carcinomas and sarcomas, as well as other solid tumors responsible for malignant effusions.

Cytoskeletal Components

The cytoskeleton is responsible for a cell's ability to keep its structural integrity. All physical properties of the cell, including its size, shape, texture, and tinctorial properties, depend on an intact cytoskeleton. Even though the individual filamentous units of the cytoskeleton cannot be visualized by light microscopy, they are responsible for preservation of crisp cytologic detail. Degeneration and necrosis involve dissolution of the orderly arrangement of cytoskeletal components. An intact cytoskeleton makes it possible for the other functions of the cells, such as secretion and storage of secretory products in vacuoles, to take place undisturbed. Integrity of the cytoskeleton is also necessary for the cell's ability to divide and multiply, two vital properties of neoplastic cells in effusions.

The filaments of the cytoskeleton fall into three major categories: (1) thin microfilaments (6 nm), mainly actin; (2) thick microtubules (25 nm), mainly tubulin; and (3) intermediate filaments (10 nm), comprising subtypes related to the tissues from which they were isolated (i.e.: neurofilaments (NF) from neurons; glial filaments (GFAP) from astrocytes; vimentin from mesenchymal cells; desmin from muscle cells; and keratin from epithelial cells. Intermediate filaments have had the greatest applicability in effusion cytology, particularly keratin, and to a lesser extent, vimentin.

Cytokeratin

A number of antikeratin antibodies have been utilized in the study of mesothelioma and carcinoma in effusions. Mesotheliomas stain the strongest with antikeratin antibodies, whereas carcinomas show variable, generally weaker intensity (Fig. 15.1). Keratin is positive in mesothelioma, regardless of the degree of differentiation. However, the degree of positivity is lower in poorly differentiated mesotheliomas (Fig. 15.2). Adenocarcinomas express only low molecular weight keratins, whereas squamous-cell carcinomas express both low and high molecular weight keratins but give a stronger reaction for the latter. Antibodies can be raised to a mixture of keratins of different molecular weights (polyclonal antibodies) or to a narrow range of molecular

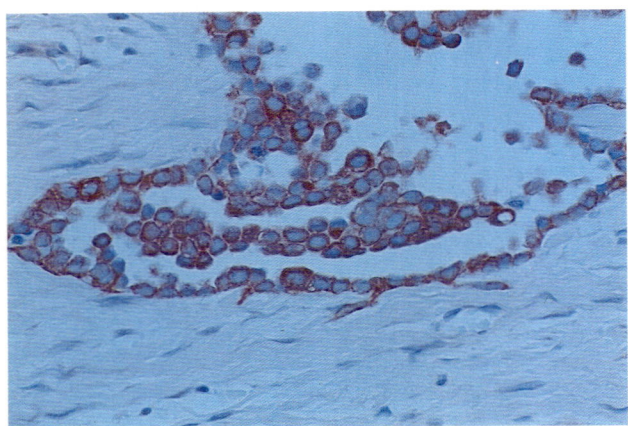

FIGURE 15.1   Mesothelioma stained for keratin. Notice perinuclear immunopositivity highlighting tumor cells lining irregular slits. (P.A.P. × 40)

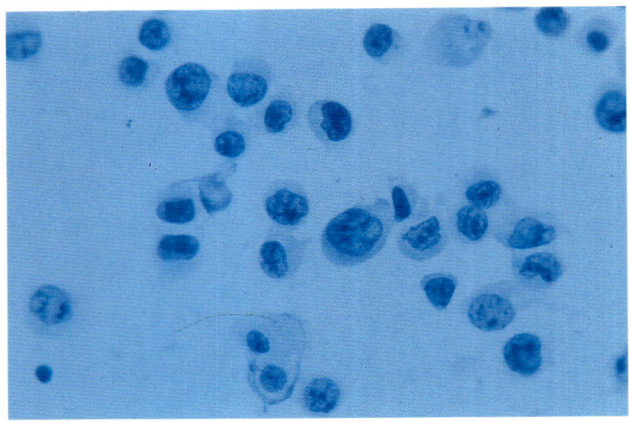

FIGURE 15.3   Pleural fluid in patient with breast carcinoma and retroperitoneal involvement by a neoplasm. Predominance of discohesive cells led to inclusion of a high grade lymphoma in the differential diagnosis in this case. (Pap × 180)

weights (monoclonal antibodies). The latter can be either utilized to recognize keratins of restricted specificity or combined in the form of a broad spectrum cocktail of monoclonal antibodies. Moll has catalogued the keratins into 19 families according to their acidic or basic properties and their molecular weight. Use of antibodies with restricted specificity has been successful in classifying neoplasms in tissue preparations and is slowly finding its way into cytologic application, including the study of effusions. A broad spectrum cocktail of keratin antibodies is helpful in differentiating carcinoma from large cell lymphoma (Figs. 15.3 and 15.4).

Mesotheliomatous effusions stained for keratin show groups of cells with their architecture well delineated by the immunostain (Fig. 15.5). In addition, the pattern of immunostain distribution within the positive cells is better appreciated than in tissue sections (Fig. 15.6). A concentric pattern of positivity for low molecular weight keratins favors a mesothelimatous rather than a carcinomatous cell origin. Carcinoma cells are negative for high molecular weight keratin, whereas mesothelial cells are positive for both high and low molecular weight keratins. Positivity for low molecular weight keratin in mesotheliomas may allow appreciation of the

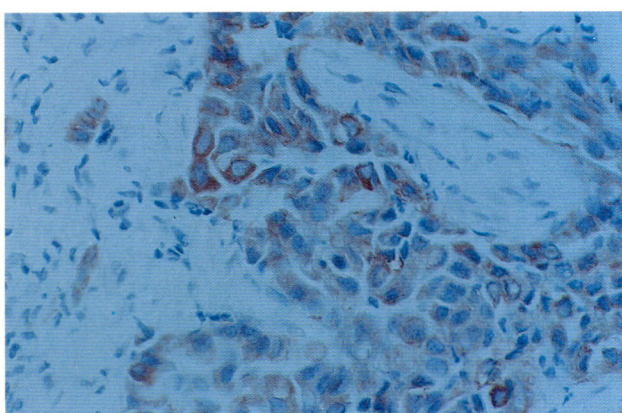

FIGURE 15.2   Mesothelioma stained for keratin. The immunostain outlines well the groups of tumor amidst a collagenous stroma (P.A.P. × 120)

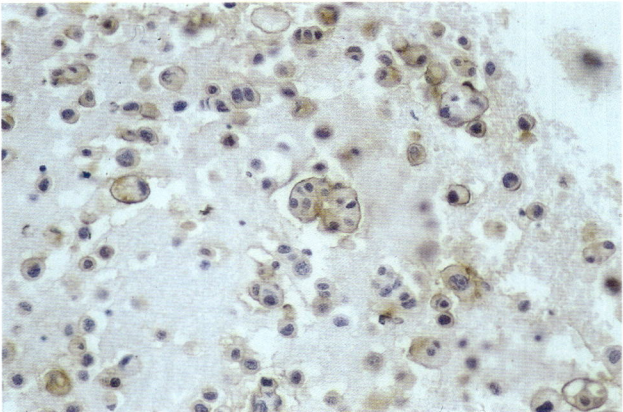

FIGURE 15.4   Cell block from same case as Fig 15.3. Keratin immunopositivity excludes lymphoma and facilitates the finding of cohesive epithelial cell groupings (P.A.P. × 60)

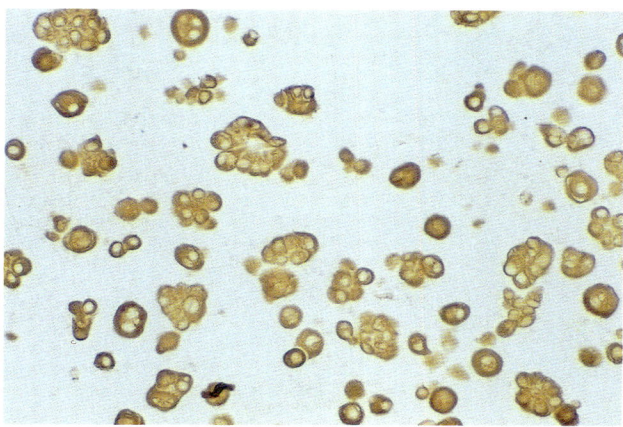

FIGURE 15.5 Pleural fluid stained for keratin without a counterstain. The mesotheliomatous groups are clearly delineated but cytologic detail cannot be appreciated. (P.A.P. × 90)

FIGURE 15.7 Breast adenocarcinoma stained for keratin. Notice absence of window between cells and short, stubby microvilli. (P.A.P. × 180)

ectoendoplasmic demarcation in their cytoplasm variably. Adenocarcinoma shows a diffuse, intense arborizing pattern of positivity throughout the cytoplasm. Individual malignant cells of squamous carcinomas stain homogeneously strong with antibodies against high molecular weight keratin. The prevalence of positivity for keratin ranges from 100% in mesotheliomas to 36% in adenocarcinomas of the pancreas. Even though keratin is an important member of the effusion panel, it cannot be relied on individually for diagnosis. Keratin, along

FIGURE 15.6 Mesothelioma stained for keratin with Lillie-Mayer's hematoxylin as a counterstain. Both nuclear morphology and distribution of the immunostain are well demonstrated (P.A.P. × 90)

with other epithelial cell markers, can be used to better define the architecture of cell groupings. For instance, the relationship between individual cells in a group can be clarified by the use of antibodies against keratin and actin, in cytologic specimens (Fig. 15.7).

Vimentin

Vimentin received a lot of attention in 1981 when it was first reported that carcinomas, which were vimentin-negative in the primary site, expressed vimentin in effusions. However, no plausible explanation has ever been set forth for this observation, except that it appears related to coexpression of vimentin and keratin by certain carcinomas. It is possible that the milieu in which the cells grow influences the physiochemical factors responsible for the cross-linking necessary for vimentin and keratin epitomes to resemble one another. The only practical importance of this phenomenon is that vimentin positivity by itself cannot be overinterpreted as evidence of a mesenchymal origin for neoplastic cells detected in the effusion.

In general, vimentin-positive malignant cells in effusions range from faint to slightly reactive; they never approach the intensity of keratin positivity found in coexpressant carcinomas. Vimentin may also be positive in reactive mesothelia and mesotheliomatous cells, but the intensity of this positivity also falls short of the keratin intensity exhibited by these cells. The list of neoplasms that coexpress keratin and vimentin has grown long over the past several years to include not only mesotheliomas but carcinomas of the salivary gland, the kidney, the lung, the thyroid, and the ovary. We have also seen sporadic examples of other primary sites coexpressing vimentin in tissue sections; an open mind should therefore be kept with regard to the ability of other carcinomas to demonstrate vimentin positivity in effusions. The possibility exists that vimentin is expressed by epithelial cells when they undergo malignant transformation. Epithelial tumors that coexpress vimentin along with keratin seem to have a worse clinical course, suggesting that vimentin may be a prognostic marker.

Epithelial Membrane Antigens

In the early 1980s, heavily glycosylated antigens were extracted from milk-fat globules derived from mammary epithelial cell lines. The resulting antibodies recognized a number of epithelial cells and sparked commercially available antibodies against epithelial membrane antigen (EMA). Initially, EMA was believed to discriminate between consistently positive epithelial cells from mesothelial cells that were either negative or show only a faint cytoplasmic positivity. Further studies, however, have demonstrated a strong apical degree of positivity for EMA in mesothelioma (Fig. 15.8). As with other markers, EMA is very helpful in defining the architecture of cell groups in mesothelioma (Fig. 15.9). The so-called "thick cell membrane" pattern of positivity corresponds to elongated microvilli and is not noted in adenocarcinoma. The latter usually shows a short,

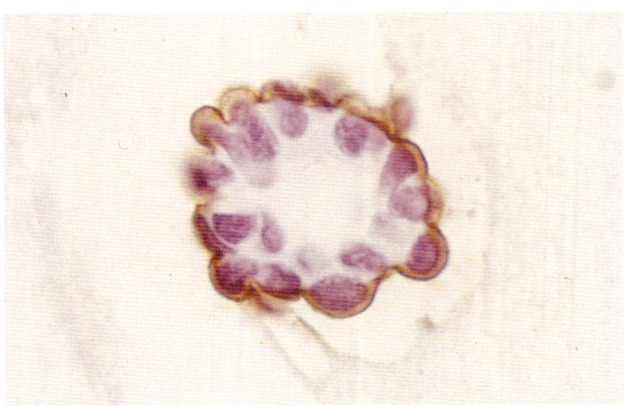

FIGURE 15.9 Scalloped group of cells stained for EMA. The thick cell membrane pattern is characteristic of mesothelioma (P.A.P. × 180)

stubby pattern of immunopositivity for EMA, demonstrable also by other stains (Fig. 15.10). Ovarian carcinomas exceptionally may present with microvilli as long as or longer than mesothelioma. In these cases, however, the microvilli are not distributed over the entire perimeter of the cell. The microvilli of mesotheliomatous cells are considerably more florid than observed in reactive mesothelial cells. Only rarely, however, this phenomenon aids in the discrimination between mesothelioma and accompanying reactive mesothelial hyperplasia by observing the pattern of immunopositivity for EMA. Most studies in the United States have utilized the commercially available antibody against EMA. Positivity ranges from 44 to 98% in mesothelioma and 62 to

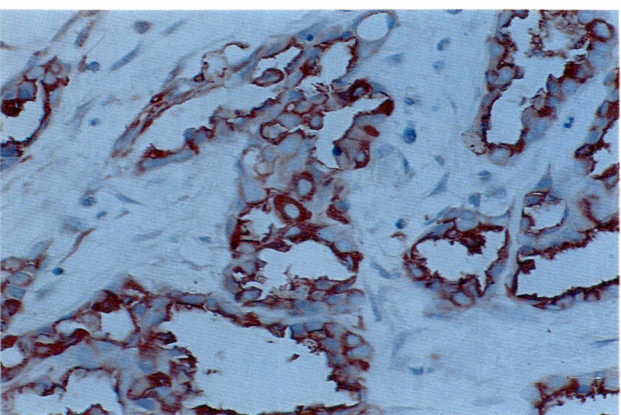

FIGURE 15.8 Mesothelioma stained for EMA. Note thick cell membrane pattern on the surface of the tumor cells. (P.A.P. × 80)

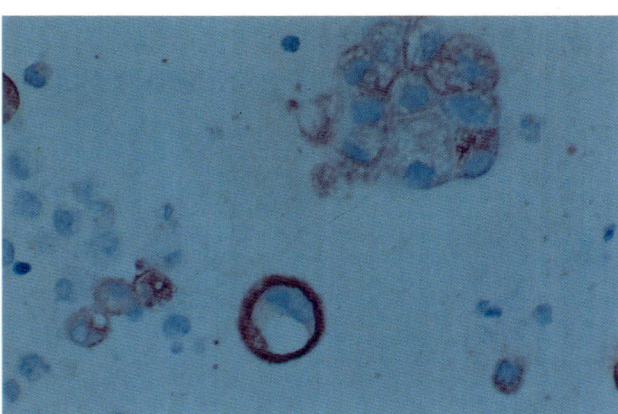

FIGURE 15.10 Individual malignant mesotheliomatous cell. Note microvilli enhanced by EMA over the entire perimeter of the cell. (P.A.P. × 90)

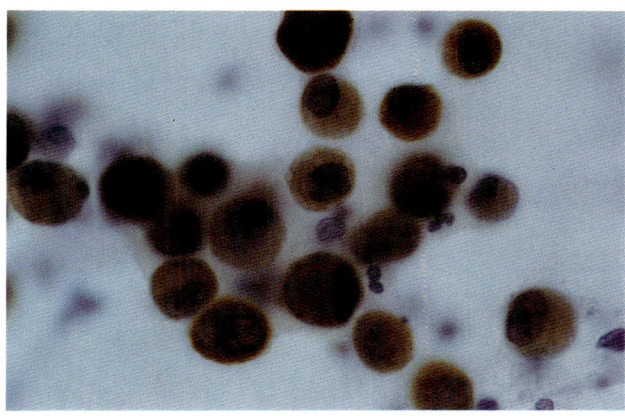

FIGURE 15.11 EMA positivity in epithelial cell. In contrast to mesothelioma, positivity of EMA in adenocarcinoma extends diffusely throughout the cytoplasm. (Pap × 90)

100% in carcinoma. In our experience, the intensity and distribution of anti-EMA positivity is variable both in epithelial and reactive mesothelial cells. Poorly differentiated carcinoma shows a diffuse generally weak pattern of positivity for EMA (Fig 15.11).

As with all immunocytochemical results, EMA has to be evaluated in the broad context of cytomorphologic and additional immunocytochemical features to achieve a more precise diagnosis. For instance, EMA may be expressed by large-cell lymphomas; it should therefore be combined with leukocyte common antigen (LCA) when the differential diagnosis is between carcinoma and lymphoma. True histiocytic lymphomas most frequently express EMA, followed by B-cell lymphomas, myeloma, and T-cell lymphomas. EMA is also expressed in epithelioid sarcomas and leiomyosarcomas, tumors that require good cytologic evaluation alongside the interpretation of immunocytochemical stains.

For instance, EMA may be expressed by large-cell lymphomas; should therefore be combined with LCA when the differential diagnosis is between carcinoma and lymphoma. True histiocytic lymphomas most frequently express EMA, followed by B-cell lymphomas, myeloma, and T-cell lymphomas. EMA is also expressed in epithelioid sarcomas and leiomyosarcomas, tumors that require good cytologic evaluation alongside the interpretation of immunocytochemical stains.

Human Milk-Fat Globule

Two antibodies prepared against human milk-fat globules (HMFG) have been applied in cytology. They rec-

ognize either large, glycosylated carbohydrate complexes (HMFG-1) or smaller molecules with a greater proportion of exposed residues of sialic acid (HMFG-2). Neither of these two antigens are demonstrated in the cytoplasm of reactive mesothelial cells but are expressed by cells derived from malignant mesotheliomas. HMFG-2, however, is identified in carcinomatous cells derived from breast, lung, ovary and gastrointestinal tract. In these cases, HMFG-2 shows a diffuse pattern of strong cytoplasmic positivity. Anti-HMFG-2 has been reported as positive in a linear pattern in mesothelioma. The antibody works better in fresh material; therefore, results in alcohol or B5-formalin–fixed effusion cell blocks have not matched results in tissue sections. In general, the thick membrane pattern in mesotheliomas appears less intense with HMFG-2 than with EMA.

Ber-Ep-4

A new antibody was described in 1990 (Ber-Ep-4) that purported to distinguish between consistently positive epithelial and consistently negative mesothelial cells. In malignant effusions, the pattern of Ber-Ep-4 staining is linear along the surface of the carcinomatous cells. However, in acinar groups, positivity is not restricted to the luminal pole but extends also to an abluminal location. This peculiarity is extremely helpful in identifying islands of bronchiolar epithelium trapped within mesotheliomas that invade the lung. In adenocarcinoma, both the tumors and any trapped normal epithelium are positive for Ber-Ep-4. Not so in mesthelioma, where nests of trapped Ber-Ep-4-positive epithelial cells appear as islands, within the mesotheliomatous tissue (Fig. 15.12). No explanation for this phenomenon is currently available due to the lack of immunoelectron microscopic studies of Ber-Ep-4-positivity. Results of controlled investigations are few but suggest high specificity and low sensitivity for identifying epithelial cells in B5-formalin–fixed material. We have utilized Ber-Ep-4 in tissue sections of mesothelioma; a few tumors showed focal immunopositivity. The small number of cells involved is not sufficient to compromise the antibody, but its true value in effusions awaits further verification of the initially promising results.

Secretory Markers

Mesothelial cells share some characteristics with epithelial cells, such as a keratin-rich cytoskeleton and a membrane system that reacts with antibodies against certain

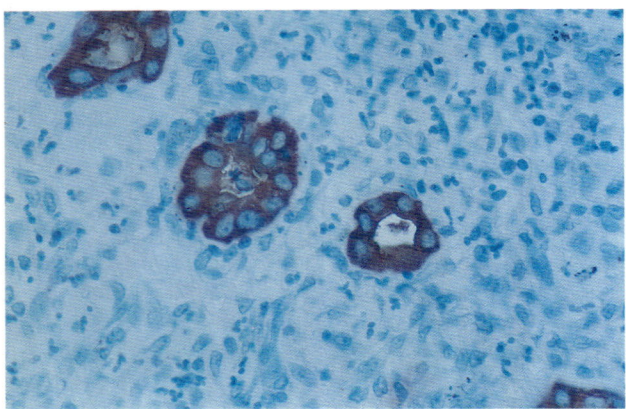

FIGURE 15.12 Trapped epithelial cells in mesothelioma highlighted by Ber Ep4. While the surrounding tumor cells are negative, the epithelial ducts are strongly positive. (P.A.P. × 60)

but not all epithelial membrane antigens. This latter finding has been observed with EMA, HMFG, and Ber-Ep-4 in a variable proportion of cases; therefore, absolute distinction between mesothelial and epithelial cells is not always possible, and interpretation depends on the pattern of immunostaining. It is obvious that a group of markers that would be negative in mesothelial cells but positive in carcinomas would be a welcome addition to the pathologist's armamentarium. No such antibody exists for all carcinomas, but a few secretory markers have been described that are consistently positive in adenocarcinomas and negative in mesothelial cells.

Leu M₁

In 1986, Leu M₁, a monoclonal antibody that recognizes monocytes, histiocytes, and activated T-lymphocytes, was found also to react with adenocarcinomatous cells but not with mesothelial cells. This property renders Leu M₁ useful in the differentiation between mesotheliomas and adenocarcinomas, particularly because the antibody shows high specificity for epithelial neoplasms. Even though Leu M₁ must be applied to fresh or frozen material to react with lymphohistiocytic cells, it works well in formalin-fixed cell blocks showing adenocarcinomas. The diffuse pattern of cytoplasmic positivity suggests that Leu M₁ localizes in the endoplasmic reticulum of carcinomatous cells, a phenomenon demonstrated by immunoelectron microscopy. Leu M₁ is positive in ovarian, mammary, pulmonary, and gastric carcinomas but negative in carcinomas of liver, kidney,

and prostate, which suggest it can discriminate between adenocarcinomas with intestinal and nonintestinal microvilli. Leu M₁ is helpful in the differential diagnosis of malignant effusions that show pleomorphic cells since it is positive in large-cell carcinomas of the lung but negative in melanomas, embryonal carcinomas, and carcinomas of the adrenal gland.

B 72-3

Great hopes were raised when an antibody (B 72-3) was developed against the TAG-72 antigen derived from a cell line of breast carcinoma. Early studies showed no reactivity for mesothelial cells and a strong specificity for breast carcinoma. Subsequent studies, however, demonstrated that only a variable proportion of breast carcinomas are positive for B 72-3, as well as other carcinomas, (e.g., colon, stomach, lung, ovary). B 72-3 may also be focally positive in tissue sections of mesotheliomas; however, this is not a problem when the findings are taken in context with the cytologic features of the cells and results obtained with other antibodies. B 72-3 will outline the boundaries of cells intracytoplasmic lumina of breast carcinoma, which makes it useful for comparison with tissue sections of the same neoplasm (Fig. 15.13). In cytologic preparations, we use B72-3 in combination with Ber-Ep-4 and Leu M1 in the differential diagnosis between mesothelioma and CEA-negative adenocarcinomas. Mesothelioma is invariably negative for all three markers, whereas adenocarcinoma is positive for at least one, if not all three antibodies.

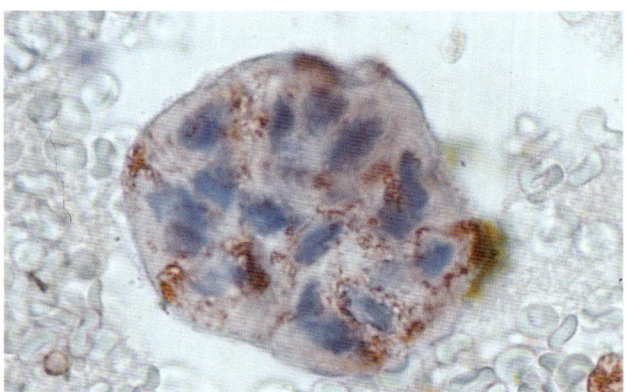

FIGURE 15.13 Breast adenocarcinoma. The immunostain for B-72-3 shows various cells surrounding a rudimentary lumen. (P.A.P. × 120)

S100

S100 protein is unique among the secretory markers because it was first described as an antigen found in tissues of neuronal derivation. Because the protein had not been characterized, its serendipitous detection in nonneuronal neoplasms was an object of great puzzlement. More recently, the chemical structure of S100 protein, composed of a two-unit chain of approximately 50 amino acids, has been deciphered, and it has been further suggested that S100 is involved in cell growth regulation. This finding explains why S100 has been detected in epithelial neoplasms such as carcinomas of lung, breast, ovary, pancreas, and gastrointestinal tract; as well as in nonepithelial tumors as diverse as melanomas, chondrosarcomas, schwanomas, and chordomas. The common denominator among all these tumors is their potential to accumulate mucin-related secretory products to the point where mucosubstances may be demonstrated histochemically in at least a small proportion of cases. We use S100 in our second-line effusion panel to distinguish between reactive mesothelial and adenocarcinomatous cells, particularly if the putative primary neoplasm was positive for S100. If the cells are consistently negative for other markers of adenocarcinomatous differentiation but positive for S100, consideration should be given to the possibility of melanoma, provided that this diagnosis is morphologically compatible. Finding of acinar structures with cytoplasmic positivity for S100 is typical of adenocarcinoma (Fig. 15.14). S100 positivity does not exclude the possibility of mesothelioma, but this tumor often presents with large papillary groups of tumor cells. Some authors have claimed that S100 is positive in mesothelioma but not in reactive mesothelial cells.

Oncofetal Antigens

During neoplastic transformation, malignant cells may revert to a primitive state and elaborate substances typical of the fetal stage of development (i.e., they mimic germ cells by expressing a number of markers not commonly found in mature tissues). These markers are differentially expressed by various tumors and have been utilized as tumor markers, tissue-specific markers, and as indicators of histogenetic derivation. Recent studies have shown oncofetal markers expressed with different prevalence and different intensity during the life of a tumor. They may, therefore, be best considered as differentiation antigens. Accordingly, some oncofetal marker (e.g., CEA) may be indicative of glandular differentiation whereas another (e.g., placental lactogen) is typical of a lesser degree of differentiation as noted in germ cell neoplasm. Oncofetal markers occur in an extreme variety of tumors, regardless of their site of origin or putative histogenesis.

Current concepts favor differentiation rather than histogenesis as the basis for the variety of histologic patterns exhibited by the same neoplasm in primary and metastatic sites. In effusions, neoplasms tend to exhibit a more homogenous appearance, which is perhaps linked to the selection mechanism that segregates the population of cells more likely to remain viable in the special milieu represented by the serous fluids. Very often, the morphologic appearance of these cells is sufficiently different from the autochthonous cell population to allow their distinction from mesothelial cells. These cells may be recognized as alien by their morphologic distinctiveness or, conversely, their misplaced character may be evident by the way they arrange themselves in comparison with mesothelial cells. However, when their morphologic resemblance to mesothelial cells is strong, immunocytochemical markers are useful in the distinction between metastatic carcinomas and mesothelial cells. CEA and other oncofetal markers expressed by carcinoma serve this purpose well.

Carcinoembryonic Antigen

CEA is one of the most useful immunocytopathology markers. Not only does it segregate epithelial from mesothelial cells, but also it frequently identifies the cells in the effusion as malignant. Furthermore, it may point

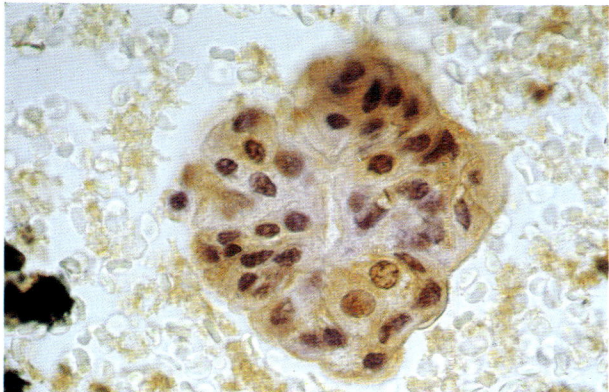

FIGURE 15.14 Same case as Fig 15.7. With an anti-S100 antibody, the texture of the cytoplasm can be appreciated. (P.A.P. × 120)

towards differentiation in the direction of adenocarcinoma. However, care should be taken not to read too much into CEA positivity when attempting to find the primary site of a neoplasm. The range of positivity for CEA is so vast that, theoretically, every carcinoma—and not only adenocarcinomas—may be positive for CEA. It is therefore important to interpret CEA in effusions in concert with (1) the clinical history, including any radiologic evidence of a neoplasm; (2) the age and sex of the patient, as well as the location of the effusion; and (3) the morphologic appearance of the malignant cells. Recognition of malignancy and tumor classification may depend on comparison of the effusion with any previous material from the tumor, including archival slides and paraffin blocks. If previous blocks are found, testing with CEA as well as a complete panel of antibodies concomitant with the new material may shed light on the primary site. There are currently broad, specific monoclonal CEA antibodies that are more specific for malignant cells and offer less cross-reactivity with non-specific cross-reactive antigen (NCA). There are also monoclonal anti-CEA antibodies of restricted specificity that allegedly discriminate between certain primary sites of adenocarcinomas. Thus, some antibodies are believed to recognize colonic and gastric carcinomas as opposed to a primary lung carcinoma.

In effusions, the pattern of CEA positivity is of some assistance in distinguishing between adenocarcinomas and other carcinomas by the way it demonstrates the texture of the cytoplasm. In adenocarcinomas, texture ranges from finely stipled to finely flocculent, reflecting the secretory nature of the cell (Fig. 15.15). CEA may also clearly delineate signet ring cells (Fig. 15.16). Poorly differentiated carcinomas lack secretory differentiation and give a more compact pattern of immunopositivity for CEA (Fig. 15.17). Single malignant cells with unclear differentiation may have their adenocarcinomatous nature revealed by CEA (Fig. 15.18). Carcinomas with multinucleated cells must be differentiated from melanoma and multiple myeloma. CEA may provide a clue as to the carcinomatous nature of these cells (Figs. 15.19 and 15.20). In squamous and transitional-cell carcinomas, texture is less foamy in appearance, which reflects increased amounts of intermediate filaments and decreased amounts of secretory vesicles. It has been demonstrated using immunoelectron microscopy that CEA localizes to the rough endoplasmic reticulum of secretory cells. CEA may be associated with a histochemical marker such as alcian blue and mucin to pinpoint the degree of secretory differentiation exhibited by the adenocarcinoma (Fig. 15.21). Such a combination may be helpful in cases with scant cellularity where

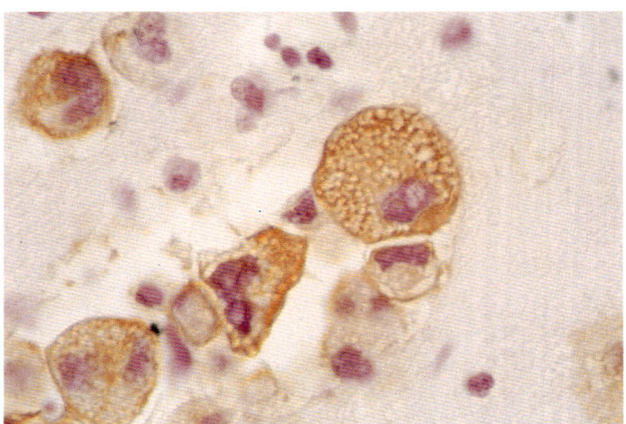

FIGURE 15.15 Gastric adenocarcinoma stained for CEA. The delicate, fluffy pattern of immunostain corresponds to the secetory apparatus of the cells. (Pap × 120)

a cell block preparation is not available. Clear cell carcinoma of cervico-vaginal origin are often positive by the alcian blue-CEA combination (Figs. 15.22 and 15.23). Well-differentiated, mucus-secreting adenocarcinomas are positive for both alcian blue and CEA, whereas poorly differentiated carcinomas are positive only for CEA. Alcian blue positivity in well differentiated tumors extends both to intracytoplasmic and extracellular mucin, whereas CEA is only positive in the cytoplasm (Fig. 15.24).

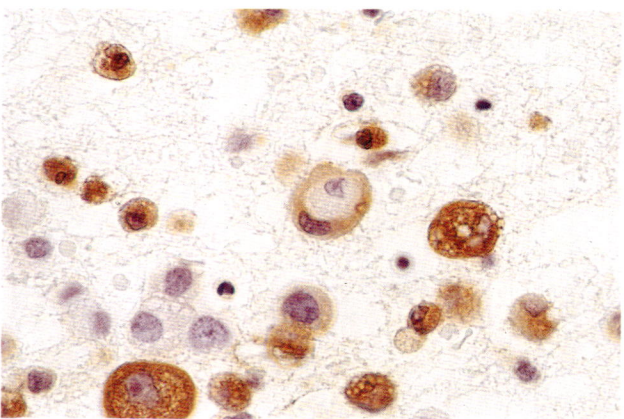

FIGURE 15.16 Adenocarcinoma of stomach stained for CEA. Notice positive pattern in tumor cells including signet rings. Mesothelial cells are either negative. (P.A.P. × 180)

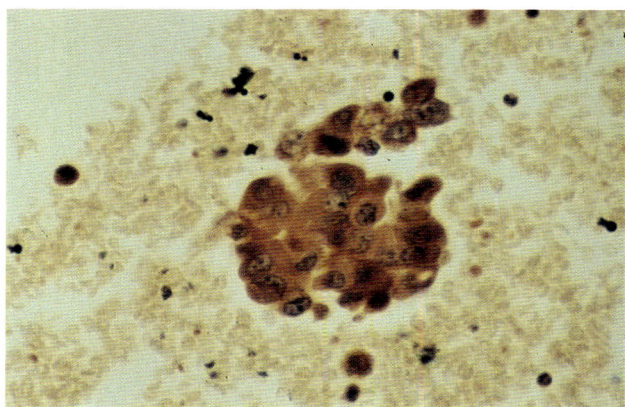

FIGURE 15.17 Poorly differentiated carcinoma of the pyriform sinus. The tumor cells show a non-textured pattern of immunopositivity for CEA. (P.A.P. × 90)

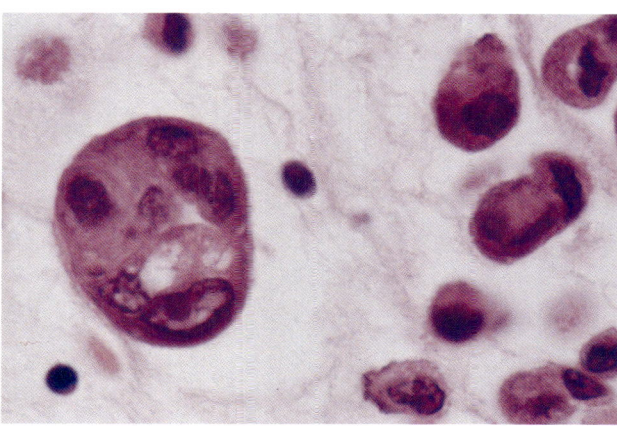

FIGURE 15.19 Cholangiocarcinoma in a cell block. The cytoplasm of the multinucleated cell suggests vacuolization. (H&E × 180)

Alpha-fetoprotein

Alpha-fetoprotein (AFP) is a sialic acid-containing protein that is structurally related to albumin and secreted in large quantities by fetuses. In adults, hepatocellular carcinomas and germ-cell tumors are accompanied by high levels of AFP in the serum, which is reflected in the immunopositivity exhibited by these same tumors. Embryonal carcinomas are positive for AFP (Fig. 15.25). This is not a specific finding, because certain adenocarcinomas also express AFP (e.g., stomach, lung, pancreas). Mesothelial cells are negative for AFP; therefore, the antibody has some application in the diagnosis of carcinoma in CEA-negative effusions. In our practice, AFP is not utilized as a member of the basic effusion panel (i.e., keratin, CEA, EMA, Leu M_1, and B 723) to rule out adenocarcinoma. AFP is reserved for those patients in whom classification of the tumor remains unresolved by the first panel, even after cytomorphologic and clinical correlations.

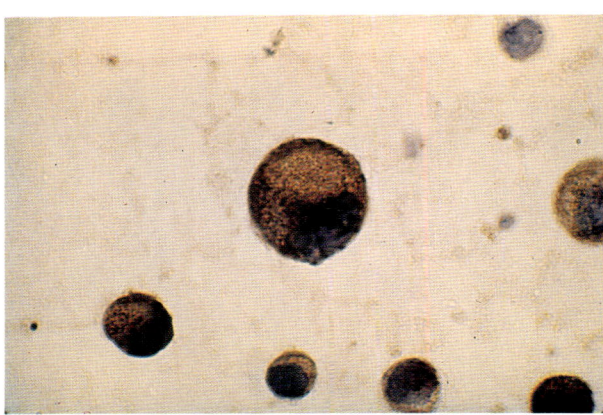

FIGURE 15.18 Adenocarcinoma initially classified as poorly differentiated. Note fluffy texture of the CEA immunostain corresponds to the rich endoplasmic reticulum of the cell. (P.A.P. × 120)

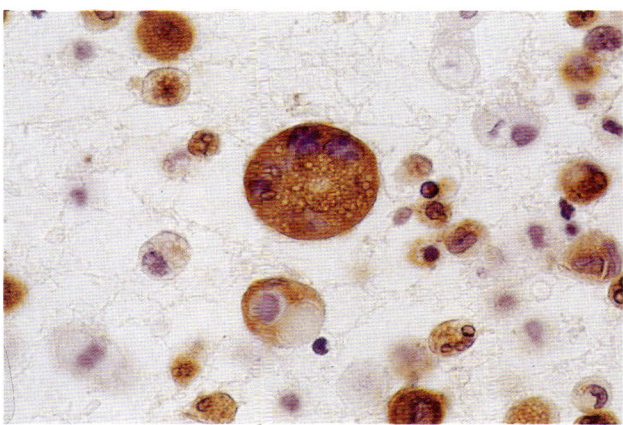

FIGURE 15.20 Same case as Fig 15.19 stained for CEA. Notice positivity of the immunostain highlighting the fine texture of the cytoplasm. (P.A.P. × 120)

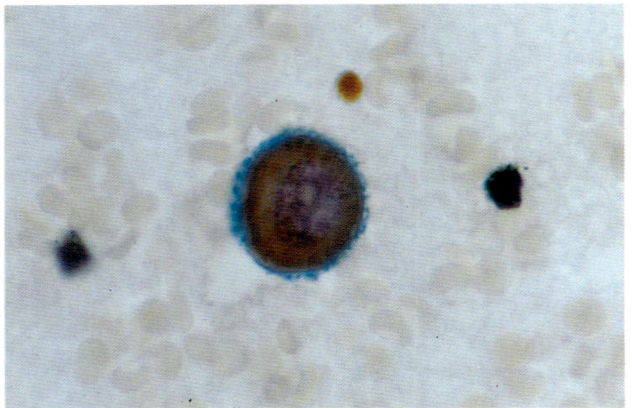

FIGURE 15.21   Adenocarcinoma double stained with Alcian blue-CEA. The CEA-positive cell shows a delicate Alcian blue staining of its apical border in a short, stubby pattern. (P.A.P./Alcian Blue)

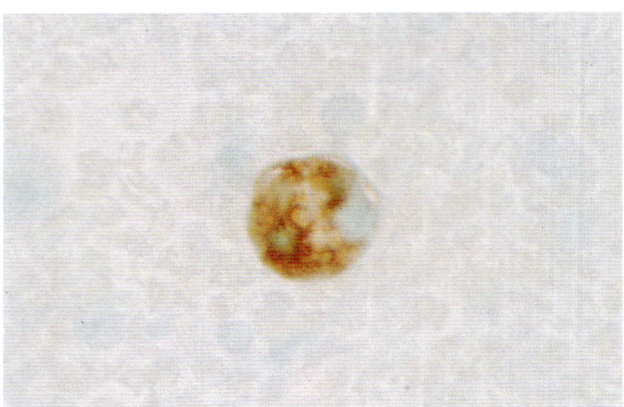

FIGURE 15.23   Same case as Fig 15.24 following immunostain. With Alcian blue-CEA, mixed positivity is indicative of glandular differentiation. (P.A.P./Alcian Blue × 180)

Placental Alkaline Phosphatase

There are six organ-specific varieties of alkaline phosphatase (i.e., bone, kidney, liver, intestine, bronchus and placenta). Placental alkaline phosphatase (PLAP) has been the most commonly used in the study of neoplasms. In contrast to AFP, PLAP is frequently positive in seminomas but almost always negative in the other subtypes of germ-cell tumors. PLAP is negative in mesothelial cells, but effusions accidentally contaminated with colonic and bronchial epithelium will show PLAP positivity. Peritoneal washes may also be positive for PLAP because cells derived from ovarian cysts are reactive for the enzyme.

PLAP is useful in identification of certain carcinomas present in effusion, including those of pulmonary, mammary, gastric, colonic, renal, endometrial, and ovarian origin (Fig. 15.26). Squamous and undifferentiated small-cell carcinomas of lung, cervix, and esophagus may also be positive for PLAP. This marker is much less frequently positive than the first line of markers of epithelial differentiation. For this reason, we reserve PLAP for those cases in which carcinoma is strongly suspected, but tumor cells fail to react to our basic epithelial cell panel.

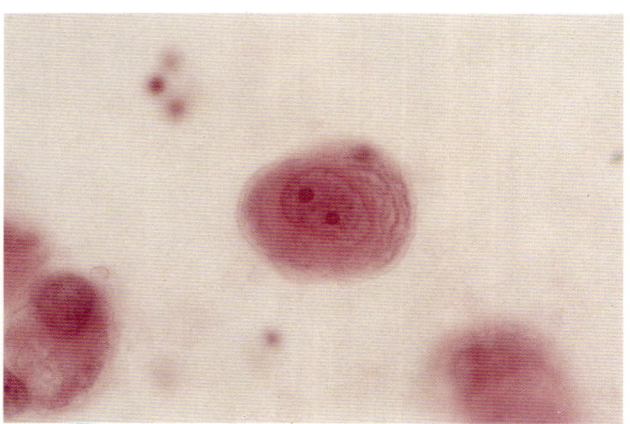

FIGURE 15.22   Clear cell carcinoma of cervix. (A) The cytoplasm shows a few clear vacuoles corresponding to glycogen accumulation. (Pap × 180)

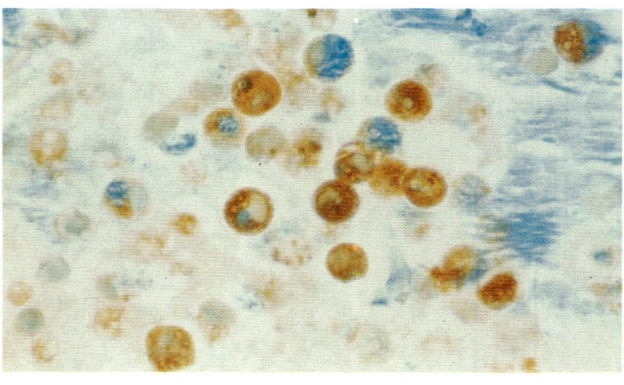

FIGURE 15.24   Adenocarcinoma of stomach double stained for Alcian blue-CEA. Notice mixture of cells positive for CEA (brown), Alcian blue or a combination of the two. (P.A.P./Alcian Blue × 90)

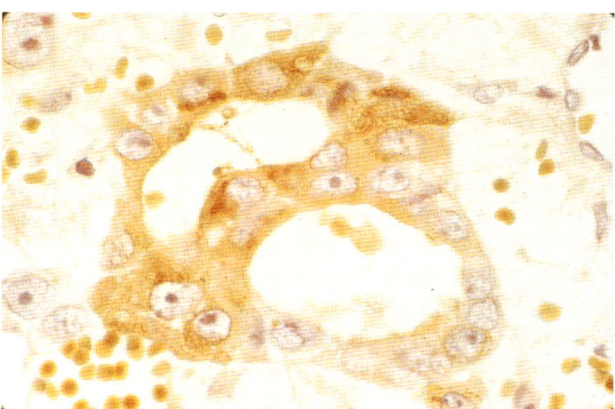

FIGURE 15.25 Alpha-fetoprotein positivity in embryonal carcinoma. Note clustering of tumor cells reminiscent of adenocarcinoma. (P.A.P. × 180)

Phenotype-Specific Markers

It is clear that cells from various neoplasms share many common immunocytochemical determinants. In the special milieu of effusions, these determinants are considered diagnostically significant because they are not shared by the autochthonous elements represented by mesothelial cells. Therefore, positivity implies the presence of alien, neoplastic elements in the serosal spaces. Because the markers discussed thus far are shared by a great number of neoplasms, they are not sufficiently specific to classify malignant effusions regarding its origin. This classification is only partially possible using

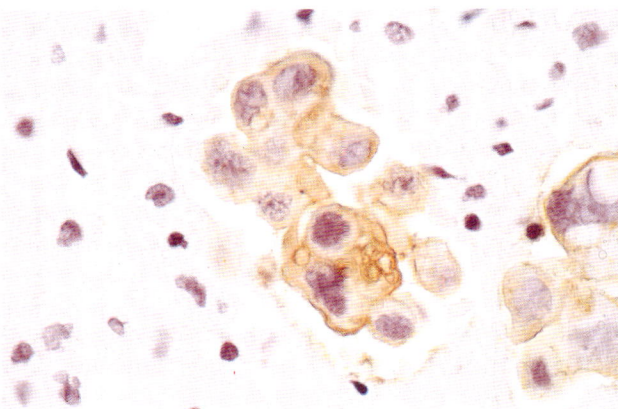

FIGURE 15.26 Adenocarcinoma stained for placental alkaline phophatase. The degree of immunopositivity is weak, in comparison to that shown by germ cell tumors. (P.A.P. × 180)

TABLE 15.2 Select Phenotypic Markers Detectable by Immunocytochemistry

Highly Specific
  Prostate PSA, PSAP
  Thyroid: TGB
  Breast: ER/PR
  Ovary: CA 125
  Lung: surfactant, Clara cell
  Melanoma: HMB 45
  Histiocytes: lysozyme
  Lymphocytic: LCA
  Vascular factor VIII
  Neuroendocrine: chromogranin
Moderately Specific
  Breast: lactalbumin,
  Neuroendocrine: NSE
  Trophoblastic: HCG
  Liver: AFP
  Mesothelial: EMA (thick membrane pattern)
  Histiocytic: A1AT, A1ACT

various markers capable of establishing the phenotypic characteristics of tumor cells not shared by other neoplasms (Table 15.2). In practice, however, no antibody is totally specific for a primary site, because tumors may take pathways of differentiation that closely mimic one another. This sharing of morphologic features is at the heart of distinction between histogenesis and differentiation. Accordingly, a tumor may originate at a given site but show differentiation toward a phenotype not commonly seen in that location or to a mixture of phenotypic expressions. The most classic example is a malignant mixed Muellerian mesodermal tumor of the uterus that may demonstrate heterologous elements; this phenomenon, however, is subtly pervasive in a number of other neoplasms. The phenotypic markers described are therefore differentiation markers grouped according to preferential differentiating pathways expressed by various neoplasms. The more narrow the pathways of differentiation are in a given primary site, the more useful immunochemical markers are for the purpose of recognizing that primary site. Likewise, the more specific antibodies are in recognizing a particular direction of differentiation, the more accurate they are in pinpointing primary sites.

Specific markers exist for carcinomas originating in the prostate, but this neoplasm is not frequently found in effusions. Both PAS and PSAP show strong specificity for prostatic tumor origin. Even though PAS and PSAP may be positive for certain nonneoplastic condi-

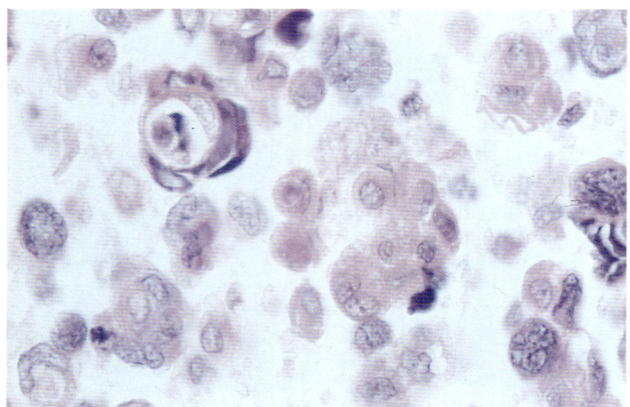

FIGURE 15.27 Oat cell carcinoma in effusion. The Pap stain demonstrates the onion-ring effect of the tumor cells. (Pap× 180)

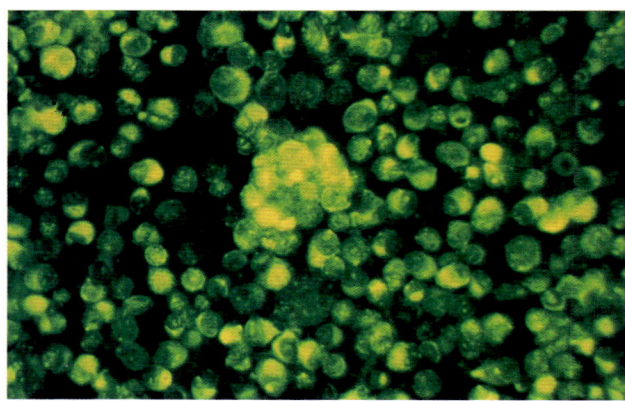

FIGURE 15.29 Breast carcinoma in pleural fluid assayed for estrogen receptor. Notice immunofluorescent positivity in over 90% of the cells. (IF× 90) (Courtesy S. Masood, MD)

tions, such as cystisis cystica and glandularis of the urinary bladder, neither of these markers are positive in the mesothelial cells or the nonprostatic neoplasms that occur frequently in malignant effusions. The same is true of thyroglobulin, a marker positive only in neoplasms of thyroid follicular origin. In contrast, calcitonin is very sensitive in detection of perifollicular thyroid neoplasms, but is also positive in neuroendocrine tumors originating outside the thyroid. Neuroendocrine differentiation is detectable by the neuron-specific enolase reaction. This marker is particularly helpful when the neuroendocrine appearance of the neoplasm is not readily appreciable in cytologic material (Fig. 15.27 and Fig. 15.28). Chromogranin is another neuroendocrine

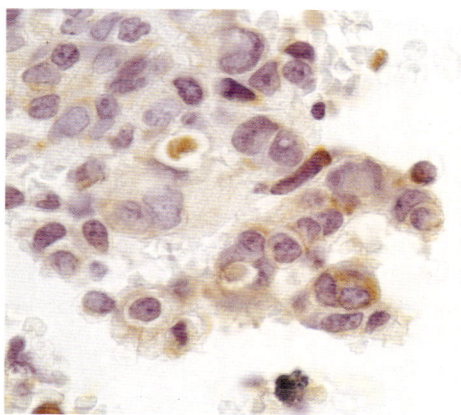

FIGURE 15.28 Oat cell carcinoma following immunostain. Positivity for NSE is characteristic of neuroendocrine neoplasms. (P.A.P. × 120)

marker, particularly useful in the recognition of carcinoids.

A cryptic effusion can be suspected to relate to breast carcinoma when the tumor cells are strongly positive for lactalbumin or estrogen and progesterone (ER/PgR) receptors. ER/PgR reactivity can be detected by immunoperoxidase or immunofluorescent methods (Fig. 15.29). Both of these can be quantitated by flow cytometry or image analysis and serve as prognostic markers. ER/PgR-positive cells occur in neoplasms other than the breast, including the uterus and the ovaries. Lactalbumin may also be positive in ovarian carcinomas; this tumor therefore is included in the differential diagnosis of lactalbumin-positive pleural effusion. Lactalbumin may rarely be positive in tumors of the skin and the salivary glands, but these tumors are rarely a source of malignant effusions. CA-125 is elevated in the serum of patients with ovarian carcinoma and may also be detected in cells from this neoplasm. A drawback, however, is that this marker works better in fresh or frozen tissue; thus, it cannot be readily applied to archival material. In cytologic specimens the marker has affinity for the surface of neoplastic cells. A few examples of CA-125 cross-reactivity have been described with neoplasms originating in the cervix and the endometrium. CA-125 is strongly positive along the microvillous surface of ovarian carcinoma cells, a very helpful phenomenon because it helps in their distinction from mesothelial cells (Fig. 15.30). This distinction is of particular interest when attempting to diagnose a benign papillary neoplasm of the peritoneum versus papillary serous carcinoma of the ovary.

A primary carcinoma of the lung is frequently the

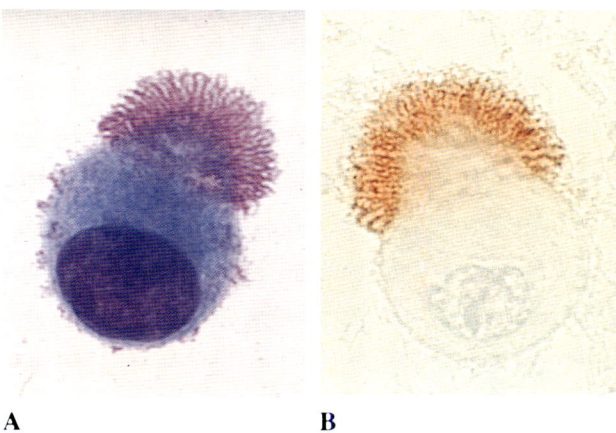

A   B

FIGURE 15.30   Microvilli in ovarian carcinoma. (A) The Diff Quik stain shows a tuft of microvilli at the apical pole of the cell. (D.Q. × 180) (B) With the CA-125 antibody the microvilli are as long as noted in mesothelioma. (P.A.P. × 180) (Courtesy of T. Kobayashi, PhD)

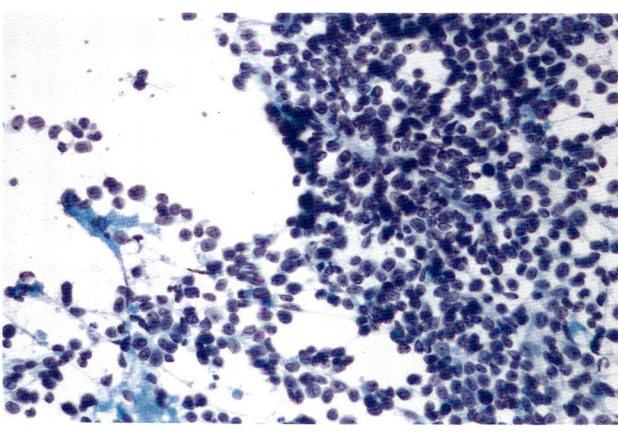

FIGURE 15.31   Melanoma in pericardial fluid. Despite the history of melanoma, doubt persisted whether these relatively small cells originated from the primary skin lesion. (Pap × 90)

source of malignant of effusions in the elderly. Unfortunately, only a small subset of lung carcinomas have a specific immunocytochemical marker. Squamous-cell carcinomas and neuroendocrine carcinomas of the lung cannot be distinguished from their counterparts arising in the oropharynx, esophagus, and other sites. The majority of adenocarcinomas are almost identical to tumors arising in the gastrointestinal tract, the pancreas, or the gallbladder, and do not express antigens for which antibodies are readily available. Only bronchioalveolar-cell carcinomas that show differentiation toward Clara cells and type II pneumonocytes are recognized by specific antibodies raised against the Clara-cell granule (SP-C) and the alveolar surfactant apoprotein (SP-A), respectively. In tumors of type II cells, positivity for apoprotein extends both to the nucleus and the cytoplasm.

Melanomas may present two sets of difficulties in effusions. First, the tumor cells may appear relatively bland and difficult to differentiate from mesothelial cells. Second, the cells may be readily recognized as malignant, but cannot be distinguished from carcinomas composed primarily of noncohesive cells (Figs. 15.31 and 15.32). HMB-45 is specific for melanomas but it has been anecdotally reported as positive in carcinoma cells. In contrast, S100 has been repeatedly reported as immunoreactive with carcinomas and other neoplasms; therefore, S100 positivity cannot be used as the sole factor to clinch the diagnosis of melanoma. Histiocytic neoplasms are rare and only infrequently the cause of malignant effusions. In poorly cellular effusions, how-

ever, these cells may be confused with degenerating malignant cells, therefore requiring exact identification. Lysozyme is specific in this regard, more so than either A1AT and A1ACT, both of which are frequently positive in carcinomas of the lung. Distinction between large lymphocytes and morphologically similar cells arising in mesothelial hyperplasia and carcinomas is easily achievable with antibodies against LCA. There are several very specific antibodies against LCA and other markers that recognize lymphocytes. Mesenchymal markers are considerably less tissue-specific than epithelial markers.

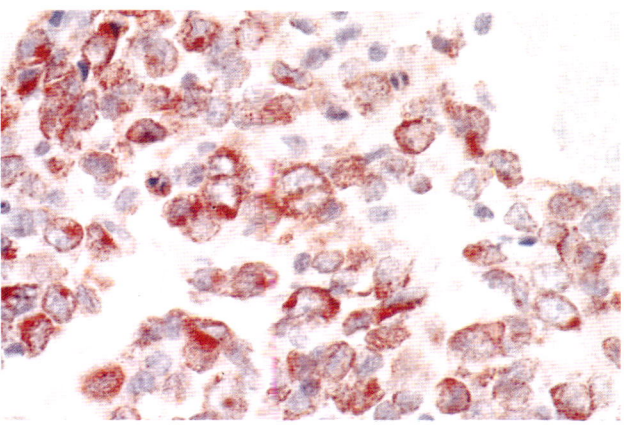

FIGURE 15.32   Same case as Fig 15.23 stained for HMB-45. The strong positivity for the immunomarker confirms the diagnosis of melanoma. (P.A.P. × 120)

The one exception is endothelial differentiation, detectable by antibodies against factor VII and Ulex europeaus antigen. Both markers are specific for vascular neoplasms; however, vascular sarcomas are not very common and are seldom the cause of malignant effusions. There are a few other markers of moderate specificity that have been utilized in the investigation of effusions due to non-epithelial malignancies as discussed in chapter 10.

TECHNICAL CONSIDERATIONS

A crucial step in the success of immunocytochemical study of effusions is to triage the specimen prior to cytopreparation. Depending on the cellularity of the specimen, cytospins or cell blocks should be prepared, both of which are suitable for immunocytochemistry. We prefer cell blocks for immunocytochemistry because recuts can be made, thus allowing comparison of various markers in the same group of cells. If lymphoma is suspected, air-dried cytospins should be made available for cell-surface markers, and a portion of the specimen should be submitted for flow cytometry. If the differential diagnosis includes mesothelioma and carcinoma, a portion of the specimen should be submitted for EM. A variety of other methods can also be utilized for specific applications on a selected basis. These ancillary techniques are often based on recent scientific technological breakthroughs that allow improved application of existing techniques, as discussed in the next chapter.

BIBLIOGRAPHY

Diagnostic Applications

Coleman D, Omerod M. Tumor markers in clinical cytology. In Koss L, Coleman D, eds. *Advances in Clinical Cytology.* New York: Masson. 1983:33–47.

Menard S, Rilke F, Della-Torre G, et al. Sensitivity enhancement of the cytologic detection of cancer cells in effusions by monoclonal antibodies. *Am J Clin Pathol.* 1985;83:571–576.

Silverman, JF. The use of immunoperoxidase panels for the cytologic diagnosis of malignancy in serous effusions. *Diagn Pathol.* 1987;3:134–140.

Ghosh AK, Butler EB. Immunocytological staining reactions of anti-carcinoembryonic antigen, Ca, and anti-human milk fat globule monoclonal antibodies on benign and malignant exfoliated mesothelial cells. *J Clin Pathol.* 1987;40:1424–1427.

Esteban JM, Yokota S, Husein S, et al. Immunocytochemical profile of benign and carcinomatous effusions—a practical approach to difficult diagnosis. *Am J Clin Pathol* 1990;94: 698–705.

Bedrossian CWM. Immunocytochemistry. In Astarita RW, ed. *Practical Cytopathology.* New York, Churchill-Livingstone, 403–457, 1989.

Nance KV, Silverman JF. Immunocytochemical panel for the identification of malignant cells in serous effusions. *Am J Clin Pathol.* 1991;95:867–874.

Mottolese A, Cianciulli I, Venturo R, et al. Selected monoclonal antibodies can increase the accuracy of cytodiagnosis of neoplastic effusions of cryptic origin expanded in a short term culture. *Diagn Cytopathol.* 1992;8:1–7.

Bedrossian CWM, Masood S. Immunocytochemistry applied to cytologic specimens in Leong AS-Y-Ed. Diagnostic Immunocytochemistry for the Surgical Pathologist. Edward Arnold, London, 1993; pp 341–376.

Cytoskeletal Components

Kahn H, Hanna W, Yeger H, Baumal R. Immunohistochemical localization of prekeratin filaments in benign and malignant cells in effusions. *Am J Pathol.* 1982;109:206–214.

Walts AE, Jonathan WS, Banks-Schlegel S. Keratin and carcinoembryonic antigen in exfoliated mesothelial and malignant cells: an immunoperoxidase study. *Am J Clin Pathol.* 1983; 80:671–676.

Miettinen M, Lehto VP, Virtanen IN. Antibodies to intermediate filament proteins in the diagnosis and classification of human tumors. *Ultrastruct Pathol.* 1984;7:83–107.

Altmannsberger M, Osborn M, Droese M, et al. Diagnostic value of intermediate filament antibodies in clinical cytology. *Klin Wochenschr.* 1984;62:114–123.

Ramaekers F, Haag D, Jap P, Vooijs P. Immunochemical demonstration of keratin and vimentin in cytologic aspirates. *Acta Cytol.* 1984;28:385–392.

Blobel GA, Moll R, Franke W, et al. The intermediate filament cytoskeleton of malignant mesotheliomas and its diagnostic significance. *Am J Pathol.* 1985;121:235–247.

Thomas P, Battifora H. Keratins versus epithelial membrane antigen in tumor diagnosis. *Hum Pathol.* 1987;18:728–734.

Epithelial Membrane Antigens

To A, Dearnsley D, Omerod M, et al. Epithelial membrane antigen—its use in the cytodiagnosis of malignancy in serous effusions. *Am J Clin Pathol.* 1982;78:214–219.

Ghosh A, Spriggs A, Taylor-Papadimitriou J, et al. Immunocytochemical staining of cells in pleural and peritoneal effusions with a panel of monoclonal antibodies. *J Clin Pathol.* 1983; 36:1154–1164.

Coleman D, Omerod M. Tumor markers in clinical cytology.

In Koss L, Coleman D, eds. *Advances in Clinical Cytology.* New York: Masson. 1983:33–47.

Hilborne L, Cheng L, Nieberg R, Lewin K. Evaluation of an antibody to human milk fat globule antigen in the detection of metastatic carcinoma in pleural, pericardial and peritoneal fluids. *Acta Cytol.* 1986;30:245–249.

Cibas ES, Corson JM, Pinkus GS. The distinction of adenocarcinoma from malignant mesothelioma in cell blocks of effusions: the role of routine mucin histochemistry and immunohistochemical assessment of carcinoembryonic antigen, keratin proteins, epithelial membrane antigen, and milk fat globule-derived antigen. *Hum Pathol.* 1987;18:67–74.

van der Kwast TH, Versnel MA, Delahaye M, et al. Expression of epithelial membrane antigen on malignant mesothelioma cells. An immunocytochemical in immunoelectron microscopic study. *Acta Cytol.* 1988;32:169–174.

Latza U, Niedobitek G, Schwarting R, Nekarda H, et al. Ber-Ep-4: A new monoclonal antibody which distinguishes epithelial from mesothelial cells. *J Clin Pathol.* 1990;43:213–219.

Leong A, Parkinson R, Milios J. Thick cell membranes revealed by immunocytochemical staining: a clue to the diagnosis of mesothelioma. *Diagn Cytopathol.* 1990;1:9–13.

Diaz-Arias AA, Loy TS, Bickel JT, Chapman RK. Utility of BER-EP4 in the diagnosis of adenocarcinoma in effusions: an immunocytochemical study of 232 cases. *Diagn Cytopathol* 1993;9:516–521.

Carcinoembryonic Antigen

O'Brien MJ, Kirkham SE, Burke B, et al. CEA, ZGM and EMA. A localization in cells of pleural and peritoneal effusion: preliminary study. *Invest Cell Pathol.* 1980;3:251–258.

Walts AE, Jonathan WS, Banks-Schlegel S. Keratin and carcinoembryonic antigen in exfoliated mesothelial and malignant cells: an immunoperoxidase study. *Am J Clin Pathol.* 1983;80:671–676.

Sehested M, Ralfkjaer E, Rasmussen J. Immunoperoxidase demonstration of carcinoembryonic antigen in pleural and peritoneal effusions. *Acta Cytol.* 1983;27:124–127.

Pinto M. An immunoperoxidase study of S-100 protein in neoplastic cells in serous effusions. *Acta Cytol.* 1986;30:240–244.

Duggan MA, Masters CB, Alexander F. Immunohistochemical differentiation of malignant mesothelioma, mesothelial hyperplasia and metastatic adenocarcinoma in serous effusions, utilizing staining for carcinoembryonic antigen, keratin and vimentin. *Acta Cytol.* 1987;31:807–814.

Silverman J. The use of immunoperoxidase panels for the cytologic diagnosis of malignancy in serous effusions *Diagn Pathol.* 1987;3:134–140.

Mason M, Bedrossian CW. Value of immunocytochemistry in the study of malignant effusions. *Diagn Cytopathol.* 1987;3:215–221.

Ghosh AK, Butler EB. Immunocytological staining reactions of anti-carcinoembryonic antigen, Ca, and anti-human milk fat globule monoclonal antibodies on benign and malignant exfoliated mesothelial cells. *J Clin Pathol.* 1987;40:1424–1427.

Osamura RY. Application of immunocytochemistry to diagnostic cytopathology. *Diagn Cytopathol.* 1989;1:55–63.

Orell SR, Dowling KD. Oncofetal antigens as tumor markers in the cytologic diagnosis of effusions. *Acta Cytol.* 1983;27:625–629.

Permanetter W, Wiesinger H. Immunohistochemical study of lysozyme, alpha 1-anti-chymotrypsin, tissue polypeptide, antigen, keratin and carcinoembryonic antigen in effusion sediments. *Acta Cytol.* 1987;31:104–112.

Pinto M, Berstein L, Brogan D, et al. Carcinoembryonic antigen in effusions. *Acta Cytol.* 1987;31:113–118.

Other Markers

Epenetos A, Canti G, Taylor-Papadimitriou J, et al. Use of two epithelium-specific monoclonal antibodies for diagnosis of malignancy in serous effusions. *Lancet.* 1982;2:1004–1006.

Martinez-Vea A, Gatell J, Segura F, et al. Diagnostic value of tumoral markers in serous effusions. *Cancer.* 1982;50:1783–1788.

Yam L, Winkler C. Immunocytochemical diagnosis of oat-cell carcinoma in pleural effusion. *Acta Cytol.* 1984;28:425–429.

Szpak C, Johnston W, Lottich A, et al. Patterns of reactivity of four novel monoclonal antibodies (B72.3, DF3, B1.1 and B6.2) with cells in human malignant and benign effusions. *Acta Cytol.* 1984;28:356–357.

Yam L, Lin D, Janckila A, Li C. Immunocytochemical diagnosis of lymphoma in serous effusions. *Acta Cytol* 1985;29:833–841.

Martin S, Moshiri S, Thor A, et al. Identification of adenocarcinoma in cytospin preparations of effusions using monoclonal antibody B72.3. *Am J Clin Pathol.* 1986;86:10–13.

Banner B, Warren W, Gould V. Cytomorphology and marker expression of malignant neuroendocrine cells in pleural effusions. *Acta Cytol.* 1986;30:99–104.

Guzman J, Costabel U, Bross K, et al. The value of the immunoperoxidase slide assay in the diagnosis of malignant pleural effusions in breast cancer. *Acta Cytol.* 1988;32:188–192.

Myers J. Development and application of immunocytochemical staining techniques: a review. *Diagn Cytopathol.* 1989;3:318–330.

Rosen-Levin E, Patil J, Watson C, Jagirdar J. Distinguishing benign from malignant pleural effusions by lectin immunocytochemistry. *Acta Cytol.* 1989;33:499–504.

Cajulis RS, Szumel R, Frias-Hidvegi D, et al. Monoclonal antibody 44-3A6 as an adjunct in cytodiagnosis of adenocarcinomas in body fluids. *Diagn Cytopathol.* 1993;9:179–182.

Loy TS, Diaz-Arias, Bickel J. Values of BCA-225 in the cytologic diagnosis of malignant effusions: an immunocytochemical study of 197 cases. *Med Pathol.* 1991;294–297.

CHAPTER SIXTEEN

Ancillary Techniques

Despite the knowledge accumulated in cytologic study of effusions, difficult cases still puzzle even those who have attained considerable expertise. Diagnosis of malignancy may remain in doubt even after careful clinical pathologic correlation, and classification of the neoplasm in an obviously malignant effusion may often be impossible to ascertain. Special stains and immunocytochemistry are becoming routine in some laboratories, and an increasing number are gaining access to an electron microscope. These methods, however, may not be sufficient to answer the clinical questions raised by effusions of unknown etiology. The need for ancillary studies has evolved from these clinical needs and as a direct extension of discoveries in the scientific arena. Cytology is gradually progressing from a purely diagnostic to a partially prognostic modality. Ancillary techniques are being used more frequently in the study of effusions in addition to classic cytomorphology.

As has been stressed throughout this book, malignant effusions are a reflection of the spread of cancer. However, advances in the management of neoplastic disease may afford a cure or at least longer survival in those patients in whom the malignant cells are responsive to emerging treatments. A number of these have been developed and others are in the process of being introduced, including new chemotherapeutic and immunotherapeutic agents, variations of radiotherapeutic protocols, and hormonal manipulation of susceptible neoplasms. The success of treatment can be enhanced by more specific diagnoses and classification of neoplasms in effusions, but it also depends on the predictions of therapeutic responses afforded by newer tests currently being developed. Among the most interesting developments are procedures that detect and measure prognostic factors in neoplastic cells. The latter include hormone receptor assays; flow cytometry and image analysis, which have already been tested in clinical trials; detection of proliferative antigens; and techniques borrowed from cell biology, such as the polymerase chain reaction (PCR), gene rearrangement detection, and molecular cytogenetics, which are currently in an experimental stage.

Table 16.1 compares these prognostic tests with other ancillary techniques employed in the study of malignant effusions for diagnostic purposes. Because malignant effusions often contain an abundant single-cell population of neoplastic cells, they are ideally suited for application of ancillary techniques. In the past, effusions were widely studied by special stains, cytogenetics, and even tissue culture, known then as "living cytology." When electron microscopy (EM) and immunocytochemistry were first used in clinical cytology, they were applied to body fluids, particularly in the study of malignant effusion. EM and immunocytochemistry are intricately intertwined and benefit from correlation with one another. In cellular samples, ultrastructural features help explain the cytomorphologic appearance and the patterns of immunopositivity noted in cells. For this reason, EM should always be correlated with observations obtained with the light microscope. The same principle applies to the emerging diagnostic and cell biology prognostic probes, which should have a firm base in cytomorphology. The study of malignant effusions is one of the most promising applications of ancillary techniques.

MORPHOMETRY

Profoundly altered cell size and shape can be good indicators of malignant transformation; however, the propensity of mesothelial cells toward reactivity make alterations of size and shape alone unreliable for the detection of malignancy. Mesothelial cells range from 7 to 8 μm in diameter to up to 70 to 80 μm in multinucle-

TABLE 16.1   Ancillary Methods to Recognize and Classify Effusions

Method	Principle	Advantage	Disadvantage
Cytogenetics	Karyotype reflecting hypo or hyperdiploidy	Inexpensive; applicable by FISH	Time consuming; cannot pinpoint primary site
DNA by flow cytometry	DNA content reflecting aneuploidy	Fast and expensive; reliable	Cannot pinpoint primary site
Image analysis	N/C ratios rapidly dividing cells	Quantitative; reproducible	Overlap between benign and malignant cells
Immunocytochemistry	Tumor-associated antigens expressed by neoplastic cells	Objective; may pinpoint primary site	Expensive, time consuming
Electron microscopy	Secretory products & other ultrastructural features revealed	Less subjective than microscopy; may pinpoint primary site	Expensive, time consuming
Proliferative antigens	PCNA (Mib-1), Ki-67	May identify low grade malignancies	Sample selection may influence results
Oncogenes, gene rearrangement	Detection by PCR and ISH	Detection of specific gene defects	High sensitivity creates problems of contamination
Hormone receptor	Detection by IF or ICC	Has prognostic value	Applicable only in selective types of tumors

FISH: fluorescent in situ hybridization; PCNA: proliferating cell nuclear antigen; PCR: polymerase chain reaction; ISH: in situ hybridization.

ated cells. Nuclear diameter is usually one third the diameter of the entire mesothelial cell but may be increased in hyperplastic cells. Measurements have been made of the cellular and nuclear diameters, the nuclear to cytoplasm (N/C) ratio, the area occupied by vacuoles, and the glycogen concentration in mesothelial cells. Morphometric measurements can be accomplished planimetrically or by point-counting, but these techniques are tedious and time-consuming. Automated planimetric devices, however, make these methods useful in the analysis of specimens containing a small number of cells. Boon noticed that the vacuoles of mesothelial cells are distributed around the nucleus, whereas they are clustered at the periphery of the cytoplasm in adenocarcinomas. The nuclear and cytoplasmic areas are increased in mesothelioma when compared with reactive mesothelial cells.

Stereology can convert two-dimensional measurements into volumetric determinations, but these are of limited value in the study of effusions. Morphometry can be accomplished by interactive instrumentation, during which cells are selected for measurements, or by automated means. The latter is fully computerized and can encompass a number of parameters, such as profile, perimeter, cluster shape, distance between clusters, texture, granularity, and more detailed features. Many of these techniques hold promise for use in the study of effusions.

CYTOPHOTOMETRY

There have been attempts to measure cellular components to establish diagnosis and to gauge the prognosis of malignant effusions. Detection and quantification of DNA occupy a prominent place among these measurements. The method includes use of a suitable dye, excitable at a specific wavelength, and quantification expressed in graph form. The biggest drawback of this method is the lack of simultaneous morphologic appreciation of cellular detail correlation is therefore difficult. This problem can be overcome when image analysis of recognizable cells is performed in combination with Feulgen cytophotometry obtained by quantification of integrated nuclear absorption. Cytophotometry is a slow method that is based on analysis of optically derived parameters. As such, this technique is less suitable for examination of thousands of cells in effusions, a task easily achieved by flow cytometry and automated image analysis. Virtually all cytophotometric methods depend on a representative and technically impeccable cellular sample. Effusions can be successfully analyzed by cytophotometry, because their cell populations tend to be less variable than, for example, cervicovaginal smears. Cytophotometry may be based on the measurement of cellular components through absorbance of transmitted light. Routinely stained preparations are analyzed for cytomorphologic features, whereas either immunoperoxidase- or immunofluorescence–stained preparations are used for quantitation of cell markers. Cytospins of malignant effusions can be analyzed this way for the presence of differentiation or proliferative markers. However, the method is capable of analyzing only a small number of cells and at a much slower pace when compared with flow cytometry. Cytophotometry, however, allows selectivity by targeting only cells of specific interest while avoiding inflammatory and other unimportant cell populations.

IMAGE ANALYSIS

Cytomorphologic changes may be so subtle in certain neoplasms that recognition of their malignant characteristics or precise classification is not possible. Alterations of size, shape, texture, and proportions of the nuclei may be the defining features of malignant transformation. Among these, the N/C ratio and complexity of the nuclear contour are well known. Measurement of these features is extremely tedious, and their estimation is not a reproducible endeavor. The emergence of analytic methods made it possible not only to recognize these subtle abnormalities but also to quantitate the changes involved. Image analysis with newer digitized technology goes beyond optical morphometric measurements into rather sophisticated, fully automated means of quantitating individual cell components (Table 16.2).

Quantitative DNA measurements to establish ploidy have enjoyed great popularity in the fields of cytogenetics and clinical cytology. Malignant effusions have been studied this way by means of cellular samples stained by the Feulgen reaction. The dye in this reaction binds stoichiometrically to DNA strands, and its absorption of light at 560 mm is directly proportional to the amount of cellular DNA, in a linear fashion. In comparison to flow cytometry, DNA ploidy determination by image analysis is a slower process, but it targets individual cells that can be selected by their morphologic features. The method is particularly advantageous in effusions with only a small proportion of aneuploid cells and in patients for whom only the cell blocks are available. Both flow cytometry and image analysis afford DNA ploidy study of archival material embedded in paraffin; however, the advantage offered by flow cytometry of examining thousands of cells per second is lost in these preparations of decidedly low cellularity. In contrast, cell image analysis is ideally suited for the

TABLE 16.2 Comparison between Flow Cytometry and Image Analysis

Feature	Flow Cytometry	Image Analysis
Basis of analysis	Fluorescence and/or light scanner	Morphology and/or cell markers through transmitted light (absorbance)
Special preparation	Single cell suspension	Cytocentrifuge preparation, imprints, fine needle aspirates, tissue sections (frozen paraffin-embedded)
Morphologic correlation	Absent	Present and will facilitate the identification of specific cells of interest
Morphometry	Limited to light scatter measurement (size, granularity)	Large numbers of direct and derived morphometric parameters

study of specimens in which malignant cells are present in tumor bank material.

A number of substances have been immunocytochemically demonstrated in cells from malignant effusions, as illustrated in Chapter 14. Some have been measured by image analysis and expressed in terms of a quantitative immunocytochemical score, particularly estrogen receptors (ER) and progesterone receptors (PgR). However, the method is adaptable to quantification of any antigen, both by immunofluorescent and immunoenzymatic detection systems. Examples include differentiation markers such as carcinoembryonic antigen (CEA), factor VIII, placental alkaline phosphatase (PLAP), and prostatic specific antigen (PSA); and prognostic factors, such as PCNA (Mib-1), Ki-67, HER-2/neu oncogene, cathepsin D, epidermal growth factor receptors, and p53.

CYTOGENETICS

The field of oncology owes much to cytogenetics, from which came the realization that chromosome abnormalities and abnormalities of the DNA content of cells are at the core of malignant transformation. Not surprisingly, karyotype analysis has been extensively utilized in the investigating of malignant effusions. Early on, studies focused on the detection of common marker chromosomes and demonstration of aneuploidy, including hyperdiploidy and hypodiploidy, in Giemsa-stained preparations, a tedious and labor-intensive method. Subsequently, the techniques of chromosome banding and flow cytometry greatly revolutionized detection of chromosome and ploidy abnormalities, respectively. Chromosome banding allows identification of specific tumor markers, including detection of the Philadelphia chromosome in leukemias and other gross chromosomal abnormalities in benign and malignant processes.

Molecular cytogenetics has opened a new era in oncologic pathology and is beginning to pay dividends in the study of malignant effusions of cryptic origin. Using fluorescent in situ hybridization (FISH), it is now possible to determine specific translocations in lymphoma and leukemia and solid tumors. Even the difficult distinction between mesotheliomas and metastatic malignancy has been facilitated by molecular cytogenetics.

FLOW CYTOMETRY

Malignant effusions in lymphoproliferative disorders are notoriously difficult to diagnose. Because the natural history of these disorders has changed drastically in the past 10 years, it is not uncommon for intercurrent effusion to develop, which may not represent relapse of their leukemia/lymphoma process. Considerable emphasis has therefore been placed on the distinction between effusions showing reactive lymphocytosis and those representing a lymphoproliferative malignancy. Such a differential can be resolved cytofluorometrically by demonstrating B-cell clonal excess in malignant effusions as opposed to polyclonality in lymphocyte-rich effusions unrelated to leukemia/lymphoma. This method can actually be superior to ploidy and cell cycle activity, particularly in low-grade lymphoproliferative disorders, where aneuploidy and S-phase fraction may be indistinguishable from reactive processes.

The most useful approach to demonstrate B-cell clonal excess is with flow cytometric light chain analysis of effusions using fluorescein-conjugated monoclonal antibodies against kappa and lambda chains. Overtly malignant lymphoproliferative disorders may be further classified with flow cytometry using antibodies against the entire CD series of surface markers, particularly CD-19 in B cells and CD-3 and CD-15 in T cells. The proportion between B and T cells in the effusion may be of diagnostic significance in recognizing reactive lymphocytosis in effusions. A prominence of T cells greater than 80% favors a reactive origin. The false-positive ratio of flow cytometric analysis in lymphoproliferative disorders is the same as for routine cytology, but flow cytometry has a much lower false-negative ratio than cytology alone. Flow cytometry is probably the best method to establish the diagnosis of leukemia/lymphoma of small lymphocytes due to their bland cytologic appearance in effusion specimens.

In large-cell lymphomas, the greatest application of flow cytometry is to distinguish them from nonlymphoid malignancies. Further classification of large-cell lymphomas is hampered by the lack of morphologic detail in immunofluorescent preparations. The same difficulty plagues classification of solid tumors, but the diagnosis of malignancy in these neoplasms may be established by cell cycle analysis and DNA ploidy determinations. In 1983, we investigated the value of flow cytometry in the study of effusions. Aneuploidy correlated well with malignancy, but both false-positive and false-negative results occurred. Not surprisingly, cirrhosis, the condition that results in strikingly atypical cells in effusions, also emerged as the most common cause of aneuploidy in the absence of malignancy. Since publication of that study, other investigators have confirmed our observations and expanded the experience with ploidy, S-phase fraction, and surface marker studies of effusions with flow cytometry.

The greatest application of flow cytometry is in recognition of malignant effusions for which cytologic criteria are insufficient to warrant an unequivocal diagnosis of malignancy. This can be accomplished by analyzing the ploidy of the cell population based on the DNA content (DI = DNA index) of the cells. Using this approach, aneuploidy has been observed in 80% of malignant solid tumors, whereas aneuploidy was absent in 96% of the benign tumors. However, another study revealed only aneuploidy in 60% of tumors and a 30% false-negative rate when aneuploidy was used as the criteria for malignancy. It is well known, however, that malignant tumors from breast, colon, endometrium, and prostate may have a considerable number of diploid cells. In low-grade lymphomas, only 33% demonstrate aneuploidy. High-grade lymphomas not only are frequently aneuploid (86% in effusions but also their DNA content can be very high (in the range of hyperdiploid). The amount of RNA expressed as RI (RNA index) also increases in association with grade and aggressiveness of the lymphoma. In contrast, reactive lymphocytes have RIs only slightly higher than normal lymphocytes despite the considerable cytologic atypia they might exhibit. The RI may also be a measure of differentiation (e.g., in a plasmacytoid lymphoma, which exhibited a very high RI in Katz's study of effusions using a morphologic, immunologic, and cytometric approach).

PROLIFERATIVE MARKERS

The proportion of cells in the proliferative phase of the cell cycle is important in the prognosis of certain tumors, particularly breast carcinomas. As noted previously, this proportion can be identified by measuring the proportion of S-phase cells with flow cytometry. Proliferative activity can also be measured by image analysis, with the advantage of identifying only tumor cells for evaluation under direct visualization. This is accomplished using antinuclear antibodies that specifically identify or exclude certain regions of the cell cycle. One example of such cell cycle–specific antibody is Ki-67, which fails to react with cells in the resting (Go) phase of the cell cycle but identifies cells in the G, S, G_2, and M phases. The proportion of cells that stain positively for Ki-67 reflects the proliferative activity of the neoplasm and may be related to prognosis and response to chemotherapy. Other markers indicative of the proliferative status include proliferating cell nucleus antigen PCNA/cyclin, which is relatively specific for the S-phase of the cycle; and the P-105 antigen, which identifies cells in mitosis. In solid tumors, poor prognosis is associated with neoplasms that have a high S-phase fraction, even though response to therapy may be better in neoplasms with a high cell turnover. It is also possible to estimate the S-phase fraction by immunostaining cells blocks with the Ki-67 antibody, considered to be a reliable marker of proliferative activity, or by measuring Ki-67 reactivity by flow cytometry. One difficulty in both Ki-67 and flow cytometric analysis of the S-phase fraction is that a small population of malignant cells in effusions may be obscured by an overwhelming number of mesothelial and inflammatory cells. This imbalance can be minimized by focussing on and studying selected abnormal nuclei by image analysis, not only for DNA content but also for a variety of proliferative markers. These include PCNA cyclin, DNA polymerase, and silver impregnation of the nucleolar organizing region (AgNOR), all of which are applicable to cytospins of malignant effusions. More elaborate methods involve measuring the uptake of gion (AgNOR), all of which are applicable to cytospins

of malignant effusions. More elaborate methods involve measuring the uptake of tritiated thymidine (^{3}H-TdR) and bromodoxyuridine (BUdR) as labeling indexes (LI). Preliminary work has shown good correlation of BRdU-LI and ^{3}TdR-LI with Ki-67. The latter appears to reflect the S-phase fraction measured by flow cytometry of fine-needle aspiration biopsies, so the potential exists for its use in malignant effusions. An even more reliable proliferative marker is MIB-1 which is rapidly replacing PCNA in the study of cytologic specimens.

RECEPTOR ANALYSIS

Malignant cells originating in breast carcinoma may be recognized on the basis of expression of steroid hormone receptors on their cell surface. Both ERs and PgRs have been detected in pleural effusions from patients with breast carcinomas. Because these substances are not expressed by mesothelial cells, ER/PgR may serve as a marker of malignancy in this setting. Their most reliable use, however, is as a prognostic marker to identify malignancies most likely to respond to hormonal manipulation. Use of ER/PgR as a differentiation marker indicative of breast origin is also problematic, because carcinomas from ovarian, endometrial, and endocervical origin may also express ER/PgR. Thus, expression of the ER/PgR marker should be interpreted in light of clinical information and cytomorphology of the malignant cells.

In general, there is good agreement between the amount of ER/PgR-positive cells in the effusion and the quantitative ER/PgR analysis of the parent neoplasm. Consequently, the ER/PgR data may obviate the need for breast surgery in inoperable tumors. This determination is also useful in monitoring the posttherapy period because pleural effusion may be the first sign of recurrent disease. Measuring ER/PgR in effusions may become more popular because it can generate staging information, in addition to its prognostic value.

ONCOGENES AND GENE REARRANGEMENT

The knowledge that mammalian cells may harbor cellular oncogenes (C-ONC) identical in every respect to viral oncogenes (V-ONC) revolutionized our grasp of cancer cell biology. These oncogenes may be altered or activated by ionizing radiation, chemical carcinogens, or biologic agents, with resultant malignant transformation. Oncogenes not only cause malignant transformation, but also they are integrated in the genome of neoplastic cells, from whence they may be responsible for formation of gene products that are detectable as abnormal cell antigens. Several of these gene products have been used as markers of malignant transformation, in combination with detection of the oncogenes themselves, or of their location in intact chromosomes and in certain abnormal chromosomal regions. This approach has opened an entire area of investigation in cancer medicine, because some oncogenes or their gene products have found diagnostic and prognostic applications.

The recent discoveries of ISH and PCR expanded even more the investigative opportunities, because a very small amount of abnormal DNA or a small number of gene copies can now be detected in cancer cells. Furthermore, certain oncogenes have histogenetic or prognostic significance that can have ready application in clinical care. For instance, amplification of certain genes has been associated with one type of neoplasm more frequently than others, including N-MYC in neuroblastomas; L-MYC and N-MYC in small-cell carcinomas of lung; cERB-B2 in breast carcinomas; and cERB-B in glioblastoma multiforme. This is a rapidly developing area, however, and these markers may yet have their specificity dispelled. Another application of oncogene analysis refers to prognostication. cERB-B2, for example, when expressed by breast carcinoma cells, carries a poorer prognosis. These and other applications of oncogenes are yet to be fully explored in the study of malignant effusions.

Lymphoproliferative neoplasms are unique in that gene rearrangements have been identified at the core of malignant transformation. These rearrangements are the result of chromosomal translocations and involve C-ONC activation frequently associated with various types of leukemias. The earliest and best known of these definitive diagnostic markers is the Philadelphia chromosome, detectable by classic cytogenetics or by identification of the protooncogen, c-abl, on chromosomes translocated to the break point cluster region (bcr) on chromosome 22. This so-called bcr/abl gene rearrangement is only one example of analogous abnormalities with potential applications in the study of effusions of suspected lymphomal/leukemia origin. Another is the bcl gene rearrangement observed in B-cell lymphomas.

DNA/RNA PROBES

DNA/RNA technology has evolved in the past several years so that methodology exists for quantitation of nucleic acids in exfoliated cells. The amount of DNA can be measured by automated means utilizing flow cytometry and image analyses. Both methods, however, lack easy correlation with cytomorphology and are not readily applicable to a very small population of abnormal cells within a large number of normal cellular components. Thus, development of in-situ hybridization (ISH) and the polymerase chain reaction (PCR) was a welcome addition. ISH is applicable to a single cell within a heterogeneous cell population and ideally suited for cytologic specimens. ISH is rather sensitive and is capable of detecting DNA and RNA target sequences that may be present only in the smallest concentration in a cytologic specimen. The product of the ISH reaction can be developed by immunocytochemistry, thus allowing for careful correlation with cytomorphology, which acts as an internal control. ISH may also be applied to archival material, including cell blocks from effusions in follow-up of a diagnosis or for comparison with new or newly discovered old material. All these advantages are also applicable to PCR, a technique that uses similar templates as ISH; however, it is much more sensitive because the hybridization reaction is amplified thousands of times. This method is particularly useful for detection of various oncogenic viruses, amplification or deletion of certain genes, expression of specific growth factors, or detection of diagnostically or prognostically significant gene products. PCR has been used for detection of low-incidence mutations of certain oncogenes, including p53 in carcinomas of the colon, lung, and other sites. Given the difficulty in establishing the primary site of origin of various carcinomas in effusion, PCR holds some promise in the study of cytologic specimens from serous effusions.

TISSUE CULTURE

Malignant effusions are teaming with live cells when first tapped, ranging from normal elements such as mesothelial cells and macrophages to a variable number of malignant cells. If the effusion is properly preserved, viable cells will resist degeneration for up to 12 hours after removal from the serous cavity. This period varies with environmental conditions, particularly temperature, and with the number of inflammatory cells present in the effusion. Likewise, the effusion has to be protected from clotting by collection in heparinized containers to minimize post-tap degeneration. If an effusion-derived cell suspension is transferred into a culture medium, the viable cells will not only survive, but also will multiply and grow through several passages. This method was utilized in the past for cytomorphologic, histochemical, and cytogenetic study of cells, and was dubbed "living cytology." A more recent application is to utilize tissue culture for immunocytochemical assay, particularly if the number of malignant cells in the effusion is small and not sufficient for adequate evaluation. Several antigenic properties are preserved through several passages, and the cultured cells are a significant source of research material. Cultured cells may also be utilized for stem-cell assays, particularly because effusions are an excellent culture medium, preserving viable cells for 24 to 48 hours in properly refrigerated conditions.

BIBLIOGRAPHY

Morphometry

Kwee WS, Veldhuizen RW, Alons CA, et al. Quantitative and qualitative differences between benign and malignant mesothelioma cells in pleural fluid. *Acta Cytol.* 1982;26:401–406.

Boon ME, Kwee HS, Alous CL, et al. Discrimination between primary pleural and primary peritoneal mesotheliomas by morphometric analysis of the vacuolization pattern of exfoliated mesothelial cells. *Acta Cytol.* 1982;26:103–108.

Van Molengraft FJJM, Van't Hot MA, Herman CJ, Vooijts PG. Quantitative light microscopy and atypical mesothelial cells and malignant cells in ascitic fluid. *Anal Quant Cytol Histol.* 1982;4:217–220.

Baak JPA, Oort J. *Morphometry in Diagnostic Pathology.* Berlin: Springer-Verlag. 1983.

Marchevsky AM, Hauptman E, Gil J, Watson C. Computerized interactive morphometry as an aid in the diagnosis of pleural effusions. *Acta Cytol.* 1987;31:131–136.

Scott N, Sutton J, Gray C. Morphometric diagnosis of serous effusions: refinement of differences between benign and malignant cases by use of outlying values and larger sample size. *J Clin Pathol.* 1989;42:607–612.

Cytophotometry

Adams LR, Dahlgren SE. Cytophotometric measurements of the DNA content of lung tumors. *Acta Pathol Microbiol Scand.* 1968;72:561–574.

Freni SC, James J, Prop FJ. Tumor diagnosis in pleural and ascitic effusions based on DNA cytophotometry. *Acta Cytol.* 1971;15:154–162.

Burger G, Ploem JS, Goertler K. *Clinical Cytometry and Histometry.* San Diego: Academic Press. 1987.

Franklin WA, Bibbo M, Doria MI, et al. Quantitation of estrogen receptor content and Ki67 staining in breast carcinoma

by the microTICAS image analysis system. *Anal Quant Cytol Histol.* 1987;9:279–286.

Mayall BH. Current capabilities and clinical applications of image cytometry. *Cytometry* 1988;3(suppl):78–84.

Mikel UV. Absolute DNA values from feulgen microspectrophotometric measurements and quantitative electron microscopy. *Anal Quant Cytol Histol.* 1987;9:13–16.

Image Analysis

Jahoda E, Bartels PH, Bibbo M, et al. Computer discrimination of cells in serous effusions. I. Pleural fluids. *Acta Cytol.* 1973;17:94–105.

Jahoda E, Bartels PH, Bibbo M, et al. Computer discrimination of cells in serous effusions. II. Peritoneal fluid. *Acta Cytol.* 1973;6:533–537.

Bedrossian CWM. Methodology. In Anderson EA, Foracker AG, eds. *Pathology of Disruptive Pulmonary Emphysema,* ed. 1. Baltimore, Maryland: Charles C. Thomas Co. 1976:9–21.

Goerttler K, Stohr M. Automated cytology: the state of the art. *Arch Pathol Lab Med.* 1982;106:657–661.

Christensen JA, Skaarland E. Nuclear and cell area measurements in the cytological evaluation of pleural effusions: A study of subjective assessments and morphometric measurements. *Diagn Cytopathol.* 1985;3:50–54.

Bacus SS, Flowers JL, Press MF, et al. The evaluation of estrogen receptor in primary breast carcinoma by computer assisted image analysis. *Am J Clin Pathol.* 1988;90:233

Gavin FM, Gray C, Sutton J, et al. Morphometric differences between benign and malignant effusions. *Acta Cytol.* 1988; 32:175–182.

Cytogenetics

Sandberg AA, Yamada K, Kikuchi Y, Takagi N. Chromosomes and causation of human cancer and leukemia. III. Karyotypes of cancerous effusions. *Cancer.* 1967;20:1099–1166.

Benedict WF, Porter IH. The cytogenetic diagnosis of malignancy in effusions. *Acta Cytol.* 1972;16:304–306.

Olinici CD, Galatir N, Lazarov P, Giurgiuman M. Chromosomes in malignant gynecological effusions. *Neoplasms.* 1973;20:311–324.

Dewald G, Dines DE, Weiland LH, Gordon H. Usefulness of chromosome examination in the diagnosis of malignant pleural effusions. *N Engl J Med.* 1976;295:1491–1500.

Hansteen IL, Hillestad L, Thomassen OK. Chromosome analysis and cell cytology in effusions: a comparative study. *Scand J Respir Dis.* 1977;58:51–56.

Carlevaro C, Rossi GA, Cerri E, Pelucco D. Cytogenetic study of pleural effusions. *Tumori.* 1978;64:335–344.

Musilova J, Michalova K, Dvorak O, et al. Cytogenetic study

of malignant and benign effusions. *Neoplasms.* 1981;28:463–471.

Falow WH, Ward RM, Brezler MR. Diagnosis of pleural effusions by chromosome analysis. *Chest.* 1982;81:193–197.

Watts KC, Boyo-Ekwueme H, To A et al. Chromosome studies on cells cultured from serous effusions: Use in routine cytologic practice. *Acta Cytol.* 1983;27:38–44.

Bousfield LR, Greenberg ML, Pacey F. Cytogenetic diagnosis of cancer from body fluids. *Acta Cytol.* 1985;29:768–774.

Meyers F, Lewis J, Marianos S. The integration of cytogenetic analysis into the evaluation of cryptic exudative effusions. *Cancer.* 1986;58:1479–1483.

Bigner SH. Cytogenetics of human neoplasia. *Cytopathol Annu.* 1992;1:1–21.

Cajulis RS, Frias-Hidvegi D. Detection of numerical chromosomal abnormalities in malignant cells on body fluids by FISH of interphase cell nuclei with chromosome-specific probes. *Diagn Cytopathol* 1992;8:627–631.

Flow Cytometry (Lymphoma-Leukemia)

Katz RL, Raval P, Manning JT, et al. A morphologic, immunologic, and cytometric approach to the classification on non-Hodgkin's lymphoma in effusions. *Diagn Cytopathol.* 1987;3:91–101

Robey SS, Cafferty LL, Beschorner We, Gupta PK. Value of lymphocyte marker studies in diagnostic cytopathology. *Acta Cytol.* 1987;31:453–459.

Ibrahim RE, Teich D, Smith BR, et al. Flow cytometric surface light chain analysis of lymphocyte-rich effusions. A useful adjunct to cytologic diagnosis. *Cancer.* 1989;63:2024–2029.

Guzman J, Bross KJ, Costabel U. Malignant lymphoma in pleural effusions; an immunocytochemical cell surface analysis. *Diagn Cytopathol.* 1991;7:113–118.

Moriarty AT, Wiersema L, Snyder W, et al. Immunophenotyping of cytologic specimens by flow cytometry. *Diagn Cytopathol* 1993;9:252–258.

Flow Cytometry (Solid Tumors)

Unger KM, Stein DA, Barlogie B, Bedrossian CWM. Analysis of pleural effusions by pulse cytophotometry. *Cancer.* 1983;52:873–877.

Hedley DW, Philips J, Rugg CA. Measurement of cellular DNA content as an adjunct to diagnostic cytology in malignant effusions. *Eur J Cancer Oncol.* 1984;20:749–752.

Hostmark J, Vigander T, Skaarland E. Characterization of pleural effusions by flow-cytometric DNA analysis. *Eur J Respir Dis.* 1985;66:315–319.

Fossa SD, Thorud E, Shoaib ME, Patterson EO. DNA flow cytometry of cells obtained from old paraffin embedded specimens. *Pathol Res Proc.* 1986;181:200.

Schneler J, Eppich E, Greenbaum E, et al. Flow cytometry

and feulgen cytophotometry in evaluation of effusions. *Cancer.* 1987;59:1307–1313.

Stonesifer KJ, Xiang J, Wilkinson EJ, et al. Flow cytometric analysis and cytopathology of body cavity fluids. *Acta Cytol.* 1987;31:125–130

Katz RL, Patel S, Sneige N, et al. Comparison of immunocytochemical and biochemical assays for estrogen receptor in fine needle aspirates and histologic sections from breast carcinomas. *Breast Cancer Re. Treat.* 1990;15:191–203.

Sinton EB, Carver RK, Morgan DL, et al. Prospective study of concurrent ploidy analysis and routine cytopathology in body cavity fluids. *Arch Pathol Lab Med.* 1990;114:188–194.

Rijken A, Dekker A, Taylor S, et al. Diagnostic value of DNA analysis in effusions by flow cytometry and image analysis. A prospective study on 102 patients as compared with cytologic examination. *Am J Clin Pathol.* 1991;95:6–12.

Zarbo RJ. Flow cytometric DNA analysis of effusions. A new test seeking validation. *Am J Clin Pathol.* 1991;95:2–4.

Proliferative Markers

Walker RA, Camplejohr RS. Comparison of monoclonal antibody Ki-67 reactivity with grade and DNA flow cytometry of breast carcinomas. *Br J Cancer.* 1983;57:281–283.

Gerdes J, Dallenbach F, Lennert K. Growth fractions in malignant non-Hodgkin's lymphomas (NHL) as determined in situ with the monoclonal antibody Ki-67. *Hematol Oncol.* 1984;2:365–371.

Clevenger CV, Epstein AL, Bauer KD. Quantitative analysis of a nuclear antigen in interphase and mitotic cells. *Cytometry.* 1987;8:280.

Mushika M, Miwa T, Suzuoki Y, et al. Detection of proliferative cells in dysplasia, carcinoma in situ, and invasive carcinoma of the uterine cervix by monoclonal antibody against DNA polymerase. *Cancer.* 1988;61:1182–1186.

Grogan TM, Limpomas BM, Spier CM, et al. Independent prognostic significance of nuclear proliferation antigen in diffuse large cell lymphomas as determined by the monoclonal antibody Ki-67. *Blood.* 1988;71:1157.

Sasaki K, Matsuma K, Tatsuo T, et al. Relationship between labeling indices by Ki-67 and BrdUrd in human malignant tumors. *Cancer.* 1988;62:989.

Garcia RL, Coltrera MD, Gown AM. Analysis of proliferative grade using anti-PCNA/Cyclin monoclonal antibodies in fixed, embedded tissue. Comparison with flow cytometric analysis. *Am J Pathol.* 1989;132:134–733.

Henry MJ, Stanley MW, Swenson B, et al. Cytologic assessment of tumor cell kinetics: applications of monoclonal antibody K-67 to fine-needle aspiration smears. *Diagn Cytol.* 1991;7:1–6.

Trevisan MS, Souza MI, Magna LA. Nucleolar organizing regions of mesothelia and carcinomatous cells in effusions. *Diagn Cytopathol* 1993;9:492–497.

Receptor Assays

McCarty KS Jr, Wortman J, Moore JO, et al. Malignant effusions in recurrent breast cancer: steroid hormone receptor analysis by effusion fluid derived cells. *Cancer.* 1980;45:1609–1614.

Murakami T, Kitamura S, Ohsawa N. A rapid, sensitive method for estrogen receptor analysis of cells from malignant pleural effusions in recurrent breast cancer. *Chest.* 1983;83:936.

Bacus S, Flowers J, Press M, et al. The evaluation of estrogen receptor in primary breast carcinoma by computerized image analysis. *Am J Clin Pathol.* 1988;90:223.

DeRosa CM, Ozzello L, Habif DV, et al. Immunohistochemical assessment of estrogen and progesterone receptors in stored imprints and cryostat sections of breast carcinomas. *Ann Surg.* 1989;212:224–228.

Redard M, Vassikos P, Weintraub J. A simple method for estrogen receptor antigen preservation in cytologic specimens containing breast carcinoma cells. *Diagn Cytol Pathol.* 1989;5:18–193.

Masood S. Use of monoclonal antibody for assessment of estrogen and progesterone receptors in malignant effusions. *Diagn Cytol.* 1991;8:1–7.

DNA/RNA Probes

Tomasi TB. Oncogenes and cancer. In Fenoglio C, Weinstein R, Kaufman N, eds. *New Concepts in Neoplasms as Applied to Diagnostic Pathology.* IAP Monographs. Williams and Wilkins, Baltimore: 1986:59–90.

Walts AE, Shintaku IP, Said JW. Diagnosis of malignant lymphoma in effusions from patients with AIDS by gene rearrangement. *Am J Clin Pathol.* 1990;94:170–175.

Saiki RK, Scharf S, Faloona F, et al. Enzymatic amplification of β-globin genomic sequences and restriction site analysis for diagnosis of sickle cell anemia. *Science.* 1985;230:1350–1354.

Mullis K, Faloona FA, Scharf S, et al. Specific enzymatic amplification of DNA in vitro: the polymerase chain reaction. *Cold Spring Harbor Symp Quant Biol.* 1986;57:263–273.

Mullis KB, Faloona FA. Specific synthesis of DNA in vitro via a polymerase-catalyzed chain reaction. *Methods Enzymol.* 1987;155:335–350.

Bresser J, Evinger-Hodges J. Comparison and optimization of in situ hybridization procedures yielding rapid, sensitive mRNA detection. *Gene Anal Techn.* 1987;4:89–104.

Marx JL. Multiplying genes by leaps and bounds. *Science.* 1988;240:1408–1410.

Cohen PS, Seeger RC, Triche TJ, et al. Detection of N-myc gene expression in neuroblastoma tumors by in situ hybridization. *Am J Pathol.* 1988;131:391–397.

Erlich HA. PCR Technology: *Principles and applications for DNA Amplification.* New York: Stockton Press, 1989:149–244.

Eisenstein BI. The polymerase chain reaction: a new method of using molecular genetics for medical diagnosis. *N Engl J Med.* 1990;322:178–183.

Anastasi J. Interphase cytogenetic analysis in the diagnosis and study of neoplastic disorders. *Am J Clin Pathol.* 1991;95(suppl 1):522–528.

Unger ER, Hammer ML, Chenggis ML. Comparison of 35-S and biotin as labels for in situ hybridization: use of an HPV model system. *J Histochem Cytochem.* 1991;39:145–150.

Tissue Culture

Monif GR, Daly JW. Living cytology in the diagnosis of intraabdominal adenocarcinoma. *Obstet Gynecol.* 1975;46:80–83.

Monif GR, Stewart BN, Block AJ. Living cytology: a new diagnostic technique for malignant pleural effusions. *Chest.* 1976;69:626–629.

Index

A

Accuracy rate (sensitivity, specificity), 11
Acini, free-floating, 205
Acute inflammation, 52–54
Adenocarcinoma, 120–121
    cytologic features, in effusion, 121
    expression of differentiation, 121
    mesothelioma, distinguished, 109–117
Adrenal, carcinoma of, 144
AgNOR, 264
Alien cell, 48–49
Allergic disease, eosinophilia, 56
Alpha-fetoprotein, 253
Amylase, pancreatic, 3, 93
Amiodarone, 89
Amyloidosis, 94
Anaplastic mesothelioma, 107–108
Anasarca, malnutrition, 3
Articulations, mesothelial cells, 37
Asbestos body, in effusion, 95–96
Ascitic fluid, clinicopathologic correlation, 12–13

B

B 72-3, 250
B-cell lymphoma, 162, 168
Bacteria
    funguslike, 75–76
    infection, 74–75
Benign papillary mesothelioma, 102–103
Ber-Ep-4, 249
Biochemical analysis, effusion, 6
Biphasic mesothelioma, 105–106
Blebs, mesothelial cells, 215, 224
Body cavity, overview, 1
Breast, carcinoma of, 121–124
Bronchogenic carcinoma, 123–130
Burkitt's lymphoma, 164–166

C

CA 125, 254
Calcitonin, 186
Carbon pigment, 192–194
Carcinoembryonic antigen, 251–252

Carcinoid tumor, 183
Carcinoma, distinction from other neoplasms, 145–146
Carcinoma
    adrenal, 144
    breast, 121–124
    colon, 137
    esophagus, 140
    kidney, 139, 141–142
    liver, 143
    lung, 123, 125–130
    ovary, 130–132
    pancreas, 137–139
    prostate, 144
    stomach, 135, 137
    thyroid, 144
    urinary bladder, 141, 142
    uterus, 132–135
Carcinosarcoma, 156–158
    Wilm's tumor, 157–158
Cardiac failure, 35
Cavity, body, overview, 1
Cell ball, solid, 198–199
Cell block technique, 19
Cell shape, categorization, of neoplasm, 191
Centrifugation, cytospins, 19
Charcot-Leyden crystals, 58
Chemotherapeutic effect, 88–90
Cholesterol effusion, crystals, 95
Choriocarcinoma, germ cell neoplasm, 156
Chylous effusion, 5
Cirrhosis, 93–94
    pancreatic ascites, 3
Classification, pathologic, effusion, 4–5
Clinicopathologic correlation, 9–15
    ascitic fluid, 12–13
    culdocentesis, 13–14
    diagnostic yield, 10–11
    follow-up, of malignant effusion diagnosis, 13–14
    pericardial fluid, 12
    peritoneal washing, 13
    pleural effusion, 11–12
    result report, 15

Clonality
kappa, 54
lambda, 54
Collagen disease
serosal membrane, 3
vascular, 58–64
Collection procedure, 18–20
Colon, carcinoma of, 136–138
Conditions confusable with, malignant mesothelioma, 108–109
Culdocentesis, clinicopathologic correlation, 13–14
Cytocentrifuge, 19
Cytogenetics, 262–263
Cytokeratin, 245–246
Cytologic features
articulations, 37
ballooning degeneration, 33
clasping, 39
discrete inclusions, 41
doublets, 39
ecto-endoplasmic demarcation, 32, 39
fuzzy border, 32
hyperchromasia, 41
intercellular cleft, 33
microvilli, 32
multinucleation, 46
perinuclear halo, 32
peripheral vacuoles, 32, 39
protrusions, 39
Cytopathology report, 13
Cytophotometry, 261–262
Cytopreparatory methods, 19
Cytoskeleton
components, immunocytochemistry, 244–250
electron microscopy, 226–228, 231
Cytotoxic drugs, 88, 89

D

Detached ciliary tufts, DCTs, 48
Diagnostic
accuracy, quality assurance, 14–15
pitfalls, 10, 96–98
yield, effusion, 10–11
Dialysis effect, 90
DNA probe, 265
Drug hypersensitivity, effusion, 3
Dyscrasias, plasma cell, 172–173

E

Echinococcus, 81
Edema formation, Starling's principle, 1, 3, 6
Effusion
biochemical analysis, 6
cause of formation, 3

of cryptic origin, 207–208
cytopreparatory techniques, chart, 20
defined, 1
differential diagnosis of malignant effusion, 145
epithelial malignancy, table, 145
metastasis, frequency of, 121
microscopic examination, 5–6
multimodal examination, overview, 20
normal cell population, 26
pathologic classification, 4–5
tumor marker, 6–7
Electron microscopy, 22–23
benign conditions, 212–213
cytoskeleton, 226–228, 231
desmosomes, 217
diagnostic applications, 237–242
endoplasmic reticulum, 225–226, 230
glycogen, 221–222
intercellular relationships, 214–218
intracytoplasmic lumina, 225, 229
lysosomes, 228
malignant tumor, 213–217
mitochondria, 228, 231
scanning, 230, 232–235
secretory granules, 222, 228
surface specializations, 218–220, 223–224
ultrastructural correlates
epithelial differentiation, 220–230
nonepithelial differentiation, 230, 232–233
Embryonal carcinoma, germ cell neoplasm, 155–156
Endodermal sinus tumor, germ cell neoplasm, 156
Endometrial cells, endometriosis, 49
Endoplasmic reticulum, electron microscopy, 225–226, 230
Eosinophilic effusion, 56, 58
Epithelial differentiation, ultrastructural correlates, electron microscopy, 220–222, 225–230
Epithelial malignancy
adenocarcinoma, 120–121
cytologic features, in effusion, 121
expression of differentiation, 121
common epithelial neoplasms, 121–138
breast, 121–124
colon, 136–138
lung, 123, 125–131
ovary, 131–133
pancreas, 138–139
stomach, 134, 137
uterus, 133–136
differential diagnosis of malignant effusion, table, 145
less common epithelial neoplasms
adrenal, 144
esophagus, 138, 140
kidney, 139, 141–142
liver, 143
prostate, 143–144

thyroid, 144
urinary bladder, 141–142
Epithelial membrane antigen, 248–249
Epithelial mesothelioma, malignant, 103–108
Epithelial neoplasms, common, 121–138
Erythrophagocytosis, 69
Esophagus, carcinoma of, 138, 140
Ewing's sarcoma, 185–187
Extraneous element in effusion
asbestos body, 95–96
diagnostic pitfalls, 96–98
foreign substance, 95–96
noncellular structure, 94–95
Exudate, transudate, contrasted, 3–4

F
Factor VIII, 254
Feulgen reaction, 262
Fibrosarcoma, spindle cell tumor, 150
Fibrous mesothelioma, localized, 108–109
Filariasis, 81
Flow cytometry, 23, 263–264
image analysis, compared, 262
Fluid extravasation, Starling's law, 6
Follow-up, of malignant effusion diagnosis, 13–14
Foreign substance, in effusion, 95–96
Free-floating acini, 206
Fungus
opportunistic, 76–77
pathogenic, 78–79
Funguslike bacteria, 75–76

G
Gastric contents, aspirated accidentally, 49
Gene/oncogene rearrangement, 264–265
Germ cell neoplasm, 155–156
choriocarcinoma, 156
embryonal carcinoma, 155
endodermal sinus tumor, 155
Giant cell inflammatory reaction, 63–65
Glycogen, electron microscopy, 220–221
Granulation tissue, 69–70
Granulomatous inflammation, 63

H
Hairy cell leukemia, 170, 171
Helminthic infection, 80–82
Heinz bodies, 69
Hemangiopericytoma, spindle cell tumor, 151
Hepatocytes, 48
Hepatocellular carcinoma, 143
Histoplasmosis, 78
Hodgkin's disease, 171–172
Human milk-fat globule, 249
Hyaluronic acid, hyaluroniclase, 111
Hydatid cyst, 81

Hyperplasia, mesothelial 36–48
Hypoproteinemia, nephrogenic effusion, 3

I
Image analysis, 262
Immunoblastic lymphoma, 169
Immunocytochemistry, 22, 244–259
alpha-fetoprotein, 253
alpha-1-antitrysin, alpha-1-antichymotrypsin, 256
Ber-Ep-4, 249
B 72-3, 250
CA-125, 255
carcinoembryonic antigen, 251–252
carcinosarcomas, 156
CD antigens, 167, 171, 175
chordoma, 154
cytokeratin, 245–247
cytoskeletal components, 244–248
in diagnosis, 244–258
epithelial membrane antigen, 248–249
germ cell tumors, 155
HMB-45, 255
human milk-fat globule, 249
lactalbumin, 255
leucocyte common antigen, 174
Leu M1, 250
lymphoma, 173
lysozyme, 256
melanoma, 197, 255
mesothelioma, 110–114, 246
myogenous markers, 153
neuroendocrine markers, 254
oncofetal antigen 251–254
phenotype-specific marker, 255–258
placental alkaline phosphatase, 254
sarcoma, 148
secretory markers, 249–251
S100, 251
SP-A (clara cell) granule, 257
SP-C (surfactant apoprotein) granule, 257
technical considerations, 258
ulex europeaus antigen, 258
vascular markers 149, 152
vimentin, 247–248
Immuno-electron microscopy, 237
Indian file, 206
Infarction, 92
Infectious disease
bacterial infection, 74–75
funguslike bacteria, 75–76
helminthic, 80–82
opportunistic fungi, 76–77
pathogenic fungi, 78–79
protozoal, 79–80
tuberculosis, 54, 75
viral infection, 73–74

Inflammatory process
  chylous effusion, 65
  collagen vascular disease, 58–64
  eosinophilic effusion, 56, 58
  giant cell reaction, 63–65
  granulation tissue, 69–70
  granulomatous inflammation, 63
  lymphocytic predominance, 54–57
  pseudochylous effusion, 68
  purulent exudate, 52–54
  serosanguinous effusion, 66–69
Intercellular relationships, electron microscopy, 213–218
Intracytoplasmic lumina, electron microscopy, 224–225, 235
Iron pigment, 21
Isolated cell, primary site, 190–192

J
Jaundice, 93
Junctional complexes, 217

K
Kaposi's sarcoma, spindle cell tumor, 151–152
Kappa, clonality, 54
Karyotype analysis, 262
Kidney, carcinoma of, 141–142

L
Lambda, clonality, 54
Lamellar bodies, 127, 222
Langhans cells, 27
Large cell lymphoma, 167–171
LE cells, 63
Leiomyosarcoma, spindle cell tumor, 150–151
Leu M1, immunocytochemistry, 250
Liposarcoma, 153, 154
Liver, carcinoma of, 141
Lobular carcinoma of breast, 123
Lung, carcinoma of, 123, 125–130
Lupus erythematosus, 62
Lymphoblastic lymphoma, 166–167
Lymphocyte, normal, 160
Lymphocytic predominance, 54–57
  kappa, staining, 54
  lambda, staining, 54
Lymphoid hyperplasia, 160–161
Lymphoma, 160–177
  Burkitt's lymphoma, 164–166
  in effusion, classification, 162–163
  large cell, 167–171
  lymphoblastic, 166–167
  lymphocyte, normal, 160
  lymphoid hyperplasia, 160–161
  markers, cytologic material, 174
  of medium-sized cells, 166
  non-Hodgkin's lymphoma, 161–163

  peripheral T-cell, 166–167
  small cell lymphoma, 163–164
Lysosomes, electron microscopy, 230
Lysozyme, 256

M
Macrophage, 26–30
Malignant cell, primary site, origin of, 190
Malignant epithelial mesothelioma, 103–108
  anaplastic mesothelioma, 107–108
  biphasic mesothelioma, 105–106
  epithelioid mesothelioma, 103–105
  sarcomatous mesothelioma, 106–107
Malignant fibrous histiocytoma, 153
Malignant histiocytosis, 171, 174
Malignant mesothelioma, conditions confusable with, 108–109
  mesothelioma, adenocarcinoma, distinguished, 109–117
  pleural fibroma, 108–109
  pleural sarcoma, 109
Malignant mixed Mullerian tumor, 156, 157
Malignant tumor, electron microscopy, 212–213
Malnutrition, anasarca, 3
May-Grünwald-Giemsa (MGG) stain, 5, 19
Megakaryocytic process, 172
Meig's syndrome, 3
Melanoma, 148–149
Membrane filter (Millipore, gelman), 19
Merkel cell neoplasm, 188–190
Mesothelial cell, overview, 30–33
Mesothelial hyperplasia, 36–46
  atypical, 46–48
  diagnosis, pitfalls, 96
Mesothelial injury/repair, 33
Mesothelial proliferation, nonmalignant, 101–102
Mesothelioma
  adenocarcinoma, distinguished, 109–117
  anaplastic, 107–108
  benign papillary mesothelioma, 102–103
  biphasic, 105–106
  epithelioid, 103–105
  fibrous, localized, 108–109
  malignant, conditions confusable with, 108–109
  nonmalignant mesothelial proliferation, 101–102
  sarcomatous, 106–107
Microscopic examination, effusion, 5–6
Milroy's disease, *see* Meig's syndrome
Mitochondria, electron microscopy, 228, 230
Mitosis, high rate, 96
Mixed mesodermal (Mullerian) tumor, 156, 157
Morphometry, 260–262
Mott cell, 95
Multimodal approach
  cell block technique, 19
  collection procedure, 18–20
  cytopreparatory methods, 19

electron microscopy, 22–23
flow cytometry, 23
immunocytochemistry, 22
routine stain, 19, 21
special stain, 20–22
transmission electron microscopy, 23
tumor marker, chart, 23
Multinucleated large cells, 195–196
Multiple myeloma, 172
Mycosis fungoides, 166

N
Nephroblastoma (Wilms' tumor), 157–158, 181–182
Nephrogenic effusion, hypoproteinemia, 3
Neuroblastoma, 180–185
Neuroendocrine carcinoma. 186, 188
Neuroendocrine markers, 188
bombesin, 188
chromagranin, 188
NSE, 188
polypeptide hormones, 188
synaptophysin, 188
Neurofibrosarcoma, spindle cell tumor, 150
Neuron-specific enolase (NSE) alpha, gamma, 189
Noncellular structure, in effusion, 94–95
talc, 94
starch, 95
Non-Hodgkin's lymphoma, 161–163
Neutrophil, PMN, 52
Nonepithelial differentiation, ultrastructural correlates, electron microscopy, 230–232
Nonepithelial neoplasm
melanoma, 148–149
sarcoma, 148–149
spindle cell tumor, 149–152
Nonmalignant mesothelial proliferation, 101–102
Nonspecific reactive cellular change, 85–92
chemotherapeutic effect, 88–90
dialysis effect, 90
peritoneal washing, 90–91
pleurodesis, 92
radiation effect, 87–88
Nonvacuolated cell cluster, 201–203
Normal cell population, effusion, 26
Nuclear, cytoplasmic (N-C) ratio, 96
Nucleolar organizing region, 264

O
Oat cell carcinoma, neuroendocrine carcinoma, 187, 189
Omental ependymoma, spindle cell tumor, 150–151
Oncofetal antigen, immunocytochemistry, 251–254
Oncogene/gene rearrangement, 264–265
Opportunistic fungus, 76–77
Organ-related process
cirrhosis, 93–94
infarction, 92

pancreatitis, 93
uremia, 92–93
Osmiophilic, lamellated inclusions, 126, 222
Osteosarcoma, 154
Ovary, carcinoma of, 130–132
teratoma of, 156

P
Pancreas
ascites, cirrhosis, 3
carcinoma of, 137–139
Pancreatitis, 93
Papanicolaou, Romanowsky, stains, compared, 21
Papillary formation, 199–201
Papillary mesothelioma, benign, 102–103
Parasites, eosinophilia 56, 58
Pathogenic fungus, 78–79
Pathologic classification, effusion, 4–5
Pathophysiology, effusions, 1–3
Perforated hollow viscera, 48, 49
Pericardial fluid, clinicopathologic correlation, 12
Periodic acid-Schiff (PAS), 21
Peripheral T-cell lymphoma, 166–167
Peritoneal
clinicopathologic correlation, 13
dialysis, 90
washings, 90, 91
Phagocytosis, 69
Phase contrast microscopy, 253–257
Phenotype-specific marker, 255–258
Phosphatase, prostatic specific alkaline, 254
Pigmented cell, 192–194
Placental alkaline phosphatase, 254
Plasma cell dyscrasias, 172
Plasmacytoma, 54
Pleomorphic cell tumor, 152–154
liposarcoma, 153
rhabdomyosarcoma, 154
skeletal sarcoma, 154
Pleomorphic large cells, 194–195
Pleural effusion, clinicopathologic correlation, 11–12
Pleural fibroma, see Fibrous mesothelioma, localized
Pleural mesothelioma See Malignant mesothelioma
Pleural membrane
histology, 1
normal anatomy, 1
Pleural sarcoma, 109
Pleurodesis, 92
Pneumothorax, pneumoperitoneum, 88, 96
Post-pneumonic effusion, 52
Preparatory methods
multimodal approach, 19
Primary site
cell size categorization, of neoplasm, 191
cell size/shape categorization, of neoplasm, 191
effusion of cryptic origin, 207

Primary site (contd.)
  free-floating acini, 205
  Indian file, 206
  isolated cell, 190–192
  large, noncohesive, tumor cell, diagnosis, 191
  malignant cell, origin of, 190
  multinucleated large cells, 195–196
  nonvacuolated cell cluster, 201–203
  papillary formation, 199–201
  pigmented cell, 192–194
  pleomorphic large cells, 194–195
  psammoma body, 201
  pseudomyxoma peritonei, 197–198
  signet ring cell, 197
  solid cell ball, 198–199
  spindle cell, 206
  tall columnar frond, 205
  vacuolated cell cluster, 203–205
Proliferative markers, 264
  AgNOR, 264
  DNA polymerase, 264
  Ki67, 264
  MIB-1, 264
  PCNA, 264
Proliferative spherules, cell balls, 96
Prostate, carcinoma of, 144
Protozoal infection, 79–80
Prussian blue stain, 21
Psammoma body, 201
Pseudoacinar formations, 47
Pseudochylous effusion, 68
Pseudomyxoma peritonei, 197
Pulmonary infarct, 69
Purulent exudate, 52–54

Q
Quality assurance, diagnostic accuracy, 14–15

R
RA cells, 59
Radiation effect, 87–88
RBCs, 70
Reactive cellular change, nonspecific, 85–92
  chemotherapeutic effect, 88–90
  dialysis effect, 90
  peritoneal washing, 90–91
  pleurodesis, 92
  radiation effect, 87–88
Reactive eosinophilic pleuritis, 56
Rearrangement, gene/oncogene, 264–265
Receptor analysis, 264
Reed-Sternberg cell, 171–173
Renal carcinoma, 139, 141
Renal failure, uremia, 92–93
Report, cytopathology results, 13
Rhabdomyosarcoma, 184, 187

Rheumatoid arthritis, effusion, 3
RNA probe, 265
Romanowsky, Papanicolaou, stains, compared, 21
Round cell tumor, 154–155
Routine stain, multimodal approach, 19, 21
Russell bodies, 95

S
S100, immunocytochemistry, 251
Sarcoidosis, 94
Sarcoma, 148–149
Sarcomatous mesothelioma, 106–107
Scanning electron microscopy, 231–233
Schwannoma, malignant, spindle cell tumor, 150
Secretory granules
  Clara cell (SP-C), 225
  electron microscopy, 222, 228
  mucosubstance, 111, 120, 121
  neuroendocrine, 189
  Surfactant apoprotein (SP-A), 255
Secretory markers, immunocytochemistry, 249–250
Seminoma, 156
Serosa, anatomy, physiology, 2
Serous cavity
  alien cell, 48–49
  effusion, normal cell population, 26
  macrophage, 26–30
  mesothelial cell, 30–33
  mesothelial hyperplasia, 36–46
    atypical, 46–48
  mesothelial injury/repair, 33
  normal cell population, effusion, 26
  reaction to injury, 49–50
  specimen collection, 18–19
Serosanguinous effusion, 66, 70
Serous membrane, 1
Signet ring cell, 197
Skeletal sarcoma, pleomorphic cell tumor, 154
SLE, 62
Small blue round cell tumor, 154–155, 177–189
  carcinoid tumor, 188
  Ewing's sarcoma, 184–186
  Merkel cell neoplasm, 188–189
  neuroblastoma, 180, 182–185
  neuroendocrine carcinoma, 186, 188
  rhabdomyosarcoma, 184, 187
  thymoma, 178–180
  Wilms' tumor, 180–181
Small cell carcinoma, oat cell, 188
Small cell lymphoma, 163–164
Solid cell ball, 198–199
Special stain, multimodal approach, 20–22
Specific gravity, 3
Specimen collection, serous cavity, 18–19
Spindle cell, 206
Spontaneous pneumothorax, 56

Spindle cell tumor, 150–152
  fibrosarcoma, 150
  hemangiopericytoma, 151
  Kaposi's sarcoma, 152
  leiomyosarcoma, 150
  neurofibrosarcoma, 150
  omental ependymoma, 150–151
  schwannoma, malignant, 150
  synovial sarcoma, 151
Squamous cell carcinoma
  cervix, 133
  esophagus, 138
  larynx, 138
  lung, 127
Starch granules, 91
Stain
  mesothelioma, adenocarcinoma, distinguished, 111
  Papanicolaou, Romanowsky, compared, 21
  routine, multimodal approach, 19, 21
  special, multimodal approach, 20–22
Starling's principle, edema formation, 1, 3, 6
Stomach, carcinoma of, 135, 137
Sudan Black, 5
Surface specializations, electron microscopy 218–220
Synovial sarcoma, spindle cell tumor, 151
Systemic lupus erythematosus (SLE), 62
Systemic process
  amyloidosis, 94
  sarcoidosis, 94

T
Talc, pleural space, 94
Tall columnar frond, 205
Tandem, arrangement, 44
T-cell lymphoma, peripheral, 166–167
T-cells, T lymphocytes, 53

Technical methods, cytopreparation, 19
Thymoma, 178–180
Thymidine, tritriated, 264
Thyroid, carcinoma of, 144
Tissue culture, 265–266
Toluidine blue, 5
Transmission electron microscopy, 23
Transudate, exudate, contrasted, 3–4
Traumatic effusion, eosinophilic, 56
Tuberculosis, 54, 75
Tubulo-papillary formations, 101
Tumor marker, effusion, 6–7
  plasma, chart, 23

U
Ultrastructural correlates
  epithelial differentiation, 220–221, 224–229
  of nonepithelial differentiation, 230–232
Ultrastructural distinction, mesothelioma, adenocarcinoma, 113
Uremia, 92–93
Urinary bladder, carcinoma of, 141
Urothelial carcinoma, 141–142
Uterine cells, 49–50
Uterus, carcinoma of, 132–137

V
Vacuolated cell cluster, 203–205
Vimentin, 246–247
Viral infection, 73–74

W
Wet-fixed smears, 5, 19
Wilms' tumor, 157–158, 180–181

Y
Yellow nail syndrome, effusion, 3